PRACTICAL APPLICATIONS FOR THE

Occupational Therapy CODE OF ETHICS (2015)

EDITED BY

Janie B. Scott, MA, OT/L, FAOTA, and

S. Maggie Reitz, PhD, OTR/L, FAOTA

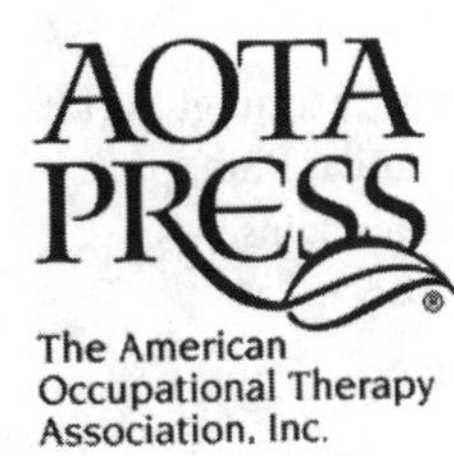

AOTA Vision 2025
Occupational therapy maximizes health, well-being, and quality of life for all people, populations, and communities through effective solutions that facilitate participation in everyday living.

Mission Statement
The American Occupational Therapy Association advances the quality, availability, use, and support of occupational therapy through standard-setting, advocacy, education, and research on behalf of its members and the public.

AOTA Staff
Frederick P. Somers, *Executive Director*
Christopher M. Bluhm, *Chief Operating Officer*

Chris Davis, *Director, AOTA Press*
Caroline Polk, *Digital Manager and* AJOT *Managing Editor*
Ashley Hofmann, *Development/Acquisitions Editor*
Barbara Dickson, *Production Editor*

Rebecca Rutberg, *Director, Marketing*
Amanda Goldman, *Marketing Manager*
Jennifer Folden, *Marketing Specialist*

American Occupational Therapy Association, Inc.
4720 Montgomery Lane
Bethesda, MD 20814
Phone: 301-652-AOTA (2682)
TDD: 800-377-8555
Fax: 301-652-7711
www.aota.org
To order: 1-877-404-AOTA or store.aota.org

ISBN: 978-1-56900387-9
Library of Congress Control Number: 2016956028

Cover design by Debra Naylor, Naylor Design, Inc., Washington, DC
Composition by Manila Typesetting Company, Manila, Philippines
Printed by Automated Graphic Systems, Inc., White Plains, MD

CONTENTS

ABOUT THE EDITORS

Janie B. Scott, MA, OT/L, FAOTA, is an occupational therapy and aging-in-place consultant and occupational therapist for the Johns Hopkins University, Center for Innovative Care in Aging, Baltimore. She earned a bachelor of science degree in occupational therapy from Wayne State University and an master's degree in legal and ethical studies from the University of Baltimore.

Ms. Scott has presented nationwide and has published in the area of health care ethics, productive aging, autism, aging in place, consultation, and mental health practice. She has been Ethics Officer, Director of Practice, and Staff Liaison to the Special Interest Sections of the American Occupational Therapy Association (AOTA). Her volunteer positions include member of the AOTA Judicial Council and Representative Assembly, chairperson of the AOTA Recognitions Committee, trustee and past president for the Maryland Occupational Therapy Association, and president and vice president of the Homes for Life Coalition of Howard County, Maryland.

S. Maggie Reitz, PhD, OTR/L, FAOTA. Prior to her roles as Vice Provost, Acting Provost, and Interim Provost, she served as chairperson and professor in the Department of Occupational Therapy and Occupational Science at Towson University, Towson, Maryland. She received both her bachelor of science and master's degrees in occupational therapy from Towson University and her doctorate in health education from the University of Maryland, College Park.

Dr. Reitz practiced as an occupational therapist in mental health and physical disabilities in the Anacostia neighborhood of Washington, DC, before beginning her academic career. She served as president of the Maryland Occupational Therapy Association and chairperson of AOTA's Ethics Commission. Her areas of interest include occupational therapy theory and philosophy, occupational science, ethics, and health promotion. She has lectured on these topics throughout the United Kingdom, as well as in Australia, Hong Kong, Ireland, Sweden, and the People's Republic of China.

ABOUT THE AUTHORS

LILIANA ALVAREZ JARAMILLO, PhD, MSc, OT
Postdoctoral Fellow and Instructor
School of Occupational Therapy, University of Western Ontario
London, Ontario, Canada

LEA CHEYNEY BRANDT, OTD, MA, OTR/L
Co-Director
MU Center for Health Ethics
Director
Missouri Health Professions Consortium Occupational Therapy Assistant Program
Associate Professional Practice Professor
School of Medicine
University of Missouri–Columbia

MARY ELLEN BUNING, PhD, OTR/L, ATP/SMS, RESNA FELLOW
Assistant Professor and Seating and Mobility Specialist
University of Louisville, School of Medicine, Department of Neurological Surgery, Division of Physical Medicine and Rehabilitation
Louisville, KY

SUSAN COPPOLA, MS, OTR/L, BCG, FAOTA
Clinical Professor
University of North Carolina–Chapel Hill

LISA CRABTREE, PhD, OTR/L, FAOTA
Associate Professor of Occupational Therapy and Occupational Science
Towson University
Towson, MD

JANET V. DELANY, DeD OTR/L, FAOTA
Dean Graduate Studies
Towson University
Towson, MD

LINDA S. GABRIEL, PhD, OTR/L
Assistant Professor of Occupational Therapy
Faculty Associate
Center for Health Policy and Ethics
Creighton University
Omaha, NE

STACEY HARCUM, MS, OTR/L, CBIS
Senior Occupational Therapist
Traumatic Brain Injury Unit
University of Maryland Rehabilitation and Orthopaedic Institute
Baltimore

TIMOTHY HOLMES, OTD, OTR/L, COMS
Clinical Specialist, Rehabilitation Services
University of North Carolina Medical Center
Chapel Hill

ELIZABETH LARSON, PhD, OTR, FAOTA
Associate Professor
University of Wisconsin–Madison
Madison

ROCHELLE J. MENDONCA, PhD, OTR/L
Assistant Professor
Department of Rehabilitation Sciences
Occupational Therapy Program
Temple University
Philadelphia

NORALYN D. PICKENS, PhD, OT
Associate Professor and Associate Director
School of Occupational Therapy
Texas Woman's University
Dallas

S. MAGGIE REITZ, PhD, OTR/L, FAOTA
Vice Provost
Towson University
Towson, MD

JANIE B. SCOTT, MA, OT/L, FAOTA
Occupational Therapist
Johns Hopkins University
Baltimore
Occupational Therapy and Aging in Place Consultant
Columbia, MD

MARY ALICE SINGER, MS, OTR/L
Private Practice
Occupational Therapy for Children
Laguna Beach, CA

ROGER O. SMITH, PhD, OT, FAOTA, RESNA FELLOW
Professor
Department of Occupational Science and Technology
College of Health Sciences
Director
Rehabilitation Research Design and Disability (R2D2) Center
University of Wisconsin–Milwaukee

SUSANNE SMITH ROLEY, OTD, OTR/L, FAOTA
Co-Founder and Chief Executive Officer
Collaborative for Leadership in Ayres Sensory Integration
Aliso Viejo, CA

JEFF SNODGRASS, PhD, MPH, OTR/L, FAOTA
Chair, Department of Occupational Therapy
Professor of Healthcare Administration & Occupational Therapy
Milligan College
Milligan College, TN
Contributing Faculty
Graduate Programs in Health Services and Public Health
Walden University
Minneapolis

SCOTT A. TRUDEAU, PhD, OTR/L
Productive Aging and Interprofessional Collaborative Practice Program Manager
American Occupational Therapy Association
Bethesda, MD

SHIRLEY A. WELLS, DrPH, OTR, FAOTA
Chair and Associate Professor
University of Texas Rio Grande Valley
Edinburg

WAYNE L. WINISTORFER, MPA, OTR
Regional Director of Rehabilitation Services
Affinity Health System/Ministry Health Care
Appleton and Oshkosh, WI
Co-Chair, Ethics Committee
St. Elizabeth Hospital
Appleton, WI
Adjunct Instructor of Occupational Therapy Assistant Program
Fox Valley Technical College
Appleton, WI
Adjunct Instructor of Occupational Therapy
Concordia University–Wisconsin
Mequon and Oshkosh

MISSI ZAHORANSKY, MSHS, OTR/L
Owner
Total Rehabilitation Specialists, Inc.
North Royalton, OH

LIST OF FIGURES, TABLES, EXHIBITS, CASE STUDIES, VIGNETTES, AND APPENDIXES

Figures

Tables

Exhibits

Case Studies

Vignettes

Appendixes

ACKNOWLEDGMENTS

We are grateful to AOTA Press and the vision of Chris Davis and her willingness to consider and discuss the concept of this book and her support of the process, including providing the stellar services of Hyde Loomis as copy editor (first edition) and Ashley Hofmann, Development and Acquisitions Editor (2015 edition). Many other people devoted their time, support, and expertise in helping this book come to fruition. First, the obvious people are the contributors, our authors: Dana Burns, Linda Gabriel, Susan Haiman, Barbara Kornblau, Elizabeth Larson, Tammy Richmond, Marian Scheinholtz, Stacey Shilling, Mary Singer, Susanne Smith Roley, and Jeff Snodgrass. These individuals pulled from their vast practice experiences and their understanding of ethics to present realistic scenarios and solutions.

Readers familiar with the first edition will notice that several of the original authors Linda Gabriel, Stacey (Shilling) Harcum, Elizabeth Larson, Mary Singer, Susanne Roley, Jeff Snodgrass, S. Maggie Reitz and Janie B. Scott updated and revised their original works and in some cases wrote new chapters. We are fortunate to receive new contributions from Lea Cheyney Brandt, Mary Ellen Buning, Sue Coppola, Lisa Crabtree, Janet DeLany, Tim Holmes, Liliana Alvarez Jaramillo, Rochelle Mendonca, Noralyn Pickens, Roger Smith, Scott Trudeau, Shirley Wells, Wayne Winistorfer, and Missi Zahoransky. These authors re-envisioned previous chapters and developed ones focused on future trends within occupational therapy practice.

Towson University supported this project by funding graduate assistants who were valuable contributors to the organization and production of this book. In the first edition these exceptional occupational therapy students included Justine Ascanio, Audrey Grant, Hollie Hatt, Stacey Harcum, Melissa Kellner, and Janell Wilson. They helped with securing research documents, formatting tables, and completing dozens of other tasks that positively contributed to this book.

Towson University undergraduate student workers in the Office of the Provost—Christy Chzajkowski, Taylor Gosnell, Mariah Grosko, and Frankie Oliveria—provided valuable assistance in their preliminary research for this edition. We are grateful for their time, energy, and helpful suggestions. We hope that they learned from their experiences as we benefitted from their efforts.

We also would like to acknowledge the support of family and friends as we journeyed through this extensive, reflective, and rewarding process. We especially would like to thank our spouses, Phil Eichmiller and Fred Reitz, for their computer expertise, completion of various domestic tasks, supply of nourishment through lengthy weekend afternoons of our joint editing and writing, and overall patience and support during these lengthy processes.

Finally, we want to acknowledge that close friendships can survive and grow while engaged in the development, writing, and editing of these editions. Opportunities for reflection and debate resulted in this current publication, which we hope will be relevant and helpful to students and occupational therapy practitioners alike.

—Janie B. Scott and S. Maggie Reitz

INTRODUCTION

Janie B. Scott, MA, OT/L, FAOTA, and S. Maggie Reitz, PhD, OTR/L, FAOTA

Practical Applications for the Occupational Therapy Code of Ethics (2015) was updated to provide occupational therapy students and practitioners with an expanded resource containing practical case studies to help promote ethical reflection and practice in their increasingly complex and varied professional roles.

Through the years the profession has had several documents to help occupational therapy practitioners consider the ethical dilemmas they encounter. However, we believed that the first edition of this book, *Practical Applications for the Occupational Therapy Code of Ethics and Ethics Standards* (Scott & Reitz, 2010), would be the first occupational therapy publication that presents ethical dilemmas in case study formats across all practice areas as designated in the *Centennial Vision* of the American Occupational Therapy Association (AOTA, 2007). We hoped that this approach would help occupational therapy practitioners, students, and others see deliberative processes that can be used when faced with complex ethical questions when it is difficult to determine a satisfactory course of action. This book was a result of our desire to meet an unmet need in our professional literature.

This new edition is titled *Practical Applications of the Occupational Therapy Code of Ethics (2015)* to reflect changes to the *Occupational Therapy Code of Ethics (2015)* (referred to throughout this book as the "Code"; AOTA, 2015). We expanded the publication by adding a Decision Table and reflective questions to each chapter, which we hope will expand the utility of the book in the classroom, in occupational therapy study groups, and for personal use. The expanded inclusion of case studies and vignettes provides readers with real-life ethical dilemmas extracted from the experiences of our expert authors.

Ethics in Occupational Therapy

The following definition of *occupational therapy practice*, developed by AOTA (2011) to describe occupational therapy to state boards of practice and external entities, highlights the profession's wide-ranging scope and settings:

> The practice of occupational therapy means the therapeutic use of occupations, including everyday life activities with individuals, groups, populations, or organizations to support participation, performance, and function in roles and situations in home, school, workplace, community, and other settings. Occupational therapy services are provided for habilitation, rehabilitation, and the promotion of health and wellness to those who have or are at risk for developing an illness, injury, disease, disorder, condition, impairment, disability, activity limitation, or participation restriction. Occupational therapy addresses the physical, cognitive, psychosocial, sensory–perceptual, and other aspects of performance in a variety of contexts and environments to support engagement in occupations that affect physical and mental health, well-being, and quality of life. (p. S81)

This definition identifies various client groups and settings in which occupational therapy services are delivered. However, the definition does not specifically address the roles of occupational therapy practitioners relative to education, research, advocacy, or volunteerism. The Principles articulated in the *Occupational Therapy Code of Ethics (2015)* can be used to guide the behaviors and ethical decision making of occupational therapy students and practitioners in their many roles.

This book provides occupational therapy practitioners and students with a resource to use in exploring the Code to promote ethical reflection and practice in their increasingly complex and varied professional roles. Occupational therapy practitioners fulfill a wide variety of roles, including those of educator, practitioner, consultant, policymaker, advocate, researcher, and volunteer. Ethical dilemmas may arise in any of these roles and across the many contexts in which occupational therapy is practiced. Practitioners can use the principles articulated in the Code as a guide for their behaviors and ethical decision making in their many roles and contexts. The overarching goal of this book is to help occupational therapy practitioners and students strive toward the aspirational principles articulated in the Code.

Content

This book is divided into four parts. Part I reviews the historical and current foundations and theories, as well as models for ethical reasoning for use in decision making in occupational therapy. This section includes a new chapter on ethical theories and perspectives to provide a more comprehensive overview. Part II discusses the six principles in the Code, and Part III illustrates applications of ethical reasoning in practice. Part IV, on trends, was added to cover areas or components of practice that are continuing to grow and evolve, frequently presenting ethical challenges. The first two sections provide the foundation on which to base an understanding of the materials presented in the final two sections.

Case studies and vignettes appear in Part I, Chapter 4 and chapters in Part II (Principles), Part III (Applications), and Part IV (Trends). The authors developed their case studies and vignettes on the basis of their experiences as occupational therapy practitioners. They wrote in their own unique voice to help readers appreciate the ethical dilemmas that arise in diverse settings and the strategies they have developed to seek good ethical outcomes. In general, the authors describe more complex ethical situations and provide more detail in the case studies than in the vignettes.

New to this edition is the inclusion of reflective questions, which can be used as a tool to promote ethical reasoning and decision-making. Chapters in Part II–Part IV include at least one decision table, which details the potential outcomes for different potential resolutions of ethical dilemmas.

Part III includes chapters on each of the six areas of practice linked to AOTA's *Centennial Vision* (AOTA, 2007) and AOTA's *Vision 2015* (AOTA, 2016). In addition, chapters are included on administration and management; education; research; interprofessional ethics; and new to this edition, a chapter on ethics and culture. Based on an analysis of current practice and ethical issues, a new section, Part IV, was added that includes chapters on international practice and internationalization, technology, autism, environment, and reimbursement. The appendices include relevant official documents and other resource materials.

An emphasis is placed on a variety of important themes, including

- Adherence to the Code, Accreditation Council for Occupational Therapy Education (2012) standards, and state regulations;
- Support of occupational therapy students' academic education and professional development for ethical practice;
- Fulfillment of state regulatory requirements;
- Promotion of occupational therapy practitioners' ethical reasoning and decision making through continuing education; and
- Compliance with continuing education mandates.

The phrase *occupational therapy practitioner* is used throughout the book to refer to both occupational therapists and occupational therapy assistants. The authors present models and approaches to help readers resolve ethical dilemmas and provide realistic case studies and vignettes to assist practitioners in identifying solutions that range from taking no action or addressing the situation at the local level to involving organizations and agencies to promote ethical practice and protect the public and the profession.

We selected the authors of this book on the basis of their expertise in the subject areas associated with their respective chapters. In Parts II and III, the authors first introduce a principle or practice area (e.g., research, children and youth) and then discuss the practical application of ethics. The authors approach their assigned ethics topic on the basis of the method best suited to sharing ethical issues in that particular practice area. The authors also include several vignettes to ensure a common thread of practical application.

A list of pertinent Internet and print resources, and appendixes with ethics-related documents by AOTA and the National Board for Certification in Occupational Therapy also are included. The Code is reprinted in Appen dix A; consult this and other documents as needed during your progress through this book.

Conclusion

Ethical dilemmas arise during the academic preparation to become an occupational therapy practitioner and continue throughout all areas of practice. Lifelong ethical education is an important part of becoming and remaining an ethical occupational therapy practitioner. One method to ensure consistent ethical practice is to use tools like this book that provide ethical decision-making models and opportunities to reflect on ethical issues and appropriate responses using the Code.

The editors and authors hope this publication will be used in academic settings and in occupational therapy practice to expand the dialogue regarding the ethical practice of occupational therapy. The purpose is to encourage occupational therapy practitioners and students to think of ethics not from a punitive perspective but rather from one that encourages learning, reflection, dialogue, and ethical behavior. Furthermore, we hope this publication helps readers make informed decisions when confronting ethical dilemmas but caution them to consult an attorney or other professional for legal or expert advice.

References

Accreditation Council for Occupational Therapy Education. (2012). 2011 Accreditation Council for Occupational Therapy Education® (ACOTE®) standards. *American Journal of Occupational Therapy, 66*(6 Suppl.), S6–S74. https://doi.org/10.5014/ajot.2012.66S6

American Occupational Therapy Association. (2007). AOTA's *Centennial Vision* and executive summary. *American Journal of Occupational Therapy, 61*, 613–614. https://doi.org/10.5014/ajot.61.6.613

American Occupational Therapy Association. (2011). Association policies: Policy 5.3.1. Definition of occupational therapy practice for state regulation. *American Journal of Occupational Therapy, 65*(Suppl. 6), S81. https://doi.org/10.5014/ajot.2011.65S80

American Occupational Therapy Association. (2015). Occupational therapy code of ethics (2015). *American Journal of Occupational Therapy, 69*(Suppl. 3), 6912310030. http://dx.doi.org/10.5014/ajot.2015.696S03

American Occupational Therapy Association. (2016). *Vision 2025.* https://www.aota.org/AboutAOTA/vision-2025.aspx

Scott, J. B., & Reitz, M. (Eds.). (2010). *Practical applications for the occupational therapy code of ethics and ethics standards.* Bethesda, MD: AOTA Press.

Part I.

FOUNDATIONS

INTRODUCTION TO PART I

Janie B. Scott, MA, OT/L, FAOTA

The historical foundations of ethical thinking that have had the greatest influence on occupational therapy and the *Occupational Therapy Code of Ethics (2015)* (hereinafter referred to as the "Code"; American Occupational Therapy Association [AOTA], 2015) are reviewed in Part I. The history of ethics is relevant to the government, philosophy, culture, and beliefs of societies and also to health care delivery in general and occupational therapy theory and practice specifically.

Part I provides glimpses of ethical constructs developed in societies around the world and across time, setting the stage for the remainder of the book by showing readers how ethical thinking in occupational therapy has been influenced by the history of ethics. Readers also will explore how this ethical legacy has been implemented within the profession of occupational therapy, from the roles of certification and state regulation of the profession as a whole to the expectations and enforcement of ethical behavior for individual occupational therapy practitioners. The section provides a structure and context for delving into the complex case studies and vignettes involving a variety of practice settings and populations that are presented in the rest of the book. The presentation of various approaches for solving ethical dilemmas will help occupational therapy students and practitioners analyze complicated situations armed with strategies for their resolution.

Chapter 1, "Ethical Theories and Perspectives," is an important addition to this edition. The author describes theories of applied ethics, metaethics, normative ethics, and others, and, through vignettes, connects readers to ways current ethical situations can be understood. The use of reflective questions here and in all later chapters encourages readers to synthesize and apply the material presented.

Chapter 2, "Historical Background of Ethics in Occupational Therapy," outlines the evolution of ethical thinking throughout history, focusing on the ancient world, medieval Europe, and the Age of Enlightenment. Taoist beliefs, the Hippocratic Oath, Socratic tradition, and medieval guilds' behaviors and values are compared with principles in the Code. Tables show how AOTA's core values and the Code's values reflect this history.

In addition, the entities and mechanisms responsible for ensuring the ethical practice of occupational therapy are described. Readers will learn when the National Board for Certification in Occupational Therapy (NBCOT) was created and how its policies and procedures and those of state regulatory boards (SRBs) ensure that occupational therapy practitioners engage in ethical practice. The jurisdictions of AOTA, NBCOT, and SRBs are presented and described, as are the disciplinary processes, enforcement procedures, and potential disciplinary actions of each. Within these contexts, the importance of continuing competence and its relationship to ethical behaviors and regulations is highlighted.

The authors of Chapter 3, "Promoting Ethics in Occupational Therapy Practice: Codes and Consequences," discuss the evolution of codes of ethics reflecting the values and standards of occupational therapy groups and organizations and the purpose of these codes in professional life. Readers will review the development of the seven core values on which the ethical practice of occupational therapy is based and see how these values were incorporated into the current Code. Through a description of AOTA's earlier codes and their parallels with the current Code, readers will gain an appreciation of how this document has evolved in response to changes in occupational therapy practice and societal beliefs.

Chapter 4, "Solving Ethical Dilemmas," introduces ethical decision-making models, drawing on the work of ethics experts and occupational therapy authors. Readers will learn a four-step decision-making process that is synthesized from the work of these authors and that provides a way to explore the ethical dilemmas practitioners face in occupational therapy practice. This Scott Four-Step Process for Ethical Decision Making, together with the resources available through their own institutions, AOTA, their SRB, and the NBCOT, will help readers address ethical situations in an appropriate manner.

Reference

American Occupational Therapy Association. (2015). Occupational therapy code of ethics (2015). *American Journal of Occupational Therapy, 69*(Suppl. 3), 6912310030. https://doi.org/10.5014/ajot.2015.696S03

Chapter 1.

ETHICAL THEORIES AND PERSPECTIVES

Lea Cheyney Brandt, OTD, MA, OTR/L

Learning Objectives

By the end of the chapter, readers will be able to

- Describe and differentiate among the terms *descriptive ethics, metaethics,* and *normative ethics;*
- Determine and understand the relationship among the profession's code of ethics, ethical theory, and ethical decision making in occupational therapy practice; and
- Apply ethical theories through vignettes depicting occupational therapy practice.

Key Terms and Concepts

✧ Applied ethics
✧ Consequentialism
✧ Deontology
✧ Descriptive ethics
✧ Ethical skills
✧ Ethics of care
✧ Metaethics
✧ Normative ethics
✧ Principlism
✧ Right action
✧ Utility
✧ Virtue ethics

This chapter on ethical theories provides readers with a basic understanding of how theory grounds ethical decision making in practice as well as the development of the profession's code of ethics. The content should not be viewed as comprehensive in nature and merely highlights a few of the most common ethical theories applied to practice. The intent is to provide perspective on how reason should guide ethical decision making to optimize the chances for a rationally supported course of action.

Each normative ethical theory explored in this chapter can be used in concert with another. Although occupational therapy practitioners may gravitate toward a particular theoretical approach, understanding the strengths and weaknesses of each theory should assist in limiting one's bias when reasoning through ethical conflicts.

Approaches to Ethical Analysis

Ethical theories relate to the study of right and wrong conduct in society and how to determine moral behavior. Approaches to ethical analysis are typically grouped into one of three categories:

(1) descriptive ethics, (2) metaethics, and (3) normative ethics.

Descriptive Ethics

Descriptive ethics is a fact-based examination of different societies or cultures using scientific inquiry to identify how people reason and act (Beauchamp & Childress, 2013). In descriptive ethics, the focus is on examining a people's beliefs about morality without judging whether that society has the "correct" ethical principles. A person who is taking a descriptive approach to determining ethical action may ask, "What do people in a society think is right?"

Metaethics

In contrast, ***metaethics*** asks questions about the meaning of moral claims, how moral knowledge might be possible, and the grounds for making the determination of right versus wrong. A metaethical theory, unlike a descriptive ethical theory, tries to define the essential meaning and nature of the problem being discussed. Instead of focusing on the action, metaethics is concerned with the status or legitimacy of ethical claims. Metaethics attempts to determine if ethical claims grounded in personal, cultural, or divine opinion are true (Shafer-Landau, 2012).

Like descriptive ethics, metaethics rarely enters into health care ethics discussions, as it does not provide guidance as to the direction to take when faced with an ethical problem. Conversely, normative ethics (discussed next) promotes a right course of action based on an established standard of morality.

Normative Ethics

A ***normative ethics*** approach is devoted to examining our moral relations with one another, and applies to occupational therapy as it guides practitioners on how they should act in consideration of their clients and colleagues. To determine the most ethical course of action, normative ethics asks, "What are our fundamental moral duties? Which character traits count as virtues, which as vices, and why? Who should our role models be? Do the ends always justify the means, or are there certain types of action that should never be done under any circumstances?" (Shafer-Landau, 2012, p. 2).

In clinical settings when ethics committees and ethics consultants engage with health care teams to determine the best course of action for their patients and clients, they are doing mainly normative ethics. Some may argue that health care practitioners are engaged in what some consider a fourth kind of ethics, applied ethics. ***Applied ethics*** is the act of applying general moral theories and principles to ethical problems arising in medical or clinical contexts (Brannigan & Boss, 2001). However, many consider applied ethics a type or subgroup of normative ethics, not a separate ethical approach; both normative and applied ethics focus on the practical task of arriving at the moral standards that should shape behavior. Applied ethics is generally focused on the application of these moral standards when examining specific ethical issues.

Normative ethical approaches dominate ethics discussions in health care, as they are linked to determining the rightness of an action. Although normative ethical approaches generally focus on either the act itself or the consequence of the action, the multiple normative theories may inform ethical decision making in practice. Understanding these theories and how they relate to practice may improve the ethical reasoning skills of practitioners and improve their ability to resolve or mitigate ethical conflicts in practice.

Ethical Theories

Theories provide a framework for addressing ethical quandaries in practice, but all theories, if applied unilaterally, may result in suboptimal outcomes (Brannigan & Boss, 2001). Ethical theories are often viewed as reductionistic. "They offer one idea as the key to morality, and attempt to reduce everything to that one idea" (Steinbock, London, & Arras, 2013, p. 9). Therefore, it is important to be familiar with the strengths and weaknesses of competing ethical theories.

Although the philosophical arguments that ground these theories do not account for this eclectic use of often diverse and competing views, in practice integrating differing approaches may better assist the practitioner to arrive at an ethically supported course of action. This is why the *Occupational Therapy Code of Ethics (2015)* (hereinafter referred to as the "Code;" American Occupational Therapy Association [AOTA], 2015; available in Appendix A) reminds personnel that familiarity with the Code is only a component of acting ethically. It is also important to recognize that resolution of "ethical issues is a systematic process that includes analysis of the complex dynamics of situations, weighing of consequences, making reasoned decisions, taking action, and reflecting on outcomes" (AOTA, 2015, p. 1). Various normative ethical theories that may assist occupational therapy practitioners to effectively analyze complex ethical problems are described below.

Although clinical ethics can be categorized as an imprecise discipline, the following ethical theories are predicated on the assumption that there are objective moral truths. Although each theory subscribes to a different approach in defining moral truth or ethically supported action, the theories presume that ethics is neither relative nor subjective and that there is such a thing as morality and, conversely, immoral action.

Occupational therapy and other health professions' ethics specifically require acceptance of the claim that ethics is objective. Although ethics contains many complex questions that may make it difficult to define an objective good, the ethical course of action is one that is supported by reason. "Moral truths are truths of reason; that is, a moral judgment is true if it is backed by better reasons than alternatives" (Rachels & Rachels, 2015, p. 41).

In occupational therapy ethics, the objective claims, or moral truths, regarding right and wrong conduct are generally linked to one of four families of theories: (1) virtue theory, (2) ethics of care, (3) consequentialism, and (4) deontology.

Virtue Ethics

The theory of ***virtue ethics*** focuses less on moral action; instead, it is concerned with the character of the *moral agent,* or the person who is completing the action. Contemporary virtue ethics can be traced back to the philosophy of the Ancient Greeks and, specifically, Aristotle's Nicomachean Ethics (Steinbock et al., 2013). According to one of the themes of virtue ethics, a ***right action*** is understood in reference to what a virtuous person would do (Shafer-Landau, 2012). Opposition to this theory stems from the subjective nature of defining *ethical action* on the seemingly arbitrary nature of why and how a "virtuous" person may choose to act.

However, in the complex world of health care, many would argue that a theory is preferred when the nuances of ethical decision making can be addressed. Proponents of virtue theory argue that, secondary to the complexity of most ethical problems, the right action "cannot be adequately captured by a set of rules" and therefore the moral agent must also rely on one's virtue, which has been cultivated in experience (Steinbock et al., 2013, p. 33). The virtuous person can use reason to support the action taken based on the facts of the situation, morally relevant variables, emotional maturity, and application of past experience. Vignette 1.1 provides an account of a virtuous practitioner.

Ethics of Care

Because ethics requires us to make decisions in consideration of others, it can be concluded that ethics, by nature, is relational. "Whether concerned with justice, character, motivation, right action or living well, ethics evaluates the implications of one's agency on others and their agency on one's self. This concept is embraced by the ethics of care" (Corcoran, Brandt, Fleming, & Gu, 2014, p. 3).

Ethics of care is a relationship-based theory, which means that it focuses on compassion and empathy rather than the character of the moral agent. It can be traced back to the work of psychologist Carol Gilligan, who objected to the notion that an

Vignette 1.1. Virtue Ethics

Corrine is an occupational therapist who has been practicing for more than 25 years. Over the course of the past 15 years, she has been working in a clinic where she is a valued mentor to her colleagues and has an impeccable reputation as a thoughtful, compassionate, and honest practitioner. During annual peer reviews her colleagues consistently praise her for "going above and beyond" when caring for her clients. When Corrine's colleagues encounter ethical dilemmas they often go to her for advice, especially when the Code does not support a clear course of action. Corrine has shown great insight when identifying which ethical principles are in conflict, applying her past experience to weigh possible consequences, and then making a reasoned decision regarding the best course of action. Her colleagues believe her to exhibit integrity and strong character; therefore, they trust she will provide them with sound advice when faced with making ethical decisions.

ethics of principles is a higher order of moral development than an ethics based on relationships (Gilligan, 1982). Ethics of care continues to be closely identified with modern feminist philosophy, as women typically respond in terms of caring, whereas men typically reason in terms of duty and justice (Rachels & Rachels, 2015).

Ethics of care is reflective of virtue ethics in that it is not focused on the action itself but rather on how we execute the action. However, it deviates from virtue ethics in that it is less focused on the character of the moral agent but rather on promotion of a caring relationship. In occupational therapy the focus would be on fostering a caring relationship between the practitioner and the client.

Although the ethics of care holds promise as a viable theory, especially in health care that is predicated on a caring relationship, there are many pitfalls associated with this theory when not tempered with an objective moral norm. Specifically, the ethics of care theory has been criticized for the following limitations: threatening to restrict the scope of the moral community, emotions related to caring relationships cloud judgment, lack of impartiality, lack of strategy in dealing with uncooperative or dangerous people, and a lack of accommodation for moral rights (Shafer-Landau, 2012). Although the ethics of care has substantial value in occupational therapy practice as it promotes an empathetic response to client needs, Vignette 1.2 outlines the limitations of the theory when not used in concert with accepted moral standards or principles.

Consequentialism

Consequentialism, also referred to as *teleological theory,* derives ethical merit by focusing on the outcome of an action. One of the most recognized consequentialist theories is utilitarianism.

Utility, or the overall usefulness of an action, is described as doing the greatest good for the greatest number of people. Ultimately, the morally right action is the one that has the best effect, either maximizing good or limiting harm. Consequentialism typically involves asking these questions:

- What will be the effects of each course of action?
- Will they be positive or negative?
- Who will benefit?
- What will do the least harm? (Pozgar, 2013, p. 7)

Consequentialism is criticized most often for its innate incompatibility with justice, especially with regard to the potential impact on the minority as well as its focus on backward-looking reasoning (Rachels & Rachels, 2015). Because this theory is concerned with the utility argument, the greatest good for the greatest number, then the theory would support committing an injustice that only affects the minority of individuals as long as the action produces benefit for the majority. Consequentialism also predicates its ethical rationale on the outcome of an action that has yet to take place. One of the strongest defenses against these criticisms is that the principle of utility should be used as a guide for choosing rules (i.e., rule utilitarianism), not as a guide for supporting individual acts (i.e., act utilitarianism). In Vignette 1.3, an occupational therapy assistant weighs the ethics of two alternative actions.

Deontology

Rule utilitarianism may seem to resolve some of the ethical critiques associated with a consequential approach, but this begs the question of how to establish the moral worth of certain rules. ***Deontology*** is a rule-based or duty-based theory. In contrast to

---

Vignette 1.2. Ethics of Care

Cory is an occupational therapist who works in a nontraditional, community-based practice that focuses on assisting young women who are homeless to find employment. One of the primary barriers for her clients is that they are unable to afford reliable transportation to different areas of the city where employers compensate at a living wage. Cory has a friend who works for the transit system. He tells Cory that he has access to free public transit passes, which he has permission to distribute to disgruntled passengers who threaten to file a complaint. He offers to give Cory a stack of passes to disseminate to her clients, stating, "Even though your clients don't technically meet the criteria for a free pass, it doesn't really hurt anything." According to the ethics of care theory, Cory would work with her friend to distribute the free passes to her clients whom she believes would benefit most. Her focus is on her relationship with the clients, not impartial rules. The act of stealing, however, is clearly unethical.

Vignette 1.3. Act vs. Rule Utilitarianism

Bobby is an occupational therapy assistant who is facing an ethical dilemma. He tends to favor a consequentialist ethic and is therefore weighing the potential outcomes of his decision. He works with children and youth, and his client's insurance will pay for intervention only after pre-authorization has occurred. Although he has never been denied for ongoing services, the front office administrator has to call for authorization monthly as the insurance company will only approve a total of 8 visits each month. Bobby just completed a session and realized that the office staff was behind, so he did not have pre-authorization. He knows that generating a bill prior to authorization will result in an out-of-pocket expense to the family that would normally be covered by insurance. The family is on a fixed income, and this will be a hardship to them.

Bobby knows that he could have the front office call and get the authorization within the hour. He could then change his documentation to reflect a later treatment time to have the session covered by insurance. Using an act-utilitarian approach Bobby may be able to ethically justify falsifying documentation to diminish the financial harm that the family could incur, even though this would violate the Code and Principle 5, Veracity. However, using a rule-utilitarian approach he could not ethically justify falsifying documentation. Even though the consequences of his actions in this case might justify the action, the consequences of supporting a rule that allows falsification of documentation would not result in the most benefit and could result in greater harm than good.

consequentialism, deontology focuses on the action as opposed to the consequence of that action.

The Ten Commandments and the Golden Rule are common examples of deontology. The primary philosophical critique of religious-based rules, or treating others as one would want to be treated, is that the rules themselves are not universal. One of the most recognized and important philosophers to refute utilitarianism and propose the idea of using universal norms to determine ethical action was Immanuel Kant.

Kant believed that people cannot be used as a means to an end and focused his work on demonstrating through reason that there are categorical imperatives that must be universally adopted (Shafer-Landau, 2012). According to Kant's categorical imperative, one should "act only according to that maxim whereby you can at the same time will that it should become a universal law" (Ellington, 1993, p. 30). By this standard, the Golden Rule falls short in health care settings; the idea that we should treat our clients as we want to be treated may, in some cases, require us to provide interventions not valued by our clients.

Although there is reasonable concern with using the Golden Rule to guide decision making in health care, ethicists such as Beauchamp and Childress argue that there are universally accepted rules that should be used to guide health care decisions—the Principles of Biomedical Ethics. Although this principles-based approach (i.e., principlism) differs from Kant's universal law theory, in the rules themselves as well as the concept of absolute duty, it still subscribes to a deontological normative theory.

Arguably, the most commonly used framework in contemporary Western health care ethics is principlism as outlined by Beauchamp and Childress (Brannigan & Boss, 2001). In 1979, Beauchamp and Childress published *Principles of Biomedical Ethics,* which was predicated on the four principles outlined in the Belmont Report and contended that the four principles of beneficence, nonmaleficence, justice, and respect for autonomy are useful in guiding ethical decision making in health care.

According to ***principlism,*** when consequences and principles conflict, the ethical act is the one in accordance with the principles. The principles are not like universal laws, as Beauchamp and Childress state, "it is a mistake in biomedical ethics to assign priority to any basic principle over other basic principles—as if morality must be hierarchically structured or as if we must cherish one moral norm over another without consideration of particular circumstances" (2013, p. ix). Principles are treated similarly in many of the health professions' codes of ethics, including our Code.

The Code (AOTA, 2015) outlines six principles and is grounded by the work completed by Beauchamp and Childress. When applying the Code to practice, the same weaknesses appear as those associated with principlism, in that there is a lack of clarity as to how to proceed when two or more principles are in conflict. Although it is important to be able to consider the context when applying ethical principles, there is again an imprecise nature to the reasoning process that can result in a flawed analysis grounded in bias, ignorance, or limited resources.

Vignette 1.4. Principlism

Jamal is an occupational therapy practitioner working in an inpatient acute care setting with **Mr. Sanjah,** an 82-year-old man recovering from a fall. Mr. Sanjah has been treated in the Emergency Department 4 times over the course of the last month, secondary to falls. This is, however, his first inpatient admission. Jamal recommends that Mr. Sanjah be discharged to a long-term-care facility with 24-hour care, secondary to his risk for falls. Later that day the social worker pages him and lets him know that Mr. Sanjah is refusing placement in a facility and demanding discharge to home. The social worker suggests having Mr. Sanjah declared incompetent and transferred to a facility, fearing that another unobserved fall at home may result in Mr. Sanjah's death.

In this case there is a clear conflict between beneficence, wanting to prevent harm from occurring, and respecting Mr. Sanjah's autonomy. There are many extenuating circumstances that must be taken into account when identifying the ethically supported course of action. Depending on how Jamal weighs and balances those factors, the decision may vary, and there are opportunities for bias to unduly influence the process.

In Vignette 1.4 an occupational therapy practitioner weighs the outcomes of following each of two competing principles.

Summary

As is true in medicine and other health professions, providing occupational therapy in an ethical manner is a practice skill. ***Ethical skills,*** like all other practice skills, are optimally learned during professional school, although occupational therapy practitioners need to continue cultivating those skills in their practice to develop a certain level of comfort and expertise in navigating ethical conflict.

There are no practices that are widely considered best when it comes to teaching occupational therapy ethics; however, minimum standards are set forth by many accreditation and regulatory agencies. The Accreditation Council for Occupational Therapy Education® (2012) requires students to "demonstrate knowledge and understanding of the [Code] and use [it] as a guide for ethical decision making" (p. 32). Although there is no consensus regarding the most effective pedagogical strategies, requiring familiarity with the Code ensures that most occupational therapy students are trained in or at least exposed to deontological or duty-based theory as a means to address ethical conflicts in practice.

The ethics curricula for most of the health professions typically focuses on a deontological approach. When using a deontological approach, an act is judged right or wrong if it is in accordance with prescribed duties or principles rather than the consequences of the act itself. Although occupational therapy's Code reflects a bias toward principlism, there are many ethical approaches that occupational therapy may draw from in order to resolve ethical conflicts.

Most practitioners would prefer to focus on case studies depicting ethical conflicts and real-life applications using the Code in place of learning the moral theory, but it is imperative for current and future practitioners to familiarize themselves with the theories and approaches that undergird ethical decision making in practice (Brannigan & Boss, 2001). By gaining a basic understanding of how to reason through complex ethical problems using theory, practitioners will be better able to develop a sound ethical argument and in turn better serve their clients' needs. To gain competence in navigating the complex environments in which occupational therapy is delivered, practitioners must cultivate skills related to ethical and clinical reasoning with equal dedication to both. In fact, it is an ethical obligation to do so.

Reflective Questions

1. Is occupational therapy ethics in need of more metaethical discussion (e.g., should we question those principles that we have identified as universally accepted)?
2. Why might there be more principles in the Code than those outlined by Beauchamp and Childress (2013)?
3. Because there is no primary principle in ethics, how should one determine the most ethical course of action when principles are in conflict?
4. Should expectations for the ethics education of future and current practitioners be modified to focus on how we execute the action rather than the action itself (e.g., incorporating feminist or virtue ethics into educational offerings)?

References

Accreditation Council for Occupational Therapy Education. (2012). *2011 Accreditation Council for Occupational Therapy Education (ACOTE) standards and interpretive guide*. Retrieved from https://www.aota.org/-/media/Corporate/Files/EducationCareers/Accredit/Standards/2011-Standards-and-Interpretive-Guide.pdf

American Occupational Therapy Association. (2015). Occupational therapy code of ethics (2015). *American Journal of Occupational Therapy, 69*(Suppl. 3), 6912310030. https://doi.org/10.5014/ajot.2015.696S03

Beauchamp, T. L., & Childress, J. F. (2013). *Principles of biomedical ethics* (7th ed.). New York: Oxford University Press.

Brannigan, M. C., & Boss, J. A. (2001). *Health care ethics in a diverse society*. Mountain View, CA: Mayfield.

Corcoran, B., Brandt, L., Fleming, D., & Gu, C. (2014). Fidelity to the healing relationship: A medical student's challenge to contemporary bioethics and prescription for medical practice. *Journal of Medical Ethics, 1,* 1–5. https://doi.org/10.1136/medethics-2013-101718

Ellington, J. W. (1993). *Immanuel Kant: Grounding for the metaphysics of morals: On a supposed right to lie because of philanthropic concerns* (3rd ed.). Indianapolis: Hackett.

Gilligan, C. (1982). *In a different voice.* Cambridge, MA: Harvard University Press.

Pozgar, G. (2013). *Legal and ethical issues for health professionals* (3rd ed.). Burlington, MA: Jones & Bartlett Learning.

Rachels, J., & Rachels, S. (2015). *The elements of moral philosophy* (8th ed.). Boston: McGraw-Hill.

Shafer-Landau, R. (2012). *The fundamentals of ethics* (2nd ed.). New York: Oxford University Press.

Steinbock, B., London, A. J., & Arras, J. D. (2013). *Ethical issues in modern medicine: Contemporary readings in bioethics* (8th ed.). New York: McGraw-Hill.

Chapter 2.

HISTORICAL BACKGROUND OF ETHICS IN OCCUPATIONAL THERAPY

S. Maggie Reitz, PhD, OTR/L, FAOTA, and Janie B. Scott, MA, OT/L, FAOTA

Learning Objectives

By the end of the chapter, readers will be able to

- Describe the historical evolution of ethics in the practice of occupational therapy,
- Contrast historical codes with the current official documents of the American Occupational Therapy Association, and
- Apply the current *Occupational Therapy Code of Ethics (2015)* to potential and future ethical dilemmas encountered in occupational therapy practice.

Key Terms and Concepts

- ✧ Ethics
- ✧ Guilds
- ✧ Hippocratic Oath
- ✧ Moral treatment
- ✧ Professional ethics
- ✧ Proto–occupational therapists
- ✧ Reason
- ✧ Taoism

History provides a lens through which occupational therapy practitioners can understand the present and a foundation on which we can wisely build the future. As Stattel (1977) noted, "We cannot accurately and professionally comprehend the present or look at the future intelligently until we become acquainted with and study the past" (p. 650).

Occupational therapy has a long history—a century in length—that is rich with practice experience, but the ethical principles governing our practice date back millennia. The history of ethics has been shaped by needs and changes within societies over time. An understanding of how this evolution has shaped society and our profession can help guide thinking and processes to ensure our conduct is consistently ethical.

After defining *ethics* and explaining its function in human society, this chapter provides a snapshot of the contributions of three eras in history—the ancient world, medieval Europe, and the Enlightenment—to the development of the ethics that govern occupational therapy. These time periods are represented in a timeline in Figure 2.1.

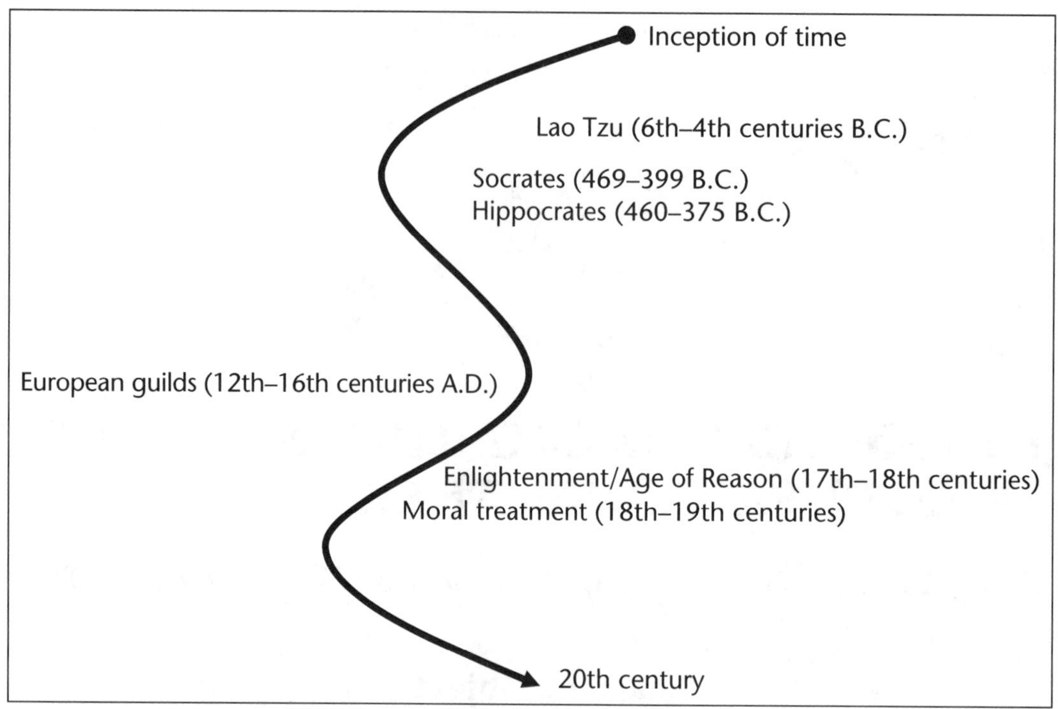

FIGURE 2.1

Milestones in the development of ethical reasoning.

Defining *Ethics*

Ethics evolved as "a systematic study of rules of conduct that is grounded in philosophical principles and theory" (Slater, 2016, p. 291). Ethics reflect societal values, morals, and norms as they are applied to the effort of communities, professions, and organizations to determine what is or is not acceptable behavior (Slater, 2016).

Codes of ***professional ethics*** articulate the duties that members of the discipline have to each other and to society, and are based on beliefs and values that a profession supports. Ethics guide behavior, and a code of ethics serves as a guide for individual practitioners and for a profession (Scott, 2007). Professional ethics reflect those morals and values that are endorsed by organizations and serve to guide the behaviors of their members. These beliefs are based on agreements about what is right or wrong in accordance with societal norms. The organization arranges its ethical beliefs into codes that reflect behavioral principles. These principles not only serve as guidelines for the profession but also inform the public of the behavioral expectations of the profession, organization, or agency (Scott, 2007; Slater, 2016).

Ethics Through Time

Humans are social beings who, since their earliest origins, have lived in groups for survival and reproductive advantages (Wilcock, 2006). To manage the challenges inherent in living in groups, people have developed increasingly complex systems over time to manage disputes and to promote behavior supportive of the group and larger society. The establishment of norms, values, and rules facilitated the aesthetics, productivity, and survival of the group as a whole and of its individual members. Scientists have proposed that early humans placed a high value on self-help and caring for kin. Once people were able to care for themselves and their kin, they would then display altruism by sharing resources with others within their larger social group (Wilcock, 2001b).

Wilcock (2001a) described ***proto–occupational therapists*** (i.e., the premodern counterparts of modern occupational therapy practitioners) as healers who used occupation as a therapeutic medium—on the basis of their instincts and observations of the results of various actions and inactions—to enhance their health and the health of their social groups. In addition, they developed "their own methods of justice to create an effective working community to meet the needs of survival" (Wilcock, 2001a, p. 15). Proto–occupational therapists included "medicine men, shamans and priests, along with . . . monks and nuns," among others (Wilcock, 2001a, p. 16). Throughout recorded history, the qualities of ethical healers have included altruism, competency, and caring (Jonsen, 2007).

Modern occupational therapy practitioners are also healers; as such, they share the common values and behaviors of those who have healed others through time. Within the fabric of these beliefs, they weave an understanding of the linkages among occupation, natural rhythms, the environment, and health.

Ethics in Society: The Ancient World

Since the earliest societies, religions have provided guidance to followers regarding appropriate behavior. For example, the Golden Rule—treat others as you wish them to treat you—is a code of conduct embraced by Brahmanism, Buddhism, Christianity, Confucianism, Islam, Judaism, and Taoism (Kornblau & Burkhardt, 2012). The first documented set of rules guiding the behavior of physicians was the Code of King Hammurabi, found chiseled into stone pillars dating to 2000 B.C. at the site of ancient Babylon (Wilcock, 2001b).

Taoism provides an example of the ethical principles of a society as distant from us in time, geography, and tradition as ancient China. The founder of Taoism, Lao Tzu, lived sometime between the sixth and fourth centuries B.C. and wrote a code of conduct, *Tao Te Ching* (Lao Tzu, 2001), which is summarized in Table 2.1. Five of the Code's six Principles, five Related Standards of Conduct (RSCs), and two of the seven core values can be recognized in Taoist beliefs.

By the time of the ancient Greeks, pragmatic decision making about survival, health, security, and happiness had evolved into organized discussions that would form the basis of Western ethics. Two early Greek philosophers, Hippocrates and Socrates, engaged in such discussions, and their thinking can be seen today in the Code. Hippocrates (460–370 B.C.) and Socrates (469–399 B.C.) were contemporaries (Wilcock, 2001c). Hippocrates is generally recognized as the father of Western medicine and is credited as the author of the ***Hippocratic Oath*** (Hippocrates, 2002), which outlines the behaviors expected of physicians in ancient Greek times. A comparison of the directives appearing in the Hippocratic Oath to the principles and RSCs in the Code is provided in Table 2.2.

The teachings of Socrates on values and their impact on human relationships and behavior—the precursor of the ethics branch of philosophy—were immortalized in his students' writings, those of Plato being the best known (Cavalier, 2002; Wilcock, 2001c). There are no known surviving written works of Socrates. Thus, it is difficult to

Table 2.1. Comparison of Taoist Beliefs to Core Values, Principles, and RSCs in the Code

Taoist Belief[a]	Core Values, Principles, and RSCs[b]
In a home it is the site that matters.	Core value—Prudence Principle 1, Beneficence
In quality of mind it is the depth that matters.	Principle 1, Beneficence Principle 2, Nonmaleficence
In an ally it is benevolence that matters.	Core value—Altruism Principle 1, Beneficence Principle 4, Justice (RSC 4C) Principle 6, Fidelity (RSC 6I)
In speech it is good faith that matters.	Principle 6, Fidelity
In government it is order that matters.	Principle 4, Justice
In affairs it is ability that matters.	Principle 1, Beneficence
In action it is timeliness that matters.	Principle 1, Beneficence (RSC 1B) Principle 5, Veracity (RSC 5C, 5G)

Source. [a]Lao Tzu (2001). [b]American Occupational Therapy Association (2015).
Note. RSCs = Related Standards of Conduct.

Table 2.2. Comparison of the Hippocratic Oath to Principles and RSCs in the Code

Hippocratic Oath[a]	Principles[b] and RSCs
To hold him who taught me this art equally dear to me as my parents, to be a partner in life with him, and to fulfill his needs when required; to look upon his offspring as equals to my own siblings, and to teach them this art, if they shall wish to learn it, without fee or contract; and that by the set rules, lectures, and every other mode of instruction, I will impart a knowledge of the art to my own sons, and those of my teachers, and to students bound by this contract and having sworn this Oath to the law of medicine, but to no others.	Principle 6, Fidelity (RSC 6I)
I will use those dietary regimens which will benefit my patients according to my greatest ability and judgment, and I will do no harm or injustice to them.	Principle 1, Beneficence Principle 2, Nonmaleficence Principle 6, Fidelity (RSCs 6H, 6I)
I will not give a lethal drug to anyone if I am asked, nor will I advise such a plan; and similarly I will not give a woman a pessary to cause an abortion.	Principle 2, Nonmaleficence Principle 4, Justice Principle 6, Fidelity (RSC 6K)
In purity and according to divine law will I carry out my life and my art.	With the removal of the word *divine:* Principle 1, Beneficence Principle 3, Autonomy Principle 4, Justice
I will not use the knife, even upon those suffering from stones, but I will leave this to those who are trained in this craft.	Principle 2, Nonmaleficence Principle 6, Fidelity (RSC 6I)
Into whatever homes I go, I will enter them for the benefit of the sick, avoiding any voluntary act of impropriety or corruption, including the seduction of women or men, whether they are free men or slaves.	Principle 2, Nonmaleficence (RSCs 2F, 2G, 2I)
Whatever I see or hear in the lives of my patients, whether in connection with my professional practice or not, which ought not to be spoken of outside, I will keep secret, as considering all such things to be private.	Principle 3, Autonomy
So long as I maintain this Oath faithfully and without corruption, may it be granted to me to partake of life fully and the practice of my art, gaining the respect of all men for all time. However, should I transgress this Oath and violate it, may the opposite be my fate.	Principle 4, Justice

Source. [a]Hippocrates (2002). [b]American Occupational Therapy Association (2015).
Note. RSCs = Related Standards of Conduct.

separate his ideas from those of his students. This has led to disagreement and debate over which ideas were Socrates' and which were those of his pupils or other writers. This lack of certainty and continued controversy has come to be called "the Socratic problem" (Nails, 2014). Despite this uncertainty, there is some general agreement regarding values and behaviors ascribed to Socrates. A comparison of these values and behaviors to core values and attitudes, principles, and RSCs in the Code is provided in Table 2.3.

Besides Socrates and Plato there were other philosophers and physicians who contributed to the development of principles and concepts related to medical ethics, including healers in the Islamic world. One of the most prominent physician–philosophers was Abu Bakr Muhammad Ibn Zakariya al-Razi, who was born in the 860s A.D. in a city near the current capital of Iran, Tehran (Elgood, 1951; Modanlou, 2008). He is often referred to as *Rhazes* in Western texts and has been credited with numerous medical advances (Modanlou, 2008; Lyons & Petrucelli, 1987), first in chemistry and pharmacy, and later in mental health and infectious diseases, among other areas of medicine (Modanlou, 2008). Razi was a rationalist who promoted the concept of a healthy mind and body union, avoided the paternalistic approaches of his time (Modanlou, 2008), and criticized charlatans (Elgood, 1951). Through his books, his work influenced teaching in major European medical schools for more than 100 years (Modanlou, 2008).

Table 2.3. Comparison of Socratic Values and Behaviors to Core Values, Principles, and RSCs in the Code

Socratic Values and Behaviors	Core Values, Principles, and RSCs[a]
"Postulated a spiritual view of knowledge and conduct . . . and the value of truth, virtue, knowledge, and appropriate action and conduct" (Wilcock, 2001c, p. 71).	Core value—Truth Principle 5, Veracity Principle 6, Fidelity
Declined to accept payment for his work, as he did not see himself as a teacher in the way it was conceptualized in his lifetime; used a conversational probing method of instruction to foster self-analysis that was not valued or accepted at the time (Nails, 2014).	Principle 1, Beneficence Principle 3, Autonomy Principle 4, Justice (RSCs 4C, 4J)
Showed greater respect for women than his contemporaries (Nails, 2014).	Core value—Justice Principle 4, Justice
Refused to escape before his planned execution because he believed "neither to do wrong or return a wrong is ever right, not even to injure in return for an injury received" (Nails, 2014).	Core value—Truth Principle 2, Nonmaleficence Principle 4, Justice

Source. [a]American Occupational Therapy Association (2015).
Note. RSCs = Related Standards of Conduct.

Ethics at Work: Medieval Guilds

During the Middle Ages (1100–1500 A.D.), people engaged in trades and crafts, including healers, organized themselves into ***guilds*** to protect their livelihoods by establishing rules about entry into the craft and requiring training and standards of work to ensure quality. The guilds held considerable power and enforced their own rules and discipline (Sox, 2007; Naylor, 1921). The standards these guilds established contributed to the later development of professionalism and codes of ethics in medicine (Sox, 2007). Later in the 19th century, social reformers in Europe called, unsuccessfully, for a return to guilds as a way to create social justice (Wilcock, 2001c). A comparison of the activities undertaken by guilds to core values, principles, and RSCs in the Code is provided in Table 2.4.

The rules and expectations for behavior set by the guilds are an early example of how people have used values as an aspirational guide for behavior. The Code is an aspirational guide in that it provides occupational therapy students and members of the profession with a description of agreed-on behavior to strive for in order to protect and promote the well-being of both themselves and society.

Ethics in Caring: The Enlightenment

Philosophers and intellectuals identified with the Age of Enlightenment (also called the *Age of Reason*) in 17th- and 18th-century Europe believed that people could improve the state of humankind by applying ***reason*** to solve problems. The goals of humans were thought to be "knowledge, freedom, and happiness" (Encyclopedia Britannica, 2011, para. 1).

Table 2.4. Comparison of Medieval Guilds' Activities to Core Values, Principles, and RSCs in the Code

Guild Activities[a]	Core Values, Principles, and RSCs[b]
Organized members to protect their livelihood	Core values—Justice, dignity, prudence Principle 6, Fidelity
Developed rules governing entry into the guild and necessary training	Core values—Justice, dignity, prudence Principle 1, Beneficence (RSCs 1D, 1G) Principle 4, Justice (RSC 4M) Principle 5, Veracity (RSCs 5A, 5I)
Instituted standards to ensure competency	Core values—Justice, prudence Principle 1, Beneficence (RSC 1E) Principle 4, Justice (RSCs 4F, 4M, 4O)
Enforced rules	Core values—Justice, prudence Principle 4, Justice (RSCs 4F, 4N)

Source. [a]Sox (2007), Naylor (1921). [b]American Occupational Therapy Association (2015).
Note. RSCs = Related Standards of Conduct.

John Locke, a prominent philosopher of the time, believed that people are born with the capacity to develop through their unique experiences, as opposed to fulfilling a prewritten destiny (Encyclopedia Britannica, 2011; Hewett, 2006). The human capacity to adapt in response to experience is foundational to occupational therapy's belief in the importance of context, doing, and recovery (Christiansen, 1991; Fidler & Fidler, 1978; Mosey, 1981; Wilcock, 2001c). Wilcock (2001b) saw a commonality in Locke's thinking and that of pragmatists who were influential during the time occupational therapy was being developed in the United States (Breines, 1986).

Moral treatment, an 18th-century social movement for asylum reform inspired by the inhumane treatment of people with mental disorders, was heavily influenced by Enlightenment philosophy (Gordon, 2009). Reformers such as Philippe Pinel in France and William Tuke in England realized the need to bring ethical care to people with mental illness. In 1798, Pinel received permission from French Revolution leaders to release people with mental illness from chains, improve their living environments, and provide some level of autonomy. Pinel's moral treatment included providing liberty and opportunities to engage in individualized, prescribed occupations tailored to the patient's diagnosis (Wilcock, 2001c).

Following the success of moral treatment in France and England, changes were implemented in many U.S. private and state mental hospitals. In 1773 in colonial Williamsburg, the Public Hospital for Persons of Insane and Disordered Minds (Zwelling, 1985)—the first public hospital built to care solely for mentally ill patients in British North America—was opened (see Figure 2.2). While serving as superintendent of the hospital from 1841 to 1861, John Galt, a physician, implemented an approach consistent with moral treatment (Zwelling, 1985). Eli Todd, a physician associated with the establishment of the Hartford (Connecticut) Retreat for the Insane in 1824, described his view of an asylum as a thoughtful combination of medicine and moral treatment:

> It should not be a jail in which for individual and public security the unfortunate are confined, nor should it be merely a hospital where they may have the benefit of medical treatment—for without moral management the most judicious course of medication is rarely successful—nor should it be merely a school where the mind is subjected to discipline while the body continues to suffer in consequences of original or symptomatic disease. (quoted in Goodheart, 2003, p. 25)

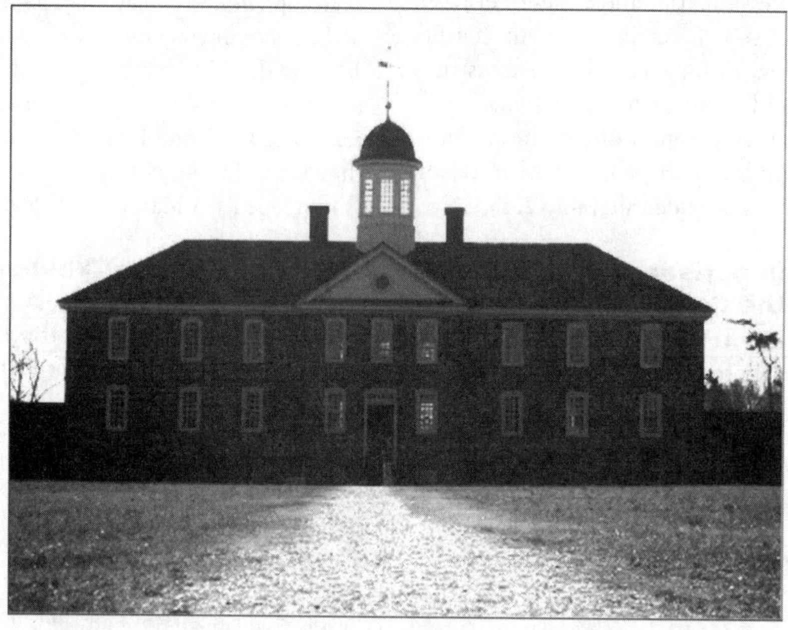

FIGURE 2.2

Public Hospital for Persons of Insane and Disordered Minds, Williamsburg, Virginia.
Source. Courtesy of Jessica Reitz Murphy. Used with permission.

Various factors contributed to the decline and later resurgent influence of moral treatment. According to Gordon (2009), the lack of scientific evidence for moral treatment, its use by nonmedical practitioners, and the high regard for the scientific method at the end of the 19th century resulted in moral treatment falling out of favor in the United States. However, Gordon argued that the core beliefs of moral treatment were not lost but became embedded in the foundation of psychiatry. Other forces beyond the preference for the scientific method also may have curtailed moral treatment (Reitz & Scaffa, 2010), including the U.S. Civil War and resulting fiscal constraints (Peloquin, 1989; Zwelling, 1985), and the push for equal access to care and resultant rapid increase in patient census without the planning and resources needed to cope with this increased volume (Kielhofner, 2004; Peloquin, 1989).

The ideals of moral treatment are ingrained in the values and ethical principles of occupational therapy. Of the six principles in the Code, the values of moral treatment can best be seen in the first four—Beneficence, Nonmaleficence, Autonomy, and Justice. Proponents of moral treatment were motivated by a desire not only to reduce suffering (i.e., Nonmaleficence) but also to bring benefits to patients (i.e., Beneficence) in an atmosphere that provided opportunities for autonomy in an equitable manner.

In his 1981 Eleanor Clarke Slagle Lecture, Robert K. Bing explored occupational therapy history. He saw moral treatment both as part of early occupational therapy for people with mental illness and as the foundation of occupational therapy. He also discussed the importance of recognizing and promoting the values of individual clients when delivering occupational therapy services. He encouraged occupational therapy practitioners to recognize and value their past as the profession moves into the future: "The history of occupational therapy is the story of ideals, deeds, hopes, and words of *individuals*" (Bing, 1981, p. 515). Bing's beliefs extend beyond the individual practitioner or student and may be seen as shared values between occupational therapy practitioners and their clients and communities.

Summary

Codes of ethics establish ideal standards that members of a group strive to achieve. Principles of ethics provide guidelines for today's occupational therapy practitioners to aspire to in their practices. Calling the Code an aspirational document underscores the challenge to practice occupational therapy ethically each day. Adhering to ethical principles is not always easy; however, the Code guides students and practitioners' actions toward ethical behavior and serves as a guidepost for examining ethical dilemmas.

Occupational therapy is a profession long concerned with providing caring, competent interventions that benefit clients and society as a whole through altruistic acts and a commitment to an aspirational code. The profession's concern with supporting ethical occupational therapy practice, as embodied in the evolving Code, reflects the long history of ethics and its application to today's societal needs.

Reflective Questions

1. Why is it important for occupational therapy practitioners to understand the historical evolution of ethics in occupational therapy practice?
2. Do you think AOTA or state associations are modern-day versions of a guild? Why or why not?
3. How do you see the Code further evolving in the next 10 years? The next 50 years?

References

American Occupational Therapy Association. (2015). Occupational therapy code of ethics (2015). *American Journal of Occupational Therapy, 69*(Suppl. 3), 6912310030. https://doi.org/10.5014/ajot.2015.696S03

Bing, R. K. (1981). Occupational therapy revisited: A paraphrastic journey (Eleanor Clarke Slagle Lecture). *American Journal of Occupational Therapy, 35,* 499–518. https://doi.org/10.5014/ajot.35.8.499

Breines, E. (1986). *Origins and adaptations.* Lebanon, NJ: Geri-Rehab.

Cavalier, R. (2002). *Introduction to ethics: Preface—Socrates (469–399 BC).* Retrieved from http://caae.phil.cmu.edu/cavalier/80130/part1/Preface/PrefaceA.html

Christiansen, C. (1991). Occupational therapy intervention: Intervention for life performance. In C. Christiansen & C. Baum (Eds.), *Occupational therapy: Overcoming human performance deficits* (pp. 1–43). Thorofare, NJ: Slack.

Elgood, C. (1951). *A medical history of Persia.* London: Cambridge University Press.

Encyclopedia Britannica. (2011). *Enlightenment.* Chicago: Encyclopædia Britannica. Retrieved from https://www.britannica.com/EBchecked/topic/188441/Enlightenment

Fidler, G., & Fidler, J. W. (1978). Doing and becoming: Purposeful action and self-actualization. *American Journal of Occupational Therapy, 32,* 305–310.

Goodheart, L. B. (2003). *Mad Yankees: The Hartford Retreat for the Insane and nineteenth-century psychiatry.* Amherst: University of Massachusetts Press.

Gordon, D. (2009). The history of occupational therapy. In E. B. Crepeau, E. S. Cohn, & B. A. B. Schell (Eds.), *Willard and Spackman's occupational therapy* (11th ed., pp. 202–215). Philadelphia: Lippincott Williams & Wilkins.

Hewett, C. (2006). *John Locke's theory of knowledge: An essay concerning human understanding.* Retrieved from http://www.thegreatdebate.org.uk/LockeEpistprnt.htm

Hippocrates. (2002). *The Hippocratic oath* (M. North, Trans.). Bethesda, MD: National Library of Medicine. Retrieved from https://www.nlm.nih.gov/hmd/greek/greek_oath.html

Jonsen, A. (2007). *Bioethics: An introduction to the history, methods, and practice* (2nd ed., pp. 3–16). Boston: Jones & Bartlett.

Kielhofner, G. (2004). The development of occupational therapy knowledge. In *Conceptual foundations of occupational therapy* (3rd ed., pp. 27–63). Philadelphia: F. A. Davis.

Kornblau, B. L., & Burkhardt, A. (2012). Introduction. In *Ethics in rehabilitation: A clinical perspective* (2nd ed., pp. 3–15). Thorofare, NJ: Slack.

Lao Tzu. (2001). Chapter 8. In *Tao Te Ching* (bilingual ed.; D. C. Lau, Trans.). Hong Kong: Chinese University Press.

Lyons, A., & Petrucelli, R. (1987). *Medicine: An illustrated history.* New York: Abradale Press.

Modanlou, H. D. (2008). A tribute to Zakariya Razi (865–925 AD), an Iranian pioneer scholar. *Archives of Iranian Medicine, 11*(6), 673–677.

Mosey, A. C. (1981). *Occupational therapy: Configuration of a profession.* New York: Raven Press.

Nails, D. (2014). Socrates. In E. N. Zalta (Ed.), *Stanford encyclopedia of philosophy.* Retrieved from http://plato.stanford.edu/archives/spr2014/entries/socrates

Naylor, E. H. (1921). Historical evolution. In *Trade associations: Their organization and management* (pp. 14–25). New York: Roland Press.

Peloquin, S. M. (1989). Moral treatment: Contexts reconsidered. *American Journal of Occupational Therapy, 43,* 537–544. https://doi.org/10.5014/ajot.43.8.537

Reitz, S. M., & Scaffa, M. E. (2010). Public health principles, approaches, and initiatives. In M. E. Scaffa, S. M. Reitz, & M. A. Pizzi (Eds.), *Occupational therapy in the promotion of health and wellness* (pp. 70–95). Philadelphia: F. A. Davis.

Scott, J. B. (2007). Ethical issues in school-based practice and early intervention. In L. Jackson (Ed.), *Occupational therapy practice in education and early childhood settings* (3rd ed., pp. 213–228). Bethesda, MD: AOTA Press.

Slater, D. Y. (2016). Glossary of ethics terms. In D. Y. Slater (Ed.), *Reference guide to the Occupational Therapy Code of Ethics* (2015 ed., pp. 291–292). Bethesda, MD: AOTA Press.

Sox, H. C. (2007). The ethical foundations of professionalism: A sociologic history. *Chest, 131,* 1532–1540. https://doi.org/10.1378/chest.07-0464

Stattel, F. M. (1977). Occupational therapy: Sense of the past—Focus on the present. *American Journal of Occupational Therapy, 31,* 649–650.

Wilcock, A. A. (2001a). A history of occupational therapy. In *Occupation for health* (Vol. 1, pp. 1–19). London: British Association and College of Occupational Therapists.

Wilcock, A. A. (2001b). Nature's regimen in primitive and spiritual times: Evolution, survival and health. In *Occupation for health* (Vol. 1, pp. 20–50). London: British Association and College of Occupational Therapists.

Wilcock, A. A. (2001c). Occupation for health in classical times. In *Occupation for health* (Vol. 1, pp. 52–97). London: British Association and College of Occupational Therapists.

Wilcock, A. A. (2006). An occupational theory of human nature. In *An occupational perspective of health* (2nd ed., pp. 50–74). Thorofare, NJ: Slack.

Zwelling, S. S. (1985). *Quest for a cure: The public hospital in Williamsburg, Virginia, 1773–1885.* Williamsburg, VA: Colonial Williamsburg Foundation.

Chapter 3.

PROMOTING ETHICS IN OCCUPATIONAL THERAPY PRACTICE: CODES AND CONSEQUENCES

Janie B. Scott, MA, OT/L, FAOTA, and S. Maggie Reitz, PhD, OTR/L, FAOTA

Learning Objectives

By the end of the chapter, readers will be able to

- Describe the jurisdictional scope for state regulatory boards (SRBs), the American Occupational Therapy Association (AOTA), and the National Board for Certification in Occupational Therapy (NBCOT);
- Analyze the disciplinary actions taken by AOTA, NBCOT, and an SRB; and
- Describe the role of the AOTA Representative Assembly (RA) in approving ethics documents.

Key Terms and Concepts

- ✧ Certification
- ✧ Core values
- ✧ Disciplinary actions
- ✧ Enforcement procedures
- ✧ Ethics Commission
- ✧ Jurisdiction
- ✧ National Board for Certification in Occupational Therapy
- ✧ NBCOT Disciplinary Action Summary
- ✧ Occupational Therapy Code of Ethics (2015)
- ✧ Preamble
- ✧ Principles
- ✧ Related Standards of Conduct
- ✧ Representative Assembly
- ✧ Stakeholders
- ✧ State regulatory boards

This chapter compares earlier versions of the occupational therapy codes to the current ***Occupational Therapy Code of Ethics (2015),*** hereinafter referred to as the "Code" (AOTA, 2015b). This chapter aims to describe the development and structure of the Code and discuss the entities that provide oversight and the mechanisms that are in place to ensure ethical behavior among occupational therapy practitioners.[1] The case studies and vignettes in future chapters of this text draw on readers' understanding of this material. Figure 3.1 is a timeline showing important milestones in occupational therapy ethics.

[1]In this text, *occupational therapy practitioners* include service providers, educators, and researchers.

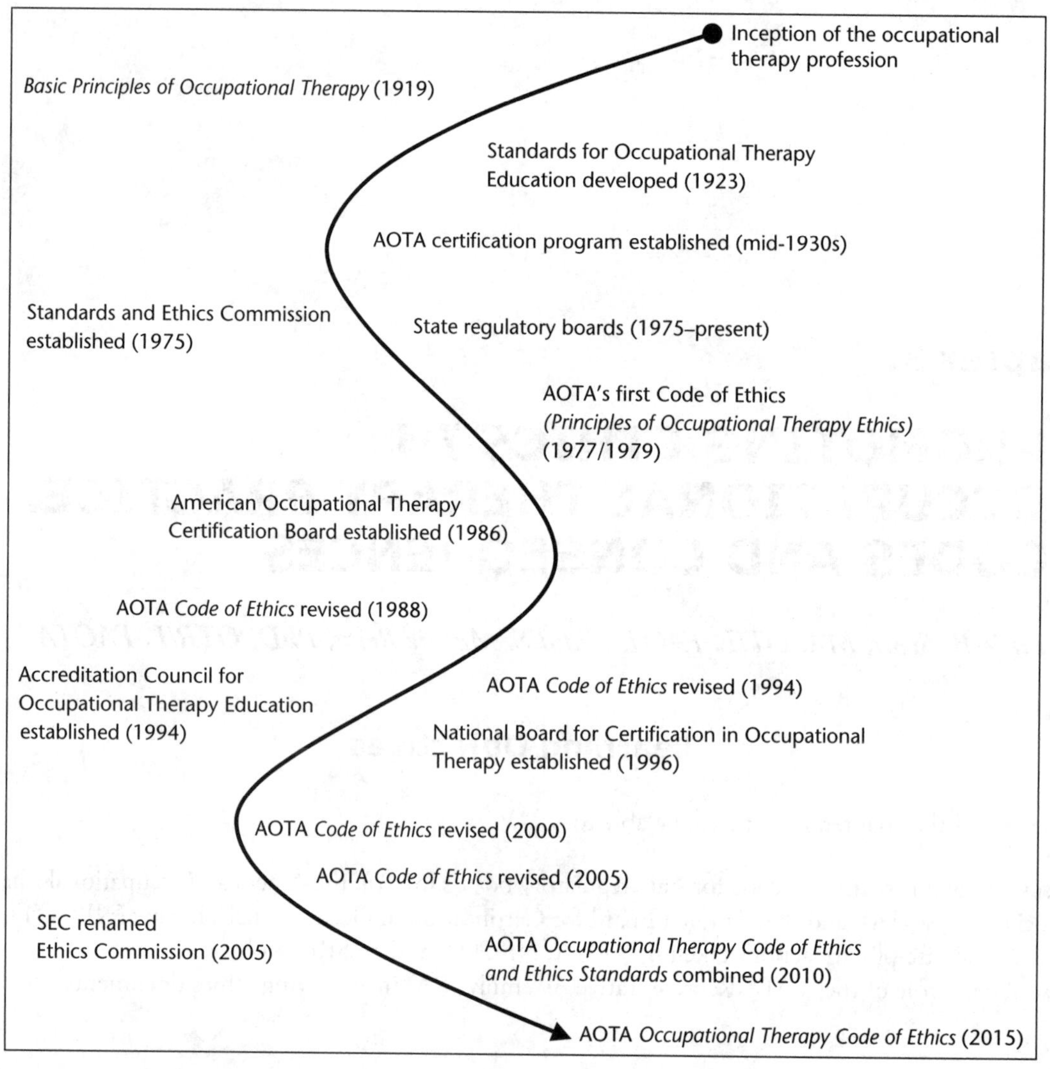

FIGURE 3.1

Milestones in occupational therapy ethics.
Note. AOTA = American Occupational Therapy Association.

Ethics Commission

The AOTA ***Ethics Commission*** (EC) serves "the Association members and public through the identification, development, review, interpretation and education of the AOTA Occupational Therapy Code . . . to provide the process whereby they are enforced" (Slater, 2016, p. 15). The EC developed *Enforcement Procedures for the Occupational Therapy Code of Ethics* (referred to as "Enforcement Procedures") in 1996 (AOTA, 1996). Possible and actual disciplinary actions from the current *Enforcement Procedures* are presented in this chapter, as are examples of disciplinary actions taken by the NBCOT and state regulatory boards (SRBs). In general, ***disciplinary actions*** are sanctions placed on eligible constituents when principles, codes of conduct, or standards are violated.

Ethics in Occupational Therapy

Two statements of principles predated the first version of the *Occupational Therapy Code of Ethics,* published in 1977. The first statement was penned in 1919 by a physician named William R. Dunton, Jr., who used occupation as a curative and preventive agent (Reed, 2011). The second statement, the Basic Principles of Occupational Therapy, was developed by a committee of the National Society for the

Promotion of Occupational Therapy (the name was changed to AOTA in 1921) that included occupational therapy pioneer Eleanor Clarke Slagle (Reed, 2011). These principles were published in 1919 and reprinted periodically until 1940 (both statements are reprinted in Reed, 2011). These documents described methods of intervention that modeled behaviors later labeled *Beneficence* and *Nonmaleficence.*

It is not known specifically why the principles were not reprinted after 1940. Initially, one possible reason could have been the disruption in life caused by World War II and the profession's focus on contributions to the war effort and returning soldiers. After World War II, the profession entered a period of great activity. This work included establishing awards such as the Eleanor Clarke Slagle Lectureship, coining definitions of occupational therapy and other professional terms, developing a variety of practice areas, and debating entry-level degrees (Reed, 2011). Given the dramatic changes in the profession, the original principles may have been viewed as outdated.

The Code was first adopted in 1977 and has been revised seven times: in 1979, 1988, 1994, 2000, 2005, 2010, and 2015 (AOTA, 1983, 1988, 1994, 2000, 2010a, 2015b; Kyler, 2016). Revisions to the Code occur in response to societal changes and AOTA's systematic review process for all of its official documents to ensure that they continue to be relevant and accurate. The current review cycle is every 5 years, unless societal changes (or a member request) indicate the need for a sooner revision. Public and AOTA member input regarding the relevance and usefulness of the Code and its related documents also helps inform the EC's revision of the Code. AOTA members are encouraged to review proposed changes, which are ultimately voted on and approved by the ***Representative Assembly*** (RA).

The principles included in the Code have changed over time, as shown in Table 3.1. Beneficence and Autonomy appeared in the first version and in each of the seven revisions, exemplifying the importance to occupational therapy practice of these timeless ethical principles. The Principle of Nonmaleficence first appeared in the 1988 version (AOTA, 1988) and has been consistently present since then, although the wording has evolved. The description of Fidelity has remained constant since 1994. Principles related to Procedural Justice were very prominent in the 1977 and 1979 versions (AOTA, 1978, 1983). The changes from the 1977 Code (AOTA, 1978) to the 1979 version (AOTA, 1983), with its emphasis on Procedural Justice, may be a reflection of increased government regulation (e.g., licensure) at that time. The principles and their descriptions in these two versions are identical except for a few wording changes and the addition of a principle regarding advertisement (e.g., Principle X. "Related to Advertising") to the 1979 version.

Although concern for Social Justice first appeared in the 1977 and 1979 Codes, it was not until the

Table 3.1. Comparison of the 2015 Code to Past Codes

	Principles of the Previous Codes[a]	
Principles of the Code	**Year**	**Wording**
Principle 1—Beneficence	1977/1979	[*Principle I.* "Related to the Recipient of Service."] Occupational therapist demonstrates a beneficent concern for the recipient of services and maintains a goal-directed relationship.
	1988	*Principle 1.* Occupational therapy personnel shall demonstrate a concern for the welfare and dignity of the recipient of their services. (Beneficence/Autonomy)
	1994	*Principle 1.* Occupational therapy personnel shall demonstrate a concern for the well-being of the recipients of their services. (Beneficence)
	2000	[Language unchanged]
	2005	*Principle 1.* Occupational therapy personnel shall demonstrate a concern for the safety and well-being of the recipients of their services. (Beneficence)
	2010	*Principle 1.* Occupational therapy personnel shall demonstrate a concern for the well-being and safety of the recipients of their services.
	2015	[Language unchanged]

(Continued)

Table 3.1. Comparison of the 2015 Code to Past Codes *(Cont.)*

Principles of the Code	Principles of the Previous Codes[a]	
	Year	Wording
Principle 2—Nonmaleficence	1977/1979	[Not addressed]
	1988	[Appears under Principle 1, Beneficence]
	1994	[Appears under Principle 1, Beneficence]
	2000	*Principle 2.* Occupational therapy personnel shall take reasonable precautions to avoid imposing or inflicting harm upon the recipient of services or to his or her property. (Nonmaleficence)
	2005	*Principle 2.* Occupational therapy personnel shall take measures to ensure a recipient's safety and avoid imposing or inflicting harm. (Nonmaleficence)
	2010	*Principle 2.* Occupational therapy personnel shall intentionally refrain from actions that cause harm.
	2015	*Principle 2.* Occupational therapy personnel shall refrain from actions that cause harm.
Principle 3—Autonomy, Confidentiality	1977/1979	[Implied under *Principle I.* "Related to the Recipient of Service."] The occupational therapist demonstrates a beneficent concern for the recipient of services and maintains a goal-directed relationship. . . . Respect shall be shown for the recipients' rights and the occupational therapist will preserve the confidence of the patient relationship.
	1988	[Autonomy and Confidentiality coupled with Beneficence]
	1994	*Principle 2.* Occupational therapy personnel shall respect the rights of the recipients of their services. (Autonomy, Privacy, Confidentiality)
	2000	*Principle 3.* Occupational therapy personnel shall respect the recipient and/or their surrogate(s) as well as the recipient's rights. (Autonomy, Privacy, Confidentiality)
	2005	*Principle 3.* Occupational therapy personnel shall respect recipients to assure their rights. (Autonomy, Confidentiality)
	2010	*Principle 3.* Occupational therapy personnel shall respect the right of the individual to self-determination.
	2015	[Confidentiality removed from title of principle but still embedded in description and RSCs] *Principle 3.* Occupational therapy personnel shall respect the right of the individual to self-determination, privacy, confidentiality, and consent.
Principle 4—Social Justice	1977	[Need to be aware of social issues addressed in Principle 12]
	1979	[Need to be aware of social issues addressed in Principle 13]
	1988	[Not addressed]
	1994	[Not addressed]
	2000	[Not addressed]
	2005	[Not addressed]
	2010	*Principle 4.* Occupational therapy personnel shall provide services in a fair and equitable manner.
	2015	[Combined with Principle 5—Procedural Justice] *Principle 4.* Occupational therapy personnel shall promote fairness and objectivity in the provision of occupational therapy services.
Principle 5—Procedural Justice	1977	[Covered under 6 of the 12 principles]
	1979	[Covered under 7 of the 13 principles]
	1988	*Principle 3.* Compliance with Laws and Regulations

(Continued)

Table 3.1. Comparison of the 2015 Code to Past Codes *(Cont.)*

Principles of the Code	Principles of the Previous Codes[a]	
	Year	**Wording**
	1994	*Principle 4.* Occupational therapy personnel shall comply with laws and Association policies guiding the profession of occupational therapy. (Justice)
	2000	[Language unchanged, now Principle 5]
	2005	[Language unchanged, now referred to as Procedural Justice]
	2010	*Principle 5.* Occupational therapy personnel shall comply with institutional rules; local, state, federal, and international laws, and AOTA documents applicable to the profession of occupational therapy.
	2015	[Combined with Principle 4, Social Justice, to become Justice]
Principle 6—Veracity	1977/1979	[Not explicitly stated but implied]
	1988	[Not explicitly stated but implied]
	1994	*Principle 5.* Occupational therapy personnel shall provide accurate information about occupational therapy services. (Veracity)
	2000	[Language unchanged]
	2005	*Principle 6.* Occupational therapy personnel shall provide accurate information when representing the profession. (Veracity)
	2010	*Principle 6.* Occupational therapy personnel shall provide comprehensive, accurate, and objective information when representing the profession.
	2015	[Now Principle 5 due to combination of Principles 4 and 5] [Language unchanged]
Principle 7—Fidelity	1977	[Covered under 3 of the 12 principles]
	1979	[Covered under 3 of the 13 principles]
	1988	*Principle 5.* Occupational therapy personnel shall function with discretion and integrity in relations with colleagues and other professionals, and shall be concerned with the quality of their services. (Professional Relationships)
	1994	*Principle 6.* Occupational therapy personnel shall treat colleagues and other professionals with fairness, discretion, and integrity. (Fidelity, Veracity)
	2000	[Language unchanged, now Principle 7]
	2005	*Principle 7.* Occupational therapy personnel shall treat colleagues and other professionals with respect, fairness, discretion, and integrity. (Fidelity)
	2010	[Language unchanged]
	2015	[Now Principle 6 due to combination of Principles 4 and 5] *Principle 6.* Occupational therapy personnel shall treat clients, colleagues, and other professionals with respect, fairness, discretion, and integrity.

Note. [a]Wording not enclosed in brackets is quoted from the source. The full citation for each version of the *Occupational Therapy Code of Ethics* appears in the reference list with "American Occupational Therapy Association" as the author and the applicable year of publication. RSCs = Related Standards of Conduct.

2010 version that it was included as a separate, distinct principle reflecting the profession's core values and roots in social activism. The Principles of Procedural Justice and Social Justice were combined in the 2015 version. This union resulted from a deliberative process between the AOTA membership, the EC, and the RA. The EC chairperson's report to the RA identified the reasons for this particular revision: "Standards which contained language that could appear ambiguous to some or more challenging to enforce were removed or modified. . . . The EC worked to strengthen language about the importance of appropriate professional boundaries and prohibition of dual relationships" (Brandt,

2015, p. 3). There were changes in the wording of each principle except Principle 1.

Development of Core Values and Code and Ethics Standards

Gilfoyle (1984) expressed the need for consistency between daily practice and professional values and believed that "values provide unity and become the underlying force in our philosophy" (p. 578). In her 1984 Eleanor Clarke Slagle Lecture, "Transformation of a Profession," Gilfoyle discussed ways occupational therapy could prepare for the future. She encouraged the examination of occupational therapy values, especially the occupation-based belief in "patients' doing" and the commitment "to provide services for severely and chronically disabled" clients (p. 576). This statement resonates with three of what would become occupational therapy's ***core values:*** (1) altruism, (2) equality, and (3) justice.

AOTA's formal effort to identify core values for the profession originated with a charge by the RA to the Commission on Practice (COP) and the Commission on Standards and Ethics (SEC) to create a list of knowledge, skills, and attitudes for the profession. The RA is the standard-setting policy-making body for AOTA and has the authority to direct the work of its commissions and committees. The COP is an advisory commission of the RA responsible for developing and updating the standards and best practices for the profession. AOTA funded the Professional and Technical Role Analysis (PATRA) Study in 1985 "to delineate entry-level practice" for occupational therapists and occupational therapy assistants:

> Knowledge, skills, and attitude statements were to be developed to provide a basis for the role analysis. The PATRA Study completed the knowledge and skills statements. The Executive Board subsequently charged the SEC to develop a statement that would describe the values and attitudes that undergird the profession. (AOTA, 1993, p. 1085)

The PATRA Study yielded a list of terms for the SEC to use in creating the *Core Values* document.

The document that resulted from these directives, *Core Values and Attitudes of Occupational Therapy Practice* (AOTA, 1993), was intended to provide the profession with a set of values flexible enough to change over time yet consistent enough to serve as the core beliefs. *Core Values and Attitudes of Occupational Therapy Practice* includes seven core values that guide occupational therapy practitioners' behaviors: (1) altruism, (2) equality, (3) freedom, (4) justice, (5) dignity, (6) truth, and (7) prudence (AOTA, 1993, 2015b). In 1993, the SEC believed that these values and beliefs of the profession were reflected in many AOTA official documents and in the occupational therapy literature. The SEC asserted that these values and beliefs should be consistent throughout the professional lives of occupational therapy students and professionals and that our professional behaviors should be based on them (AOTA, 1993). The *Core Values* document provides users with a resource to support daily professional ethical behavior and to aid in the resolution of conflicting professional values. Actions that demonstrate the core values are detailed in Table 3.2.

The Code was built on the foundation of the seven core values articulated by the SEC in 1993. The *Core Values* document was never revised and was rescinded in 2010 when it was incorporated into the Code and Ethics Standards (AOTA, 2010b). The SEC originally believed that the document might evolve to reflect the changing values of the profession (AOTA, 1993); indeed, its grounding in professional and societal values has stood the test of time. The current Code continues to refer to the core values—for example, altruism appears in Principle 4, equality in Principle 2, justice in Principle 4, and truth in Principle 5.

The EC considered input from AOTA members who reported that the existence of three separate documents—the *Occupational Therapy Code of Ethics,* the *Core Values and Attitudes of Occupational Therapy Practice,* and the *Guidelines to the Occupational Therapy Code of Ethics* (AOTA, 2006)—was confusing (D. Slater, personal communication, June 13, 2012). The *Guidelines* document referred to the professional behaviors of honesty, communication, ensuring the common good, competence, confidentiality and protected information, conflict of interest, impaired practitioners, payment for services and other financial arrangements, and resolution of ethical issues with principles from the Code (AOTA, 2006).

In 2010, the RA rescinded the *Core Values* and *Guidelines* documents and incorporated the constructs and some of the language into the 2010

Table 3.2. Behaviors That Exemplify Occupational Therapy Core Values

Value	Description
Altruism	Demonstrates "unselfish concern for the welfare of others" (AOTA, 1993, p. 1085) Places the needs of others first (AOTA, 2010a) "Involves demonstrating concern for the welfare of others" (AOTA, 2015b, p. 2)
Equality	Perceives and acts on belief that all people "have the same fundamental human rights and opportunities" (AOTA, 1993, p. 1085; AOTA, 2010a) "Refers to treating all people impartially and free of bias" (AOTA, 2015b, p. 2)
Freedom	Promotes choice for individuals, families, and communities Helps recipients of services "find a balance between autonomy and societal membership that is reflected in the choice of various patterns of interdependence with" people and the environment (AOTA, 1993, p. 1085) "Freedom and personal choice are paramount in a profession in which the values and desires of the client guide our interventions" (AOTA, 2015b, p. 2).
Justice	Provides "occupational therapy services for all individuals who are in need of these services" (AOTA, 1993, p. 1086) Respects "the legal rights of individuals receiving occupational therapy services" (AOTA, 1993, p. 1086) Abides by the local, state, and federal laws governing practice (AOTA, 1993) "Justice expresses a state in which diverse communities are inclusive; diverse communities are organized and structured such that all members can function, flourish, and live a satisfactory life. Occupational therapy personnel, by virtue of the specific nature of the practice of occupational therapy, have a vested interest in addressing unjust inequities that limit opportunities for participation in society" (AOTA, 2015b; Braveman & Bass-Haugen, 2009, p. 2).
Dignity	Demonstrates "an attitude of empathy and respect for self and others" (AOTA, 1993, p. 1086) Treating the client with "respect in all interactions" (AOTA, 2015b, p. 2)
Truth	Is "faithful to facts and reality . . . [and] accountable, honest, forthright, accurate, and authentic in . . . attitudes and actions" (AOTA, 1993, p. 1086) "In all situations, occupational therapy personnel must provide accurate information in oral, written, and electronic forms" (AOTA, 2015b, p. 2)
Prudence	Exercises "judiciousness, discretion, vigilance, moderation, care, and circumspection in the management of one's affairs" (AOTA, 1993, p. 1086) Use of "clinical and ethical reasoning skills, sound judgment, and reflection to make decisions in professional and volunteer roles" (AOTA, 2015b, p. 2)

Note. AOTA = American Occupational Therapy Association.

Code and Ethics Standards (AOTA, 2010b). That new document and the 2015 Code detail the ethical expectations of occupational therapy students and practitioners relative to ethical reasoning throughout occupational therapy practice.

Code Structure

Preamble

The Code begins with a ***Preamble*** that discusses the scope and objectives of the document. According to the Preamble, the Code's purpose is to provide "aspirational Core Values that guide members toward ethical courses of action in professional and volunteer roles" and delineate "enforceable Principles and Standards of Conduct that apply to AOTA members" (AOTA, 2015a, p. 1).

Thus, preventive education is the primary desired outcome of the Code. Through time, this document also has become a tool with which the occupational therapy profession communicates its values and standards to the public, including regulatory bodies and recipients of services.

Principles

The body of the Code consists of descriptions of each of six ***Principles*** and lists of ***Related Standards of Conduct*** (RSCs), which are proactive behaviors that are in alignment with a specific principle and that are identified immediately after each principle.

The EC and AOTA members review the Code regularly and the language is updated to reflect current values and beliefs, ensuring that this document remain relevant to the practice of occupational therapy as a valuable tool for practitioners and the public as they attempt to solve the ethical dilemmas they may encounter.

Oversight of Ethical Practice in Occupational Therapy

To oversee occupational therapy practitioners' adherence to their respective codes of ethics and conduct, AOTA and other organizations charged with ensuring the ethical practice of occupational therapy have established enforcement procedures. When occupational therapy practitioners become licensed or certified, or join a professional organization, they agree to adhere to the code of ethics or conduct of the appropriate body and to abide by its enforcement procedures. ***Enforcement procedures*** help ensure that practitioners under a specific jurisdiction (i.e., under an entity's authority to take disciplinary action) who do not adhere to the appropriate code of ethics or guidelines for professional behavior become subject to a process of complaint and investigation that will result in disciplinary action if the complaint is determined to have merit.

If someone (e.g., client, fellow professional) believes that an occupational therapy practitioner has engaged in unethical behavior, enforcement procedures outline the requirements for filing a formal complaint and the investigatory steps that will follow. Typically, a special committee examines the testimonies of the complainant, the respondent, and any witnesses and considers facts and supporting evidence. The nature of the complaint and the surrounding facts determine whether the committee dismisses the complaint, or assesses a fine, takes disciplinary action, or both. The organizations concerned with ethical occupational therapy practice and their enforcement procedures are briefly described in the sections that follow.

American Occupational Therapy Association

The most recent version of AOTA's *Enforcement Procedures* (AOTA, 2015a) was revised in 2015, after the new Code was adopted (available in Appendix B). Jurisdiction, potential disciplinary actions, complaint timeline and processes, and the appeal process are specified in the *Enforcement Procedures.*

A consumer, another occupational therapy practitioner, or any member of the public may file a complaint against an occupational therapy practitioner who is an AOTA member or was a member at the time of the alleged incident. The EC reviews each complaint according to a specified process and, when warranted, issues a disciplinary action against the member. Four of the five disciplinary actions are public and one is private (e.g., reprimand, which is between the EC and the people involved). The disciplinary actions are defined in Table 3.3. A summary of AOTA's public disciplinary actions for a recent 1-year period appears in Table 3.4. In addition to disciplinary actions, the EC may write an educative letter, which is private. An educative letter is used when available evidence is insufficient to determine that an ethics violation has occurred

Table 3.3. Possible Disciplinary Actions in AOTA Enforcement Procedures

Action	Description
Reprimand	"A formal expression of disapproval of conduct communicated privately by letter from the EC Chairperson that is nondisclosable and noncommunicative to other bodies (e.g., SRBs, NBCOT). Reprimand is not publicly reported" (AOTA, 2015a, p. 2)
Censure	"A formal expression of disapproval that is publicly reported" (AOTA, 2015a, p. 2)
Probation of membership subject to terms	"Continued membership is conditional, depending on fulfillment of specified terms. Failure to meet terms will subject an Association member to any of the disciplinary actions or sanctions." (AOTA, 2015a, p. 2)
Suspension	"Removal of Association membership for a specified period of time" (AOTA, 2015a, p. 2)
Revocation	"Permanent denial of Association membership" (AOTA, 2015a, p. 2)

Note. AOTA = American Occupational Therapy Association; EC = AOTA's Ethics Commission; NBCOT = National Board for Certification in Occupational Therapy; SRB = state regulatory board.

Table 3.4. Examples of AOTA Disciplinary Actions in a 1-Year Period

Principles Violated in Each Case	Disciplinary Action
Principle 6B—Refrain from false statements or claims. *Principle 7A*—Respect self, colleagues, institutions, and agencies by maintaining competence, traditions, responsibilities, and competencies.	Revocation of membership
Principle 1B—Provide assessments and interventions appropriate to client needs. *Principle 1E*—Provide services within level of competence and scope of practice. *Principle 1F*—Use evidence and adhere to scope of practice in all phases of service delivery. *Principle 2J*—Avoid exploitation. *Principle 3G*—Ensure confidentiality and right to privacy. *Principle 3H*—Maintain the confidentiality of all communications. *Principle 5G*—Verify that all duties and responsibilities assigned to others are within their skill level, experience, and scope of practice. *Principle 5O*—Be fair and equitable in fees charged, and adhere to standards. *Principle 6B*—Refrain from false statements or claims. *Principle 6C*—Adhere to standards and regulations when documenting professional activities. *Principle 6D*—Ensure that documentation for reimbursement is accurate and complies with standards. *Principle 6E*—Accept responsibility for professional actions that reduce the public's trust in occupational therapy. *Principle 6F*—Ensure that advertising and marketing materials are accurate.	Revocation of membership
Principle 2E—Avoid causing harm to others by recognizing and caring for personal problems when they arise. *Principle 2J*—Avoid placing one's self-interest above others in a way that may cause harm. *Principle 3B*—Obtain consent from the client or representative before initiating services and keep the client or their representative updated about progress. *Principle 4E*—Endeavor to advocate for clients' occupational therapy needs *Principle 5G*—Verify that all duties and responsibilities assigned to others are within their skill level, experience, and scope of practice. *Principle 6A*—Represent credentials, qualifications, education, experience, training, and competence accurately. *Principle 6B*—Refrain from false statements or claims. *Principle 6C*—Adhere to standards and regulations when documenting professional activities. *Principle 6D*—Ensure that documentation for reimbursement is accurate and complies with standards.	Revocation of membership
Principle 2A—Avoid exploiting the recipient of services. *Principle 2C*—Avoid exploitative relationships that conflict with objectivity or professional judgment. *Principle 2D*—Avoid sexual relationships with clients, their families, or supervisee when professional relationships exist. *Principle 2J*—Avoid relationships that exploit others for personal gain.	Revocation of membership
Principle 6B—Refrain from false statements or claims. *Principle 6D*—Ensure that documentation for reimbursement is accurate and complies with standards.	Censure
Principle 5E—Maintain appropriate credentialing (national, state, other) consistent with services provided.	Censure
Principle 5O—Be fair and equitable in fees charged, and adhere to standards. *Principle 6B*—Refrain from false statements or claims. *Principle 6D*—Ensure that documentation for reimbursement is accurate and complies with standards. *Principle 7*—Fidelity.	Suspension of membership 4 months

(*Continued*)

Table 3.4. Examples of AOTA Disciplinary Actions in a 1-Year Period *(Cont.)*

Principles Violated in Each Case	Disciplinary Action
Principle 5—Procedural Justice. *Principle 5O*—Be fair and equitable in fees charged, and adhere to standards. *Principle 6B*—Refrain from false statements or claims. *Principle 6C*—Adhere to standards and regulations when documenting professional activities. *Principle 6D*—Ensure that documentation for reimbursement is accurate and complies with standards.	Revocation of membership
Principle 5—Procedural Justice. *Principle 6A*—Represent credentials, qualifications, education, experience, training, and competence accurately.	Censure

Source. AOTA (2015c).
Note. AOTA = American Occupational Therapy Association. Reflects the most current summaries of the AOTA EC's disciplinary actions at the time of writing. The 2010 Code (AOTA, 2010a) was the version in place at the time the infractions occurred.

but sufficient to indicate a failure to engage in best practice (AOTA, 2015a).

If an individual whose Association membership was suspended or revoked was recognized as a member of the Roster of Fellows (ROF) or Roster of Honor (ROH), the individual would lose the ability to use these credentials (FAOTA or ROH) for as long as the discipline was specified. The Chairperson for the Board for Advanced and Specialty Certification is also notified through the Association's EC staff liaison of these disciplinary actions and the opportunity to apply for or renew their certification would be deemed ineligible (AOTA, 2015a).

The EC reviews the behaviors that result in disciplinary actions and may develop advisory opinions to help occupational therapy practitioners avoid similar outcomes by understanding the ethical implications of challenging situations. The primary purposes of advisory opinions are to inform and educate occupational therapy practitioners regarding strategies to address ethical issues that arise in everyday practice. These opinions also may be developed in response to themes identified in other communications with AOTA's EC. Advisory opinions are made available to AOTA members via the website and through AOTA educational products.

National Board for Certification in Occupational Therapy

In the mid-1930s, the AOTA established a certification program for occupational therapists; in the 1960s, a similar program was instituted for occupational therapy assistants. ***Certification*** is a process that agencies use to determine that a professional may "use a certain title if that person has attained entry-level competence" (Willmarth, 2011, p. 455). In 1986, AOTA transferred responsibility for certification of occupational therapy practitioners to a newly formed independent organization, the American Occupational Therapy Certification Board, which was renamed the ***National Board for Certification of Occupational Therapy*** (NBCOT) in 1998 (Willmarth, 2011). NBCOT has less authority over certificants than the SRBs that license occupational therapy practitioners.

Since 2006, AOTA has also made available board and specialty certifications in certain practice areas. These certifications are awarded once the practitioner submits an application and fee and their submitted evidence is reviewed and recognized as having met specified qualifications and standards (M. L. Louch, personal communication, June 14, 2012).

NBCOT administers certification exams to graduates of accredited occupational therapy programs who have passed all education and fieldwork components. Candidates who pass an exam and meet other NBCOT requirements are entitled to use the Occupational Therapist Registered (OTR®) or Certified Occupational Therapy Assistant (COTA®) designation. State laws governing occupational therapy practice require that occupational therapists and occupational therapy assistants pass the entry-level certification examination administered by NBCOT (C. Willmarth, personal communication, November 23, 2015). In addition to administering the certification examinations, NBCOT offers a voluntary recertification program that requires practitioners to attest to having earned the minimum number of professional development units to maintain currency in their practice area (NBCOT, 2015a). Most SRBs do not require occupational therapy practitioners to renew their NBCOT certification (Moyers, 2009; Willmarth, 2011).

The NBCOT has its own code, called the *Candidate/Certificant Code of Conduct* (NBCOT, 2014; available in Appendix C). Exam candidates, occupational therapy practitioners who hold initial certification, and those who renew their certification agree to abide by this code. The *NBCOT's Candidate/Certificant Code of Conduct* (NBCOT, 2014) comprises eight principles:

- *Principle 1* requires accuracy and truthfulness in all information submitted to NBCOT (consistent with Principle 4, Justice, and Principle 5, Veracity, of the Code).
- *Principle 2* requires cooperation with NBCOT's investigation process in case of a complaint (consistent with Principle 4, Justice, and Principle 6, Fidelity, of the Code).
- *Principle 3* requires accuracy and truthfulness in all professional communications (consistent with Principle 1, Beneficence, and Principle 5, Veracity, of the Code).
- *Principle 4* requires compliance with the legal requirements of occupational therapy practice (consistent with Principle 4, Justice, and Principle 6, Fidelity, of the Code).
- *Principle 5* disqualifies from certification those convicted of crimes related to the practice of occupational therapy (consistent with Principle 2, Nonmaleficence, and Principle 4, Justice, of the Code).
- *Principle 6* forbids practitioners from threatening the health, well-being, or safety of recipients of occupational therapy services (consistent with Principle 2, Nonmaleficence, of the Code).
- *Principle 7* prohibits the practice of occupational therapy while the practitioner's ability to practice is impaired because of legal or illegal drug or alcohol use (consistent with Principle 2, Nonmaleficence, of the Code).
- *Principle 8* forbids sharing information or photos of recipients of occupational therapy services via electronic means (consistent with Principle 3, Autonomy, of the Code).

The *NBCOT Candidate/Certificant Code of Conduct* (NBCOT, 2014) and the *Procedures for the Enforcement of the NBCOT Candidate/Certificant Code of Conduct* (NBCOT, 2015c; available in Appendix D) are available on the NBCOT website (www.nbcot.org). Breaches of the *NBCOT Candidate/Certificant Code of Conduct* (NBCOT, 2014) may result in sanctions. Each specific situation is reviewed, and if a violation is found, the candidate or certificant may receive one or more sanctions, including ineligibility for certification, reprimand, censure, probation, suspension, and revocation (NBCOT, 2015a). These sanctions mirror AOTA's except that AOTA's disciplinary actions relate to the person's membership in AOTA (AOTA, 2014). A summary of NBCOT disciplinary actions for a recent 1-year period is displayed in Table 3.5. A brief comparison of the disciplinary sanctions that might be applied by AOTA, NBCOT, and SRBs appears in Table 3.6.

State Regulatory Boards

SRBs have the legislative authority to license occupational therapy practitioners when they meet specific conditions. The purpose of licensure is to regulate occupational therapy practice and protect the public from injury by incompetent or unqualified practitioners. Licensees are recognized as having met the requirements established by a government agency for a profession (Willmarth, 2011). Occupational therapists were first licensed in 1975 in two states—Florida and New York. All 50 states, the District of Columbia, and Puerto Rico have passed a licensure law for occupational therapists and occupational therapy assistants. Hawaii's regulation of occupational therapy assistants will become effective on January 1, 2017 (C. Willmarth, personal communication, November 23, 2015). Many SRBs have adopted part or all of AOTA's Code and require licensees to adhere to these tenets (Willmarth, 2011).

In addition to regulating the practice of occupational therapy, SRBs publish standards to inform licensees and the public about what constitutes acceptable practice. SRBs also inform the public about what to do in case of a complaint and, in many instances, publish summaries of disciplinary actions taken. The majority of states also require licensees to meet competence standards (see Appendix E, "Ethics Resources"). SRBs have the authority to discipline occupational therapy practitioners under their jurisdiction or fine licensees, or both, for violations of laws and regulations. Occupational

Table 3.5. Summary of NBCOT Principle Violations During a 1-Year Period

Number of Cases	Principle Violated
3	*Principle 1.* Certificants shall provide accurate and truthful representations to NBCOT concerning all information related to aspects of the Certification Program, including, but not limited to, the submission of information • On the examination and certification renewal applications, and renewal audit form; • Requested by NBCOT for a disciplinary action situation; or • Requested by NBCOT concerning allegations related to: Test security violations and/or disclosure of confidential examination material content to unauthorized parties; Misrepresentations by a certificant regarding his/her credential(s) and/or education; The unauthorized use of NBCOT's intellectual property, certification marks, and other copyrighted materials, including all NBCOT exam preparation tools (e.g., practice exams).
1	*Principle 2.* Certificants who are the subject of a complaint shall cooperate with NBCOT concerning investigations of violations of the NBCOT Practice Standards, including the collection of relevant information; and *Principle 4.* Certificants shall comply with state and/or federal laws, regulations, and statutes governing the practice of occupational therapy.
4	*Principle 4.* Certificants shall comply with state and/or federal laws, regulations, and statutes governing the practice of occupational therapy.
1	*Principle 5.* Certificants shall not have been convicted of a crime, the circumstances of which substantially relate to the practice of occupational therapy or indicate an inability to engage in the practice of occupational therapy safely and/or competently.
1	*Principle 6.* Certificants shall not engage in behavior or conduct, lawful or otherwise, that causes them to be, or reasonably perceived to be, a threat or potential threat to the health, well-being, or safety of recipients or potential recipients of occupational therapy services.
1	*Principle 6.* Certificants shall not engage in behavior or conduct, lawful or otherwise, that causes them to be, or reasonably perceived to be, a threat or potential threat to the health, well-being, or safety of recipients or potential recipients of occupational therapy services; and *Principle 4.* Certificants shall comply with state and/or federal laws, regulations, and statutes governing the practice of occupational therapy.

Source. Data courtesy of NBCOT (2015d). Table reflects the summaries of NBCOT's recent disciplinary actions at the time of publication.
Note. NBCOT = National Board for Certification in Occupational Therapy.

Table 3.6. Disciplinary Sanctions by AOTA, NBCOT, and SRBs

AOTA	NBCOT	SRBs
Educative letter	Ineligibility for certification	Civil penalty/disciplinary costs
Reprimand	Reprimand	Reprimand
Censure	Censure	Suspension of license[a]
Probation of membership subject to terms	Probation	Probation[a] Suspension with probation subject to terms
Suspension of membership	Suspension of certification	Revocation of license
Revocation of membership	Revocation of certification	Permanent surrender of license

Note. AOTA = American Occupational Therapy Association; NBCOT = National Board for Certification in Occupational Therapy; SRBs = state regulatory boards.
[a]Conditions may apply (e.g., seek psychiatric or substance abuse treatment, attend additional continuing education, complete jurisprudence exam, receive supervision through a mentor, perform community service). At the time of publication, table reflects a summary of disciplinary actions from the following organizations and agencies: American Occupational Therapy Association (2015a); National Board for Certification in Occupational Therapy (2015a); Maryland Department of Health and Mental Hygiene, Board of Occupational Therapy Practice (2015); and North Carolina Board of Occupational Therapy (2015).

Table 3.7. Summary of SRB Disciplinary Actions in One State During a 1-Year Period

Failed to renew license on time, resulting in practicing with an expired license for 4 days.	Letter of reprimand. Assessed civil penalty.
Failed to renew license on time, resulting in practicing with an expired license for 2 days.	An order was issued. Licensee reprimanded. Assessed civil penalty and disciplinary costs.
Failed to renew license on time, resulting in holding herself out as an OT/L and practicing with an expired license.	An order was issued. Licensee reprimanded. Assessed civil penalty and disciplinary costs.
Failed to renew license on time, resulting in practicing with an expired license.	Letter of reprimand. Assessed civil penalty.
Attempted to obtain payment by fraud or deceit, convicted of attempting to defraud an insurance company and failed to notify the Board within 30 days of conviction of a felony that involved moral turpitude.	An order was issued. License revoked. Assessed civil penalty and disciplinary costs.
Obtained or attempted to obtain payment by fraud or deceit and documented services or treatments not performed.	A consent order was issued. License put on probation for 1 year. Assessed disciplinary costs. Complete the jurisprudence exam.
Attempted to obtain payment by fraud or deceit, documented services or treatments not performed, and improper documentation.	A consent order was issued. License put on probation for 1 year. Assessed civil penalty and disciplinary costs. Complete the jurisprudence exam. Additional CCA points required for 2015 renewal.
Failed to renew license on time, resulting in practicing with an expired license.	Letter of reprimand. Assessed civil penalty.
Failed to provide documentation of completion of the required continuing competence activities necessary to renew license for the 2014–2015 licensure period.	A consent order was issued. License put on probation for 1 year. Provide documentation of CCAs for 2014–2015 license renewal. Complete the jurisprudence exam. Assessed civil penalty and disciplinary costs.
Documented services or treatments not performed.	A consent order was issued. License put on probation for 1 year. Complete the jurisprudence exam. Assessed civil penalty and disciplinary costs.
Failed to renew license on time, resulting in practicing with an expired license.	Letter of reprimand. Assessed civil penalty.
Obtained or attempted to obtain payment by fraud or deceit and documented services or treatments not performed.	A consent order was issued. License put on probation for 1 year. Complete the jurisprudence exam. Assessed civil penalty and disciplinary costs.
Failed to complete continuing competence activity in a timely manner for 3 renewal periods.	Letter of reprimand. Assessed civil penalty. Complete the jurisprudence exam.
Failed to report practicing occupational therapy in another State with an expired license.	Letter of reprimand. Assessed civil penalty and disciplinary costs.

Source. Data provided by the North Carolina Board of Occupational Therapy (2015). At the time of publication, table reflects the summaries of the NCBOT's recent disciplinary actions.
Note. CCA = Continuing Competence Activities.

therapy practitioner behaviors that warranted disciplinary action by one state's SRB in a 1-year period are presented in Table 3.7. Some SRBs publish additional details regarding disciplinary cases on their websites.

Jurisdiction

Because AOTA, NBCOT, and SRBs are all concerned with the ethical practice of occupational therapy, confusion can arise regarding the ***jurisdiction*** of each organization (e.g., authority to take disciplinary action) for a specific complaint. As shown in Figure 3.2, jurisdiction depends on the degree of authority that the organization or agency has over the certificant applicant, occupational therapy practitioner, or AOTA member.

The consequences of ethical and legal misconduct vary across jurisdictions. ***Stakeholders*** (e.g., AOTA members, NBCOT certificants, consumers, professionals) may report unethical practice to any of the three entities; however, the complaint would move forward for review only if it fell under the jurisdiction of the entity. If the board or organization reviewing the complaint determines that the complaint is not within its jurisdiction, the complainant is notified in writing.

Some actions subject to disciplinary action by one organization also are within the jurisdiction of another; for example, an SRB action may also result in discipline through NBCOT or AOTA if the practitioner is under its jurisdiction. In addition, situations in which client harm occurred may result in legal action against the practitioner and a claim to a liability insurance company.

Reporting on Disciplinary Actions

Systems are in place to gather and report data on occupational therapy practitioners who are found

QUESTION	JURISDICTION		
	NBCOT	SRB	AOTA
1. Who should I call if I have questions about the following?			
a. Ethical violations that could cause harm or have potential to cause harm to a consumer or the public	X	X	X
b. Violations that do not cause harm or have a limited potential for causing harm to a consumer or the public			X
c. Violations of professional values that do not relate directly to potential harm to the public			X
2. Where did the alleged violation occur, and who was involved in the alleged incident?			
a. Took place in a state with rules, regulations, and disciplinary procedures in place	X	X	X
b. Was committed by an AOTA member	X	X	X
c. Was committed by a person who is not an AOTA member	X	X	
3. What is the disciplinary action that you wish as a consequence of filing a complaint?			
a. Restrict or revoke licensure		X	
b. Restrict or revoke certification	X		
c. Restrict or prohibit membership in AOTA			X

FIGURE 3.2

Disciplinary jurisdiction.

Source. Adapted from "Overview of the Ethical Jurisdictions of AOTA, NBCOT, and SRBs," by R. A. Hansen & D. Y. Slater. In *Reference Guide to the Occupational Therapy Code of Ethics (2015),* edited by D. Y. Slater, 2016, Bethesda, MD: AOTA Press, p. 44. Copyright © 2016 by the American Occupational Therapy Association. Reprinted with permission.

Note. AOTA = American Occupational Therapy Association; NBCOT = National Board for Certification in Occupational Therapy; SRB = state regulatory board.

to be in violation of ethics and competence requirements. Publishing the results of disciplinary actions is intended to notify and protect the public by identifying practitioners who have violated laws, regulations, or best practices. Ultimately, these initiatives also protect the occupational therapy profession by identifying these practitioners and preventing their actions that might harm the public and the image of occupational therapy. In addition, public notification serves to remind current practitioners about the importance of legal, ethical, and competent practice.

NBCOT gathers and makes publicly available the outcomes of its disciplinary actions through its ***NBCOT Disciplinary Action Summary,*** which is available on the NBCOT website. This final list of disciplinary actions serves as "a national resource for consumers of occupational therapy services, the general public, regulatory agencies, employers, and others" (NBCOT, 2015b, para. 1).

AOTA, NBCOT, and SRBs have a legal mandate under Title IV of the Health Care Quality Improvement Act of 1986 to monitor complaints; to gather data regarding disciplinary actions; and to communicate the outcomes of their disciplinary actions publicly on their websites, in official publications, or both.

AOTA, NBCOT, and SRBs also may report disciplinary actions to government-sponsored data collection agencies. For example, the National Practitioner Data Bank (NPDB), a quality assurance division within the U.S. Department of Health and Human Services (DHHS), is also a database with information about all licensure actions taken against all health care practitioners and health care entities, as well as any negative actions or findings against health care practitioners or organizations by peer review and private accreditation organizations. The NPDB is a confidential clearinghouse responsible for collecting and releasing information about, for example, medical malpractice payments, adverse licensure actions, adverse professional society membership actions, and negative actions by state licensing or certification authorities (DHHS, n.d.). Its legal authority is greater than that of NBCOT and AOTA because its mandates are driven by state or federal regulations, and some of the regulations may affect an individual's ability to practice occupational therapy. Notices of health care provider violations are available to states under specific conditions and may further affect a practitioner's ability to practice.

The number of disciplinary actions taken by AOTA, NBCOT, and the SRBs during a 1-year period is typically larger than that reported in the NPDB. This discrepancy is attributable to several possible reasons; for example, a person reported in more than one state would appear only once in the NPDB, entities incur no legal consequences for not reporting to the NPDB and may not take the time to do so, budget cuts may prevent some states from reporting, and some SRBs publish their disciplinary actions on their own websites rather than on the NPDB.

Summary

The profession of occupational therapy protects both the public and its practitioners by developing and enforcing its core values through the Code. As the needs of society evolve, new interventions, grounded in evidence, are developed that respond to these changing needs; the core values of the profession, however, remain constant as they have since the inception of the profession (AOTA, 2015b). These core values will continue to inform revisions of the Code as principles and RSCs are modified, providing occupational therapy practitioners with the guidance they need to practice with pride and ethical behavior.

Reflective Questions

1. Correlate the values found in the Code to the Principles and RSCs.
2. Describe the similarities and differences of disciplinary actions among AOTA, NBCOT, and SRBs.
3. Theresa identified herself as an OTR/L, however, she had not renewed her certification with NBCOT. Theresa was licensed to practice occupational therapy in her state. The state board of occupational therapy practice received a complaint from the place of Theresa's employment that she had entered private residences, provided interventions, and submitted fraudulent billing.

   Review Figure 3.2; Appendix B, "Enforcement Procedures for Occupational Therapy Code of Ethics; and Appendix C, "NBCOT Candidate/Certificant Code of Conduct" to determine who has jurisdiction in Theresa's situation.

References

American Occupational Therapy Association. (1978). Principles of occupational therapy ethics. In H. L. Hopkins & H. D. Smith (Eds.), *Willard and Spackman's occupational therapy* (5th ed., pp. 709–710). Philadelphia, PA: Lippincott.

American Occupational Therapy Association. (1983). Principles of occupational therapy ethics (1979 version). In *Reference manual of the official documents of the American Occupational Therapy Association* (pp. 127–134). Rockville, MD: Author.

American Occupational Therapy Association. (1988). Occupational therapy code of ethics. *American Journal of Occupational Therapy, 42,* 795–796. https://doi.org/10.5014/ajot.42.12.795

American Occupational Therapy Association. (1993). Core values and attitudes of occupational therapy practice. *American Journal of Occupational Therapy, 47,* 1085–1086. https://doi.org/10.5014/ajot.47.12.1085

American Occupational Therapy Association. (1994). Occupational therapy code of ethics. *American Journal of Occupational Therapy, 48,* 1037–1038. https://doi.org/10.5014/ajot.48.11.1037

American Occupational Therapy Association. (1996). Enforcement procedures for occupational therapy code of ethics. *American Journal of Occupational Therapy,* 50(10), 848–852. https://doi.org/10.5014/ajot.10.848

American Occupational Therapy Association. (2000). Occupational therapy code of ethics (2000). *American Journal of Occupational Therapy, 54,* 614–616. https://doi.org/10.5014/ajot.54.6.614

American Occupational Therapy Association. (2005). Occupational therapy code of ethics (2005). *American Journal of Occupational Therapy, 59,* 639–642. https://doi.org/10.5014/ajot.59.6.639

American Occupational Therapy Association. (2006). Guidelines to the occupational therapy code of ethics. *American Journal of Occupational Therapy, 60,* 652–658. https://doi.org/10.5014/ajot.60.6.652

American Occupational Therapy Association. (2010a). Occupational therapy code of ethics and ethics standards (2010). *American Journal of Occupational Therapy, 64*(Suppl. 6), S17–S26. https://doi.org/10.5014/ajot.2010.64S17

American Occupational Therapy Association. (2010b). Rescind OT code of ethics (2005), core values and guidelines to ethics. In *Draft minutes of the American Occupational Therapy Association, Inc., Representative Assembly.* Retrieved from http://www.aota.org/-/media/corporate/files/secure/governance/ra/minutes/draft%202010%20ra%20minutes%20_7-7-10_.pdf

American Occupational Therapy Association. (2014). Enforcement procedures for the Occupational Therapy Code of Ethics and Ethics Standards. *American Journal of Occupational Therapy, 64*(Suppl. 6), S4–S16. https://doi.org/10.5014/ajot.2010.64S4

American Occupational Therapy Association. (2015a). Enforcement procedures for the Occupational Therapy Code of Ethics. *American Journal of Occupational Therapy, 69*(Suppl. 3), 6913410012p1–6913410012p13. https://doi.org/10.5014/ajot.2015.696S19

American Occupational Therapy Association. (2015b). Occupational therapy code of ethics (2015). *American Journal of Occupational Therapy, 69*(Suppl. 3), 6913410030. https://doi.org/10.5014/ajot.2015.696S03

American Occupational Therapy Association. (2015c). *Resources: Disciplinary action.* Retrieved from http://www.aota.org/About-Occupational-Therapy/Ethics/Enforce.aspx

Braveman, B., & Bass-Haugen, J. D. (2009). Social justice and health disparities: An evolving discourse in occupational therapy research and intervention. *American Journal of Occupational Therapy, 63,* 7–12. https://doi.org/10.5014/ajot.63.1.7

Brandt, L. C. (2015). *Report of the chairperson of the Ethics Commission (EC) to the Representative Assembly.* Retrieved from https://www.aota.org/-/media/corporate/files/secure/governance/ra/2015-spring/ethics.pdf

Gilfoyle, E. M. (1984). Transformation of a profession (Eleanor Clarke Slagle Lecture). *American Journal of Occupational Therapy, 38,* 575–584. https://doi.org/10.5014/ajot.38.9.575

Hansen, R. A., & Slater, D. Y. (2016). Overview of ethical jurisdictions of AOTA, NBCOT, and SRBs. In D. Y. Slater (Ed.), *Reference guide to the Occupational Therapy Code of Ethics (2015)* (pp. 39–45). Bethesda, MD: AOTA Press.

Health Care Quality Improvement Act of 1986, Pub. L. 99–660, 42 U.S.C. §§ 11101–11152.

Kyler, P. (2016). Reference guide to the *Occupational Therapy Code of Ethics.* In D. Y. Slater (Ed.), *Reference guide to the Occupational Therapy Code of Ethics* (2015 ed., pp. 3–5). Bethesda, MD: AOTA Press.

Maryland Department of Health and Mental Hygiene, Board of Occupational Therapy Practice. (2015). *Disciplinary actions.* Retrieved from www.dhmh.maryland.gov/botp/SitePages/discipline.aspx

Moyers, P. (2009). Occupational therapy practitioners: Competence and professional development. In E. B. Crepeau, E. S. Cohn, & B. A. B. Schell (Eds.), *Willard and Spackman's occupational therapy* (11th ed., pp. 240–251). Philadelphia: Lippincott Williams & Wilkins.

National Board for Certification in Occupational Therapy. (2014). *NBCOT practice standards/code of conduct.* Retrieved from http://www.nbcot.org/certificant-code-of-conduct

National Board for Certification in Occupational Therapy. (2015a). *NBCOT certificant attestation.* Retrieved from http://www.nbcot.org/certification-renewal-process

National Board for Certification in Occupational Therapy. (2015b). *NBCOT disciplinary action summary.* Retrieved from http://www.nbcot.org/disciplinary-action-info

National Board for Certification in Occupational Therapy. (2015c). *Procedures for the enforcement of the NBCOT Candidate/Certificant Code of Conduct.* Retrieved http://www.nbcot.org/assets/regulatory-pdfs/enforcement_procedures

National Board for Certification in Occupational Therapy. (2015d). *Your guide to continuing competency. Certification matters.* Retrieved from http://www.nbcot.org/newsletter

North Carolina Board of Occupational Therapy. (2015). *Disciplinary actions.* Retrieved from http://www.ncbot.org/otpages/disciplinary_actions.html

Reed, K. L. (2011). Occupational therapy values and beliefs: The formative years, 1904–1929. In D. Y. Slater (Ed.), *Reference guide to the Occupational Therapy Code of Ethics and Ethics Standards* (2010 ed., pp. 57–72). Bethesda, MD: AOTA Press.

Slater, D. Y. (Ed.). (2016). *Reference guide to the Occupational Therapy Code of Ethics (2015).* Bethesda, MD: AOTA Press.

U.S. Department of Health and Human Services. (n.d.). *About us.* Rockville, MD: Health Resources and Services Administration Data Bank. Retrieved from https://www.npdb-hipdb.hrsa.gov/topNavigation/aboutUs.jsp

Willmarth, C. (2011). State regulation of occupational therapists and occupational therapy assistants. In K. Jacobs & G. L. McCormack (Eds.), *The occupational therapy manager* (5th ed., pp. 455–467). Bethesda, MD: AOTA Press.

Chapter 4.

SOLVING ETHICAL DILEMMAS

Janie B. Scott, MA, OT/L, FAOTA

Learning Objectives

By the end of the chapter, readers will be able to

- Describe a model for ethical decision making as applied to occupational therapy practice,
- Apply the Scott Four-Step Process for Ethical Decision Making to an ethical dilemma through the use of the Decision Table, and
- Analyze a situation to determine whether an ethical dilemma exists.

Key Terms and Concepts

- ✧ Decision Table
- ✧ Ethical dilemma
- ✧ Framework for ethical decision making
- ✧ Morris Ethical Decision-Making Model
- ✧ Nurses' Ethical Reasoning Skills model
- ✧ Primary stakeholder
- ✧ Purtilo and Doherty Six-Step Model for Solving Ethical Dilemmas
- ✧ Scott Four-Step Process for Ethical Decision Making
- ✧ Secondary stakeholders
- ✧ Tertiary stakeholders

An ***ethical dilemma*** is a conflict between two divergent moral challenges that one must resolve in deciding on the proper course of action. Some have defined an ethical dilemma as a struggle in deciding between good and evil (Beauchamp & Childress, 2013; Hansen, 1988; Purtilo & Doherty, 2011), but most situations health care practitioners face involve subtler distinctions: "As occupational therapists we face dilemmas in day-to-day practice that may not be as dramatic as those discussed in the media, however, to the individual patients and families involved they are crucial" (Hansen, 1988, p. 279).

When occupational therapy practitioners identify an ethical situation that is difficult to resolve, a decision-making model can help them analyze the situation, determine the appropriate course of action, and reach an equitable solution. A four-step process for use in solving ethical dilemmas is described in this chapter. This process draws from models that reflect both thinking within occupational therapy and perspectives from medicine and nursing. The Decision Table assists occupational therapy practitioners and students in weighing the positive outcomes and negative consequences of potential choices when solving ethical challenges encountered in the vast expanse of occupational therapy practice.

Background

A variety of decision-making models are available in the literature to assist occupational therapy practitioners and other health professionals in resolving ethical dilemmas. This section briefly examines a selection of the many available models.

Occupational Therapy Ethical Decision-Making Models

The ***Morris Ethical Decision-Making Model*** (Morris, 2016) established a three-step approach for evaluating ethical dilemmas in occupational therapy practice:

1. Ascertain whether an ethical dilemma is being faced.
2. Analyze possible courses of action to arrive at a proposed course of action.
3. Evaluate the proposed course of action at different levels of moral reasoning (see Exhibit 4.1).

Purtilo and Doherty (2011) defined the ***Puritio and Doherty Six-Step Model for Solving Ethical Dilemmas:***

- *Step 1:* Gather relevant information.
- *Step 2:* Identify the type of ethical problem.
- *Step 3:* Analyze the problem using ethics theories or approaches.
- *Step 4:* Explore the practical alternatives.
- *Step 5:* Act.
- *Step 6:* Evaluate the process and outcome.

Purtilo and Doherty's and Morris's models are similar; both underscore the importance of gathering all relevant data, articulating which ethical issues may apply following a review of ethical principles, defining a plan of action, and evaluating the potential outcomes of the plan. However, Purtilo and Doherty's model includes a final step of evaluating the process and outcomes after action has been taken. This evaluative component can promote a practitioner's competence in solving future ethical dilemmas.

Brandt and Slater (2011) developed a ***framework for ethical decision making*** (see Exhibit 4.2) that consists of an eight-step decision-making process with specific questions to help practitioners address situations that contain ethical dilemmas. Because this framework has more detail than the previously described models, it may help some practitioners better understand the full context of a dilemma, consider additional options for action, evaluate potential consequences of an action, analyze outcomes, and use the experience to improve future decisions.

Ethical Decision-Making Models From Other Professions

Fairchild (2010) developed an ethical decision-making model to assist nurses in processing ethical dilemmas. The ***Nurses' Ethical Reasoning Skills*** (NERS) ***model*** includes "reflection (critically reflective consciousness), reasoning (dialectic reasoning), and review of competing values" (Fairchild, 2010, p. 356). The NERS model highlights the importance of using intuition and reflection to support the process of ethical decision making. Fairchild discussed the responsibility nurses have to be moral, particularly in complex health care environments in which there are multiple duties (e.g., to administration, patient, family). She acknowledged that although caring comes from within individual practitioners, caring also is expected from leadership and the health care delivery system itself.

In addition, she noted, practitioners evaluate each situation as a whole, examining the context and the values, motivations, and perspectives of the stakeholders in making decisions or evaluating complex situations. The ultimate outcome of the process is to avoid conflict and open a dialogue to promote understanding between the parties involved.

Hundert (1987) proposed an ethical problem-solving model for use within medicine in response to an identified lack of models available to physicians:

> The model . . . attempts to fill this void by developing a conceptual understanding of the nature of moral dilemmas that can be applied to both theoretical and practical problems in medicine. . . . A difficult problem becomes a "dilemma" when we are quite sure that we will be making a big mistake regardless of whatever path we choose. (p. 839)

Exhibit 4.1. Morris Ethical Decision-Making Model

Morris's approach analyzes whether an ethical dilemma exists and presents a straightforward strategy to determine ways to address a challenging situation. For example, Gayle, the student in Vignette 4.1, sought a resource to help her resolve whether a course of action suggested by her classmates was ethical.

Am I facing an ethical dilemma?

1. What are the relevant facts, values, and beliefs?

2. Who are the key people involved?

3. State the dilemma clearly.

Analyze

1. What are the possible courses of action?

2. What conflicts could arise from each action?

3. Proposed course of action:

Evaluate

1. Code and Ethics Standards, Level III

2. Social Roles, Level II

3. Self-Interests, Level I

Does your proposed course of action lead to *consensus*? If yes, then proceed. If no, contact the appropriate resource for guidance: AOTA, NBCOT, or your State Regulatory Board.

Source. From "Is It Possible to Be Ethical?" by J. Morris, February 24, 2003, *OT Practice*, *8*(4), 18–23. Copyright © 2003 by the American Occupational Therapy Association. Adapted with permission.
Note. AOTA = American Occupational Therapy Association; NBCOT = National Board for Certification in Occupational Therapy.

Vignette 4.1. Student Collaboration: Is It Ethical?

Keisha, Rachel, Dillon, and **Gayle** were members of a cohort in their occupational therapy program. They frequently worked together on in- and out-of-class assignments. While out on their Level I internships (at different sites), they were each asked to complete an independent project that would benefit a client at their site. The students discussed the assignment offline and decided to work together to complete the individual assignments to save time and effort.

Although Gayle liked the idea of saving time like anyone else, she became concerned that if her academic fieldwork educator or clinical instructor became aware of the plan, they might not approve. Gayle wondered if she could continue to work with her group and avoid violating academic and ethical principles. She wasn't sure if their group project, which was designed to be individualized, might ultimately harm the identified clients due to the lack of specificity of their initiatives. Gayle was also perplexed about how or whether to share her concerns with her group, the faculty, or her clinical instructor. She wanted to process these questions before moving forward. Gayle wanted to feel confident when deciding if an ethical dilemma existed. Using the Morris Ethical Decision-Making Model helped Gayle analyze this dilemma and determine an ethical course of action.

Exhibit 4.2. Framework for Ethical Decision Making

- What is the nature of the perceived problem (e.g., ethical distress, ethical dilemma), and what is the specific problem (i.e., "name and frame" the problem)?
- Who are the players—not just those immediately involved but others who may be influenced by the situation or any decision that is made?
- What information is known, and what additional information is needed to thoroughly evaluate the situation and formulate options?
- What resources are available to assist?
- What are the options and likely consequences of each option?
- How are values prioritized (e.g., prioritize moral values, despite potential negative personal repercussions, to act on best decision)?
- Good intentions do not always bring about good deeds (Kanny & Slater, 2008).
- What action is being taken, and is defensible?
- Was the outcome expected? Would one make a different decision if confronted with a similiar situation in the future?

Source. Brandt and Slater (2011, p. 478). Used with permission.

Hundert's descriptive model for balancing conflicting values or moral principles involves the following steps:

- Identify conflicting values (e.g., make lists of values or issues in question).
- Balance values, that is, weighting of each value (e.g., consider the consequences of actions; weigh legal responsibilities, cultural expectations, and institutional policies; identify personal vs. professional values).
- Practice reflective equilibrium (e.g., ensure close adherence to values).
- Review actions taken for consistency with stated moral principles.

As Hundert noted, decision making provokes anxiety in many people because it involves weighing their own values against competing perspectives (e.g., moral principles). He recommended retaining lists of conflicting values and decisions and reviewing them to help understand and expand the ethical reasoning process.

Scott Four-Step Process for Ethical Decision Making

The ***Scott Four-Step Process for Ethical Decision Making*** outlines four actions that occupational therapy practitioners can take when confronted with a potential ethical dilemma:

1. Gather the facts, and specify the dilemma.
2. Analyze possible courses of action, taking into account both a set of principles and potential consequences.
3. Select and implement a course of action.
4. Evaluate the results of the action. Regardless of the specific ethical decision-making model one uses, it is beneficial to use the same model

whenever dilemmas arise; consistent use of one model can help practitioners gain competence and ensure that their decisions are ethical.

Step 1: Gather the Facts, and Specify the Dilemma

The first step is to reflect on the facts of the situation and decide whether they constitute an ethical dilemma as opposed to a misunderstanding, a potential legal issue, or a personnel issue (Morris, 2016). It is useful at this stage to identify the personal values and beliefs of the key people involved and their bearing on the dilemma. These key people, or stakeholders, could include the client and his or her family members, internal influencers (e.g., supervisor, institutional rules), and external influencers (e.g., third-party payers, state regulatory boards; see Chapter 20, "Interprofessional Ethics with Internal and External Communities").

It is important to identify the primary, secondary, and tertiary stakeholders and examine their relationships and obligations. The ***primary stakeholder*** may be a company, agency, or organization around whom the ethical situation pivots. The primary stakeholder is the key figure who is directly affected by the ethical dilemma. ***Secondary stakeholders*** are close to the situation and indirectly affected. Finally, ***tertiary stakeholders*** may be affected by the actions of other stakeholders from a more distant relationship.

Step 2: Analyze Possible Courses of Action

Evaluating the facts of a dilemma against existing principles and regulations helps occupational therapy practitioners analyze their options and select the appropriate course of action. In addition to the *Occupational Therapy Code of Ethics (2015)*, hereinafter referred to as the "Code" (American Occupational Therapy Association [AOTA], 2015a), practitioners are obligated to abide by federal and state laws, the policies of their employers, and regulations established by *state regulatory boards* (SRBs) governing practice in their state or jurisdiction. State regulations, national certifications, and organizational policies help guide practitioners in their behaviors, choices, and approaches to ethical decision making (see Chapter 3, "Promoting Ethics in Occupational Therapy Practice: Codes and Consequences").

For example, the responsibilities of occupational therapy assistants are dictated by SRB practice acts and the profession's standards of practice. Occupational therapy assistants may contribute to a client's evaluation, but an occupational therapist has the primary responsibility to evaluate clients, interpret the findings, and develop a plan of intervention (AOTA, 2014a, 2014b, 2015b; see Appendix G, "Guidelines for Supervision, Roles, and Responsibilities During the Delivery of Occupational Therapy Services"). An occupational therapy assistant who is asked to complete an evaluation would know that refusing to complete the evaluation is both legally and ethically correct.

Step 3: Select and Implement a Course of Action

Once the best way to resolve the ethical dilemma is clear, the occupational therapy practitioner takes action. For example, he or she may attempt to remediate the problem locally (e.g., through direct communication with the person involved), or file a complaint through the SRB, National Board for Certification in Occupational Therapy (NBCOT), or AOTA (jurisdiction guidelines are provided in Figure 3.2 of Chapter 3).

The "best" course of action is situation specific; what works in one situation may be ineffective in another. In general, the best course of action may be for the stakeholders to discuss the situation, the issues that are involved, and ways to identify a satisfactory resolution. This step may include the primary stakeholder agreeing to take an ethics course or engage in other remediation activities to reduce the potential of reoccurrences. This strategy is most likely to be effective when no one was harmed and no laws or regulations were broken.

Step 4: Evaluate the Results of the Action

Purtilo and Doherty (2011), Hundert (1987), Morris (2016), and others include a step in their models focusing on the importance of evaluating the conclusions that were drawn at the end of a deliberative process. During reflection, the practitioner should review whether the recommendations made were consistent with ethical standards, laws, and institutional policies; were reached by consensus; and stood the test of time. The final question to consider is, if disciplinary actions were recommended, were they consistent with actions taken previously when similar infractions occurred? In Case Study 4.1, an

Case Study 4.1. Addressing Duty to Report vs. Right to Privacy

Keith was hospitalized following a stroke and received occupational therapy and physical therapy services. Before his stroke, Keith had led an active life working part time, socializing with friends, providing transportation for family and friends, and maintaining his own apartment. Keith shared with his occupational therapist, **Carolyn,** that he believed he was ready to return to his "old life" and to reestablish familiar routines.

Carolyn was committed to supporting Keith's health and participation in familiar and meaningful occupations, a role consistent with that described in AOTA's *(2014b) Occupational Therapy Practice Framework: Domain and Process*. She and Keith agreed to complete a series of formal and informal assessments to determine his level of occupational performance before he returned to his previous occupations, including driving. These assessments raised concerns about Keith's readiness to return to driving, and Carolyn recommended a comprehensive driving evaluation through a driver rehabilitation program.

Carolyn believed that her primary duty was to Keith, but she was uncertain about her ethical obligation to report her misgivings about his driving to the state motor vehicle administration (MVA), to her employer (who might be liable if Keith caused a car crash following discharge), and to Keith's family. Carolyn used the Scott Four-Step Process for Ethical Decision Making to analyze the situation and determine a course of action.

Step 1: Gather the facts and specify the dilemma. Keith had had a stroke. Carolyn's assessment revealed possible deficits in Keith's judgment, reaction time, and attention. Carolyn recommended a comprehensive driver evaluation because she believed Keith or the community might be at risk if he returned to driving now, and she also believed that she could collaborate with Keith to enable his return to his prior roles in the community. The key people involved included Keith, Keith's family, Carolyn, her employer, the state medical advisory board, and the community. Carolyn identified her dilemma as the following: Did she have an ethical obligation to inform others about her concerns regarding Keith's ability to drive safely?

Step 2: Analyze possible courses of action. Carolyn considered the following possible actions:

- Inform Keith of the outcome of the formal and informal assessments and reiterate her recommendations.
- Investigate state regulations, Health Insurance Portability and Accountability Act of 1996 (HIPAA; P. L. 104–191) guidelines, the Code, and institutional rules that might relate to this situation. Contact the medical advisory board (MAB) of the MVA regarding their reporting requirements.
- Inform Keith's family of her concerns.
- Do nothing.

Carolyn also considered the potential consequences of these actions. Carolyn might discover that legal, ethical, and policy rules obligated her to report her doubts about Keith's driving. If she fulfilled this obligation, Keith might discontinue his occupational therapy intervention. If Keith failed to obtain a comprehensive driver evaluation, his family might take away his car keys without justifiable evidence. If Carolyn reported Keith, he might claim that she had violated HIPAA provisions (i.e., that Carolyn had no right to discuss the outcome of her evaluations with third parties). Doing nothing, however, had the potential to cause harm and to violate laws and ethical principles.

Carolyn reviewed the Code and discovered that the following principles were relevant: Principle 1, Beneficence, especially Related Standards of Conduct (RSCs) 1A ("Provide appropriate evaluation and a plan of intervention for recipients of occupational therapy services specific to their needs"); Principle 3, Autonomy, especially RSC 3A ("Respect and honor the expressed wishes of recipients of service"); and 3H (maintain confidentiality of all communications); and Principle 5, Veracity, especially RSC 5A ("Represent credentials, qualifications, education, experience, training, roles, duties, competence, contributions, and findings accurately in all forms of communication"); and 5B ("Refrain from using or participating in the use of any form of communication that contains false, fraudulent, deceptive, misleading, or unfair statements or

(Continued)

Case Study 4.1. Addressing Duty to Report vs. Right to Privacy *(Cont.)*

claims"). At the social roles level, Keith's family and friends relied on him to live independently, do errands for others, and give friends rides as needed.

Carolyn's social roles involved her professional membership and identity. She had an obligation to practice occupational therapy ethically and competently. Carolyn also was a member of the same community as Keith and wanted to maintain her reputation. Carolyn's self-interest was focused on her desire to be respected in the workplace and the community. The outcome of this was important to her for altruistic reasons, for employment security, and as an opportunity to give occupational therapy increased public visibility.

Step 3: Select and implement a course of action. Carolyn contacted her state MVA's MAB. She learned that people with certain conditions (e.g., epilepsy, dementia, stroke) must notify the MVA when they have a new occurrence of one of these conditions or when applying for or renewing a driver's license (Code of Maryland Regulations, 2016). The MAB receives reports from physicians and health care providers when they provide services to a patient who has one of the reportable conditions. Carolyn decided to present Keith with the results of the assessments and reiterate her recommendation to obtain the comprehensive driver evaluation. She explained to him that she had ethical and legal responsibilities to act on his and the community's behalf, particularly if he did not follow her recommendations. Carolyn revealed the outcome of her research with the MVA, which created an obligation for her to report her concerns to the state for their action. She also reinforced that following through with the driver assessment did not necessarily mean he would have to retire from driving. Carolyn let Keith know that assessment and intervention might result in several years of continued driving, continuation of his role as driver for his friends, and reassurance to his family of his confirmed safe driver status.

Step 4: Evaluate the results of the action. At the conclusion of this analytical process, Carolyn was confident that her proposed course of action was ethical and in compliance with state regulations. She provided Keith, the primary stakeholder, encouragement to act on his own behalf in a way that would ensure that he and the community would be safe and that he could maintain his roles with family and friends. Reaching a collaborative decision with Keith to have the driver evaluation enabled Carolyn to stay within ethical guidelines, state MVA requirements, and federal HIPAA regulations.

occupational therapist must disentangle her obligation to safeguard the client's right to privacy from her duty to report a potential danger to the community.

Decision Table

Another approach to analyzing the situation in Case Study 4.1 is through the use of a ***Decision Table*** (see below in Table 4.1; a blank version of the Decision Table is available in Appendix G). The Decision Table is separate from the Scott Model as it presents a template for analyzing what to do when one has determined that there is a dilemma. This correlates to action taken after processing through Step 2 of the Scott Model.

Once the ethical dilemma has crystallized, the Decision Table establishes a method for an occupational therapy practitioner to analyze their possible actions in a straightforward manner. This table is simple as it asks the person with the dilemma to consider the situation from three different perspectives: What are the possible courses of action that the individual can take? Once that is determined, consider the positive outcomes and negative consequences for each action.

By weighing the major issues and consulting the Code, regulations, and institutional policies and procedures, and the roles or scopes of practice for other team members, one should be able to make an informed decision. Table 4.1 uses the current case study of Carolyn's dilemma as a sample of how to effectively use the Decision Table.

Case Study 4.2 describes the conflict between the duty to maintain appropriate professional boundaries and the desire to avoid harming the client, and uses the Scott Four-Step Process for Ethical Decision Making to determine a course of action.

In Vignette 4.2, occupational therapy practitioners must take immediate steps to rectify an ethics breach involving competence. Questions are

Table 4.1. Decision Table for Case Study 4.1

Possible Action	Positive Outcomes	Negative Consequences
Take no action	Carolyn would avoid the stress of presenting her clinical views and ethical duties.	Without appropriate intervention, Keith may continue to drive and injure himself or members of the community. Carolyn would have breached her duty to Keith, his family, the community, and regulators.
Review assessment results with Keith, and make recommendations.	Carolyn would adhere to best practices. Carolyn becomes informed and able to be thoughtful and ethical in her decision making.	Keith might discontinue occupational therapy. Carolyn may realize that her past and current actions could possibly violate ethical standards.
Research legal and ethical requirements for reporting.	Carolyn's knowledge of reporting requirements would increase, enabling her to act based on her research.	Carolyn may feel obligated to take action in ways that may alienate her relationship with Keith.
Comply with the MAB and other reporting requirements.	Carolyn would be in compliance with state and federal regulations, and association and institutional policies. Carolyn might be more confident in her communication with Keith and his family.	The time required to provide the necessary documentation takes away from Carolyn's productivity.
Inform family of concerns.	Family may support Keith, encouraging him to take action. If necessary, other family and friends may offer to help solve transportation issues (e.g., errands, rides).	Family may take Keith's car keys away based on emotions, not data.

Note. MAB = medical advisory board.

Case Study 4.2. Protecting Professional Boundaries

Diego was an occupational therapy assistant employed at a rural community hospital. His primary responsibility was service delivery to an inpatient rehabilitation population. Diego was occasionally asked to work with outpatient clients when there were staff shortages. Diego enjoyed the opportunity to work in both areas because he was able to work with clients over a longer period of time and observe their progress.

One client with whom Diego was familiar was **Petra,** who had been treated for a brain injury. She had been a client on both the inpatient and outpatient physical rehabilitation caseloads and later for depression on the behavioral health unit. Diego had implemented the intervention plan for Petra in both settings. Because he had worked with Petra for so long, they usually chatted when they saw each other. Diego shared some of his personal history with Petra, part of which he considered to be a therapeutic use of self. He tried to stay within the boundaries of professional behavior.

Diego terminated his employment with the community hospital and began to work at an outpatient rehabilitation facility nearby. Before leaving the hospital, Diego said good-bye to the clients and staff with whom he was most familiar, including Petra, and wished them well. After he left, to his surprise, Petra stopped by his new job to say hello on several occasions. Diego attempted to handle the situation by professionally greeting Petra and letting her know that his new job kept him busy. Shortly thereafter, however, Petra began calling and driving by Diego's house. The phone calls disturbed Diego's spouse. Petra also had left a note for Diego on his front door and tried to reach him through social media.

He did not want to be friends with Petra and was uncertain how to appropriately end contact with her without hurting her feelings. His spouse grew concerned about his safety and urged him to take action, but he had difficulty deciding whether this was a personal, professional (ethical), or legal situation. He decided to take the time to use the

(*Continued*)

Case Study 4.2. Protecting Professional Boundaries *(Cont.)*

four-step ethical decision-making process to determine his next steps.

Step 1. Gather the facts and specify the dilemma. Petra was visiting Diego's place of employment and contacting him at home. Diego valued his privacy. He also valued equality and wanted to treat Petra and himself fairly. Diego had an obligation to adhere to applicable laws and regulations that governed his practice. Finally, he did not want to act precipitously and violate Petra's dignity. The key people involved were Diego, Petra, Diego's employer, and Diego's family. Diego's dilemma was as follows: Did Diego owe Petra a duty to protect her from disappointment, which might exacerbate her behavioral health condition, by taking assertive steps to get her to stop visiting him at home and at work without invitation?

Step 2. Analyze possible courses of action. Diego considered the following courses of action:

- Tell Petra again, verbally and in writing, to cease contacting him.
- Contact his new supervisor at work for guidance because Petra's visits were disruptive at his place of employment.
- Consult the Code to see whether ethical principles apply to his situation.
- Contact the local police and report his concerns that Petra was stalking him.
- Do nothing and hope Petra would get bored or find another love interest.

Diego also considered the potential consequences of these actions. Petra might not understand Diego's intention and might feel that he was harassing her. Diego's supervisor might say that, because Petra is not one of their clients, Diego needs to take care of this problem quickly or his probationary status might be jeopardized. Diego reviewed the Code to attempt to clarify whether, under these values and guidelines, he owed a duty to Petra since she was no longer his client.

Step 3: Select and implement a course of action. The next time Diego saw Petra, he told her directly that they no longer had a therapeutic relationship and that he did not want to be her friend. He also stated clearly that if she did not stop contacting him, he would contact the police and obtain a restraining order.

Step 4: Evaluate the results of the action. After delivering the communication to Petra, Diego decided to evaluate the effectiveness of his direction within a limited (e.g., 2 week) time period. If Petra continued her undesirable behaviors, then Diego would notify his supervisor for guidance.

Vignette 4.2. Taking Responsibility for Ensuring Competence

Diane was a registered occupational therapist with 3 years of experience in hospital-based physical rehabilitation. The census at the hospital had decreased in the past year because of downsizing in local industries. Diane's position changed from full-time to part-time. To supplement her income, she began working in an outpatient clinic.

When Diane first accepted the position at the outpatient clinic, she was unaware that many of the clients needed hand therapy. During a typical session with a client requiring hand therapy, Diane used electrical and superficial (e.g., hot packs) physical agent modalities (PAMs; e.g., hot packs). During a weekly supervision meeting, Diane asked whether the clinic would pay for her to take classes so she could learn the proper administration of PAMs. **Jayne,** Diane's supervisor, was shocked to learn that Diane hadn't already taken these courses as required by the SRB. She told Diane to see no more hand clients until she had taken the appropriate courses and had the required credentials in place.

Jayne reflected on her conversation with Diane and felt conflicted about whether further action was appropriate and necessary. Fortunately, no one had been injured by Diane's use of PAMs; however, the potential for injury had existed. Was educating Diane about the licensure requirements regarding PAMs enough? Because Diane was an AOTA member, possessed current certification through NBCOT, and was licensed through the SRB, did Jayne have an obligation to report her discovery to the organizations and to the SRB? Moreover, did Jayne have an obligation to verify Diane's competence in the use of PAMs before assigning her to see hand clients? If so, what is the appropriate course of action for her to take?

Vignette 4.3. Addressing Failure to Maintain Ethical Principles in Private Practice

Pamela Pediatrics, a company owned by **Pamela,** an occupational therapist, provided occupational therapy services to preschool children with special needs. Pamela had been a clinical fieldwork supervisor for 8 years, and although the practice was busy and the clinic's staffing level was low, she currently had 3 Level I fieldwork students. The students were concerned that the children were receiving inadequate care and that the students themselves were receiving inadequate supervision.

The students consulted the Code and discovered that Principle 1, Beneficence, was violated because understaffing could lead to a lack of safety for both the children and the students. Principle 4, Justice, and RSC 4H, regarding the provision of appropriate supervision by those with supervisory responsibility, also were relevant as was RSC 4N. The students realized Pamela was held to the same obligations to her clients and fieldwork students in her private practice as she would be in an institution. Pamela was responsible both for providing competent services to the children—who may have been at increased risk for injury—and for supervising the students according to relevant guidelines (e.g., Accreditation Council for Occupational Therapy Education, 2012). The students contacted their university for guidance.

Note: RSC = Related Standard of Conduct.

provided to prompt readers to analyze the ethical dilemmas themselves.

Vignette 4.3 describes a scenario in which occupational therapy students and pediatric clients may be receiving inadequate care and supervision. The students researched their situation using the Code and Decision Table to determine the most appropriate courses of action.

Summary

A variety of approaches to solving ethical dilemmas are available to occupational therapy practitioners using models that have been proposed within occupational therapy, medicine, and nursing. These models, a four-step process, and a Decision Table discussed in this chapter, can help practitioners analyze ethical dilemmas to find the solution that best matches the context.

Some ethical dilemmas are easy and straightforward to resolve. Others, however, involve reflection, research, and thoughtful analysis. Practitioners should remember that, in difficult situations, resources are available through the SRB, AOTA, and NBCOT. For dilemmas that cannot be solved on the local or direct levels, these organizations and agencies function as stakeholders to protect the professional and the public.

The question "Is it possible to be ethical?" (Morris, 2016) has no easy answer. Each ethical dilemma is unique; the people, stakeholders, and nuances differ from case to case. With this in mind, consistent use of a decision-making model will help occupational therapy practitioners and students identify potential courses of action. There are no black-and-white answers to most ethical dilemmas, but with patience, research, and objectivity, occupational therapy practitioners will successfully solve their difficult ethical questions.

Reflective Questions

1. Refer to Vignette 4.2. Use the Decision Table to help Jayne
   - Determine which agency or organization has primary jurisdiction in this situation,
   - Identify 2–3 courses of action that Jayne has available to her, and
   - Specify the positive outcomes and negative consequences for each identified course of action.
2. Refer to Case Study 4.2 and complete the Decision Table in Appendix G, "Decision Table," to help identify the best course of action based on the positive outcomes and negative consequences associated with each potential course of action.
   - What values and principles apply to this situation?
   - How might Diego's social roles be affected by his actions?
   - Whose self-interests are being served?
   - Does the proposed course of action lead to consensus? If not, what resource is most appropriate to contact for guidance—AOTA, NBCOT, or SRB?

References

Accreditation Council for Occupational Therapy Education. (2012). 2011 Accreditation Council for Occupational Therapy Education (ACOTE®) standards. *American Journal of Occupational Therapy, 66*(Suppl. 6), S6–S74. https://doi.org/10.5014/ajot.2012.66S6

American Occupational Therapy Association. (2014a). Guidelines for supervision, roles, and responsibilities during the delivery of occupational therapy services. *American Journal of Occupational Therapy, 68*(Suppl. 3), S16–S22. https://doi.org/10.5014/ajot.2014.686S03

American Occupational Therapy Association. (2014b). Occupational therapy practice framework: Domain and process (3rd ed.). *American Journal of Occupational Therapy, 68*(Suppl. 1), S1–S48. https://doi.org/10.5014/ajot.2014.682006

American Occupational Therapy Association. (2014c). Scope of practice. *American Journal of Occupational Therapy, 68*(Suppl. 3), S534–S540. https://doi.org/10.5014/ajot.2014.686S04

American Occupational Therapy Association. (2015a). Occupational therapy code of ethics. *American Journal of Occupational Therapy 69*(Suppl. 3), 6913410030. https://doi.org/10.5014/ajot.2015.696S03

American Occupational Therapy Association. (2015b). Standards of practice for occupational therapy. *American Journal of Occupational Therapy, 69*(Suppl. 3), 6913410057p1. https://doi.org/10.5014/ajot.2015.696S06

Beauchamp, T. L., & Childress, J. F. (2013). *Principles of biomedical ethics* (7th ed.). New York: Oxford University Press.

Brandt, L. C., & Slater, D. Y. (2011). Ethical dimensions of occupational therapy. In K. Jacobs & G. L. McCormack (Eds.), *The occupational therapy manager* (5th ed., pp. 469–483). Bethesda, MD: AOTA Press.

Code of Maryland Regulations. (2016). *Disorders reported by applicant or licensee [COMR 11.17.03.02-1].* Retrieved from http://www.dsd.state.md.us/comar/comar.html/11/11.17.03.02-1.htm

Fairchild, R. M. (2010). Practical ethical theory for nurses responding to complexity in care. *Nursing Ethics, 17,* 353–362. https://doi.org/10.1177/0969733010361442

Hansen, R. A. (1988). Nationally speaking: Ethics is the issue. *American Journal of Occupational Therapy, 42,* 279–281. https://doi.org/10.5014/ajot.42.5.279

Health Insurance Portability and Accountability Act of 1996, Pub. L. 104–191, 110 Stat. 1936.

Hundert, E. M. (1987). A model for ethical problem solving in medicine, with practical applications. *American Journal of Psychiatry, 144*(7), 839–846. https://doi.org/10.1176/foc.1.4.427

Kanny, E. M., & Slater, D. Y. (2008). Ethical reasoning. In B. A. Boyt Schell & J. W. Schell (Eds.), *Clinical and professional reasoning in occupational therapy* (pp. 188–208). Philadelphia: Wolters Kluwer/Lippincott Williams & Wilkins.

Morris, J. (2003). Is it possible to be ethical? *OT Practice, 8*(4), 18–23.

Morris, J. F. (2016). Is it possible to be ethical? In D. Y. Slater (Ed.), *Reference guide to the Occupational Therapy Code of Ethics* (2015 ed., pp. 83–89). Bethesda, MD: AOTA Press.

Purtilo, R., & Doherty, R. F. (2011). *Ethical dimensions in the health professions* (5th ed.). St. Louis: Elsevier.

Part II.

PRINCIPLES

INTRODUCTION TO PART II

Janie B. Scott, MA, OT/L, FAOTA

Now that groundwork has been laid for understanding the history of the American Occupational Therapy Association's (AOTA's) *Occupational Therapy Code of Ethics (2015)* (hereinafter referred to as the "Code;" AOTA, 2015), Part II proceeds to an examination of its principles. Readers will gain an in-depth understanding of the elements of each ethical principle and its relationship to occupational therapy practice. Through case studies and vignettes, readers will explore the practical applications of each principle—including analytical processes to use in resolving ethical dilemmas—in the context of current occupational therapy practice. A Decision Table is introduced and used throughout this publication, providing readers with a straightforward way to assess possible actions and their outcomes when an ethical dilemma is identified.

The six Principles reviewed in Part II are as follows:

- *Principle 1: Beneficence.* The Principle of Beneficence requires occupational therapy practitioners to work for the well-being and safety of the recipients of their services. The importance of continuing competence in occupational therapy practices that benefit consumers and promote evidence-based practice is highlighted in Chapter 5. The expectation of continuing competence for occupational therapy practitioners has been articulated by AOTA in its standards of practice, by the National Board for Certification in Occupational Therapy, and by state regulatory boards.
- *Principle 2: Nonmaleficence.* The Principle of Nonmaleficence reinforces the obligation of occupational therapy practitioners to avoid exploitation of and prevent harm to recipients of services. Chapter 6 also focuses on the importance of practitioners' own self-care, including vigilance against conflicts of commitment or interest.
- *Principle 3: Autonomy.* Occupational therapy practitioners' legal and ethical responsibility to respect the client's right to privacy, self-determination, confidentiality, and consent is the focus of Chapter 7. Practitioners are encouraged to become culturally sensitive to support service recipients' autonomy and to focus on supporting client self-determination by engaging in client-centered practice.
- *Principle 4: Justice.* The Principle of Justice, presented in Chapter 8, embraces occupational therapy's responsibility to be fair and equitable in practice and to those served. Respect is encouraged toward individuals (e.g., clients, colleagues, communities) and the laws, regulations, and policies that govern occupational therapy practice. Justice includes the important role for students and occupational therapy practitioners to advocate for access to their services by reducing economic and other barriers to services through policy changes and available means. This Principle is germane to all occupational therapy roles, including those of educator, researcher, volunteer, and practitioner. Requirements for credentialing and documentation and the importance of informing supervisees, colleagues, and administrators about occupational therapy practitioners' ethical and regulatory responsibilities also are discussed.

- *Principle 5: Veracity.* The Principle of Veracity emphasizes truth, honesty, and respect in communication with others (e.g., clients, colleagues, the public). As discussed in Chapter 9, these expectations extend to oral communication and written documentation and include providing proper attributions to the works of others.
- *Principle 6: Fidelity.* The Principle of Fidelity involves the constructs of respect, fairness, and integrity. Chapter 10 discusses the importance of balancing obligations to stakeholders (e.g., clients, colleagues, and other professionals) and provides strategies for preventing breaches of this Principle.

The chapters in Part II closely examine one of the Code's six ethical Principles. The use of vignettes and case studies will help readers apply the knowledge about one or more Principles to actual situations where ethical dilemmas presented themselves.

Reference

American Occupational Therapy Association. (2015). Occupational therapy code of ethics (2015). *American Journal of Occupational Therapy, 69*(Suppl. 3), 6912310030. https://www.doi.org/10.5014/ajot.2015.696S03

Chapter 5.

PRINCIPLE 1: BENEFICENCE

Janie B. Scott, MA, OT/L, FAOTA

Learning Objectives

By the end of the chapter, readers will be able to

- Describe how competence affects knowledge and skills in all areas of occupational therapy practice;
- Analyze the relationship of evidence-based knowledge with clinical expertise, reimbursement, and client preferences; and
- Apply the Related Standards of Conduct for Principle 1, Beneficence, to decisions that occupational therapy practitioners should arrive at when making referrals or discontinuing services.

Key Terms and Concepts

✧ Assessments
✧ Beneficence
✧ Competence
✧ Evidence-based practice
✧ Personal reflection

Beneficence

Principle 1. Occupational therapy personnel shall demonstrate a concern for the well-being and safety of the recipients of their services.

Beneficence includes all forms of action intended to benefit other persons. The term *beneficence* connotes acts of mercy, kindness, and charity (Beauchamp & Childress, 2013). Beneficence requires taking action by helping others, in other words, by promoting good, by preventing harm, and by removing harm. Examples of beneficence include protecting and defending the rights of others, preventing harm from occurring to others, removing conditions that will cause harm to others, helping persons with disabilities, and rescuing persons in danger (Beauchamp & Childress, 2013).

Related Standards of Conduct

Occupational Therapy Personnel Shall

A. Provide appropriate evaluation and a plan of intervention for all recipients of occupational therapy services specific to their needs.
B. Reevaluate and reassess recipients of service in a timely manner to determine if goals are being achieved and whether intervention plans should be revised.
C. Use, to the extent possible, evaluation, planning, intervention techniques, assessments, and therapeutic equipment that are evidence based, current, and within the recognized scope of occupational therapy practice.
D. Ensure that all duties delegated to other occupational therapy personnel are congruent with credentials, qualifications, experience, competency, and scope of practice with respect to service delivery, supervision, fieldwork education, and research.
E. Provide occupational therapy services, including education and training, that are within each practitioner's level of competence and scope of practice.
F. Take steps (e.g., continuing education, research, supervision, training) to ensure proficiency, use careful judgment, and weigh potential for harm when generally recognized standards do not exist in emerging technology or areas of practice.
G. Maintain competency by ongoing participation in education relevant to one's practice area.
H. Terminate occupational therapy services in collaboration with the service recipient or responsible party when the services are no longer beneficial.
I. Refer to other providers when indicated by the needs of the client.
J. Conduct and disseminate research in accordance with currently accepted ethical guidelines and standards for the protection of research participants, including determination of potential risks and benefits.

Source. From *Occupational Therapy Code of Ethics (2015)* (American Occupational Therapy Association, 2015b, pp. 2–3).

The concept of *Beneficence*, the first principle of the *Occupational Therapy Code of Ethics (2015)* (hereinafter referred to as the "Code"; American Occupational Therapy Association [AOTA], 2015b), has been explored by religious leaders, philosophers, and ethicists, as well as by occupational therapy practitioners. Although the exact wording of their definitions varies, the focus on being helpful to others is consistent. For example, Veatch and Flack (1997) described beneficence in the allied health professions as "the state of doing or producing good . . . [and] the moral principle that actions are right insofar as they produce good" (p. 277).

Beneficence in occupational therapy has similarly been defined as "doing good for others or bringing about good for them" (Slater, 2016, p. 291). Occupational therapy practitioners promote positive outcomes and prevent harm when they adhere to the behavioral expectations described in Principle 1 of the Code.

This chapter focuses on two such expectations: (1) maintaining competence and (2) engaging in evidence-based practice. The material presented underscores the importance of meeting these expectations along with personal reflection leading the occupational therapy practitioner to recognize when a client no longer benefits from services (Related Standard of Conduct [RSC] 3H) and the need to refer the client to another when the skill set does not match the client's needs (RSC 3I).

Beneficence Through Competence

Competence is possession of the knowledge base, skill level, and clinical reasoning ability to deliver occupational therapy services in a safe and consistent manner (Wilson, 1977). State regulatory boards, AOTA, the National Board for Certification in Occupational Therapy (NBCOT), and other organizations and agencies external to occupational therapy each define specific requirements for competence in occupational therapy practitioners (e.g., AOTA, 2015c; see also Appendix E, Procedures for the Enforcement of the NBCOT *Candidate/Certificant Code of Conduct,* and Chapter 3, "Promoting Ethics in Occupational Therapy Practice: Codes and Consequences").

Reed, Ashe, and Slater (2009) reviewed cases considered by the AOTA Ethics Commission, including those that focused on breaches of ethics related to competence. They identified the following components of competence related to Principle 1 that practitioners need to support the ideal of Beneficence:

- Qualifications and experience
- Evidence base
- Self-assessment
- Expert education
- Current knowledge.

To maintain the ethical obligation of beneficence, occupational therapy practitioners have a duty to continually maintain their competence by building their knowledge and skills and applying these to clinical, academic, and research practice. The expectation of competence, articulated by AOTA, NBCOT, and state regulatory boards, emphasizes the importance of occupational therapy practitioners' developing and maintaining the requisite skills needed to serve clients safely. Therefore, competence is a value and a standard that encourages high levels of skills and abilities throughout the profession.

Continuing education, research, independent reading, attendance at workshops and conferences, and many other vehicles are available to expand the occupational therapy practitioner's knowledge base. Vignette 5.1 describes an example of beneficent practice by a practitioner who has maintained and improved his competence over time.

Competence is important to clients, the profession, and individual occupational therapy practitioners. Most important, high-quality and competent occupational therapy services benefit the recipients, be they individuals or communities (McConnell, 2001). According to the Preamble of the Code, "AOTA members are committed to promoting inclusion, participation, safety, and well-being for all recipients in various stages of life, health, and illness and to empowering all beneficiaries of service to meet their occupational needs" (AOTA, 2015b, p. 1).

Moyers (2002) pointed out that unsatisfactory competence can manifest in several ways, including increased expenditures of time and resources. Additionally, practitioner incompetence may worsen clients' condition or cause additional secondary conditions, which may lead to discontent with or poor quality of life (Moyers, 2002). By maintaining competence, occupational therapy practitioners are better able to prevent the consequences of incompetent practice.

The occupational therapy profession benefits from practitioner competence when practitioners deliver the highest quality services to clients. As stated in Vision 2025, "Occupational therapy maximizes health, well-being, and quality of life for all people, populations, and communities through effective solutions that facilitate participation in everyday living" (AOTA, 2016, para. 1). This vision of the profession

Vignette 5.1. Using Expertise to Benefit Clients

Darius, an occupational therapist, had worked in the construction industry before entering occupational therapy school. He wanted to integrate his construction experience with occupational therapy and establish his own business once he developed competence in providing occupational therapy rehabilitation services to people recovering from traumatic injuries and neurological and orthopedic conditions. He maintained his entrepreneurial vision through school and during his first 4 years of practice. While gaining his occupational therapy expertise, he continued working part-time on a construction job. He realized that, when he began his private practice, his referral base would potentially be greater if he obtained his AOTA Specialty Certification in Environmental Modifications.

After Darius had been in private practice 2 years, he was awarded a consultant contract to assess the internal and external environments of a community center and identify potential hazards that could harm people with disabilities who attended programs in the center. As part of his contract, Darius also provided recommendations and evidence-based practice guidelines to address the deficiencies he identified. Darius's high level of competence in environmental assessment and redesign strengthened his ability to provide beneficent occupational therapy services by advocating to reduce potential harm to people with disabilities. The resources and continuing education he took advantage of through AOTA and other vendors helped ensure his competence in both practice areas.

is dependent on recognition by consumers, providers, and payers that occupational therapy practitioners deliver valuable services with a high level of competence.

Finally, professional competence benefits the practitioner. Continuing education can add meaning to one's professional career; as Bush, Powell, and Herzberg (1993) stated, "therapists must independently navigate their career paths in directions that are personally satisfying and productive" (p. 932). By engaging in continuing education pertaining to one's current position or to new topics of interest, practitioners are able to direct their professional growth in a meaningful way.

Personal reflection, including that gained through continuing education, can assist occupational therapy practitioners in developing a meaningful and gratifying career, thus ensuring benefits to themselves and their clients (Crist, Wilcox, & McCarron, 1998). The process of personal reflection is similar to developing a strategic or intervention plan, but this one is for the individual occupational therapy practitioner. Personal reflection involves assessing a baseline of where one is now (e.g., position, income, job satisfaction) and forecasting where he or she wants to be as a future professional (i.e., mission).

For example, do you want to specialize in your current practice area, or switch to a different one (i.e., vision)? Whatever is decided, identify what continuing education or certifications will help achieve these objectives.

A personal reflection plan may also include a timeline to help attain short- and long-term goals. If this process results in needing to find a mentor, or learning that you have the competencies to become a mentor, it can be added to your professional plan. Finally, this process should be regularly reviewed and updated to ensure continued competence and efforts toward lifelong learning.

According to Wilcox (2005), "Continuing professional development is the means to keep you up to date, safe and competent as a practitioner. It can keep you interested and satisfied in your work, and it can certainly keep you in employment" (p. 44) by opening career opportunities.

In Case Study 5.1, Azure's use of the Decision Table (Table 5.1) helped her to consider the best course of action to benefit novice occupational therapy practitioners and their clients, choosing to advocate for the resources novice practitioners needed to increase their competence.

Case Study 5.1. Developing Competence in Novice Practitioners

Azure, an occupational therapist with 10 years of experience, provided physical rehabilitation to clients in hospital settings and in their homes. Azure had worked in home care for the past 5 years and enjoyed the independence, flexibility, and personal client care this setting offered. She had no administrative or supervisory responsibilities for the home care agency.

Three novice occupational therapists working for the same home care agency approached Azure to ask for her assistance in negotiating home care as a practice environment and learning intervention strategies that promote good client care. Although Azure's official role did not include supervision, the novice practitioners sought her assistance to reduce potential harm and optimize care (i.e., promote beneficent practice). Azure stated that her schedule was too busy and her caseload too high to permit her to provide this kind of supervision and support.

The novice occupational therapists wondered if this refusal constituted a breach of Principle 1, Beneficence. They wondered whether Azure's refusal to provide them with the remediation they needed and share the responsibility for their clients' safety conflicted with the duty of providing beneficent care.

Azure, for her part, was concerned about the novice practitioners' lack of knowledge and experience in a practice area that demands independence and highly competent practice. She consulted the Code and found RSC1E, which clearly states that occupational therapists shall provide services within the practitioners' level of competence, to be relevant to her concerns. Azure also reviewed her contract and the *Reference Guide to the Occupational Therapy Code of Ethics* (Slater, 2016) for strategies she could use to clarify expectations, roles, and responsibilities for her and the novice practitioners in a way that would promote client care and safety and well-being.

(Continued)

Case Study 5.1. Developing Competence in Novice Practitioners *(Cont.)*

In the *Reference Guide,* she found "Combating Moral Distress" (Slater & Brandt, 2016) and "Is It Possible to Be Ethical?" (Morris, 2016) to be particularly helpful. She determined that the most effective approach would be to encourage the occupational therapists to review Principle 1 of the Code to understand their responsibilities for continuing competence. She also recommended they contact the home care company's account manager and ask the company to provide either leave time for continuing education or paid supervision until their competence improved to a level at which clients would be more likely to benefit from and less likely to be harmed by their services.

On the basis of Azure's recommendations, the novice occupational therapists set up a meeting with the company's representative to discuss their concerns. They thanked Azure for her patience and guidance and for her ability to serve as a good advocate for both clients and colleagues. Table 5.1 demonstrates the analytic process used to review the primary issues, actions, and outcomes of this situation.

Table 5.1. Decision Table for Case Study 5.1

Possible Action	Positive Outcomes	Negative Consequences
Azure could decline to provide supervision to the novice occupational therapists.	Azure avoids a conflict of commitment (RSC 6C).	Novice occupational therapists would be left to provide services with skills they had yet to attain (violation of RSC 1E).
Azure could help the novice occupational therapists understand what their responsibilities are in becoming competent practitioners.	If the novice occupational therapists heed Azure's advice they would take steps to comply with RSC 1F.	Azure might be faced with the difficult option of referring clients to other providers who had the necessary competencies (RSC 1I).
Azure could collaborate with the novice occupational therapists and advocate for their supervision and training.	Advocating for the novice occupational therapists would increase their employer's awareness of AOTA's official documents concerning continuing education, training, and supervision in compliance with RSC 4F and novice therapists' compliance with RSC 1E.	Azure's lack of more immediate action may ultimately put the novice occupational therapists and their clients at risk (violation of RSC 6B).

Note. AOTA = American Occupational Therapy Association; RSC = Related Standard of Conduct.

Beneficence Through Evidence-Based Practice

Understanding the evidence base provided by occupational therapy research and incorporating it into a methodology lead to effective and beneficent practice. According to AOTA (2015a), ***evidence-based practice*** (EBP) "is based on the integration of critically appraised research results with the clinical expertise, and the client's preferences, beliefs, and values" (para. 1). Further, RSC 1C urges occupational therapy practitioners to "use, to the extent possible, evaluation, planning, intervention techniques, and therapeutic equipment that are evidence-based and within the recognized scope of occupational therapy practice" (AOTA, 2015b, p. S2; see Appendix H, "Scope of Practice"). Occupational therapy practitioners must keep abreast of current research outcomes relevant to their practice areas to increase the beneficence of their practice (see Vignette 5.2). Craik and Rappolt (2006) suggested that occupational therapy practitioners invest in professional development to ensure they obtain the skills necessary to understand and use research findings.

One important area of evidence-based practice is the use of assessments in occupational therapy

Vignette 5.2. Beneficence Through Evidence-Based Practice

Nina has been a practicing occupational therapy practitioner for 21 years. She worked for the first 16 years in different positions within a major health system. Nina left that position 5 years ago to work independently as a consultant and contractor. When she worked within the health care system, she had access to in-service education and was able to keep up with practice updates, including evidence-based practice publications relevant to her positions.

Once she left her full-time employment, her adherence to the licensure laws related to continuing education diminished. Nina's license became in jeopardy due to her inability to acquire the required continuing education units. If Nina could not keep abreast of practice trends and evidence-based research, her practice would suffer and she would be out of compliance with state licensure requirements and the Code, specifically Principles 1 and 4.

evaluation and intervention. ***Assessments*** are typically face-to-face evaluations of individuals' occupations in the context of their daily performance and ability to interact with their environments. These standardized measures are based on evidence-based research and practice that require the integration of knowledge into practice (Coster, 2008). Occupational therapy practitioners use assessment results to assist in making decisions for intervention planning (Portney & Watkins, 2009), and they are ethically obligated to use assessments in ways that are supported by the evidence base.

Practitioners have a responsibility to conduct re-evaluations of their clients' progress toward their goals in a timely manner (RSC 1B) and use evidence-based and current assessments that are within their competence (RSC 1E). The practitioner's obligation to use standardized assessments according to administration and scoring standards exists regardless of setting. As Law and Baum (2006) noted,

> measurement is used to improve our decisions regarding specific clients or programs. As professionals, occupational therapists have an obligation to measure the need for service, design interventions based on knowledge gained from measurement, and evaluate the results of interventions. (p. 15)

Occupational therapy practitioners' obligation in appropriately using assessments to measure client capacities and limitations begins with being knowledgeable about each assessment instrument used. Practitioners must locate the appropriate assessment, master the correct administration procedures, and be sure never to offer test items for practice (Asher, 2014). Using assessments as intended provides valid data regarding clients that can be used to document the value of occupational therapy services. As Law and Baum (2006) affirmed, "as occupational therapists develop evidence-based practice, a valid measurement process is essential in providing evidence of the effectiveness and efficiency of our services" (p. 16). Practitioners also must "review the validity features of the measure to be sure that the test is designed to offer the kind of information the professional desires" (Dunn, 2006, p. 23).

If assessments are not used according to the developers' instructions and the evidence regarding their use, the client may not receive the full benefit of occupational therapy services because intervention has been planned and implemented on the basis of incomplete, inaccurate, or missing data about important limitations or potential capabilities (Reed, 2016).

Reitz, Pizzi, and Scaffa (2010) stated that "working expediently can be a positive attribute, but it can also lead to unethical behavior if sufficient care is not taken to select the best available assessment, to properly administer the assessment, and to properly report results" (p. 167). Any deficiencies in the application of the test or assessment instrument should be noted in the assessment summary and allowances made for inaccurate interpretation (Reed, 2016), and the client's performance should not be compared with standard scores. Case Study 5.2 describes an occupational therapist's efforts to ensure that assessments are used correctly in her setting. In a similar situation, a hospital-based occupational therapist's understanding of competence is challenged in Vignette 5.3.

Case Study 5.2. Using Assessments Appropriately

Julie practiced as an occupational therapist for 1 year in an urban hospital. She provided care to clients with a variety of physical and cognitive disabilities in both acute care and acute rehabilitation services. She believed she was competent in evaluating clients, planning interventions, and discharging clients appropriately.

Julie attended a session at an occupational therapy conference on the appropriate and ethical use of assessments. Julie remembered studying and learning current administration procedures during her recent academic preparation. Her coworkers and mentors at her current institution, however, used practices that conflicted with what Julie had learned in academic study and at the conference session. She weighed what she was taught in school and what she learned through continuing education activities against the guidance she received from her coworkers.

For example, it was common practice among Julie's coworkers to use portions of a standardized assessment, rather than the entire assessment, and to ignore scoring guidelines. When Julie questioned a coworker about this type of assessment use, the coworker responded, "I don't record that I am using the assessment. I am just basing my evaluation on how they do on those portions of the assessment. It's not like I am saying they are performing at this level, based on this assessment." In addition, Julie observed several occupational therapy practitioners using assessments as an intervention. When Julie asked her coworkers about this practice, one responded, "No one uses the assessments anyway, so why does it matter?"

Julie confirmed that competent assessment administration means documenting when standardized assessments are used. She also concluded that the use of assessments as interventions potentially reduces the validity of the standardization if, in the future, another practitioner were to administer the tool with the same client. Julie determined that administering and using assessments in this manner violated RSCs 1A and 1B of the Code. She decided to discuss the matter with her immediate supervisor during a private meeting.

Julie and her supervisor agreed that Julie would provide an educational in-service to her peers regarding appropriate and current assessment administration and scoring. After the in-service was held, facility leadership created mandatory competencies for occupational therapy practitioners to ensure their competence in the administration of assessments. Julie believed her presentation was well received by her superiors and peers.

Note. Written with contributions from Dana Burns Dukehart. Used with permission.

Vignette 5.3. Making Referrals to Community Practitioners

Morgan, an occupational therapist and care coordinator at a pediatric rehabilitation hospital, was responsible for helping families identify and order assistive devices and environmental modifications for children and youth. Her duties also included tracking the client's transition back to home and community and providing education and support to the family regarding the child or youth's adjustment following their illness, disability, or exacerbation of their condition.

This was demanding work that required Morgan to develop and sustain relationships with providers in the community for referral purposes. Morgan had a good network in the occupational therapy community and primarily made referrals to **Justin,** an occupational therapy assistant who performed home evaluations. There were occupational therapy practitioners in the community, one who held an AOTA Specialty Certification in Environmental Modifications, another who was a Certified Aging in Place Specialist through the National Association of Home Builders, and several experienced contractors. Many questions arose regarding Morgan's referral procedures, particularly relating to the awareness of professional boundaries and the ethics principle and RSC of Beneficence.

Summary

The emphasis on continuing competence and evidence-based practice reflects the commitment of the occupational therapy profession to the principle of Beneficence. Maintaining professional competence is a lifelong obligation for all occupational therapy practitioners. A prescribed path for pursuing professional competence does not exist; it is up to each practitioner to identify his or her strengths and needs and create a plan for professional development. As Law and Baum (2006) noted, "What is best practice today evolves into standard practice in the future. This is how knowledge advances in our discipline. The standard practices of today were best practices of the past that have influenced practice" (pp. 9–10). Therefore, occupational therapy practitioners must constantly critique best practices and incorporate those worthy into their practice. State regulations, the Code, and other official documents help guide us to occupational therapy practice that is ethical, beneficent, competent, and evidence based.

Reflective Questions

1. Identify the relevant RSCs in Vignette 5.3 associated with Principle 1, Beneficence.
2. Describe what alternative referral procedures Morgan could use that would not put her professional ethics in question.
3. When reviewing Morgan's referral relationship with Justin, the Quality Improvement staff person discovered that Justin frequently took Morgan out to lunch or dinner as a thank you for the referral. Review the Code and determine if this is acceptable ethical behavior, and if not, what principles and RSCs might have been violated.

Acknowledgments

The author acknowledges Dana Burns Dukehart's contributions from the previous edition of this text.

References

American Occupational Therapy Association. (2015a). *Evidence-based practice and research.* Retrieved from http://www.aota.org/Practice/Researchers.aspx

American Occupational Therapy Association. (2015b). Occupational therapy code of ethics (2015). *American Journal of Occupational Therapy, 69*(Suppl. 3), 6912310030. https://doi.org/10.5014/ajot.2015.696S03

American Occupational Therapy Association. (2015c). *Occupational therapy profession—Continuing competence requirements.* Retrieved from http://www.aota.org/-/media/corporate/files/advocacy/licensure/stateregs/contcomp/continuing%20competence%20chart%20short%208-2015%20cw.pdf

American Occupational Therapy Association. (2016). *Vision 2025.* Retrieved from http://www.aota.org/aboutaota/vision-2025.aspx

Asher, I. E. (Ed.). (2014). *Asher's assessment tools: An annotated index for occupational therapy* (4th ed.). Bethesda, MD: AOTA Press.

Beauchamp, T. L., & Childress, J. F. (2013). *Principles of biomedical ethics* (7th ed.). New York: Oxford University Press.

Bush, J. V., Powell, N. J., & Herzberg, G. (1993). Career self-efficacy in occupational therapy practice. *American Journal of Occupational Therapy, 47,* 927–933. https://doi.org/10.5014/ajot.47.10.927

Coster, W. J. (2008). Embracing ambiguity: Facing the challenge of measurement. *American Journal of Occupational Therapy, 62,* 743–752. https://doi.org/10.5014/ajot.62.6.743

Craik, J., & Rappolt, S. (2006). Enhancing research utilization capacity through multifaceted professional development. *American Journal of Occupational Therapy, 60,* 155–164. https://doi.org/10.5014/ajot.60.2.155

Crist, P., Wilcox, B. L., & McCarron, K. (1998). Transitional portfolios: Orchestrating our professional competence. *American Journal of Occupational Therapy, 52,* 729–736. https://doi.org/10.5014/ajot.52.9.729

Dunn, W. (2006). Measurement issues and practices. In M. Law, C. Baum, & W. Dunn (Eds.), *Measuring occupational performance: Supporting best practice in occupational therapy* (2nd ed., pp. 21–32). Thorofare, NJ: Slack.

Law, M., & Baum, C. (2006). Measurement in occupational therapy. In M. Law, C. Baum, & W. Dunn (Eds.), *Measuring occupational performance: Supporting best practice in occupational therapy* (2nd ed., pp. 3–20). Thorofare, NJ: Slack.

McConnell, E. A. (2001). Competence vs. competency. *Nursing Management, 32*(5), 14.

Morris, J. F. (2016). Is it possible to be ethical? In D. Y. Slater (Ed.), *Reference guide to the Occupational Therapy Code of Ethics* (2015 ed., pp. 83–89). Bethesda, MD: AOTA Press.

Moyers, P. A. (2002). Continuing competence and competency: What you need to know. *OT Practice, 7*(9), 18–22. Retrieved from http://www1.aota.org/pdt/MoyersOTArticle.htm

Portney, L. G., & Watkins, M. P. (2009). Principles of measurement. In L. G. Portney & M. P. Watkins (Eds.), *Foundations of clinical research: Applications to practice* (3rd ed., pp. 63–75). Upper Saddle River, NJ: Pearson Education.

Reed, K. L. (2016). Outdated and obsolete tests and assessment instruments. In D. Y. Slater (Ed.), *Reference guide to the Occupational Therapy Code of Ethics* (2015 ed., pp. 217–221). Bethesda, MD: AOTA Press.

Reed, K. L., Ashe, A. M., & Slater, D. Y. (2009, April). *Everyday ethics: Ethical challenges inemerging practice.* Slide show presented at the AOTA Annual Conference & Expo, Houston.

Reitz, S. M., Pizzi, M. A., & Scaffa, M. E. (2010). Evaluation principles in health promotion practice. In M. E. Scaffa, S. M. Reitz, & M. A. Pizzi (Eds.), *Occupational therapy in the promotion of health and wellness* (pp. 157–172). Philadelphia: F. A. Davis.

Slater, D. Y. (Ed.). (2016). *Reference guide to the Occupational Therapy Code of Ethics (2015 ed.).* Bethesda, MD: AOTA Press.

Slater, D. Y., & Brandt, L. C. (2016). Combating moral distress. In D. Y. Slater (Ed.), *Reference guide to the Occupational Therapy Code of Ethics* (2015 ed., pp. 117–123). Bethesda, MD: AOTA Press.

Veatch, R. M., & Flack, H. E. (1997). *Case studies in allied health ethics.* Upper Saddle River, NJ: Prentice Hall.

Wilcox, A. (2005). How to succeed as a lifelong learner. *Primary Health Care, 15*(10), 43–50. https://doi.org/10.7748/phc2005.12.15.10.43.C564

Wilson, M. A. (1977). A competency assurance program. *American Journal of Occupational Therapy, 31,* 573–579.

Chapter 6.

PRINCIPLE 2: NONMALEFICENCE

S. Maggie Reitz, PhD, OTR/L, FAOTA

Learning Objectives

By the end of the chapter, readers will be able to

- Describe professional behavior that upholds the Principle of Nonmaleficence;
- Determine potential conflicts of interests within their professional roles; and
- Apply Principles and Related Standards of Conduct to potential ethical dilemmas related to the prevention of harm to clients, their family, students, research participants, or employees.

Key Terms and Concepts

- ✧ Abandonment
- ✧ Analysis of occupational performance
- ✧ Avoiding exploitation
- ✧ Client abandonment
- ✧ Conflict of commitment
- ✧ Nonmaleficence
- ✧ Preventing harm
- ✧ Self-reflection

Nonmaleficence

Principle 2. Occupational therapy personnel shall refrain from actions that cause harm.

Nonmaleficence "obligates us to abstain from causing harm to others" (Beauchamp & Childress, 2013, p. 150). The Principle of Nonmaleficence also includes an obligation to not impose risks of harm even if the potential risk is without malicious or harmful intent. This Principle often is examined under the context of due care. The standard of due care "requires that the goals pursued justify the risks that must be imposed to achieve those goals" (Beauchamp & Childress, 2013, p. 154). For example, in occupational therapy practice, this standard applies to situations in which the client might feel pain from a treatment intervention; however, the acute pain is justified by potential longitudinal, evidence-based benefits of the treatment.

Related Standards of Conduct

Occupational Therapy Personnel Shall

A. Avoid inflicting harm or injury to recipients of occupational therapy services, students, research participants, or employees.
B. Avoid abandoning the service recipient by facilitating appropriate transitions when unable to provide services for any reason.
C. Recognize and take appropriate action to remedy personal problems and limitations that might cause harm to recipients of service, colleagues, students, research participants, or others.
D. Avoid any undue influences that may impair practice and compromise the ability to safely and competently provide occupational therapy services, education, or research.
E. Address impaired practice and, when necessary, report to the appropriate authorities.
F. Avoid dual relationships, conflicts of interest, and situations in which a practitioner, educator, student, researcher, or employer is unable to maintain clear professional boundaries or objectivity.
G. Avoid engaging in sexual activity with a recipient of service, including client's family or significant other, student, research participant, or employee, while a professional relationship exists.
H. Avoid compromising rights or well-being of others based on arbitrary directives (e.g., unrealistic productivity expectations, falsification of documentation, inaccurate coding) by exercising professional judgment and critical analysis.
I. Avoid exploiting any relationship established as an occupational therapy clinician, educator, or researcher to further one's own physical, emotional, financial, political, or business interests at the expense of recipients of services, students, research participants, employees, or colleagues.
J. Avoid bartering for services when there is the potential for exploitation and conflict of interest.

Source. From the *Occupational Therapy Code of Ethics (2015)* (American Occupational Therapy Association, 2015, pp. 3–4).

Nonmaleficence, Principle 2 of the *Occupational Therapy Code of Ethics (2015)* (hereinafter referred to as the "Code"; American Occupational Therapy Association [AOTA], 2015), is closely linked to Principle 1, Beneficence. The difference is subtle but important; according to Beauchamp and Childress (2013), "while beneficence requires action to incur benefit, nonmaleficence requires non-action to prevent harm" (as cited in AOTA, 2010, p. S19). Nonmaleficence first appeared as a separate principle in the 2000 version of the *Occupational Therapy Code of Ethics* (AOTA, 2000).

The Principle of Nonmaleficence addresses four categories of behavior: (1) avoidance of exploitation, (2) prevention of harm, (3) self-reflection and mindfulness to avoid harm, and (4) self-care (i.e., the protection of one's own health). Although these categories are not mutually exclusive, they constitute a framework for further exploring the complexity of the Principle of Nonmaleficence. Early action, de-escalation, and collaboration are all strategies occupational therapy practitioners can use to ensure they do not engage in unethical actions. Good people can make bad decisions. The Code is not punitive but rather aspirational, intended to help occupational therapy practitioners as a collective be responsible for protecting the people they serve.

Avoidance of Exploitation

Half of the 10 Related Standards of Conduct (RSCs) in Principle 2 address the need for ***avoiding exploitation,*** which is taking advantage of a client, therapeutic situation, student, colleague, or business relationship for personal gain. Four of these RSCs (2C, 2D, 2F, 2G) relate to exploitation in relationships. The fifth, RSC 2I, is associated with business exploitation.

The ability to develop and engage in therapeutic relationships is an essential quality of competent occupational therapy service provision; when these relationships are not in place, intentional and unintentional harm can result. Engaging in bartering that exploits businesses, vendors, or others in the organization can damage the reputation of the profession and employer or institution.

The profession has long paid attention to the importance of relationships within occupational therapy practice. Taylor (2008) described the evolution of thought regarding the optimal use of relationships in occupational therapy practice, including the principles of therapeutic use of self proposed by Frank in 1958 and conscious use of self, encouraged by Mosey in 1981. After a review of contemporary literature, Taylor identified two themes in regard to the therapeutic use of relationships in occupational therapy practice: (1) collaboration and client-centeredness, and (2) caring and empathy. In addition, Taylor discussed the use of narrative and clinical reasoning as valued intervention approaches to develop therapeutic relationships.

Case Study 6.1 shows that exploitation can involve employees, not only clients and students, and exemplifies three important considerations in ethical resolution:

1. Validating perceptions before assuming a violation has occurred
2. Addressing ethical concerns and perceptions as soon as possible
3. Handling concerns locally whenever possible.

Case Study 6.1. Avoiding Exploitation

Christina, an occupational therapist, was looking forward to being assigned her first new employee to supervise and mentor. She wanted both to share her expertise in evidence-based practice and to help educate the next generation of occupational therapy practitioners. **Serge,** the employee assigned to Christina, was similarly looking forward to starting his first job as an occupational therapist.

Christina took Serge to lunch in the hospital cafeteria on his first day to get to know him better and to review the policy manual with him. After reviewing the manual, Christina switched the conversation to more personal topics. During this portion of the conversation, Christina found out that Serge was single and lived with his mother, who ran a house-cleaning service; Serge worked for her on Saturdays. She responded to this news by saying, "I've been looking forever for someone to clean my house but can't find an affordable person. Can your mom give me a deal?"

Serge did not know what to do. He felt bad for his supervisor because he knew that hospital employees had been furloughed because of state budget cutbacks. He also felt guilty that Christina had bought him lunch. However, Serge did not want to undermine the livelihood of the four women who worked for his mother by offering discounted service. He went home and told his mother, **Olga,** about the conversation he had had with Christina. Olga, a first-generation U.S. resident, was anxious for her son to do well. She offered to discount the rate, provided he did the cleaning on a twice-a-month schedule. Olga contacted Christina, and they scheduled the first cleaning. Christina was overjoyed at the deeply discounted rate she had been provided.

As soon as Serge entered Christina's townhouse the following Saturday, he felt uneasy; this feeling intensified over the coming weeks. Christina's large-screen, high-definition television and upscale furnishings contrasted with his assumption that she was financially vulnerable. When he arrived for the second scheduled cleaning session, Christina was just getting out of the shower. He left immediately and waited in his car, reviewing his textbooks in preparation to evaluate a client the following Monday.

When Christina left, he reentered the townhouse to complete the cleaning job. He shrugged off her behavior, knowing how easy it was to lose track of time. However, 2 weeks later, when he next went to clean, Christina had left negligées around the townhouse. Serge cleaned around the clothes, being careful not to touch any of them. Although he was feeling increasingly uncomfortable, he did not share his feelings with Christina or anyone else.

Two weeks later, when Serge arrived to clean, Christina had set the table for lunch and was provocatively dressed. She apologized, saying that she had forgotten Serge was scheduled to clean that day. Serge left, but 2 hours later she called and asked if he could return as her lunch date had

(*Continued*)

Case Study 6.1. Avoiding Exploitation *(Cont.)*

unexpectedly been cancelled. When he arrived, she was still dressed for her date and asked him to stay for lunch after he had finished cleaning. He politely said he could not because he was scheduled to clean other homes that afternoon. Hearing this, she then asked him if he was available for dinner. At this point Serge, feeling truly troubled, told Christina that he needed to leave. He called his mother and asked her to schedule one of the other women for future cleanings, stating that he would pay her the money that the cleaner would lose because of the discounted rate.

Serge was worried that Christina would seek revenge for his rejection of the dinner invitation when she completed his probation report, which was due the following month. After a 2-mile run to clear his head, he remembered that, in one of his occupational therapy classes, they had reviewed frameworks that could be used when facing an ethical challenge. He found the course material and reviewed the Code. From this review, he determined that Christina had possibly violated RSCs 2A, 2C, 2F, and 2I. Serge realized, on reflection, that he did not know for certain whether Christina was flirting with him and attempting to engage in a sexual relationship or not, so at this time he did not believe RSC 2G had been violated. However, it became clear to him that the request for discounted cleaning services was inappropriate and that he should not have agreed to ask his mother's cleaning company to work for Christina.

When Serge returned to work on Monday, he asked if he could meet with Christina. At the start of the meeting, he told her that he had become uncomfortable with the house-cleaning arrangement and that he would no longer be able to clean her house. He also shared his concerns that, by offering her the discounted cleaning rate, he had unwittingly put her in possible violation of RSCs 2A, 2C, 2F, and 2I. At first, Christina became defensive, saying, "I am an extremely competent occupational therapist. The Code is to protect clients. I have never harmed a client!" Serge remained calm and responded that she was one of the most competent occupational therapists he had ever had the honor to work with and that he had learned a great deal from watching her work. He then showed her a copy of the Code. As Christina read Principle 2, she became visibly more upset. She apologized, saying she had not been aware that her actions were in violation of the Code.

Serge then shared that he felt uncomfortable with her invitations for lunch and dinner. At this, Christina started to laugh. Serge became tense. Christina, seeing his anxiety, stopped laughing and explained that, although Serge was an attractive young man, she was in a committed relationship. In fact, she said she had been preparing a wardrobe for her wedding and honeymoon and apologized for leaving the garments around the townhouse. She further explained that she had offered him the invitation to lunch and dinner because she did not wish to waste the food she had prepared for her fiancé. She shared that although she was now financially comfortable, she had grown up in a family that needed to use food stamps, and she remained very conscious of wasting food.

Serge believed that he could continue to learn a great deal from Christina. He also was proud they had worked through a challenging ethical situation together in a positive way. Therefore, he decided to continue their current professional relationship but end the house-cleaning arrangement. Christina agreed, saying this decision also would make her most comfortable, and she encouraged Serge to continue to be forthright with her as he had done that day. Other possible actions that Serge could have considered for addressing this ethical issue are detailed in Table 6.1.

Serge, by following the last option in Table 6.1, addressed all three considerations in ethical resolution. His approach to the first two, validating perceptions and addressing concerns as soon as possible, is readily apparent. The third consideration, handling issues locally, was demonstrated by Serge's speaking directly to Christina rather than reporting her behavior to the department head. Handling issues locally does not preclude using resources such as the staff liaison to AOTA's Ethics Commission or a professional mentor to discuss strategies for approaching the situation, as long as confidentiality is maintained.

Case Study 6.1. Avoiding Exploitation *(Cont.)*

Table 6.1. Decision Table for Case Study 6.1

Possible Action	Positive Outcomes	Negative Consequences
No action.	Serge avoids conflict and maintains a comfortable relationship with his supervisor.	Serge allows for possible exploitation of self or others.
Explain, when first asked for the discounted services, that entering into such a business relationship could be viewed as a conflict of interest and promote the possible or perceived exploitation of each party; refer Christina to another reputable cleaning company; and suggest that Christina read the book *Nickel and Dimed: On (Not) Getting By in America* (Ehrenreich, 2011), so she understands the economic and social justice issues of her looking for deeply discounted services.	Serge avoids possible exploitation of self or others. Serge promotes Principle 4: Justice.	This action could result in possible conflict and an uncomfortable relationship with his supervisor.
Share his discomfort over the lunch invitation with Christina and clarify the expectations of their relationship.	Serge promotes transparency and honest communication earlier in the scenario, preventing further miscommunication. Serge avoids possible exploitation of self.	This action could result in possible conflict and an uncomfortable relationship with his supervisor.
Ask the department head to reassign him to another supervisor and mentor while Christina continues to be a customer of Olga's cleaning service, paying the full cost of services.	Serge avoids possible exploitation of Olga and Olga's employees.	Principle 1, Beneficence, could be a factor if the new mentor is not a good match for Serge's professional growth.
Continue their current professional relationship, and seek a referral from Olga for another reputable cleaning company for Christina.	Serge supports Principle 2, Nonmaleficence; Principle 4, Justice; and Principle 6, Fidelity.	None foreseen.

Prevention of Harm

Benjamin Franklin is credited with saying, "an ounce of prevention is worth a pound of cure" (Independence Hall Association, 2010, para. 1). The truth of this saying is as evident in ethics as it is in other areas of life. ***Preventing harm*** involves being vigilant to avoid circumstances with the potential to evolve into situations in which harm occurs.

Prevention of harm is detailed in RSCs 2A, 2B, 2C, and 2H. Specifically, RSC 2B relates to ***client abandonment,*** which is the "premature termination of the professional treatment relationship by the health care provider without adequate notice or the patient's consent" (*Taber's Cyclopedic Medical Dictionary,* 2005, p.1). Thus, occupational therapy practitioners must avoid situations in which clients are harmed by being restricted from access to needed services, thereby impacting clients' progress toward their goals.

Vignettes 6.1–6.3 directly relate to Nonmaleficence, in which occupational therapy practitioners are guided to avoid inflicting harm. These vignettes also show how behaviors associated with the prevention of harm can be related to the avoidance of exploitation.

Self-Reflection to Avoid Harm

RSC 2H involves the use of the analysis of occupational performance and ***self-reflection*** (i.e., introspective examination of one's motivations and performance) to avoid harm. According to AOTA (2014), ***analysis of occupational performance*** is the

> step in the evaluation process in which the client's assets and problems or potential problems are more specifically identified through assessment tools designed to observe, measure, and inquire about factors that support or hinder

Vignette 6.1. Preventing Academic Dishonesty

Heather and **Lynn** were best friends in different sections of the same graduate course. They were assigned to complete presentations on the same topic. In the week before the presentation, when Lynn had planned on preparing her presentation, her boyfriend broke their engagement and moved to London for a job opportunity. The same day, Lynn lost her wallet, and the next day she was laid off from her job. Overwhelmed, Lynn asked Heather to send her a copy of her draft PowerPoint slides so that she could make a few changes then submit them as her own work.

Heather knew that such an action would put both her and Lynn in violation of the Code. Although Lynn did not put Heather in danger of physical injury, she jeopardized both her own and Heather's status as occupational therapy students and their future professional careers. Instead of agreeing to Lynn's request, Heather suggested that Lynn talk to her professor and adviser about getting an extension on the assignment, seek help from the university counseling center to deal with her personal turmoil, and accept help from a group of volunteers Heather organized to walk Lynn's dog and bring dinner over so that Lynn could catch up on her schoolwork.

Vignette 6.2. Avoiding Potential Harm to Colleagues

The patient census in a skilled nursing facility was low. **Ginger,** an occupational therapist at the facility, decided it was an opportune time to reorganize her office to improve her efficiency and comfort. She went to find **Cliff,** an occupational therapy assistant, and **Sarah,** an occupational therapy student, to help her move some of her office furniture. She was unable to locate either of them. **Sandy,** another occupational therapist, asked Ginger why she needed Cliff and Sarah. When Ginger explained her plan, Sandy suggested to Ginger that she should get the plan approved by their supervisor, **Bob.** Ginger rolled her eyes and yelled, "Is this really necessary? It's making a mountain out of a molehill!" Ginger reflected on this exchange for a few minutes and went to find Bob to complain.

Bob commended Ginger for using the low patient census time to enhance her work environment to increase productivity and comfort. However, he communicated to Ginger that it was inappropriate to ask a coworker and student to perform tasks that were not within their job descriptions and that put them at risk for incurring injury. Ginger continued to protest until he asked her if it would be appropriate for him to ask her to make him a cup of coffee. She responded, "Certainly not!" She then smiled and said, "OK, whose job is this?" Bob and Ginger talked and were able to schedule the appropriately trained staff to assist her in her office reorganization project the next day.

Vignette 6.3. Analyzing Risks and Benefits in Research

Brianna was an occupational therapy educator working with a group of occupational therapy master's degree students on examining the link between sports engagement and successful aging among community-dwelling older adults. The research team decided to conduct a focus group with older adults to determine the meaning sports had played in their lives and their current level of engagement in sports. Several students were concerned that if a potential participant was no longer able to engage in favorite sports, their research might provoke sadness and depression.

The concerns of these students led to a lively and reflective discussion. The group decided to take extra care to be explicit in both the marketing and informed consent materials to ensure that potential participants knew the topic of the research and could make their own decisions as to whether to attend the focus group. Originally, the students had planned to conduct the focus groups in pairs, with one student asking the questions and the other being responsible for the informed consent form process and taking handwritten notes during the group. They decided to adjust their plans and have an additional student available in an adjoining room to talk with anyone who became upset during the focus group and to refer them to predetermined support services. The students also reviewed Principle 2; they believed that the potential risk to participants was low in comparison to the more likely positive social benefits gained from their project. After taking these actions, and knowing that their project would be reviewed by the university's institutional review board prior to initiating their study, the students felt more comfortable.

> occupational performance and in which targeted outcomes are identified. (p. S41)

Occupational therapy practitioners are adept in using this analysis in direct client care, but the application in the course of administrative responsibilities and volunteer roles may be less evident. Case Study 6.2 and Vignette 6.4 address the need to exercise thoughtful analysis and self-reflection when carrying out administrative roles and responsibilities.

Self-Care

Gilfoyle (1986) urged occupational therapists to take care of themselves to prevent harm. She believed that "our future depends on our ability to take care of ourselves both personally and

Case Study 6.2. Engaging in Self-Reflection to Avoid Harm When Making Decisions

Juan, an occupational therapy assistant in a skilled nursing facility, was approached by **Mildred** and **Bernice,** residents of the facility who shared a room. Mildred and Bernice were receiving similar occupational therapy for hip fractures from **Ann,** their occupational therapist. Mildred and Bernice wanted to switch their afternoon occupational therapy times. Mildred was currently scheduled at 1 p.m., when her daughter was available to bring Mildred's dog to visit during her lunch hour each day. Bernice was scheduled at 4 p.m., when her favorite television show aired.

Juan thought this was a logical request and approached Ann to ask permission to make the schedule switch. Ann was having a challenging day because one of the other occupational therapists had called in sick. She responded in an agitated voice that she didn't have the time to deal with this change and was concerned that, even if she did, it would "open the floodgates" for other similar requests. She then said she needed Juan to return another client to his room right away, effectively ending the conversation.

After Ann's long day ended, she went home and reflected on the day's events. She realized she had made an arbitrary decision because of the stresses of that particular day. The next day, she directed Juan to change Mildred's and Bernice's schedules. In addition, she asked if he was aware of any other clients who were dissatisfied with their current schedule. Juan said he was not but offered to ask each client for the next month and log the time needed to inquire and modify the schedule. Ann commended Juan for his logic and initiative.

One month later, Ann remarked to Juan that the head of Rehabilitation Services had been pleased with the increase in client satisfaction scores with occupational therapy services. She further commented that she believed this increase was attributable, in large part, to Juan's client advocacy efforts and the department's willingness to reconsider previous administrative procedures. Juan had found that only a few clients desired therapy schedule changes. Thus, Ann's concern about needing to spend extra time rearranging schedules was unfounded. In addition, the department realized actual benefits (i.e., an increase in client satisfaction scores) with relatively little effort.

Pleased by the results, Ann asked Juan if he would like to submit a joint proposal for a presentation to the state occupational therapy conference. Juan was excited about this opportunity and readily agreed. Ann thought it would be good to cite their experience of improving client satisfaction through communication and advocacy efforts in their presentation. While reviewing the Code for wording about respecting client autonomy, she found RSC 2H, which guides practitioners to "avoid compromising rights or well-being of others based on arbitrary administrative directives" (AOTA, 2015, p. 4). After an initial reaction of "Oh, my!" Ann whispered to herself, she smiled and was thankful that, through self-reflection and Juan's efforts, her actions avoided a potential violation of the Code and resulted in several positive outcomes.

Vignette 6.4. Avoiding Conflicts of Interest

After relocating to a new state, **Joan** joined the state's occupational therapy conference committee to meet other occupational therapy practitioners. She was excited about the new friendships she made and wanted to be a contributing member of the committee. The conference planning went well, and the committee was ready to print the conference brochure. Joan's uncle, **Jim,** lived in the area and owned a printing business. His business had been losing money, so Joan hoped that she could guide the committee toward using his services. She volunteered to find a printer without disclosing that she had a relationship with one of the potential vendors.

After arriving home from the meeting, she called Jim to see if he would like the business. Jim asked her who else was bidding on the opportunity. She said, "No one else—it's yours for the taking." There was a period of silence on the phone, after which Jim asked whether Joan was aware of the term *conflict of interest.* Joan responded, "Not really." Jim then described what conflict of interest is and told Joan that, although he greatly appreciated her efforts, she should get bids from at least two other printers. If the committee determined that his company offered the best value (i.e., quality for cost) of the three, he would be happy to perform the work. He also asked if the occupational therapy profession had ethical guidelines for situations such as this.

Joan went online and located the Code on the AOTA webpage. She found RSCs 2F and 6D, both pertaining to the inappropriate use of relationships. Joan also noted that RSCs 2F and 6C directly relate to conflict of interest, with 6C and 6D specifically referring to volunteer roles. Joan completed the bid process, provided the information to the conference committee, and recused herself from the vendor selection process after disclosing her relationship to one of the bidders, without indicating which business. The conference committee was impressed with her ethical behavior and thanked her for her efforts.

Vignette 6.5. Avoiding Undue Influences

Stella was attending her state conference many miles away from the university where she taught. After one of the afternoon workshops, a group of local occupational therapy practitioners organized a happy hour outing, suggesting several places with 2-for-1 drink specials. Not knowing anyone else at the conference, Stella at first decided to go along with the group. She set her phone alarm to be sure she would get back to the hotel room in time to teach her synchronous online class at 6 p.m.

As Stella reflected on her plan, she became concerned that she might be tempted to take advantage of the drink specials and, as a result, not be in her best form for class that evening. She therefore chose to have an early dinner by herself and skip happy hour. Realizing that she did not trust herself in this situation, she pledged to discuss this self-reflection and her current drinking habits with her physician to determine if she needed to take further action to protect her health.

Stella's actions were consistent with the behavior required by RSCs 2C and 2D. At a minimum, she avoided the potential embarrassment of a poor performance while conducting class. She also eliminated the students' potential need to report her performance if it became evident that she was under the influence of alcohol while conducting class. Her actions also show that she was actively reflecting on her behavior and planned to seek assistance to determine if she needed to further examine her drinking habits to ensure they did not affect either her health or her professional performance.

professionally. Taking care of ourselves is the positive force that promotes the ability to seize opportunities for the future" (p. 387). RSCs 2C and 2D both involve taking care of ourselves. Vignette 6.5 features an occupational therapy practitioner with a potential alcohol problem and thus relates to both of these RSCs.

Conflict of Commitment

Nonmaleficence can occur when conflicts of commitment interfere with the prevention of harm. ***Conflict of commitment*** "arises when outside activities substantially interfere with the person's obligation to students, colleagues, or the institution" (University System of Maryland, 2003, para. 5). Conflict of commitment can be thought of broadly as accepting too many professional responsibilities for the available energy and time.

Vignette 6.6 describes a potential conflict of commitment situation that needs to be avoided to uphold the spirit of RSC 2C: the need to "recognize and take appropriate action to remedy personal problems and limitations that might cause harm to recipients of service, colleagues,

Vignette 6.6. Preventing Conflicts of Commitment

After receiving her doctoral degree, **Sally** was excited to be hired as a new tenure-track faculty member at the university from which she had graduated the previous month. She took on this position with gusto, tackling all the responsibilities associated with this new role. Knowing that she had to perform in the areas of teaching, advising, scholarship, and service to obtain tenure, she volunteered to advise the new entering class of occupational therapy students and to revise the course on clinical reasoning. **Jennifer,** the program director, greeted Sally's contributions with relief and appreciation, as they had been short staffed for several years.

Later that fall, Jennifer was surprised to hear that Sally was running for president of the state occupational therapy association, given all of her university commitments and the stresses of a first-year teaching appointment. Jennifer did not voice any concerns, however, until Sally asked Jennifer to nominate her for a leadership position in AOTA. Jennifer, out of concern for Sally's ability to meet her increasing workload, declined to nominate Sally for the opportunity.

Sally was offended at first. Jennifer explained her action, stating that this particular AOTA committee required a great deal of work. She also shared that she was concerned about Sally's potential conflict of commitment and the possible impact on her health and professional success. Jennifer offered to meet with Sally the following week to lay out a 4-year strategy to gradually increase service contributions, both within and outside the university, as Sally became more experienced in teaching and disseminating her scholarly work.

students, research participants, or others" (AOTA, 2015, p. 3).

Summary

Occupational therapy practitioners have the necessary prerequisite knowledge and skills to work through challenging ethical situations and avoid actions that may result in harm to patients, themselves, or the profession. Occupational performance analysis, activity analysis, self-reflection, and a willingness to confront colleagues in a spirit of collaboration are important tools that can help occupational therapy practitioners protect the people they serve.

Reflective Questions

1. Refer to Vignette 6.1 and respond to the following questions.
   a. Which ethical RSCs did Heather exhibit?
   b. Which ethical RSCs did Lynn exhibit in accepting Heather's course of action?
2. Review and reflect on your current professional roles. Are you at risk of a conflict of interest?
3. Review and reflect on your current professional responsibilities. Are you at risk of a conflict of commitment?

References

American Occupational Therapy Association. (2010). Occupational therapy code of ethics (2000). *American Journal of Occupational Therapy, 54,* 614–616. https://doi.org/10.5014/ajot.54.6.614

American Occupational Therapy Association. (2010). Occupational therapy code of ethics and ethics standards (2010). *American Journal of Occupational Therapy, 64*(Suppl.), S17–S26. https://doi.org/10.5014/ajot2010.32S17

American Occupational Therapy Association. (2014). Occupational therapy practice framework: Domain and Process (3rd ed.). *American Journal of Occupational Therapy, 68*(Suppl. 1), S1–S48. https://doi.org/10.5014/ajot.2014.682006

American Occupational Therapy Association. (2015). Occupational therapy code of ethics (2015). *American Journal of Occupational Therapy, 69*(Suppl. 3), 6912310030. https://doi.org/10.5014/ajot.2015.696S03

Beauchamp, T. L., & Childress, J. F. (2013). *Principles of biomedical ethics* (7th ed.). New York: Oxford University Press.

Ehrenreich, B. (2011). *Nickel and dimed: On (not) getting by in America.* New York: Metropolitan Books.

Frank, J. D. (1958). Therapeutic use of self. *American Journal of Occupational Therapy, 8,* 215–225.

Gilfoyle, E. M. (1986). Nationally Speaking—Taking care of ourselves as health care providers. *American Journal of Occupational Therapy, 40,* 387–389. https://doi.org/10.5014/ajot.40.6.387

Independence Hall Association. (2010). *The electric Ben Franklin: The quotable Franklin.* Retrieved from http://www.ushistory.org/franklin/quotable/

Mosey, A. C. (1981). *Occupational therapy: Configuration of a profession.* New York: Raven Press.

Taber's Cyclopedic Medical Dictionary (20th ed.). (2005). Philadelphia: F.A. Davis.

Taylor, R. R. (2008). Changing landscape of therapeutic use of self. In R. R. Taylor, *The intentional relationship: Occupational therapy and use of self* (pp. 3–18). Philadelphia: F. A. Davis.

Taylor, R. R. (2008). Changing landscape of therapeutic use of self. In R. R. Taylor, *The intentional relationship: Occupational therapy and use of self* (pp. 3–18). Philadelphia: F. A. Davis.

University System of Maryland. (2003). *II–3.10—Policy on professional commitment of faculty.* Retrieved from http://www.usmd.edu/regents/bylaws/SectionII/II310.html

Chapter 7.

PRINCIPLE 3: AUTONOMY

Janie B. Scott, MA, OT/L, FAOTA

Learning Objectives

By the end of the chapter, readers will be able to

- Describe potential courses of action that occupational therapy practitioners or students can take when faced with ethical dilemmas concerning autonomy or confidentiality;
- Determine how the Principle of Autonomy applies to expanding areas of community-based practice; and
- Apply Principles and Related Standards of Conduct from the *Occupational Therapy Code of Ethics (2015)* to communication with recipients of service, including research participants.

Key Terms and Concepts

- ✧ Autonomy
- ✧ Collaboration
- ✧ Communication
- ✧ Confidentiality
- ✧ Consent

Autonomy

Principle 3. Occupational therapy personnel shall respect the right of the individual to self-determination, privacy, confidentiality, and consent.

The Principle of Autonomy expresses the concept that practitioners have a duty to treat the client according to the client's desires, within the bounds of accepted standards of care, and to protect the client's confidential information. Often, respect for Autonomy is referred to as the *self-determination principle*. However, respecting a person's autonomy goes beyond acknowledging an individual as a mere agent and also acknowledges a person's right "to hold views, to make choices, and to take actions based on [his or her] values and beliefs" (Beauchamp & Childress, 2013, p. 106). Individuals have the right to make a determination regarding care decisions that directly affect their lives. In the event that a person lacks a decision-making capacity, his or her autonomy should be respected through involvement of an authorized agent or surrogate decision maker.

Related Standards of Conduct

Occupational Therapy Personnel Shall

A. Respect and honor the expressed wishes of recipients of service.
B. Fully disclose the benefits, risks, and potential outcomes of any intervention; the personnel who will be providing the intervention; and any reasonable alternatives to the proposed intervention.
C. Obtain consent after disclosing appropriate information and answering any questions posed by the recipient of service or research participant to ensure voluntariness.
D. Establish a collaborative relationship with recipients of service and relevant stakeholders, to promote shared decision making.
E. Respect the client's right to refuse occupational therapy services temporarily or permanently, even when that refusal has potential to result in poor outcomes.
F. Refrain from threatening, coercing, or deceiving clients to promote compliance with occupational therapy recommendations.
G. Respect a research participant's right to withdraw from a research study without penalty.
H. Maintain the confidentiality of all verbal, written, electronic, augmentative, and non-verbal communications, in compliance with applicable laws, including all aspects of privacy laws and exceptions thereto (e.g., Health Insurance Portability and Accountability Act, Family Educational Rights and Privacy Act [FERPA]).
I. Display responsible conduct and discretion when engaging in social networking, including but not limited to refraining from posting protected health information.
J. Facilitate comprehension and address barriers to communication (e.g., aphasia; differences in language, literacy, culture) with the recipient of service (or responsible party), student, or research participant.

Source. From the *Occupational Therapy Code of Ethics (2015)* (American Occupational Therapy Association, 2015b, pp. 4–5).

Principle 3 of the *Occupational Therapy Code of Ethics (2015)* (hereinafter referred to as the "Code"; American Occupational Therapy Association [AOTA], 2015b) addresses the value of Autonomy. In this chapter, ***Autonomy*** is defined to provide a foundation for the exploration of four related ethical issues that support Principle 3: (1) confidentiality, (2) communication, (3) consent, and (4) collaboration.

According to Fremgen (2012), "*autonomy* means that people have the right to make decisions about their own life" (p. 21). To make such decisions, clients or their representatives need to understand both what is involved in the intervention and its risks and potential benefits. In their roles as service providers, researchers, educators, and students, occupational therapy practitioners must ensure that this information is delivered in a manner that is clear, unbiased, and culturally and linguistically appropriate.

Confidentiality

Occupational therapy practitioners and others who have access to confidential information must strictly comply with the preferences of clients; doing less is a breach of ethics and potentially the law. As defined by Fremgen (2012), ***confidentiality***

> refers to keeping private all information about a person (patient) and not disclosing it to a third party without the patient's written consent. . . . Information such as test results, patient histories, and even the fact that a person is a patient cannot be passed on to another person without the patient's consent. (p. 62)

Occupational therapy practitioners must be aware of the influence of clients' family and cultural traditions relative to autonomy. Some clients want practitioners to share all information about their condition, intervention options, and recovery both with the entire health care team directly involved with the provision of care and with their family and friends. Other clients want information about their current status and projected needs to be shared with only one or two designated people, whereas others may ask that only information about their participation in therapy be shared with specified people or with no one at all. Taylor (2008) recommended, "As a general guideline, when talking about a client to any other individual, even a family member, always obtain permission from the client before disclosing any information to anyone" (p. 210). By adhering to the client's needs, beliefs, wishes, customs, and rights regarding confidentiality, practitioners support their autonomy.

When speaking about confidentiality, Taylor (2008) encouraged occupational therapy practitioners to be cautious about what information they document in client, student, research participant, colleague, or employee records. Records should include only information that is relevant, not extraneous, to the situation to ensure adherence to standards of confidentiality. For example, occupational therapy practitioners with significant experience in occupational therapy practice may serve as expert witnesses in cases that are reviewed for compliance with laws or policies. As Vignette 7.1 illustrates, when testifying or submitting requested materials, practitioners must make sure to provide only the information specifically requested; any information outside of the scope of the request must be kept confidential (Fremgen, 2012).

In addition, practitioners must ensure that client records are not left in view of unauthorized people and that confidential information cannot be overheard in conversation. Such carelessness constitutes a violation of Principle 3 and of government regulations, including HIPAA and the Patient Protection and Affordable Care Act of 2010 (P. L. 111–148); as in other areas, the law and ethical mandates are in agreement when it comes to confidentiality. Case Study 7.1 describes the consequences of a therapist's failure to safeguard confidentiality.

Vignette 7.1. Maintaining Confidentiality in Testimony

Jansen provided occupational therapy services to **Marcus** as part of a work rehabilitation program following a back injury. Jansen was subpoenaed to testify on behalf of Marcus's employer about his recovery and fitness to return to work. He was careful to ensure compliance with HIPAA regulations as well as Principle 3 and RSCs 3H and 5C of the Code. In fact, RSC 3H specifically addresses confidentiality and the person's right to privacy, and it underscores the importance of adhering to laws and regulations. Moreover, RSC 5C reminds occupational therapy practitioners that privacy and confidentiality laws and regulations require the practitioner to remain current regarding changes to laws, policies, and procedures governing practice; failure to keep up to date can result in a violation of ethical principles and established laws. Jansen ensured the confidential information Marcus had shared with him that was unrelated to his care was not a part of the medical record he provided or discussed.

Case Study 7.1. Addressing Inadvertent Violation of Confidentiality

Natasha, a licensed occupational therapist, worked in a behavioral health hospital. She had 15 years of experience and was passionate about her work and occupational therapy's role in mental health. Natasha and her friend **Claudia** went out to dinner at a local restaurant after a particularly long and stressful day for Natasha. As she and Claudia unwound over a pre-dinner drink, Natasha began describing her day to Claudia. She talked about the repeated absence of one of the occupational therapists and having to cover his caseload as well as her own and offer supervision to a student, **Erin,** in her third week of Level II fieldwork. Natasha shared that she had had to attend 2 case conferences, run 3 groups by herself that were usually co-led with the absent therapist, complete an evaluation on a new client, and meet with Erin to discuss some behavioral issues she had observed on the unit and in group that day.

Natasha was feeling better when her second drink and dinner arrived. They returned to casual conversation during dinner, and while Claudia was having dessert, Natasha was having her third drink. Toward the end of dessert, Natasha began to discuss work again. She was a good storyteller,

(Continued)

Case Study 7.1. Addressing Inadvertent Violation of Confidentiality *(Cont.)*

and Claudia found her reports of work events to be entertaining. Natasha told her about a client, **Latoya,** whom she had evaluated after being admitted following a suicide attempt. Latoya had some standing in the community as a volunteer and advocate. Natasha relayed the efforts that were taken to keep the client safe on the unit and in the hospital. She also told Claudia in some detail what Latoya had reported to her were the stressors that prompted her admission.

Unknown to Natasha, the parents of the fieldwork student, Erin, were sitting behind Natasha and Claudia and overheard the entire conversation. When Erin's parents returned home, they repeated the conversation to Erin. Erin was distressed to learn that her supervisor had breached hospital policies, HIPAA, and Principle 3 of the Code by discussing confidential client information in a public place. She wondered what course of action she should take. Should she do nothing? This situation involved her supervisor, who had significant influence over her future as an occupational therapy practitioner. Should she present the information she had learned directly to her supervisor or to the department director? Finally, should she report Natasha's alcohol use? Erin had previously noted on a few occasions that Natasha had returned from lunch smelling of alcohol. Table 7.1 reviews some of the courses of action available to Natasha and their consequences.

Erin's review of the Code identified several RSCs that might have been breached or were at risk of being breached through Natasha's behaviors. In addition to RSC 3H (maintain confidentiality in compliance with HIPPA and other laws), she realized, her actions also depended on her and Natasha's obligations under

- RSC 2A (avoid inflicting harm on clients),
- RSC 2C (take action to remedy personal problems that might cause harm),

Table 7.1. Decision Table for Case Study 7.1

Possible Action	Positive Outcomes	Negative Consequences
Take no action.	Erin would avoid dealing with an uncomfortable situation.	Erin's silence would violate RSC 2E. Natasha's behaviors would likely continue and endanger others.
Present information to the academic fieldwork advisor.	Natasha's understanding of her obligations under RSC 3H would increase. Erin would be compliant with the Code.	Erin would feel vulnerable. Natasha would be unaware of the concerns about alcohol use and potential harm to patients (RSCs 2A, 2C, 2D, 2F).
Present information to the department director.	The director has responsibility to patients, the hospital, Natasha, and the profession. The director would fulfill RSC 2C by taking action to confront the situations revealed to her and avoid harm (RSC 2A). The director would review legal and ethical responsibilities with Natasha (RSC 4E).	None. Erin would behave in a professional and ethical way.
Support Natasha's decision to enter treatment to help her control her alcohol use.	Erin would fulfill RSC 6L. Natasha would comply with a remediation plan developed in collaboration with the department director, which would help her integrate RSCs 4K, 6A, and 6B.	Erin's inaction could result in job loss and disciplinary actions from the licensure board, the hospital, and AOTA's EC. Natasha might increase her criticism of Erin on her performance evaluation as retribution.

Note. AOTA = American Occupational Therapy Association; EC = Ethics Commission; RSC = Related Standard of Conduct.

Case Study 7.1. Addressing Inadvertent Violation of Confidentiality *(Cont.)*

- RSC 2D (avoid undue influences),
- RSC 2E (address impaired practice and report to the authorities when necessary),
- RSC 4K (report breaches in practice, education, or research), and
- RSC 6L ("refrain from any actions that reduce the public's trust in occupational therapy;" AOTA, 2015b, p. 7).

In addition, Erin reflected on the potential impacts of her action or inaction. She identified three RSCs—4E (be aware of laws and the profession's official documents that guide practice), 4K (report unethical acts to the appropriate authorities), and 6A (respect private information about colleagues)—that specifically relate to her decision making.

Erin decided that keeping this information to herself would potentially do more harm than good. She understood that, under optimal circumstances, it is best to discuss ethical dilemmas directly with the person involved. As a student, however, Erin felt she was not on sufficiently equal ground to do this, so she decided to have a confidential conversation with her faculty fieldwork advisor. She hoped that they would present the situation to the department director together and, if the director believed it would be helpful, then both Erin and her faculty advisor would meet with Erin's clinical fieldwork supervisor. Erin was confident that she was addressing this sensitive situation in the most ethical way possible.

Communication

Communication is a dialogue (written, spoken, electronic, nonverbal) that exchanges ideas between the occupational therapy practitioner and client, student, or community. Client-centered care must be based on the needs and preferences expressed by the client, whether the client is an individual (e.g., patient, research participant, or student) or community. The Code's RSCs 3A, 3C, 3E, 3G, 3H, 3J, 5I, and 6A specifically address the importance of clear communication between occupational therapy practitioners and others.

RSC 3A specifies occupational therapy practitioners' responsibility to "respect and honor the expressed wishes of recipients of service (AOTA, 2015b, p. 3)." In addition, RSCs 3C and 3E address the need to obtain client consent from individuals who receive occupational therapy services and from research participants, and individuals' right to refuse services. Moreover, RSC 3G reminds occupational therapy practitioners to respect a research participant's ability to withdraw from a study without consequence, and RSC 3H establishes the responsibility to keep all forms of communication compliant with applicable laws. As noted by the U.S. Department of Health and Human Services (n.d.),

> Effective health communication is as important to health care as clinical skill. To improve individual health and build healthy communities, health care providers need to recognize and address the unique culture, language and health literacy of diverse consumers and communities. (para. 1)

Whether presenting the information verbally, in writing, or electronically, practitioners have an obligation to provide information that is clear and at a level of linguistic intelligibility that recipients can understand (RSC 3J). Schwab (2006) noted "obstacles to good decision making by patients are a serious concern in health care," and cited lack of information as one of those obstacles (p. 575). Ethical practitioners need to be vigilant for other obstacles to effective communication, especially those under their control.

Personal biases of the health care provider, time constraints for making decisions, and other barriers may influence communication in ways that limit the client's decision-making processes. It is important to take time for self-reflection to separate one's personal values from clients' wishes. Ethical practitioners must be client advocates and take the necessary steps to ensure the clients' understanding of presented information. Software programs can help analyze the reading levels of written materials. In addition, real-time, in-person, or telephonic translation programs are available that can help to bridge language barriers.

Occupational therapy practitioners need to ensure that communication with clients and their families is complete and thorough, which means ensuring that clients have an accurate understanding of data and research outcomes to avoid confusion and harm. For example, when discussing the possible use of constraint-induced therapy with a stroke survivor, the practitioner should describe the evidence available for both this approach and the other interventions used in stroke recovery.

Likewise, practitioners' communication with parents who request sensory integration as the primary intervention for their child on the basis of stories they read on an online autism chat room also should draw on evidence-based reviews of sensory interventions with this population.

Communication style (e.g., tone, pace, gearing the message to the listener's language and educational level) influences how the client and family make decisions about the client's care, so occupational therapy practitioners have a responsibility to communicate recommendations to clients in a fair and unbiased way—for example, by providing clients with a review of the literature on the effectiveness of the range of available interventions. Communicating in a culturally appropriate way is exemplified in Case Study 7.2.

Terrance thus developed a plan that he thought was viable and ethically grounded that would help him continue to expand his cultural competence

Case Study 7.2. Exploring Health Communication Across Cultures

Terrance was an occupational therapist working with Hispanic clients with psychiatric disorders in a prevocational program. When he first began work with this population, he recognized that if he wanted to engage in client-centered, community-based practices, he would need to understand the issues unique to people in the Hispanic community. The first and most obvious issue was communication. Terrance needed to decide whether he would rely on an interpreter, learn the Spanish language, or use a combination of approaches. He ultimately used a combination of approaches depending on the situation and his increasing level of Spanish proficiency.

After 5 years of practice in this area, Terrance was ready for a new experience. He had learned much about himself and the issues that occupational therapy practitioners and other service providers face when working with the cultural issues embedded in the Hispanic community. He believed that he had developed the sensitivity to expand his interventions to immigrant populations with even greater cultural diversity.

To improve his confidence, Terrance decided to review the available literature on communication and cultural competence. He discovered the work of Wells, Black, and Gupta (2016) in *Culture and Occupation: Effectiveness for Occupational Therapy Practice, Education, and Research,* which explored concepts of cultural competence in depth. This work expanded Terrance's understanding of the importance of good communication and cultural effectiveness.

In addition, several chapters in *Occupational Therapy Without Borders: Learning from the Spirit of Survivors* (Kronenberg, Algado, & Pollard, 2005) expanded his understanding of how communication influences the therapeutic process and were helpful to his journey. For example, Kronenberg and Pollard (2005) note that language gaps and barriers make it difficult to fully understand a person's needs in his or her cultural context and that family members should not be relied on to serve as translators because they may not accurately transmit the client's needs and desires, potentially leading to failed interventions. Thibeault (2005) observed that "occupational therapy is best practiced in a context where specific cultural environments are understood and respected, even if this translates into service delivery that is almost entirely defined and controlled by local stakeholders" (p. 236).

Terrance also discovered a book—*Race, Culture, and Disability* (Balcazar, Suarez-Balcazar, Taylor-Ritzler, & Keys, 2010)—that he found

(Continued)

Case Study 7.2. Exploring Health Communication Across Cultures *(Cont.)*

helpful in making a connection between people with multicultural backgrounds and respecting their needs for autonomy and confidentiality. He located a program in his community that provided transition, counseling, and support services to immigrants, refugees, asylees, and other foreign-born people, some of whom had persistent mental illnesses (FIRN, n.d.). Terrance also learned from Cook, Razzano, and Jonikas (2010) that "different cultures have different likelihoods of help-seeking for mental illness and these may influence ways in which programs and providers handle engagement and the forging of effective therapeutic relationships" (p. 120).

Per RSCs 2J and 3J of the Code, occupational therapy practitioners need to appreciate cultures and gain cultural competence. Occupational therapy practitioners can assist individuals in need of services to facilitate access directly or through referrals in compliance with RSCs 4B and 4C. Terrance understood that he and others have a responsibility to advocate for systematic changes that enable underserved and culturally diverse populations to gain the opportunity to receive occupational therapy (RSC 4D). Terrance was confident that, after taking these steps, he would be better equipped to provide competent and ethical occupational therapy services that recognized each person's right to autonomy and confidentiality. He also recognized that to serve these communities well and ensure his credibility, he must strictly adhere to Principle 3, Autonomy, when visiting or working in community programs.

Cultural competence is particularly important to professionals serving diverse communities of people with psychiatric disorders. Terrance found through his reading of Cook et al. (2010) that methods of identifying and intervening with people with psychiatric disorders vary across cultures, necessitating education of professionals in the belief systems of the people and families served. He also learned that, to expand his practice to work with diverse populations, he needed to network with multicultural groups and organizations like the one he found in his community and gain additional knowledge and credibility. This learning needed to be a two-way street: Terrance also had to have something to offer the communities he was learning from. Finally, he reached out to AOTA's Multicultural Networking Groups (AOTA, 2015a) to learn more about cultural diversity from an occupational therapy perspective.

through reading, networking, and volunteering with diverse individuals and organizations in and around his community and through developing relationships with Multicultural Networking Groups. In this way, he was able to increase his understanding of cultural differences and occupational therapy interventions in community-based settings. A further discussion of the importance of cultural competence is presented in Chapter 21, "Ethics and Culture."

Communication that has sometimes been neglected is presented in the Code in RSC 5I, which focuses on students' unobstructed access to the educational requirements in college and university policies and procedures. In addition, RSC 6A advises protecting information about students, employees, and colleagues while maintaining compliance with current laws.

Consent

Consent means "assent or approval" (Merriam-Webster, 2011, para. 1). Occupational therapy practitioners have an ethical obligation to obtain consent from clients or their representatives before initiating an evaluation or intervention, enrolling in research, or making information about their care available to third parties. Local, state, and federal regulations, and institutional policies governing these activities, reinforce this ethical obligation. Supporting the client's wishes, sometimes over the preferences of family members, is of prime importance as long as the client's safety and well-being are not in jeopardy. Vignette 7.2 describes an occupational therapist's efforts to obtain parents' consent

Vignette 7.2. Obtaining Consent for Consultation

Elliott, an occupational therapist, was asked by the middle school where he delivered occupational therapy services to make recommendations for **Tara's** 504 plan (Section 504 of the Rehabilitation Act of 1973 ensures that schools provide students who have disabilities with reasonable accommodations to access educational materials; U.S. Department of Education, 2015). Although Elliott had worked in school-based practice for 4 years, he was unfamiliar with how to contribute to a 504 plan for a student with developmental coordination disorder (DCD). Elliott reviewed the student's record carefully and obtained brief information from team members, including Tara's parents. He continued to be unsure about assessing Tara's needs and making useful recommendations.

Elliott reviewed textbooks, read journal articles, and attended a webinar on DCD. In addition, he had general discussions with colleagues working with children and youth in other settings. He continued to believe that he needed more information to be helpful. Elliott consulted the Code, reading RSC 1E that reminds occupational therapy practitioners to have competence in the services they deliver. He also noted in 3D his obligation to keep the team, including Tara's parents, informed about his efforts and to obtain the parents' consent before discussing Tara's specific needs with another occupational therapy practitioner who had expertise in recommending assistive technology for students with DCD. Elliott knew this step was important in respecting Tara's and her family's confidentiality, which is supported by RSC 3H. All of these efforts demonstrated Elliott's clinical reasoning processes, which were consistent with the guidance provided in the *Occupational Therapy Practice Framework: Domain and Process* (AOTA, 2014).

to discuss their child's occupational therapy priorities with his professional colleagues in order to meet the child's accessibility needs.

A corollary of the practitioner's obligation to obtain consent is the client's right to refuse intervention. Clients and research participants have the right to refuse an intervention or withdraw from research studies, as supported by RSCs 3E and 3G. Although occupational therapy clients have the right to refuse an intervention (e.g., by informing the practitioner that they do not want to participate in occupational therapy for that session or day), the practitioner's ethical obligation to respect the clients' wishes does not preclude encouraging clients to participate in therapy as a way to achieve their established goals. Likewise, a practitioner should not attempt to restrain a client from leaving a session unless his or her departure could potentially harm the client or others or is against hospital or agency policies.

Clients who freely consent to participate in a research study (RSC 3G) may decide during the course of the study that they wish to withdraw. They may feel, for example, that participation requires too much time, that the benefit is not worth the risk, or simply that the process is boring. Although withdrawal from a research study may make life more complicated for the researcher, it is the participant's right to withdraw at any time for any reason.

Collaboration

Occupational therapy practice emphasizes collaboration between the occupational therapy practitioner and the client (AOTA, 2014, 2015b). This partnership can extend to the immediate family, significant others, caregivers, or agencies as designated by the client or the law. AOTA (2014) presents this ***collaboration*** as a dynamic process between the occupational therapy practitioner and client: "Occupational therapy practitioners develop a collaborative relationship with clients in order to understand their experiences and desires for intervention" (p. S12).

The Code's RSC 3D obligates occupational therapy practitioners to establish collaborative relationships with clients and, as appropriate, their families, significant others, and caregivers. Before collaborating on setting goals and priorities, practitioners need to make sure they fully inform the client and designated others about the purpose of the intervention; benefits, risks, and potential outcomes, as well as any reasonable alternatives; the personnel who will provide the intervention; and time frames for goal attainment (RSC 3B). Vignette 7.3 describes an occupational therapy practitioner's efforts to involve the client and her family in learning about what the fall prevention assessment and intervention process has to offer and their available options.

Vignette 7.3. Balancing Autonomy and Collaboration

Clinton, an occupational therapist in private practice, had an exhibit at a senior expo in his county. He presented a poster and information focused on fall prevention and provided a screening tool for expo participants. **Felicia** was one of the older adults who visited Clinton's booth.

Felicia told Clinton that she'd had a recent fall that had shaken her confidence even though she wasn't seriously injured. She had reluctantly told her son and daughter-in-law about the incident, and she reported that they were now feeling very protective of her, even suggesting that she move in with them or to assisted living. Felicia asked Clinton whether there was anything among his materials or in his practice experience that might help her. Clinton gave Felicia some fall prevention materials and links to evidence-based Web sites with additional information. He also told Felicia that most falls occur within the home and that sometimes an environmental assessment can identify human and environmental factors that contribute to falls. Felicia was excited to hear about this and wanted Clinton to come to her home the next day.

Clinton suggested that Felicia review the materials he had provided her and share this information with her son and daughter-in-law. He said that if, after reviewing this material, she still wanted him to conduct a home visit and environmental assessment, he would be pleased to work with her. Felicia called Clinton a few days later to say that she had discussed their conversation with her son and daughter-in-law and that they all agreed to move forward with the home visit.

Clinton's approach to work with Felicia respected her autonomy by establishing a collaborative relationship (RSC 3D) and explaining possible interventions (RSC 3B), and by obtaining her consent regarding the proposed assessment (RSC 3C). She was also apprised of her option to share information with family members (RSC 3D). Clinton was pleased that Felicia had discussed fall prevention and an environmental assessment with her family; he had suggested having this discussion to encourage their collaboration and support for this potential process. Clinton also suggested that Felicia invite her son and daughter-in-law to their session, if Felicia wished, so they could learn more about the assessment process and what he might propose in terms of Felicia's safety and ability to age in place.

Summary

Adherence to Principle 3, Autonomy, of the Code helps occupational therapy practitioners ensure the services they provide are client centered and interactions with clients are clear, without bias, and allow the exercise of personal freedoms. Respect for the autonomy and confidentiality of both individual and collective clients is necessary to establish a sense of partnership, honesty, and understanding in occupational therapy practice.

Reflective Questions

1. **Alicia** is majoring in occupational therapy. She received services and supports through campus Disability Student Services as she self-identified as a person on the autism spectrum. Alicia is doing her first internship in behavioral health. Now at the 3-week mark, she is beginning to display greater difficulty when communicating with clients; staff; and her clinical supervisor, **Frank.** Alicia's need for supervision, direction, and emotional support had not lessened and Frank is becoming concerned. He shares his concerns with Alicia, who became quieter and more anxious as a result of this supervision session. Frank decides to contact Alicia's fieldwork educator, **Denise,** express his concerns, and ask for guidance. Alicia had informed Denise about her disability, but she had not told Frank, afraid that the information might bias him and her student experience. Denise wants Alicia to succeed and believes that information about Alicia's disability might help Frank in his role as supervisor. Use the Decision Table, found in Appendix G, to
   - Determine at least 3 possible courses of action Denise could take, including their positive outcomes and negative consequences.
   - Identify relevant RSCs from Principle 3, Autonomy, to support your identified positive outcomes and negative consequences.
2. **Sam** is an occupational therapist on contract to provide services primarily to middle school students. He encounters challenges meeting with teachers, scheduling students, and meeting the goals and objectives for students with individualized education plans in his contractual role. Review Principle 3, and select the primary RSCs that apply to Sam's situation.

References

American Occupational Therapy Association. (2014). Occupational therapy practice framework: Domain and process (3rd ed.). *American Journal of Occupational Therapy, 68*(6 Suppl. 1, S1–S48). https://doi.org/10.5014/ajot.2014.682006

American Occupational Therapy Association. (2015a). *Multicultural networking groups.* Retrieved from http://www.aota.org/practice/manage/multicultural/groups.aspx

American Occupational Therapy Association. (2015b). Occupational therapy code of ethics (2015). *American Journal of Occupational Therapy, 69*(Suppl. 3), 6912310030. https://doi.org/10.5014/ajot.2015.696S03

Balcazar, F. E., Suarez-Balcazar, Y., Taylor-Ritzler, T., & Keys, C. B. (Eds.). (2010). *Race, culture, and disability: Rehabilitation science and practice.* Sudbury, MA: Jones & Bartlett.

Beauchamp, T. L., & Childress, J. F. (2013). *Principles of biomedical ethics* (7th ed.). New York: Oxford University Press.

Cook, J. A., Razzano, L. A., & Jonikas, J. A. (2010). Cultural diversity and how it may differ for programs and providers serving people with psychiatric disabilities. In F. E. Balcazar, Y. Suarez-Balcazar, T. Taylor-Ritzler, & C. B. Keys (Eds.), *Race, culture and disability: Rehabilitation science and practice* (pp. 115–135). Sudbury, MA: Jones & Bartlett.

Family Educational Rights and Privacy Act of 1974, Pub. L. 93–380, 20 U.S.C. 1232g.

FIRN. (n.d.) *What is FIRN?* Retrieved from http://www.firnonline.org/?page_id=4

Fremgen, B. F. (2012). *Medical law and ethics* (5th ed.). Upper Saddle River, NJ: Pearson Education.

Health Insurance Portability and Accountability Act of 1996, Pub. L. 104–191, 110 Stat. 1936.

Kronenberg, F., Algado, S. S., & Pollard, N. (Eds.). (2005). *Occupational therapy without borders: Learning from the spirit of survivors.* Philadelphia: Elsevier.

Kronenberg, F., & Pollard, N. (2005). Overcoming occupational apartheid: A preliminary exploration of the political nature of occupational therapy. In F. Kronenberg, S. S. Algado, & N. Pollard (Eds.), *Occupational therapy without borders: Learning from the spirit of survivors* (pp. 158–186). Philadelphia: Elsevier.

Merriam-Webster. (2011). *Consent.* Retrieved from http://www.merriam-webster.com/dictionary/consent

Patient Protection and Affordable Care Act, Pub. L. 111–148, § 3502, 124 Stat. 119, 124 (2010).

Rehabilitation Act of 1973, Pub. L. 93–112, 29 U.S.C. § 701 *et seq.*

Schwab, A. P. (2006). Formal and effective autonomy in healthcare. *Journal of Medical Ethics,* 575–579. https://doi.org/10.1136/jme.2005.013391

Taylor, R. L. (2008). *The intentional relationship: Occupational therapy and use of self.* Philadelphia: F. A. Davis.

Thibeault, R. (2005). Connecting health and social justice: A Lebanese experience. In F. Kronenberg, S. S. Algado, & N. Pollard (Eds.), *Occupational therapy without borders: Learning from the spirit of survivors* (pp. 232–244). Philadelphia: Elsevier.

U.S. Department of Education. (2015). *Protecting students with disabilities.* Retrieved from http://www2.ed.gov/about/offices/list/ocr/504faq.html

U.S. Department of Health and Human Services. (n.d.). *Culture, language and health literacy.* Retrieved from http://www.hrsa.gov/culturalcompetence/index.html

Wells, S. A., Black, R. M., & Gupta, J. (Eds.). (2016). *Culture and occupation: Effectiveness for occupational therapy practice, education, and research* (3rd ed.). Bethesda, MD: AOTA Press.

Chapter 8.

PRINCIPLE 4: JUSTICE

Janie B. Scott, MA, OT/L, FAOTA; S. Maggie Reitz, PhD, OTR/L, FAOTA; and Stacey Harcum, MS, OTR/L, CBIS

Learning Objectives

By the end of the chapter, readers will be able to

- Describe how the Principle of Justice relates to occupational therapy practice;
- Analyze the relationship of regulations to ethical practice; and
- Apply the Related Standards of Conduct for Principle 4, Justice, to decisions that occupational therapy practitioners should make to protect clients and the profession.

Key Terms and Concepts

- ✧ Advocacy
- ✧ Competency
- ✧ Compliance
- ✧ Duty
- ✧ Health disparities
- ✧ Injustice
- ✧ Justice
- ✧ Occupational justice
- ✧ Procedural justice
- ✧ Professional boundaries
- ✧ Regulatory body or agency
- ✧ Reimbursement
- ✧ Reprimand
- ✧ Social justice
- ✧ Supervision
- ✧ Transparency

Justice

Principle 4. Occupational therapy personnel shall promote fairness and objectivity in the provision of occupational therapy services.

The Principle of Justice relates to the fair, equitable, and appropriate treatment of persons (Beauchamp & Childress, 2013). Occupational therapy personnel should relate in a respectful, fair, and impartial manner to individuals and groups with whom they interact. They should also respect the applicable laws and standards related to their area of practice. Justice requires the impartial consideration and consistent following of rules to generate unbiased decisions and promote fairness. As occupational therapy personnel, we work to uphold a society in which all individuals have an equitable opportunity to achieve occupational engagement as an essential component of life.

Related Standards of Conduct

Occupational Therapy Personnel Shall

A. Respond to requests for occupational therapy services (e.g., referral) in a timely manner as determined by law, regulation, or policy.
B. Assist those in need of occupational therapy services in securing access through available means.
C. Address barriers in access to occupational therapy services by offering or referring clients to financial aid, charity care, or *pro bono* services within the parameters of organizational policies.
D. Advocate for changes to systems and policies that are discriminatory or unfairly limit or prevent access to occupational therapy services.
E. Maintain awareness of current laws and AOTA policies and Official Documents that apply to the profession of occupational therapy.
F. Inform employers, employees, colleagues, students, and researchers of applicable policies, laws, and Official Documents.
G. Hold requisite credentials for the occupational therapy services they provide in academic, research, physical, or virtual work settings.
H. Provide appropriate supervision in accordance with AOTA Official Documents and relevant laws, regulations, policies, procedures, standards, and guidelines.
I. Obtain all necessary approvals prior to initiating research activities.
J. Refrain from accepting gifts that would unduly influence the therapeutic relationship or have the potential to blur professional boundaries, and adhere to employer policies when offered gifts.
K. Report to appropriate authorities any acts in practice, education, and research that are unethical or illegal.
L. Collaborate with employers to formulate policies and procedures in compliance with legal, regulatory, and ethical standards and work to resolve any conflicts or inconsistencies.
M. Bill and collect fees legally and justly in a manner that is fair, reasonable, and commensurate with services delivered.
N. Ensure compliance with relevant laws, and promote transparency, when participating in a business arrangement as owner, stockholder, partner, or employee.
O. Ensure that documentation for reimbursement purposes is done in accordance with applicable laws, guidelines, and regulations.
P. Refrain from participating in any action resulting in unauthorized access to educational content or exams (including but not limited to sharing test questions, unauthorized use of or access to content or codes, or selling access or authorization codes).

Source. From the *Occupational Therapy Code of Ethics (2015)* (American Occupational Therapy Association, 2015b, pp. 5–6).

Principle 4 of the *Occupational Therapy Code of Ethics (2015)* (American Occupational Therapy Association [AOTA], 2015b)—referred to as the "Code" hereinafter—focuses on ***justice.*** This chapter addresses obligations that govern the practice of occupational therapy as directed by the Principle of Justice. These obligations have been grouped into the following five categories: (1) promoting access to services (RSCs 4A–4D), (2) fulfilling credentialing and supervisory duties according to regulations (RSCs 4G, 4H, 4L), (3) maintaining current knowledge of regulations and official AOTA documents and informing others about these materials (RSCs 4E, 4F, 4N, 4O, 4P), (4) developing and adhering to institutional policies and procedures to ensure ethical practice (RSCs 4D, 4I, 4K, 4L, 4N), and (5) ensuring that financial and business relationships abide by the regulations (RSCs 4J, 4K, 4M, 4N, 4O). These categories facilitate the exploration of how the Principle of Justice relates to all occupational therapy practice.

Types of Justice

Social justice "includes ethical concepts related to fair opportunity, unfair discrimination, and whether there is a right to healthcare, as well as appropriate criteria for rationing care when there are limits to availability" (Ashe, 2016, p. 235). ***Procedural justice*** is ensuring that policies and laws are implemented, adhered to, and enforced in a fair and equitable manner (Maiese, 2004). (To review why and when procedural and social justice were merged, please see Chapter 3, "Promoting Ethics in Occupational Therapy Practice: Codes and Consequences.")

The other five Principles of the Code all relate in some way to promoting procedural and social justice and, at times, occupational justice. ***Occupational justice*** reflects the desire for full inclusion in everyday meaningful activities for individuals, groups, or communities regardless of age, sex, gender identity, race, socioeconomic status, or degree of ability (Nilsson & Townsend, 2010; Townsend, 2012; Townsend & Wilcock, 2004). Related Standard of Conduct (RSC) 1A states, "provide appropriate evaluation and a plan of intervention for recipients of occupational therapy services specific to their needs" (AOTA, 2015b, p. 2). This obliges occupational therapy practitioners to customize services to meet clients' needs, which also can address occupational justice when the client is a community and the services assist with building a capacity for increased participation in or access to occupations. Such services could take the form of facilitating engagement in occupations previously denied to members of a community or supporting the development of policies that enable the return of freedoms forcibly removed such as the ability to engage in roles, routines, habits, or rituals as a community (AOTA, 2014b).

Principle 4 also details the responsibility to provide access to occupational therapy services; resolve conflicts; follow institutional rules; comply with local, state, federal, and international laws (referred to collectively throughout this chapter as "regulations"); and refer to AOTA's applicable documents. More specifically, to meet the ethical obligation of justice, occupational therapy practitioners are required to

- Provide timely service;
- Advocate for access;
- Maintain knowledge of regulations and AOTA official documents;
- Obtain and maintain credentialing;
- Comply with relevant laws, standards, policies, and procedures;
- Abide by requirements established by third-party payers;
- Refrain from cheating in any form; and
- Meet specific expectations related to ethical conduct as established by AOTA, the National Board for Certification in Occupational Therapy (NBCOT), and state regulatory boards (SRBs).

Access

The first four RSCs address access to services, and one, RSC 4A, specifically focuses on the timeliness of service delivery, which is the topic of Vignette 8.1. Promoting access to services is consistent with the occupational therapy profession's roots in social activism. These RSCs encourage occupational therapy practitioners to continue the commitment of the profession to those who need our services regardless of personal attributes or ability to pay. Case Study 8.1 explores how discrimination affects access to services.

Credentialing and Supervisory Duties

Occupational therapy practitioners are obligated to have the appropriate credentials to practice in a particular state or jurisdiction and to keep these credentials current (RSC 4G). For example, practitioners are responsible for notifying the SRB

Vignette 8.1. Timely Response to Request for Services

Sergei manages and works as an occupational therapist in an outpatient hand therapy clinic. About a year ago, the clinic began a marketing campaign targeting postsurgical patients from several local hospitals to boost referrals. The campaign was a huge success, and the clinic was now the number one outpatient provider for several local surgeons. The clinic worked hard to build a relationship with these physicians in order to ensure quality services and continuity of care.

Within the past month, 1 of the clinic's 4 certified hand therapists resigned unexpectedly and a second went out on maternity leave. Subsequently, the wait for an initial evaluation has skyrocketed to over 2 months. Sergei knows that the postsurgical patients should not wait 2 months to be seen based on their physicians' protocols, but he doesn't want the clinic to lose out on the potential ***reimbursement*** (fees or other remuneration collected in exchange for clinical services) they had marketed for just because they are a bit short-staffed at the moment. Other than RSC 4A, what other Principles and RSCs would guide Sergei's action? An AOTA advisory opinion by Ashe (2016) is an additional resource to help explore other potential actions for Sergei.

when they change their residence. In addition, occupational therapy practitioners have the duty to verify the backgrounds, skill sets, and expertise of those they supervise (Reed, Ashe, & Slater, 2009). In providing adequate ***supervision*** (i.e., observation, monitoring, and oversight for students or practitioners in accordance with legal standards), practitioners both adhere to regulations (RSC 4H) and fulfill the public trust (RSC 6L). In addition, many third-party payers have rules regarding not only what services they reimburse but also whom they consider as qualified to provide those services and with what level of supervision (RSC 4M). Case Studies 8.2 and 8.3 and Vignette 8.2 describe how failure to meet supervision responsibilities can affect clients, employers and institutions, students, and the profession.

Knowledge of Regulations and AOTA Official Documents

Principle 4 of the Code obligates occupational therapy practitioners not only to maintain current knowledge regarding regulations governing occupational therapy practice but also to inform employers and occupational therapy employees, students, and others about those regulations and any changes to them. To meet this obligation, occupational therapy practitioners must continually update their knowledge about the regulations that pertain to practice. Occupational therapy practitioners also are advised, whether they are AOTA members or not, to stay current with AOTA official documents that address their practice area and responsibilities. In Vignette 8.3, an occupational therapist and occupational therapy assistant inform a supervisor about the regulations regarding the supervision of an occupational therapy assistant.

Develop and Adhere to Institutional Policies

The Principle of Justice emphasizes the duty of occupational therapy practitioners to comply with the documentation requirements of third-party payers and their employers' institutional policies. Occupational therapy documentation should accurately reflect the services delivered and their outcomes and should be of the kind and quality that satisfy the scrutiny of peer reviews, legal proceedings, and accrediting agencies. Inaccurate documentation is a violation of the Code, which states that occupational therapy practitioners should not use any form of communication that is false, fraudulent, or deceptive (RSC 5B). Vignette 8.4 describes an occupational therapist's efforts to inform herself and her supervisor about regulations regarding documentation. Vignette 8.5 involves collaboration to cheat.

Financial and Business Relationships

Financial accountability extends to all work roles and contexts involving the delivery of occupational

Case Study 8.1. Fairness and Advocacy for Ethical Care

Dante, an occupational therapist, was the director of an acute inpatient rehabilitation unit in a large rural hospital. A physician admitted a young man named **Andrew** for an anticipated 3-week stay for occupational therapy and physical therapy services after a high-speed car crash. Andrew had sustained poly-traumatic injuries, including a moderate traumatic brain injury, multiple fractures, and some mild burns.

Sally was the occupational therapist assigned to complete Andrew's initial evaluation. On beginning the activities of daily living part of her evaluation, Sally realized that Andrew was a transgender person who identified as male. Unsure of how to proceed, Sally shared Andrew's gender identity with the rest of the rehabilitation team, and his identity became a topic of much discussion. The issue was brought to Dante's attention by a nurse on the unit who was aware of the ***health disparities*** (i.e., discrepancy or imbalance in health care and wellness based on access, availability, or client factors) associated with being transgender and worried about the quality of Andrew's care.

Concerned about potential ***injustice*** (i.e., the application of that which is prejudicial, unfair, or discriminatory), Dante began to investigate the situation immediately. On reviewing the medical record, Dante found that documentation in the medical record fluctuated between referring to Andrew as "he" or "she" and often made reference to his gender identity, even when it was not relevant in the context of the note. In discussing the matter with his staff, he received reports that some members of the team were very curious and had asked Andrew questions about his gender unrelated to his medical care, while other staff had become wary of interacting with Andrew at all. Sally, the occupational therapist, also shared with Dante that Andrew's mother was openly unsupportive of his transgender status and even requested that Sally call Andrew by his female birth name and train him to dress in the women's clothes she had brought in. Andrew had cried and argued with her about this, but due to his cognitive deficits he was not yet deemed to have decision-making capacity by his attending physician; his mother was his surrogate decision maker.

Dante demonstrated ***advocacy*** (i.e., promotion of or support for a client, program, or policy) for Andrew by elevating these complex issues to his supervisor, the hospital's vice president of clinical services. They jointly agreed on three actions. First, the supervisor suggested that Dante contact Human Resources, which had excellent staff who could provide the rehabilitation team with in-service training regarding cultural competency, patient privacy, and patients' rights. Second, they replaced Andrew's primary treatment team with staff that had a history of a high level of cultural competence and professionalism to ensure that Andrew would receive superior quality of care and allow them time to remediate or discipline other staff as appropriate. Third, they engaged the hospital's ethics and risk management teams to address the issue of Andrew's capacity and future as a decision maker for his care.

therapy services. This obligation exists for practitioners in clinics, long-term care facilities, independent practice, and any other setting in which monetary compensation is involved. There is a strong correlation between the Principles of Justice and Veracity. Both Principles embody the expectation that occupational therapy practitioners will follow established policies and procedures to accurately document and bill.

Many occupational therapy practitioners with an entrepreneurial spirit establish a private practice based on their expertise, often with children and youth, injured workers, or older adults who wish to age in place. Other practitioners are employed part-time and contractually across practice areas (AOTA, 2015c; Bureau of Labor Statistics, U.S. Department of Labor, 2015; Herz, Bondoc, Richmond, Richman, & Kroll, 2005). RSC 4N guides private

Case Study 8.2. Addressing Failure to Maintain Credentials

Mary Jo had been an occupational therapist for 3 1/2 years when she took maternity leave. Soon after the baby was born, she notified her employer that she would not be returning to her previous position in the near future. When the baby was age 6 months, Mary Jo and her new family moved to a larger home. Later that year, she applied for a new position with her previous employer and returned to work.

She had been back to work for almost a year when the time came for her annual performance review. Mary Jo had to provide evidence of her continuing education activities, a list of goals and accomplishments, and a copy of her current license to her supervisor, **Bill.** As Mary Jo and Bill reviewed her performance and related documentation covering the past year, they noticed that Mary Jo's license to practice occupational therapy had expired a year and a half ago and that she had been practicing with a lapsed license. Mary Jo realized that, in the chaos of caring for a young child and moving, she had neglected to inform her state ***regulatory body or agency*** (i.e., an organization established to govern, maintain standards, or legally circumscribe practice) about her change of address and consequently did not receive her license renewal notice. Although Mary Jo had renewed her membership in AOTA, her membership in the state occupational therapy association had lapsed, and she missed the notices this organization also had provided about licensure renewal.

An analysis of the consequences, potential actions, and outcomes of Mary Jo's failure to maintain her credentials is summarized in Table 8.1. Can you identify other potential actions?

Mary Jo and Bill were aware that occupational therapy practitioners are required to adhere to all state and national rules governing practice, including the principles of ethical practice. Mary Jo had a ***duty*** (i.e., ethical or legal accountability) to practice occupational therapy in full ***compliance*** (i.e., meeting all legal and regulatory standards for occupational therapy practice and licensure) with her licensure law, which included language from the Code regarding ethical conduct. In addition, as an AOTA member, she had the duty to uphold the Principles articulated in the Code. Mary Jo was in violation of RSCs 4G, 5A (represent credentials accurately), and 5B (refrain from making false claims).

Although Mary Jo's actions were not intentional, her neglect had serious consequences. Mary Jo's employer had billed Medicare and other third-party payers for services she had provided that required occupational therapy services to be delivered by qualified therapists who meet ***competency*** (i.e., ability to demonstrate the knowledge, capacity, and skills for practice and meet legal standards for credentialed practitioners) requirements and adhere to the licensure regulations. The facility was at risk of being fined, required to repay the reimbursed funds, and charged with fraudulent billing.

When Mary Jo approached her SRB to renew her occupational therapy license, the board reviewed her situation, placed her on probation for 1 year, and issued her a substantial fine. Once informed of these actions, AOTA's Ethics Commission (EC) reviewed the circumstances surrounding Mary Jo's lapsed license. The EC issued her a ***reprimand,*** "a formal expression of disapproval of conduct communicated privately by letter . . . that is nondisclosable and noncommunicative to other bodies" (AOTA, 2015a, p. 2). Hospital administrators subjected Bill to disciplinary action for his failure, as Mary Jo's supervisor, to verify Mary Jo's licensure on her return to work.

(Continued)

Case Study 8.2. Addressing Failure to Maintain Credentials *(Cont.)*

Table 8.1. Decision Table for Case Study 8.2

Action	Positive Outcomes	Negative Consequences
Take no action—a failure to notify the SRB of address change.	None. A lack of action produces no positive results. Mary Jo remains out of compliance with the SRB and AOTA's Code.	The SRB reviews Mary Jo's application for licensure renewal because she had been practicing without a license. RSC 4G requires practitioners to hold appropriate credentials. The SRB issues Mary Jo a license to practice occupational therapy but places her on 1 year of probation and issues her a fine. Mary Jo agrees to provide occupational therapy staff with an in-service regarding the SRB's requirement to notify the practice board of changes in personal information.
Bill's failure to verify Mary Jo's credentials.	Bill and Mary Jo recognize their responsibilities and the violation of RSC 4G.	Bill and Mary Jo develop a tracking and notification system to help occupational therapy practitioners at the facility keep abreast of license renewal dates and continuing education credits.
Mary Jo's use of the OT/L credential.	None	The AOTA Ethics Commission reviews Mary Jo's case for violations of RSCs 4G, 5A, and 5B and issues her a letter of reprimand. Signing documentation as an OT/L was a misrepresentation in communications to the public and third-party payers and thus a violation of RSC 5A. The administration at Mary Jo's facility instructs her to review all policies and procedures related to credentialing and documentation as well as the code of conduct. Mary Jo agrees to take continuing education courses on ethics.
Use of inaccurate information in billing to Medicare and third-party payers.	None	The facility agrees to work with Medicare and Mary Jo to negotiate a settlement. This action violated RSCs 4O and 5B.
Bill's failure to adhere to the *Guidelines for Supervision, Roles, and Responsibilities During the Delivery of Occupational Therapy Services* (AOTA, 2014a).	Bill reviews the *Guidelines* document and attends continuing education courses related to supervision.	Bill's lack of familiarity with policies and guidelines of the profession. Bill, his staff, and ultimately, the hospital violate organizational policies and federal regulations.

Note. AOTA = American Occupational Therapy Association; RSCs = Related Standards of Conduct; SRB = state regulatory board.

Case Study 8.3. Addressing Failure to Provide Adequate Supervision

Paul, an occupational therapy student in a fieldwork placement, was concerned about the limited supervision he was receiving. He reviewed the Code and found that, by failing to provide him with adequate supervision, his immediate supervisor may have breached RSCs 4G and 4H. Paul's supervisor also may have violated state laws and regulations that address the responsibilities of a licensed occupational therapist in supervising occupational therapy assistants, students, and other personnel. According to RSCs 4K and 6B, Paul had an obligation under the Code to address reporting the suspected breaches of his supervisor's ethical conduct. These RSCs helped him to understand the importance of reporting the potentially illegal and unethical conduct (RSC 4K) and to recognize that these behaviors need to be addressed to protect clients, the student experience, and the team (RSC 6B).

Paul considered the appropriate lines of communication to follow. He decided that a meeting with his immediate fieldwork supervisor to discuss his concerns and needs was the first step, so he made an appointment with her. If this conversation did not result in the desired outcome, he resolved to consult with university faculty. If these efforts did not result in additional supervision, Paul would contact his academic fieldwork coordinator to see whether she would agree to provide more regular and direct supervision to enhance Paul's educational experience and to help safeguard the clients on his caseload.

If all of these strategies failed, Paul discovered he could file a complaint with the SRB, NBCOT, or AOTA. His SRB had specific regulations addressing supervision of nonlicensed personnel. If his occupational therapy fieldwork supervisor held current certification with NBCOT, he could file a complaint with that organization based on his concerns that the lack of supervision violated the public interest and safety. Finally, if Paul's fieldwork supervisor was an AOTA member, he could file an ethics complaint citing the Principles and RSCs of the Code that he believed were violated (Scott, 2002a).

Vignette 8.2. Addressing Failure to Maintain Ethical Principles in Private Practice

Pamela Pediatrics, a company owned by **Pamela,** an occupational therapist, provided occupational therapy services to preschool children with special needs in a clinic setting. Pamela had been a clinical fieldwork supervisor for 8 years, and although the practice was busy and the clinic's staffing level was low, she currently had 3 Level I fieldwork students. The students were concerned that the children were receiving inadequate care and that they were receiving insufficient supervision.

The students consulted the Code and discovered that Pamela had violated Principle 1, Beneficence, because understaffing could lead to a lack of safety for both the children and students. Specifically, RSC 4H, regarding the provision of appropriate supervision by those with supervisory responsibility, also was relevant. They realized RSC 4N held Pamela to the same obligations to her clients and fieldwork students in her private practice as she would have in an institution. Pamela was responsible both for providing competent services to the children, who may have been at increased risk for injury, and for supervising the students according to relevant guidelines (e.g., Accreditation Council for Occupational Therapy Education, 2012). The students contacted their school for guidance.

practitioners to "ensure compliance with relevant laws, and promote transparency when participating in a business as owner, stockholder, partner, or employee" (AOTA, 2015b, p. 6). Vignette 8.2, describes a situation in which an occupational therapist in private practice fails to meet these obligations. Vignette 8.6 addresses the receipt of a gift that conflicts with the employer's policy.

Vignette 8.3. Fulfilling Duty to Inform Others

Connie, an occupational therapy supervisor, submitted her resignation to her immediate supervisor. Connie located an occupational therapist who was willing to contract with the hospital to supervise the department's occupational therapy assistant, **Kelly,** and communicated this information to the assistant program director before leaving her position. Months later, Connie learned that Kelly had not received supervision by an occupational therapist since her departure.

Connie communicated the seriousness of the situation to the assistant program director on at least two occasions and offered suggestions and solutions. Connie no longer wanted to be involved, but she wanted to be responsible and ethical. She obtained copies of the supervision requirements from the SRB and the *Guidelines for Supervision, Roles, and Responsibilities During the Delivery of Occupational Therapy Services* (AOTA, 2014a) and mailed them to Kelly and the assistant program director. She also telephoned Kelly to discuss the situation and her concerns directly with him, noting that Kelly might jeopardize his license if he continued to practice without adequate supervision. She suggested to Kelly that he consider contacting the state board of occupational therapy practice and reporting the situation and that he investigate whether third-party payers had rules about whom they considered to be qualified to provide services. Kelly gathered the results of his research and met with the assistant program director to reiterate his need for supervision by an occupational therapist under the Code, state licensure laws, and third-party payer requirements. As a result, an occupational therapist was hired.

Vignette 8.4. Complying With Institutional Regulations

Amelia recently passed the NBCOT certification exam and began working at a state facility serving people with developmental disabilities. Her supervisor, **José,** who was also new to the facility, discovered that many of the client records did not have any occupational therapy progress notes. José suggested that he and Amelia re-create notes for all of the charts using the sign-in sheets documenting client attendance.

Amelia wanted to please José and keep her new job, but she was uncertain whether she should comply with José's request. She was concerned about whether her compliance would be legal and ethical and, if so, whether to take time away from client care or come in on the weekends to complete the documentation.

Amelia reviewed the Code for guidance. In addition to RSCs 4F, 4K, 4L, and 4N, all of which address adherence to regulations and educating others about regulatory compliance, she discovered that Principle 5, Veracity, also applied—particularly RSCs 5A (accuracy in all types of communication), 5B (refrain from participating in deceptive communication), and 5C (record and report accurately and timely). She also reviewed institutional policies regarding coming in to work when not scheduled and denying current clients the services they need and expect. She decided that it would be inappropriate and unprofessional to comply with José's request and made an appointment to discuss her concerns with José (Scott, 2002b).

Vignette 8.5. Refraining From Unauthorized Access to Educational Materials

Stefan was an occupational therapy student entering the final year of his academic program. He found a great new apartment for his final year with 2 other occupational therapy students who were entering their first year. They all quickly became friends and study buddies. Stefan wanted his new roommates to do well, so he passed along to them all of his notes and papers from his first year in the program, which included his graded tests. He also shared his login information to a few professional journals he had subscribed to so that they could have the benefit of looking at the latest research. His roommates were very grateful for Stefan's help and thanked their new friend.

Vignette 8.6. Accepting Gifts and Adhering to Employer Policy

Alicia is an occupational therapist in the intensive care unit of a large trauma center. Alicia recently worked with a patient with significant occupational therapy needs from complications following a stroke, and she devoted a great deal of time with the patient's family conducting education and training as well as providing general support. When the patient was ready for discharge, Alicia completed her paperwork and said her goodbyes to the patient and family. The patient's spouse handed Alicia a small card in an envelope when thanking her for the care she provided. Alicia often received thank you notes from families, which was always very touching.

However, when she returned to her work area and opened the card, she was shocked to find that the thank you card contained two hundred dollars in cash. Hospital policy states that staff should not accept any gift greater than thirty dollars cash value. In the interest of ***transparency*** (i.e., open, honest, and unambiguous behavior or communication) and ***professional boundaries*** (i.e., ethical limits on the relationship between practitioner and client, payer, employer, or other entity), Alicia went back to the patient's bedside to explain the hospital's policy and return the money, but the patient and family were already gone.

Summary

The creation of laws, rules, and guidelines helps to ensure that unqualified practitioners do not harm the public. Justice, Principle 4 of the Code, outlines the duty of occupational therapy practitioners to abide by regulations established to protect consumers of occupational therapy services, employers, third-party payers, students, the profession, and society at large. This Principle also emphasizes the important role of the occupational therapy practitioner in reducing barriers to clients' access to needed services. This responsibility extends to facilitating system change through advocacy. Practitioners also must continually update their knowledge about applicable laws, rules, and regulations governing practice, including billing practices. In addition, practitioners are obligated to appropriately bill for services and to advocate for access to services.

Reflective Questions

1. Justice has just been described relative to occupational therapy practice. Identify the RSC that address procedural justice and those focused on ideas of social justice.
2. Review Vignette 8.5 and identify which Principles and RSCs were relevant in this situation. Describe the positive and negative consequences to Stefan, his roommates, and their academic program.
3. Vignette 8.6 focuses on accepting gifts. Discuss what you would do in this situation. Apply Principles and RSCs from the Code that support your decisions.

References

Accreditation Council for Occupational Therapy Education. (2012). 2011 Accreditation Council for Occupational Therapy Education (ACOTE®) standards. *American Journal of Occupational Therapy, 66*(Suppl. 6), S6–S74. https://doi.org/10.5014/ajot.2012.66S6

American Occupational Therapy Association. (2014a). Guidelines for supervision, roles, and responsibilities during the delivery of occupational therapy services. *American Journal of Occupational Therapy, 68,* S16–S22. https://doi.org/10.5014/ajot.2014.686S03

American Occupational Therapy Association. (2014b). Occupational therapy practice framework: Domain and process (3rd ed.). *American Journal of Occupational Therapy, 68*(Suppl. 1), S1–S48. https://doi.org/10.5014/ajot.2014.682006

American Occupational Therapy Association. (2015a). Enforcement procedures for the Occupational Therapy Code of Ethics and Ethics Standards. *American Journal of Occupational Therapy, 68,* S3–S15. https://doi.org/10.5014/ajot.2014.686S02

American Occupational Therapy Association. (2015b). Occupational therapy code of ethics (2015). *American Journal of Occupational Therapy, 69*(Suppl. 3), 6912310030. https://doi.org/10.5014/ajot.2015.696S03

American Occupational Therapy Association. (2015c). *2015 AOTA salary & workforce survey.* Bethesda, MD: Author.

Ashe, A. M. (2016). Social justice and meeting needs of clients. In D. Y. Slater (Ed.), *Reference guide to the Occupational Therapy Code of Ethics* (2015 ed., pp. 235–238). Bethesda, MD: AOTA Press.

Beauchamp, T. L., & Childress, J. F. (2013). *Principles of biomedical ethics* (7th ed.). New York: Oxford University Press.

Bureau of Labor Statistics, U.S. Department of Labor. (2015). *Occupational outlook handbook, 2016–2017 Edition, occupational therapists*. Retrieved from http://www.bls.gov/ooh/healthcare/occupational-therapists.htm

Herz, N., Bondoc, S., Richmond, T., Richman, N., & Kroll, C. (2005, March). Becoming an entrepreneur. *Administration and Management Special Interest Section Quarterly, 21*, 1–3.

Maiese, M. (2004). *Procedural justice*. Retrieved from www.beyondintractability.org/essay/procedural_justice/

Nilsson, I., & Townsend, E. (2010). Occupational justice—Bridging theory and practice. *Scandinavian Journal of Occupational Therapy, 17*(1), 57–63. Retrieved from http://www.tandfonline.com/doi/abs/10.3109/11038120903287182?journalCode=iocc20

Reed, K. L., Ashe, A. M., & Slater, D. Y. (2009, April). *Everyday ethics: Ethical challenges in emerging practice*. Slide show presented at the AOTA Annual Conference & Expo, Houston.

Scott, J. B. (2002a, January 14). Everyday ethics: Clarifying concerns and remedies. *OT Practice, 7*(1), 9.

Scott, J. B. (2002b, May 13). Everyday ethics: Recreating notes. *OT Practice, 7*(5), 7.

Townsend, E. (2012). Boundaries and bridges to adult mental health: Critical occupational and capabilities perspectives of justice. *Journal of Occupational Science, 19,* 8–24. https://doi.org/10.1080/14427591.2011.639723

Townsend, E., & Wilcock, A. (2004). Occupational justice and client-centered practice: A dialogue in progress. *Canadian Journal of Occupational Therapy, 71*(2), 75–87. https://doi.org/10.1177/000841740407100203

Chapter 9.

PRINCIPLE 5: VERACITY

Janie B. Scott, MA, OT/L, FAOTA

Learning Objectives

By the end of the chapter, readers will be able to

- Describe the harm that can occur when veracity in communication is not upheld,
- Analyze the range of behaviors that can lead to the perceptions of plagiarism, and
- Apply Related Standards of Conduct associated with the Principle of Veracity to situations where materials presented are inaccurate.

Key Terms and Concepts

- ✧ Attribution
- ✧ Communication
- ✧ Documentation
- ✧ Moral courage
- ✧ Plagiarism
- ✧ Veracity

Veracity

Principle 5. Occupational therapy personnel shall provide comprehensive, accurate, and objective information when representing the profession.

Veracity is based on the virtues of truthfulness, candor, and honesty. The Principle of Veracity refers to comprehensive, accurate, and objective transmission of information and includes fostering understanding of such information (Beauchamp & Childress, 2013). Veracity is based on respect owed to others, including but not limited to recipients of service, colleagues, students, researchers, and research participants.

In communicating with others, occupational therapy personnel implicitly promise to be truthful and not deceptive. When entering into a therapeutic or research relationship, the recipient of service or research participant has the right to accurate information. In addition, transmission of information is incomplete without also ensuring that the recipient or participant understands the information provided.

Concepts of veracity must be carefully balanced with other potentially competing ethical principles, cultural beliefs, and organizational policies. Veracity ultimately is valued as a means to establish trust and strengthen professional relationships. Therefore, adherence to the Principle of Veracity also requires thoughtful analysis of how full disclosure of information may impact outcomes.

Related Standards of Conduct

Occupational Therapy Personnel Shall

A. Represent credentials, qualifications, education, experience, training, roles, duties, competence, contributions, and findings accurately in all forms of communication.
B. Refrain from using or participating in the use of any form of communication that contains false, fraudulent, deceptive, misleading, or unfair statements or claims.
C. Record and report in an accurate and timely manner, and in accordance with applicable regulations, all information related to professional or academic documentation and activities.
D. Identify and fully disclose to all appropriate persons errors or adverse events that compromise the safety of service recipients.
E. Ensure that all marketing and advertising are truthful, accurate, and carefully presented to avoid misleading recipients of service, research participants, or the public.
F. Describe the type and duration of occupational therapy services accurately in professional contracts, including the duties and responsibilities of all involved parties.
G. Be honest, fair, accurate, respectful, and timely in gathering and reporting fact-based information regarding employee job performance and student performance.
H. Give credit and recognition when using the work of others in written, oral, or electronic media (i.e., do not plagiarize).
I. Provide students with access to accurate information regarding educational requirements and academic policies and procedures relative to the occupational therapy program or educational institution.
J. Maintain privacy and truthfulness when utilizing telecommunication in delivery of occupational therapy services.

Source. From the *Occupational Therapy Code of Ethics (2015)* (American Occupational Therapy Association, 2015, pp. 6–7).

Principle 5, ***Veracity,*** is detailed the *Occupational Therapy Code of Ethics (2015)* (hereinafter referred to as the "Code"; American Occupational Therapy Association [AOTA], 2015). This obligation extends to all areas of professional and public communication, including marketing, "professional relationships, documentation standards, billing practices, risk management, peer review, community relations, and regulatory reporting and compliance" (Bennett-Woods, 2005, p. 11).

According to Beauchamp and Childress (2013), neither the Hippocratic Oath (see Chapter 2, "Historical Background of Ethics in Occupational Therapy") nor the early versions of the *Principles of Medical Ethics* (the first version of the American Medical Association's [AMA's] code of ethics) made reference to veracity. AMA created the *Code of Medical Ethics* in 1847, and the title was changed to the *Principles of Medical Ethics* in 1903 (AMA, n.d.). Beginning in the 1980s, however, the *Principles of Medical Ethics* began to include language regarding the duty to be honest with both patients and colleagues.

As Beauchamp and Childress (2013) observed, "veracity in health care refers to accurate, timely, objective, and comprehensive transmission of information" (p. 303). Principles of Veracity, Trust, Autonomy, and Fidelity are closely linked, particularly as they relate to the relationships and obligations that occupational therapy practitioners have involving their clients, colleagues, students, and the public. This chapter discusses the three primary categories of behavior covered by Principle 5, Veracity: (1) truthful communication with others (i.e., public duty), (2) documentation, and (3) attribution (AOTA, 2015).

Communication With the Public

Occupational therapy practitioners have a public duty to be honest in all oral and written communication within the profession and with external audiences, including students, colleagues, clients, and the public (AOTA, 2015). All areas of occupational therapy practice rely on ***communication,*** which is the transmission of information (e.g., assessment results, intervention proposals and plans, and research findings). When practitioners present information in a way that is unclear or dishonest, harm may occur to the recipient, and the public perception of the occupational therapy profession may be damaged.

Related Standards of Conduct (RSCs) 5A, 5B, 5D, 5E, 5G, 5H, and 5I address Veracity as a public duty. Conducting oneself in a way that deviates from these standards is a violation of Principle 5 of the Code, as well as of many requirements established by state occupational therapy regulatory boards (SRBs) and the National Board for Certification in Occupational Therapy (NBCOT). As physician and social work pioneer Richard Clark Cabot (1915) observed a century ago, "To fool a patient is tyranny, not guidance" (p. ix).

An example from the medical literature serves to illustrate the harm caused by failure to uphold the Principle of Veracity. Wakefield and his colleagues (1998) published research in *Lancet* purporting to provide evidence of a connection between the measles, mumps, and rubella (MMR) vaccine and the onset of autism. The veracity of Wakefield's claims could not be substantiated, and he was required to retract his reports of study outcomes (Godlee & Smith, 2011), was convicted of misconduct and ethics breaches, and had his medical license revoked (General Medical Council, 2010). Because of the fraudulent information he communicated to the public, rates of immunization with the MMR vaccine dropped, potentially leading to a public health problem. Wakefield continued to stand behind his fraudulent reporting, meaning that his miscommunication has continued to spread fear. Wakefield violated his public duty to be honest and truthful in his communications, a major violation of the ethical Principle of Veracity.

This example highlights the ethical obligation of all health care professionals to fulfill the public duty of Veracity to avoid direct or indirect harm to patients. RSC 1C enlists occupational therapy practitioners to make sure that interventions are evidence based to the extent possible, and RSC 1F obligates the insurance of competence to avoid inflicting harm directly or indirectly. Occupational therapy practitioners have an obligation to be aware of retracted research by staying current with developments in the literature and to debunk myths and prevent further harm by ensuring that clients have up-to-date knowledge. The Code also places the expectation on practitioners to be objective in their practice (RSC 2F) and to maintain high standards of competence (RSC 1E) to ensure the safety and well-being of those served. Adherence to these RSCs helps occupational therapy practitioners remain alert to innovations in practice and ensures that they deliver competent services so that information and interventions provided are efficacious.

In her 2011 American Occupational Therapy Foundation's Breakfast with a Scholar lecture, Ruth Purtilo spoke about ***moral courage***—the importance of having confidence in one's decisions and a reasonable belief that the course of action one takes is the correct one. Moral courage is required when facing an ethical dilemma and is possible only when one has the competence and the confidence to make the best possible judgment or decision. For example, an occupational therapy practitioner who receives a referral for a client whose condition is unfamiliar must assess his or her skills and abilities in the context of the client's needs and determine whether it would be in the client's best interest to refer him or her to another practitioner with expertise in that practice or specialty area. Occupational therapy practitioners must have the moral courage to make the best choice for the client, which is ultimately the best choice for the practitioner as well. In Case Study 9.1, the practitioners have the moral courage to review their behaviors and choose ethical actions.

Occupational therapy students have reported observations from their Level II fieldwork experiences about clients who received a doctor's referral for occupational therapy but who were not aware of why they were referred and the outcomes they should expect from these interventions. When occupational therapists do not review the evaluation results, plan of care, expected length of intervention, and anticipated outcomes with their patients, the patients' trust in the services and providers wavers. In Case Study 9.2 and Vignette 9.1, occupational therapists must take steps to fulfill the duty of Veracity in communicating with patients.

Documentation

All facets of occupational therapy practice, research, and education require documentation, and RSCs 4O, 5C, and 5F refer specifically to documentation. ***Documentation,*** relative to occupational therapy practice, is the process of recording data into records, or materials to communicate ideas, outcomes, projections, and education. The information occupational therapy practitioners and students supply to local, state, and federal agencies must be accurate and in accordance with stated regulations. Failure to ensure veracity in documentation violates Principle 5, as well as laws and regulations established to govern occupational therapy and protect clients.

Billing and Reimbursement

Ethical practice requires the documentation of assessments, progress, and number of minutes or units spent in interventions for billing purposes. Those whose practice includes consultation must provide documentation according to the specifications of the agreed-on work. Whether documentation is

Case Study 9.1. Exhibiting Moral Courage to Address Lack of Veracity

Joel and **Monica** were occupational therapists who had worked together for 4 years with older adults in an inpatient subacute unit of a long-term care facility. They had had limited opportunities to provide caregiver education to their clients' families to help them anticipate the needs of the family member after discharge and adapt their home environment for greater accessibility. Joel and Monica thought their clients and families needed these services to experience successful transitions back home.

Joel and Monica began planning a business venture that would enable them to provide caregiver education, environmental assessment, and care coordination for clients being discharged from hospital and acute care settings to home and to their families. They planned a transition from full-time employment to private practice. Joel and Monica constructed a business plan, conducted a needs assessment, created an office location initially in one of their homes, and promoted their practice through brochures directed to clients and families and to the professional community (e.g., doctors, rehabilitation professionals, area agencies on aging). As part of the process, Monica investigated AOTA's Specialty Certification in Environmental Modification and Joel planned to obtain a Certified Aging-in-Place Specialist designation through the National Association of Home Builders (NAHB). They understood that to be successful in their business, they had to fulfill a need that wasn't currently being met in their community and promote themselves as experts in the area of aging in place (Scott, 2009).

The promotional materials Joel and Monica developed listed the services they would offer, including aging-in-place consultation, environmental assessments, caregiver education, and care coordination. In their bios, they listed the following skills and experience: 8 years of experience in inpatient occupational therapy service delivery, discharge planning with clients and families, caregiver education and training, and home safety evaluations. They included the following certifications: certification by NBCOT, state licensure in occupational therapy, and certification in home modifications. Joel and Monica knew, as they were creating these materials, that they had initial certification by NBCOT; however, this certification was not current, and the certification in home modifications they listed was what they hoped to acquire before they officially opened their business.

Joel and Monica decided to get a head start on their outreach campaign and shared their publicity materials with the agency's social worker, a physical therapist who was a friend, and staff at the local area agency on aging. Once the information was released, however, people began to question the veracity of the statements they made in their materials. Joel and Monica knew with moral certainty that they needed to review the misstatements they had made in the brochures and other documents they had distributed, examine the ramifications and impact of having this information go public, and develop strategies to retract the materials. They also realized that they would have to re-examine their entire plan of implementation.

Joel and Monica used the Code to help structure their reflection on the facts in their situation and begin their remediation plan. Their reflection led to the following realizations:

- Joel and Monica had misrepresented their credentials—NBCOT certification, AOTA specialty certification, and NAHB certification—in violation of RSC 5A. In particular, they realized, their use of a federally registered trademark with NBCOT could potentially involve

(Continued)

Case Study 9.1. Exhibiting Moral Courage to Address Lack of Veracity *(Cont.)*

them in fraud litigation, which could be communicated to their SRB and the National Practitioner Data Bank (see Chapter 3, "Promoting Ethics in Occupational Therapy Practice").

- They had published information suggesting that they had far more experience than was accurate, violating RSC 5B.
- They made a commitment to revise their materials and their business plan in an effort to restore the public's trust in them as practitioners and in the profession in general. Failure to do so would have resulted in a violation of RSC 5E.

Joel and Monica were overwhelmed by the scope of their errors, but they had the moral courage to face and rectify them. They decided to personally contact each person and agency that had received their material with a written apology and a request that the recipient destroy the brochures they had received. They thought this was an important step in respecting their public duty to be ethical. In addition, Joel and Monica decided to delay publicizing their private practice until they had obtained the certifications and gained the expertise they needed to be successful, competent, and ethical occupational therapists.

Case Study 9.2. Improving Veracity in Client Communication

Caroline was an occupational therapist with 20 years of experience specializing in interventions for clients recovering from hand surgery and traumas of the hand and upper extremity. After undergoing hand surgery and 4 occupational therapy sessions, **Deborah,** a client, asked Caroline about her prognosis. Although Caroline was aware of the outcomes that would likely result from the intervention, she told Deborah, "I'm really not sure; you should ask your doctor."

Later, Caroline reflected on her actions regarding sharing information with this client and others. She realized she was afraid that, if she replied honestly, Deborah might terminate care early, reducing the potential benefits of the intervention. Caroline also questioned whether she had been operating from a position of paternalism by taking away Deborah's opportunity to make decisions about her care. Caroline consulted the Code and found direction that would be helpful in her client interactions.

Under RSC 3B, Caroline found her obligation to fully disclose to Deborah the benefits, risks, and potential outcomes of the interventions offered. She also understood her responsibility to keep Deborah informed about her progress toward established goals. Caroline identified the ethical duty articulated in RSC 1H regarding her responsibility to terminate occupational therapy services in collaboration with Deborah or when Deborah had achieved maximum benefits. If Caroline had any doubts about whether Deborah could understand the information regarding the assessments, interventions, and potential risks and benefits (RSC 3D), Caroline would need to take steps to make sure that this information was clear and delivered in a way that Deborah could comprehend (RSC 3J). Regarding the duty of Veracity, if Caroline withheld information or provided Deborah with communication that was vague, false, or deceptive, she would be in violation of RSC 5B. Caroline recognized that she needed to be clear and accurate when presenting information to Deborah and her other clients. Finally, Caroline reflected that if she did not share her assessment of Deborah's progress with her, it might reduce Deborah's belief in the benefits of the interventions she was receiving.

Caroline decided to contact the referring doctor and explain Deborah's concerns regarding her care and prognosis. She also informed the doctor of her own intention to more fully share her assessment and anticipated outcomes with Deborah during their next session. They agreed that Caroline would encourage Deborah to speak with the surgeon if she had any additional questions. Caroline felt freer after sharing her dilemma with the surgeon and clarifying her responsibilities to her patient. These actions helped her maintain compliance with the Code.

Vignette 9.1. Ensuring Veracity in Multiple Roles

Bruce worked for a pediatric inpatient rehabilitation facility and provided services to survivors of brain and spinal cord injuries. He also made and sold pediatric furniture and adaptive equipment through his home business. Bruce wanted to know whether it would be ethical for him to tell his patients' parents about his business and the opportunity for them to buy furniture or adaptive equipment created especially for them. Bruce knew he had an obligation to adhere to the policies and guidelines of the institution in which he worked and to federal and state laws and regulations. He also consulted Principle 5 of the Code, his employer's guidelines on employees' referrals to their own businesses (RSCs 2F, 5B, 5E), and an advisory opinion for the Ethics Commission by Austin (2016). Austin described the ethical conflicts that can exist when occupational therapists provide direct service to clients and also sell products to them from a company in which they have invested or from which they receive a commission.

required for the purposes of billing, recording gains and losses, or supplying evidence to standard setters, compliance is required on a consistent basis.

Third-party payers (e.g., Medicare) have specific stipulations about the type and timing of documentation that must be submitted to receive reimbursement. Documentation standards and requirements established by Medicare are often followed by other payers. In addition, the SRBs (see Chapter 3, "Promoting Ethics in Occupational Therapy Practice") and NBCOT (2014) have established standards requiring the professionals they regulate to be accurate and truthful and to respect the privacy of the clients they serve. The *NBCOT Code of Conduct* articulates two principles that are consistent with the language and expectations in the Code:

- *Principle 3.* Shall be accurate, truthful, and complete in any and all communications, direct or indirect, with any client, employer, regulatory agency, or other parties as relates to their professional work, education, professional credentials, research and contributions to the field of O.T. (NBCOT, 2014, p. 2).
- *Principle 4.* Certificants shall comply with state and/or federal laws, regulations, and statutes governing the practice of occupational therapy (NBCOT, 2014, p. 2).

As described in Case Study 9.3, the accuracy of documentation for billing purposes (RSC 4O) has both ethical and legal implications.

Research

Occupational therapy practitioners involved in research also must abide by the ethical Principle of Veracity. They must obtain approval from the appropriate institutional review board and secure consent from research participants. If occupational therapy practitioners misrepresent their research and outcomes, they potentially endanger both their clients and the profession. Chapter 19, "Ethics in Occupational Therapy Research," discusses the need for concern about the accuracy and veracity of reports of findings in occupational therapy research, including ensuring that the work reported is accurate and reflects the author's own work unless specified otherwise.

Education

Occupational therapy educators are bound by the Principle of Veracity in developing a syllabus that articulates performance expectations by which student and faculty are judged and that provides guidelines for integrity. In addition, syllabi should be constructed to meet the standards approved by the Accreditation Council for Occupational Therapy Education (ACOTE). Faculty must be honest and forthcoming regarding course-specific details such as learning activities, and more broadly communicate how a particular course is related to the curriculum design to be in compliance with the following standard:

> The program must have written syllabi for each course that include course objectives and learning activities that, in total, reflect all course content required by the Standards. Instructional methods (e.g., presentations, demonstrations, discussion) and materials used to accomplish course objectives must be documented. Programs must also demonstrate the consistency between course syllabi and the curriculum design. (ACOTE, 2012, p. S32)

Case Study 9.3. Ensuring Veracity in Documentation

Madison was an occupational therapist working in a not-for-profit teaching hospital on an inpatient rehabilitation unit. The pace was fast, and the productivity requirements kept all of the rehabilitation professionals moving quickly to meet the established standards. On a regular basis, however, patients were not ready or available or refused to come to the unit for their therapy sessions. When this occurred, the competition for patients increased between occupational therapy and physical therapy; whoever could get to the patient first was able to complete their minutes. Madison and **Jonah,** a physical therapist, agreed that when schedules got tight and it was feasible, they would co-treat so that patients would get some amount of services and the therapists' productivity numbers wouldn't be too low, which would get them into trouble.

Jonah approached Madison at lunch one day when their workloads were particularly heavy. Jonah proposed that they co-treat **Mr. Pitts** in the afternoon and each bill for the standard 3 units of service. By the time Jonah and Madison saw Mr. Pitts, though, it was late in the day, and there wasn't enough time for them to see him for the full 3 units. Even though Madison was able to provide only 2 units of occupational therapy service to Mr. Pitts, Madison and Jonah agreed that they would each bill for the full 3 units of time, and Madison would make up the time with Mr. Pitts the next day. Madison wasn't totally comfortable with this plan but didn't want to get in trouble with their supervisor, so she documented the intervention as 3 units. This same situation occurred several times over a period of 3 months until Jonah was reassigned to another unit. During all of this time, Madison neglected to think about the legal and ethical implications of her actions.

Late one evening, Madison reflected on her day and became uncomfortable with the decisions she and Jonah had been making regarding billing. At first she told herself not to worry about it, that occupational therapists and physical therapists did this kind of thing all the time and it wasn't a big deal. However, she remembered that she had recently read about Medicare fraud investigations and worried that she could fall into this legal and ethical abyss. Madison consulted the Code and went to Medicare.gov, the Centers for Medicaid and Medicare Services website, to review how her behaviors might be interpreted. Madison searched the site for "fraud" and found hundreds of informational articles on the topic. Also, at the bottom of the home page she discovered STOPMedicareFraud.gov that led to the sections About Fraud, Prevent Fraud, and For Providers (U.S. Department of Health and Human Services, n.d.). The more she read, the more she realized that what she and Jonah had done had placed them, their licenses, and the hospital in jeopardy.

Madison's review of the Code led her to see that her behaviors violated RSC 4O, "ensure that documentation for reimbursement purposes is done in accordance with applicable laws, guidelines, and regulations" (AOTA, 2015, p. 6). She also found that Principle 4, Justice, had been violated: "Occupational therapy personnel shall promote fairness and objectivity in the provision of occupational therapy services" (AOTA, 2015, p. 5).

Madison realized that, in the worst-case scenario, she could lose her job along with her license to practice occupational therapy and could be sued. She considered her potential courses of action, which included saying and doing nothing, contacting the family lawyer to get guidance on the situation, or making an appointment to meet with her supervisor and be honest about what had happened then work with her toward resolution. Madison chose the last option. Some of the options and the possible results she considered are reflected in Table 9.1.

Madison met with her supervisor, and then they met with the hospital's legal counsel. Under the Code, her supervisor had an ethical obligation (RSCs 4F, 4H, 4K) to report this situation to the AOTA and the SRB. Madison shared all of the information she had discovered in the Code, at Medicare.gov, and STOPMedicareFraud.gov in an effort to be transparent. At the end of many meetings, Madison wasn't fired; however, she was

(Continued)

Case Study 9.3. Ensuring Veracity in Documentation *(Cont.)*

disciplined by the AOTA Ethics Commission as an AOTA member and by the SRB. In addition, she arranged a way to achieve financial restitution with the hospital and Medicare. All agencies involved were somewhat lenient because Madison voluntarily came forward to disclose her actions rather than waiting to see whether her actions would be discovered.

Table 9.1. Decision Table for Case Study 9.3

Possible Action	Positive Outcomes	Negative Consequences
No action.	Madison avoids discomfort and embarrassment.	Madison continues the behaviors and places her license in jeopardy. Jonah continues his billing practices. Madison violates state and federal laws and hospital policies. Madison violates her responsibility as an AOTA member to uphold ethics Principles (Principle 5, RSC 4O).
Cease behavior but take no additional action.	Madison avoids discomfort and embarrassment. Madison avoids committing additional fraudulent billing.	Jonah continues his billing practices. Madison and Jonah continue to violate state and federal laws and hospital policies. Madison violates her responsibility as an AOTA member to uphold ethics Principles (Principle 5, RSC 4O).
Discuss the issues with her supervisor.	Madison feels relief from her emotional tension when she discloses her behaviors and concerns to her supervisor. Both Madison and her supervisor have an obligation to report to the authorities any acts that appear unethical or illegal (RSC 4K). Madison's supervisor also contacts Jonah's supervisor to provide information and seek appropriate legal and ethical action (Principle 4, RSC 6B).	Madison's supervisor is obligated under RSCs 4F and 4H to prevent breaches of the Code. The hospital may fire or discipline Madison and her supervisor. Jonah may be angry that he is also disciplined. Medicare may fine the hospital. Madison may face civil penalties from Medicare and the SRB, may lose her license to practice, and may be disciplined by AOTA's Ethics Commission.
Inform Medicare.	Madison upholds her duty under RSCs 4K, 4N, and 4O to address her violations of these Principles. Madison gains a greater understanding of her legal and ethical obligations regarding billing and reimbursement.	Medicare reports these breaches of policy and ethics to the National Practitioner Data Bank. Madison negotiates repayment of debt with Medicare. The SRB disciplines Madison by placing her on probation and requiring her to pay a fine and take ethics education courses.

Note. AOTA = American Occupational Therapy Association; RSCs = Related Standards of Conduct; SRB = state regulatory board.

Vignette 9.2 considers a situation in academia and the responsibility to students in the development of a fieldwork program.

Continuing Education

Requirements exist for faculty, practitioners, and all occupational therapy personnel under RSC 5C to accurately document the continuing education they obtain for licensure or certification renewal and for continuing competence (AOTA, 2015). Practitioners must maintain a record of continuing education courses and activities in accordance with the standard-setting body, typically to include the name of the course, dates, number of contact hours, and evidence of attendance or participation. The

Vignette 9.2. Truthfulness in Academic Program Marketing

Latisha accepted a position as an AFWC in a growing occupational therapy assistant (OTA) program. She was a clinical instructor in her recent position at a hospital-based behavioral health unit before moving to a new state and accepting this position. The OTA program was new, and Latisha would be responsible for getting certification as a fieldwork educator, using the ACOTE Standards to establish fieldwork at the school, and networking with local sites where students may intern.

Terry, the department chair for the OTA program, promised to help Latisha with implementing the ACOTE standards and familiarizing her with the occupational therapy community. The only problem that soon became apparent was that Terry was overwhelmed with her own program development responsibilities and her availability was quite limited. Latisha was frustrated with her situation; however, she deeply wanted to be successful in this position and develop quality fieldwork experiences for students.

In an attempt to make the development of a fieldwork program a manageable process, Latisha began by outlining the resources that were available. Her first step was to visit the AOTA website (www.aota.org), where she found information under Education & Careers → Fieldwork. She was relieved to discover useful materials in this section, including guidelines for Level I and Level II fieldwork, directions on establishing specific objectives, information on obtaining a Fieldwork Educator's Certificate, and more. As she perused these materials she also wondered where ethics figured into the picture. One of her primary concerns was to be in compliance with the Code. Also on the AOTA website Latisha found the Code and reviewed it carefully. She created a table reflecting the Code's RSCs related to students (see Table 9.2). Finally, Latisha made connections with other AFWCs in local academic programs and through the AOTA Education Special Interest Section.

Armed with the outcomes of her research, Latisha made an appointment to see Terry to get help establishing goals and timelines to develop fieldwork education in the OTA program. Both Latisha and Terry were relieved by the progress Latisha had made and felt satisfied that they had a plan to move forward.

Table 9.2. Accuracy in Fieldwork Program Development

Principle	Description	RSCs
1. Nonmaleficence	Occupational therapy personnel shall refrain from actions that cause harm.	2A, 2C, 2F, 2G, 2I
2. Autonomy	Occupational therapy personnel shall respect the right of the individual to self-determination, privacy, confidentiality, and consent.	3J
3. Justice	Occupational therapy personnel shall promote fairness and objectivity in the provision of occupational therapy services.	4F
4. Veracity	Occupational therapy personnel shall provide comprehensive, accurate, and objective information when representing the profession.	5F, 5G, 5I
5. Fidelity	Occupational therapy personnel shall treat clients, colleagues, and other professionals with respect, fairness, discretion, and integrity.	6A

Note. AFWC = academic fieldwork coordinator; RSCs = Related Standards of Conduct.

organization or SRB may require that these records be submitted at the time of license or certification renewal or in the event of an audit. Practitioners should be aware of documentation retention policies; those whose documentation is reviewed and considered to be incomplete may face disciplinary action, including fines or a delay in license or certification renewal.

Attribution

RSCs 5A, 5B, 5C, and 5H focus on ***attribution,*** or the explicit recognition of others as the originators of ideas. Occupational therapy students and practitioners have a duty to provide attribution when they use the words and thoughts of others. This topic is relevant not only for students and researchers but also for clinicians who develop in-services, policy manuals, and screening tools and for consultants who create surveys and reports for people, communities, organizations, and agencies. This obligation applies both to word-for-word duplications and to summaries of others' ideas that are incorporated into one's own work.

Ashe and Kornblau (2016) wrote in the advisory opinion *Avoiding Plagiarism,* "the concept of *plagiarism* encompasses not only material that has been

Vignette 9.3. Failing to Ensure Veracity in Attribution

Lisa, an occupational therapist, and **Peter,** an occupational therapy assistant, received funding from the occupational therapy department where they worked to attend a national conference. As a condition of receiving this funding, their supervisor, **Dominique,** made two requests. First, they were to attend sessions relevant to the hospital's interest in increasing its health promotion programming, particularly sessions focused on mental health; productive aging; and rehabilitation, participation, and disability. Second, after the conference, they were to provide a series of 5 staff in-services about the sessions they attended and recommend ways the department could translate this new information into innovative health promotion programming to be offered to outpatients and the community. Lisa and Peter enthusiastically agreed to these requirements and appreciated the opportunity they had been offered.

Lisa and Peter had an excellent time at the conference. They attended a variety of sessions and special events and were reunited with many of their friends from occupational therapy school, past positions, and recent conferences. Unfortunately, Lisa and Peter lost their focus on Dominique's assignment. They attended a couple of sessions on health promotion but none on mental health or rehabilitation, participation, and disability. Lisa and Peter decided to download the handouts from the sessions they had missed from the conference website and combine this information to develop several of their in-services. They also put together a presentation for staff about health promotion activities they had learned about relative to productive aging. In putting together their in-service presentations, however, they neglected to provide reference citations to the content they shared or otherwise credit the conference presenters.

copyrighted and published but also unpublished works, speeches, tweets, blog posts, photographs, drawings, and the like" (p. 229, *italics added*). They acknowledge that these thefts can be intentional or unintentional and occur at the hands of students, educators, occupational therapy clinicians, researchers, volunteers, and others. The authors underscore the responsibility "to maintain professional integrity and support appropriate ethical conduct, as delineated in the Code" (p. 233).

Howard (2016) wrote specifically about the issue of ***plagiarism*** in *Clinical Plagiarism and Copyright Violations.* She advised readers to be mindful about the reproduction of ideas, images, and forms (e.g., assessments, handouts) when developing or distributing materials for articles, in-services, and use with clients. RSC 5H addresses these issues, as does copyright law.

When reproducing the words and thoughts of others, ignorance is not a legitimate defense. All students and occupational therapy practitioners have a responsibility under the Code, institutional rules, and copyright law to clearly state when ideas, words, and images are not their own. A circumstance in which occupational therapy practitioners decide to use others' work without attribution is described in Vignette 9.3.

Summary

Occupational therapy students and practitioners have an obligation to be truthful when they present information to their clients, organizations, agencies, and the public. Veracity is an ethical Principle that helps occupational therapy practitioners focus on the ongoing importance of candor in their written and oral communications to fulfill their public duty of truthful communication, be honest in documentation, and ensure that attributions are accurate.

Reflective Questions

1. Refer to Vignette 9.1 and respond to the following questions.
   - What RSCs of Principle 5, Veracity, of the Code are applicable to this situation?
   - Are there any potential problems if Bruce bills a third party (e.g., the state Medical Assistance program) for these contractual services?
   - In addition, what is the answer to the question, as Austin (2016) asked, "Would the objective therapeutic relationship be compromised?" (p. 163).
2. Refer to Vignette 9.3 and respond to these questions.
   - If Lisa and Peter downloaded mental health session slides from the conference Web site and presented this information to staff as if they had been in attendance, was this a violation of the ethical principle of Veracity? If yes, what RSCs are applicable?

- Did the fact that their presentation materials did not provide full attributions to their sources constitute an ethics violation? If yes, what RSCs are applicable?
- What is your responsibility if you became aware of Lisa and Peter's inactions and actions?
- List the conflicts of interest that practitioners may be involved with that would violate Principle 5.

References

Accreditation Council for Occupational Therapy Education. (2012). 2011 Accreditation Council for Occupational Therapy Education (ACOTE®) standards. *American Journal of Occupational Therapy, 66*(Suppl. 6), S6–S74. https://doi.org/10.5014/ajot.2012.66S6

American Medical Association. (n.d.). *Ethics timeline: 1847–1940.* Retrieved from www.ama-assn.org/ama/pub/physician-resources/medical-ethics/code-medical-ethics/history-ama-ethics/ethics-timeline-1847-1940.page

American Occupational Therapy Association. (2015). Occupational therapy code of ethics (2015). *American Journal of Occupational Therapy, 69*(Suppl. 3), 6912310030. https://doi.org/10.5014/ajot.2015.696S03

Ashe, A. M., & Kornblau, B. L. (2016). Avoiding plagiarism. In D. Y. Slater (Ed.), *Reference guide to the Occupational Therapy Code of Ethics* (2015 ed., pp. 229–234). Bethesda, MD: AOTA Press.

Austin, D. (2016). Ethical considerations when occupational therapists engage in business transactions with clients. In D. Y. Slater (Ed.), *Reference guide to the Occupational Therapy Code of Ethics* (2015 ed., pp. 161–165). Bethesda, MD: AOTA Press.

Beauchamp, T. L., & Childress, J. F. (2013). *Principles of biomedical ethics* (7th ed.). New York: Oxford University Press.

Bennett-Woods, D. (2005). *Ethics at a glance: Veracity.* Denver: Regis University. Retrieved from http://rhchp.regis.edu/HCE/EthicsAtAGlance/Veracity/Veracity.pdf

Cabot, R. C. (1915). *Social service and the art of healing.* New York: Moffat, Yard.

General Medical Council. (2010, May 24). *Determination on serious professional misconduct (SPM) and sanction.* Retrieved from http://briandeer.com/solved/gmc-wakefield-sentence.pdf

Godlee, F., & Smith, J. (2011). Wakefield's article linking MMR vaccine and autism was fraudulent. *British Medical Journal,* 342, c7452. https://doi.org/10.1136/bmj.c7452

Howard, B. S. (2016). Clinical plagiarism and copyright violations. In D. Y. Slater (Ed.), *Reference guide to the Occupational Therapy Code of Ethics* (2015 ed., pp. 145–148). Bethesda, MD: AOTA Press.

Medicare.gov. (n.d.). *Fraud and abuse.* Retrieved from https://www.medicare.gov/site-search/search-results.html?q=fraud%20and%20abuse

National Board for Certification in Occupational Therapy. (2014). *NBCOT code of conduct.* Retrieved from http://www.nbcot.org/code-of-conduct

Purtilo, R. (2011, April). *A conversation about moral courage.* Lecture presented at the AOTA Annual Conference & Expo, Philadelphia.

Scott, J. B. (2009). Consultation. In E. B. Crepeau, E. S. Cohn, & B. A. B. Schell (Eds.), *Willard and Spackman's occupational therapy* (11th ed., pp. 964–972). Philadelphia: Lippincott Williams & Wilkins.

U. S. Department of Health and Human Services. (n.d.). *Stop Medicare fraud.* Retrieved from https://www.stopmedicarefraud.gov/

Wakefield, A. J., Murch, S. H., Anthony, A., Linnell, J., Casson, D. M., Milik, M., . . . Walker-Smith, J. A. (1998). Ileal-lymphoid-nodular hyperplasia, nonspecific colitis, and pervasive developmental disorder in children. *Lancet, 351,* 637–641.

Chapter 10.

PRINCIPLE 6: FIDELITY

S. Maggie Reitz, PhD, OTR/L, FAOTA

Learning Objectives

By the end of the chapter, readers will be able to

- Describe professional behaviors consistent with Fidelity,
- Determine mechanisms to resolve conflicts within an interdisciplinary team, and
- Apply Principles and Related Standards of Conduct to ethical situations involving working with clients and all colleagues in a fair manner consistent with the profession's and employer's expectations.

Key Terms and Concepts

- ✧ Civility
- ✧ Fidelity
- ✧ Fiduciary
- ✧ Occupational potential
- ✧ Professional relationships

Fidelity

Principle 6. Occupational therapy personnel shall treat clients, colleagues, and other professionals with respect, fairness, discretion, and integrity.

The Principle of Fidelity comes from the Latin root *fidelis,* meaning loyal. *Fidelity* refers to the duty one has to keep a commitment once it is made (Veatch, Haddad, & English, 2010). In the health professions, this commitment refers to promises made between a provider and a client or patient based on an expectation of loyalty, staying with the client or patient in a time of need, and compliance with a code of ethics. These promises can be implied or explicit. The duty to disclose information that is potentially meaningful in making decisions is one obligation of the moral contract between provider and client or patient (Veatch et al., 2010).

Whereas respecting Fidelity requires occupational therapy personnel to meet the client's reasonable expectations, the Principle also addresses maintaining respectful collegial and organizational relationships

(Purtilo & Doherty, 2011). Professional relationships are greatly influenced by the complexity of the environment in which occupational therapy personnel work. Practitioners, educators, and researchers alike must consistently balance their duties to service recipients, students, research participants, and other professionals as well as to organizations that may influence decision making and professional practice.

Related Standards of Conduct

Occupational Therapy Personnel Shall

A. Preserve, respect, and safeguard private information about employees, colleagues, and students unless otherwise mandated or permitted by relevant laws.
B. Address incompetent, disruptive, unethical, illegal, or impaired practice that jeopardizes the safety or well-being of others and team effectiveness.
C. Avoid conflicts of interest or conflicts of commitment in employment, volunteer roles, or research.
D. Avoid using one's position (employee or volunteer) or knowledge gained from that position in such a manner as to give rise to real or perceived conflicts of interest among the person, the employer, other AOTA members, or other organizations.
E. Be diligent stewards of human, financial, and material resources of their employers, and refrain from exploiting these resources for personal gain.
F. Refrain from verbal, physical, emotional, or sexual harassment of peers or colleagues.
G. Refrain from communication that is derogatory, intimidating, or disrespectful and that unduly discourages others from participating in professional dialogue.
H. Promote collaborative actions and communication as a member of interprofessional teams to facilitate quality care and safety for clients.
I. Respect the practices, competencies, roles, and responsibilities of their own and other professions to promote a collaborative environment reflective of interprofessional teams.
J. Use conflict resolution and internal and alternative dispute resolution resources as needed to resolve organizational and interpersonal conflicts, as well as perceived institutional ethics violations.
K. Abide by policies, procedures, and protocols when serving or acting on behalf of a professional organization or employer to fully and accurately represent the organization's official and authorized positions.
L. Refrain from actions that reduce the public's trust in occupational therapy.
M. Self-identify when personal, cultural, or religious values preclude, or are anticipated to negatively affect, the professional relationship or provision of services, while adhering to organizational policies when requesting an exemption from service to an individual or group on the basis of conflict of conscience.

Source. From the *Occupational Therapy Code of Ethics (2015)* (American Occupational Therapy Association, 2015b, pp. 7–8).

Fidelity has been defined as the "faithful fulfillment of vows, promises, and agreements" (Slater, 2016, p. 291). Principle 6, Fidelity, of the *Occupational Therapy Code of Ethics (2015)* (referred to hereafter as the "Code,"; (American Occupational Therapy Association [AOTA], 2015b) focuses on professional relationships and exhibiting faithfulness and loyalty within these relationships. ***Professional relationships*** include those with clients, colleagues across the institution, employers, and institution administrators (AOTA, 2010; Purtilo & Doherty, 2011).

When examining any ethical issue, it is important to review all Principles and then weigh the possible conflicting values before taking action. Within the Principle of Fidelity, balance also is stressed; occupational therapy practitioners have a duty to balance loyalty to clients with loyalty to colleagues, employers, and institutions.

After an historical overview of fidelity in occupational therapy ethics, this chapter applies the Principle to various aspects of occupational therapy practice through two case studies and several vignettes. These applications address respect, civility, transparency, and the stewardship of resources. In addition, the duty to prevent ethical breaches and resolve them in an appropriate manner is reviewed.

Although occupational therapy practitioners are obligated to their clients as well as their colleagues and students, the focus of Principle 6 is on the importance of maintaining and nurturing professional relationships to facilitate the ultimate goal of enhanced client care. Professional behaviors related to the Principle of Fidelity can be categorized via the associated Related Standards of Conduct (RSCs) as respect (RSCs 6A, 6F, 6G, 6I), prevention and analysis of potential ethical breaches (RSCs 6B, 6H, 6J, 6L, 6M), prevention of possible conflicts (RSCs 6C, 6D), and stewardship of resources (RSCs 6E, 6I, 6K).

Overview of Fidelity

Fidelity centers on relationships. As stated above, professional relationships are greatly influenced by the complexity of the environment in which occupational therapy personnel work.

> Practitioners, educators, and researchers alike must consistently balance their duties to service recipients, students, research participants, and other professionals as well as to organizations that may influence decision making and professional practice. (AOTA, 2015b, p. 7)

In discussions of fidelity, the term *fiduciary* often appears. ***Fiduciary*** refers to

> a person, often in the position of authority, who obligates himself or herself to act on the behalf of another and assumes a duty to act in good faith and with care, candor, and loyalty in fulfilling the obligation. (Slater, 2016, p. 291)

In ways beyond merely managing physical objects or money, occupational therapy practitioners are obligated to clients, students, peers, employers, and employees, as well as fellow board members and fellow volunteers on professional committees or commissions or in other groups. We are obligated to their care and the fulfillment of their ***occupational potential,*** defined by Wilcock (2006) as the "future capability to engage in occupation toward needs, goals, and dreams for health, material requirement, happiness, and well-being" (p. 343).

History of Fidelity in Occupational Therapy

The focus of the ethical principles articulated by the profession at its founding was on the provision of ethical and competent care, not on professional relationships. The profession addressed the value and importance of professional relationships at a later date. The spirit of the current Principle 6 first appeared in *Principles of Occupational Therapy Ethics* (AOTA, 1978) under two separate principles:

- *IV. Related to intraprofessional colleagues:* The occupational therapist shall function with discretion and integrity in relations with other members of the profession and shall be concerned with the quality of their services. Upon becoming aware of objective evidence of a breach of ethics or substandard service, the occupational therapist shall take action according to established procedure.
- *V. Related to other personnel:* The occupational therapist shall function with discretion and integrity in relations with personnel and cooperate with them as may be appropriate. Similarly, the occupational therapist expects others to demonstrate a high level of competence. Upon becoming aware of objective evidence of a breach of ethics or substandard service, the occupational therapist shall take action according to established procedure (p. 710).

When the principles were organized into the *Occupational Therapy Code of Ethics* in 1988, only one of these two principles remained: Principle 5, which was renamed "Professional Relationships" (AOTA, 1988). Six years later, when the Code was again revised, the term *fidelity* first appeared in Principle 6 (AOTA, 1994, p. 1038): "Occupational therapy personnel shall treat colleagues and other professionals with fairness, discretion, and integrity (fidelity, veracity)." In the 2000 revision of the Code, *veracity and fidelity* were separated into two distinct principles. Principle 6 focused on truthfulness, whereas Principle 7 primarily addressed fidelity; the wording of the Principle remained the same except for the removal of the term *veracity* (AOTA, 2000).

In the 2005 revision, the term *respect* was added to Principle 7 (AOTA, 2005), and that language remained in effect in the next version: "Occupational therapy personnel shall treat colleagues and other professionals with respect, fairness, discretion, and integrity" (AOTA, 2010, p. S24). The word *client* was added to what is now Principle 6 in the current version of the Code to emphasize the dual responsibility to treat both clients and fellow professionals with civility; "occupational therapy personnel shall treat clients, colleagues, and other professionals with respect, fairness, discretion, and integrity" (AOTA, 2015b, p. 7).

Respect

Calls for ***civility,*** an outward display of respect, have been increasing in recent times in business, politics, education, and health care and within communities. The American Medical Association (2011) recently announced that about 20% of graduating medical students reported being mistreated and that the Association would take action to lower this figure. The most frequent type of mistreatment medical students reported was humiliation and belittlement by faculty, residents, and fellow students. Respect is the topic of Vignette 10.1, which takes place in an occupational therapy education classroom, and Vignette 10.2, which unfolds in the hallway of an academic department. Situations similar to those described in these vignettes could easily occur in other practice settings.

Prevention and Analysis of Potential Ethical Breaches

The need to be vigilant in identifying potential ethical issues and preventing breaches if at all possible is one of the themes woven throughout Principle 6. However, if an ethical breach has already occurred, then occupational therapy practitioners need to take steps to resolve the issue directly without escalating the issue to other levels unless necessary. Sometimes the behavior warrants the involvement of other entities. Vigilance is required

Vignette 10.1. Showing Respect

Carmen was excited about starting her first faculty position. The semester was going well, and she felt well prepared to share her expertise with her students. A few weeks later, however, she became concerned when a student, **Mary,** started leaving the class for 10-minute intervals on a regular basis. Carmen thought this unusual and was concerned about Mary's inability to remain seated and concentrate for the 50-minute lectures. She also was concerned because Mary's frequent departures caused Carmen to lose her focus and disrupted the other students' attention. Carmen could tell by observing their nonverbal communication, including unprofessional behaviors such as rolling their eyes and making sidebar comments, that the rest of the class was frustrated by Mary's behavior. Carmen knew she needed to take action before the situation further deteriorated, but she was unsure what to do.

After class, Carmen scheduled a meeting to discuss the situation with the program director, **Kurt.** At the meeting, they both agreed that Mary's and the other students' behaviors were disrespectful but that Mary's behavior should be addressed first. Carmen e-mailed Mary and asked her to meet before class. Carmen told Mary that her behavior of frequently leaving class was disruptive and disrespectful to both the class and to her as the professor. Mary was mortified and said that she had not realized how her behavior affected others and that she was not intentionally being disrespectful. Using the problem-solving and activity analysis skills she was learning, Mary determined that she needed to wake up earlier so she had time to find a parking spot and visit the restroom before class. Mary thanked Carmen for bringing this to her attention and asked if she could apologize to the class. Carmen agreed, and they went to class together.

Vignette 10.2. Promoting a Climate of Civility

Amanda was a graduate assistant for **Dr. Howell.** She was working on a literature review for a project of Dr. Howell's and had a question. Amanda approached the faculty office hallway and overheard Dr. Howell and another faculty member talking about a third faculty member in very disparaging terms. Amanda coughed to alert them to her presence, but after acknowledging her presence they continued their conversation in a similar manner. She then returned to the graduate assistant office and sat there feeling awkward, wondering what she should do.

In the days that followed, Amanda was frozen in non-action and felt ill and distracted. She started missing classes, calling in sick, and missing work hours with Dr. Howell. Dr. Howell became frustrated because she was working on a deadline for a complex grant application, and she fired Amanda. Amanda considered warning Dr. Howell's newly hired graduate assistant about the inappropriate behavior of the faculty. Amanda was concerned, however, that this behavior, like Dr. Howell's, would be disrespectful, so she abandoned that plan.

Instead, Amanda sought out the program director, **Dr. Casey,** and reported her observations and her concern that if she reported Dr. Howell's behavior, it might appear to be in retaliation for being fired. Although not excusing Dr. Howell's behavior, Dr. Casey shared that the faculty were under a great deal of stress because of statewide budget cuts and that she was planning to address the level of stress and adaptive versus maladaptive coping strategies at the next faculty meeting. Dr. Casey also reminded Amanda that if she saw a repeat of Dr. Howell's behavior, she should be prepared to address her concerns directly with Dr. Howell. Dr. Casey offered to mentor Amanda on how to approach Dr. Howell if this situation was to recur.

Dr. Casey followed through with her plan to discuss adaptive stress reduction techniques at the faculty meeting and reminded faculty about the importance of role modeling professional behavior and collegiality. Which Principles are supported by this action? Does this action violate any of the Principles? What other actions could or should Amanda or Dr. Casey take?

to see and address unethical behaviors before they become entrenched in individuals or organizations. Addressing potential unethical behavior can be challenging and uncomfortable but is the necessary and preferred action because it can prevent harm to clients, coworkers, the institution, and the profession. An example of how an occupational therapist identified a potential problem and addressed it without escalation is provided in Case Study 10.1.

Prevention of Possible Conflicts

Although open communication and transparency can assist in preventing conflicts, not all conflicts can or should be prevented. For example, failure to confront an individual or group regarding unethical behavior because of fear of a potential conflict is a violation of the Code, specifically RSCs 2E, 2F, 4F, 4K, 4L, 6J, 6K, and 6L. However, if the potential for a conflict is known, occupational therapy practitioners can take steps to resolve it quickly before the conflict has a chance to expand and take important time away from other institutional priorities. (Avoidance of conflicts of interest and commitment was discussed in Chapter 6 on Nonmaleficence; see Vignettes 6.4 and 6.6.) In Case Study 10.2, an occupational therapist deals with conflict provoked by a lack of transparency.

Stewardship of Resources

Occupational therapy personnel in supervisory positions are stewards of a variety of resources, including equipment, supplies, and time. The largest expense in an occupational therapy department budget is usually salaries. Occupational therapy practitioners and their supervisors must be ethical in their time usage because this is a valuable (and therefore expensive) resource. Depending on the circumstances, misuse of time may constitute mere inefficiency, or it may constitute fraud.

Social interaction among team members while on the job is essential to team building and collaboration. Occupational therapy practitioners need

Case Study 10.1. Analyzing and Preventing a Potential Ethics Breach

Noemi, the occupational therapy supervisor at a skilled nursing facility, was excited to learn that **Bonnie,** one of the occupational therapy staff, was presenting at the state association conference. Noemi arrived early to the session to be sure to get a good seat and wish Bonnie well, but Bonnie was not in the room. As time passed, Noemi double-checked her conference schedule to make sure she was in the correct room. Finally, Bonnie arrived. Noemi overheard someone in the audience say, "Oh, the presenter was in that group having so much fun in the bar last night with that guy **Don.** I could never drink before presenting; I would wait to celebrate after I had presented! If she partied that hard last night, I wonder what she will do tonight?"

When it was time for Bonnie to begin her presentation, she dropped her notes, became flustered, and stated, "I wish someone would bring me a drink to settle my nerves." She continued with the presentation, frequently apologizing for not being prepared. After the presentation was over, Noemi waited for the other audience participants to leave and approached Bonnie. Bonnie said, "I am glad that's over; let's go get drinks." Noemi agreed to go with Bonnie but said that she wanted to talk to her about her presentation. Although Noemi was worried about the health and well-being of Bonnie, she also was concerned for the reputation of her staff and facility.

Once they were seated, Noemi asked Bonnie some open-ended questions to have Bonnie reflect on her performance. As the conversation unfolded, Bonnie told of unexpectedly meeting a group of occupational therapy school alums the night before and losing track of time as she enjoyed the impromptu reunion and reconnected with Don, an "old flame." Noemi then shared the comment she had heard before the presentation started about Bonnie's behavior at the bar. Bonnie was embarrassed and declined an offer of a second drink from the server, saying she needed to get home.

When Noemi returned to work the following week, she reviewed the Code, particularly Principle 2, Nonmaleficence, and Principle 6, Fidelity. She was concerned that Bonnie might have an evolving substance abuse problem or other personal issues that could affect both client care and Bonnie's own well-being. Noemi reviewed the time records and productivity measures for all 5 occupational therapists who reported to her. She discovered that Bonnie had a pattern of arriving late to work most Fridays.

When Noemi met with Bonnie, Bonnie at first was angry and wanted to know why she was being picked on. Noemi explained that she had reviewed the attendance records of all 5 therapists. Bonnie then admitted that she regularly went to a happy hour on Thursday nights at a bar that was a favorite among out-of-town, young businessmen. The happy hours and related socialization kept her up quite late. The businessmen only had to fly home the next day, but Bonnie had to wake up early and go to work. Noemi was sympathetic about Bonnie wanting a social life; however, Noemi told Bonnie that her attendance pattern had to be modified if she wanted to keep her job. In addition, she provided Bonnie with materials from human resources about their employee assistance program.

The following Friday, Bonnie reported to work early, brought Noemi her favorite muffin, and thanked her for taking the time to address the issue before it escalated further. If Bonnie's behavior had continued and adversely affected client care, Noemi had been prepared to report Bonnie to the appropriate institution officials and, if needed, the appropriate professional regulatory bodies. Soon thereafter, Noemi was relieved to see that Bonnie was making adjustments to ensure that her personal lifestyle did not affect her punctuality and job performance.

to network and spend time communicating with colleagues both within and external to the department. They are obligated, however, to ensure that this networking supports both collegiality and client care. Frequent socialization at the expense of the performance of other job duties or persistent use of work time to perform personal life tasks is inappropriate and unethical. An incident involving the fraudulent use of time by an employee is detailed in Vignette 10.3.

Case Study 10.2. Preventing Conflict by Promoting Transparency

Candace was a 30-year-old computer programmer with chronic schizophrenia. Following an acute episode of psychosis and subsequent hospitalization, Candace lost her job. When she got out of the hospital, she joined a local clubhouse to ease back into community responsibilities and find a new job. There she met **Eleanor,** a clubhouse staff member and occupational therapist, who provided her with an orientation to the clubhouse model and a tour of the facility.

At the end of the orientation, Eleanor asked Candace how she had learned about the program and whether she had any questions. Candace explained that her inpatient occupational therapist had recommended the clubhouse. She also said that she had been very reluctant to join the clubhouse but that the occupational therapist had convinced her to join by telling her that she could get paid for duties such as assisting with upgrading the computers at the facility and that they would find her a permanent full-time job. Eleanor had to inform Candace that it was not possible for the clubhouse to pay members for their duties at the facility; however, she also explained that they could train her and find her a temporary position, but it was up to Candace to find permanent employment for herself with the support of clubhouse staff.

Eleanor was familiar with many of the occupational therapists at the hospital where Candace disclosed she had been admitted, so Eleanor decided to call and make sure the hospital staff had accurate information about the clubhouse model and available services. She spoke with **Hannah,** the director of the occupational therapy department, which provided services to clients with both mental illness and physical dysfunctions. Hannah explained that sometimes they chose to misinform clients or exaggerate what the clubhouse offered to get people to become members. In the course of the conversation, it became apparent that Hannah, who specialized in stroke rehabilitation, did not have much concern for or knowledge about the importance of transitional mental health services. When Eleanor suggested to the director that exaggerating the services offered at the clubhouse might raise ethical concerns, Hannah became very defensive and stated that she was more experienced and had a more advanced degree than Eleanor. She told Eleanor to "forget the whole thing."

Eleanor had followed the guidance of Principle 6 and had attempted to handle the situation locally without escalating the situation and involving more people than needed. Hannah, however, chose to be confrontational and obstructive. Instead of forgetting about the whole thing as Hannah had directed, Eleanor reflected on the options available to her to ensure that clients were told the truth about the clubhouse and the available services while minimizing potential conflict, if possible. After a period of reflection and review of the Code, Eleanor considered her options. The potential actions and an analysis of the pros and cons of each appear in Table 10.1.

Table 10.1. Decision Table for Case Study 10.2

Possible Action	Positive Outcomes	Negative Consequences
No action.	Eleanor avoids potential conflicts with Hannah and the occupational therapy staff.	Patients continue to be lied to at the hospital. This action does not uphold Principle 6 and also fails to uphold Principles 1, 2, and 5.
Review the MOU between the clubhouse and the hospital and discuss with Hannah.	Eleanor seeks to bring hospital policies into line with ethical practice. Hannah may provide more accurate information to potential clients.	Patients may continue to be lied to at the hospital. Eleanor may cause conflict with Hannah and hospital staff. This action does not uphold Principle 6 and also fails to uphold Principles 1, 2, and 5.

(Continued)

Case Study 10.2. Preventing Conflict by Promoting Transparency *(Cont.)*

Table 10.1. Decision Table for Case Study 10.2 *(Cont.)*

Possible Action	Positive Outcomes	Negative Consequences
Review current clubhouse marketing materials, both printed and on the website, work with clubhouse members to make edits to ensure clarity, and send updated materials to Hannah.	Eleanor seeks to bring hospital policies into line with ethical practice. Hannah may provide more accurate information to potential clients. This action upholds Principles 3 and 5, especially RSC 5B.	Patients may continue to be lied to at the hospital. This action fails to uphold Principles 1, 2, and 5.
Request a formal meeting with Hannah and a clubhouse member to review the current MOU and to review the updated marketing materials.	Eleanor opens an honest dialogue that is client centered. If the meeting is successful, this action upholds all Principles.	Hannah could refuse to meet, and this might distress the clubhouse member. If the meeting is not held, Eleanor fails to uphold Principles 1, 2, 5, and 6. Patients would continue to be lied to at the hospital, resulting in failure to uphold Principles 1, 2, and 5.
Request a meeting with the clubhouse executive board for guidance.	Because of the care taken to try other local, direct strategies first, this action upholds RSC 6I. Eleanor's action follows the chain of command at the clubhouse.	Eleanor may cause conflict with other hospital employees. Patients may continue to be lied to at the hospital.
Report Hannah to appropriate regulatory bodies.	Eleanor seeks to bring hospital occupational therapy practices into line with the Code. Eleanor's action follows the chain of command at her place of employment. This action may encourage the upholding of all Principles.	Eleanor may cause conflict with Hannah and other hospital employees.

Note. MOU = memorandum of understanding; RSCs = Related Standards of Conduct.

Vignette 10.3. Addressing Resources Misuse

Ralph, an occupational therapy supervisor for the past 5 years, was proud of his department's productivity and ability to positively influence clients' lives. **Miranda,** a head nurse, stopped him in the hall one day and asked to speak to him. He was surprised when she reported that the new graduate they had just hired, **Tim,** was playing online poker and flirting at the nursing station. Although Ralph was aware that Tim spent a good deal of time networking on the nursing units, he believed this to be a positive behavior. Now he was concerned that Tim's behavior was having a negative impact on clients.

Ralph decided to collect more information because he did not want to confront Tim on the basis of only one person's perception. Unfortunately, the 3 unit head nurses reported similar behavior. In addition, as Ralph left the office of one of the head nurses, he saw Tim playing a video. Because it was near lunchtime, Ralph asked Tim if he would like to join him for lunch.

Ralph opened the lunchtime discussion by asking Tim how he was balancing the need for productivity with his enjoyment of the social milieu of the hospital. As the discussion unfolded, Tim confirmed that he was having difficulty with that balance. He had been rounding up his documented productivity minutes, as he had seen done while at his Level II fieldwork placement.

Ralph informed Tim that this was unethical behavior, as was his use of work time to play games, and that he would be placed on a more intensive mentoring program. Ralph further explained that charging patients for services not rendered was fraud and could jeopardize both Tim's job and his license. Ralph also informed Tim that he would arrange a meeting with the hospital's accountant and lawyer to determine what corrective actions were needed. Ralph then strongly encouraged Tim to report his actions and planned remediation to the state regulatory board as soon as possible, because it would be in his best interest to self-report his behavior than for Ralph to contact the board.

Summary

Occupational therapy practitioners are human and, therefore, fallible. Principle 6, Fidelity, encourages practitioners to acknowledge this fact and seek to minimize ethical violations and their repercussions through preventive action. Occupational therapy practitioners need to be proactive and strengthen collegiality to promote the well-being of our clients, colleagues, and employers.

By concentrating on developing a positive, respectful climate and instituting other preventive strategies, practitioners can diminish the severity and frequency of unprofessional behaviors. However, if unprofessional behaviors are evidenced and are egregious or frequent, Principle 6, together with the Code (AOTA, 2015a), provides guidance as to the necessary next steps.

Reflective Questions

- How do you define fidelity in your personal life? How do you define fidelity in your professional life? Are the definitions different, and if so, why?
- Review Vignettes 10.1 and 10.2. Describe how these could play out in another practice area and what actions you would take to prevent or address the issues.
- How could students or coworkers find themselves in a conflict of interest situation? What is the responsibility of students, employees, and employers to prevent this from occurring?

References

American Medical Association. (2011). One in five medical school grads report mistreatment; AMA taking action. *AMA MedEd Update*. Retrieved from www.ama-assn.org/ama/pub/meded/2011-august/2011-august.shtml

American Occupational Therapy Association. (1978). Principles of occupational therapy ethics. In H. L. Hopkins & H. D. Smith (Eds.), *Willard and Spackman's occupational therapy* (5th ed., pp. 709–710). Philadelphia: Lippincott.

American Occupational Therapy Association. (1988). Occupational therapy code of ethics. *American Journal of Occupational Therapy, 42,* 795–796. https://doi.org/10.5014/ajot.42.12.795

American Occupational Therapy Association. (1994). Occupational therapy code of ethics. *American Journal of Occupational Therapy, 48,* 1037–1038. https://doi.org/10.5014/ajot.48.11.1037

American Occupational Therapy Association. (2000). Occupational therapy code of ethics (2000). *American Journal of Occupational Therapy, 54,* 614–616. https://doi.org/10.5014/ajot.54.6.614

American Occupational Therapy Association. (2005). Occupational therapy code of ethics (2005). *American Journal of Occupational Therapy, 59,* 639–642. https://doi.org/10.5014/ajot.59.6.639

American Occupational Therapy Association. (2010). Occupational therapy code of ethics and ethics standards (2010). *American Journal of Occupational Therapy, 64*(Suppl. 6), S17–S26. https://doi.org/10.5014/ajot2010.62S17

American Occupational Therapy Association. (2015a). Enforcement procedures for the occupational therapy code of ethics. *American Journal of Occupational Therapy, 69*(Suppl. 3), 6913410012. https://doi.org/10.5014/ajot.2015.696S19

American Occupational Therapy Association. (2015b). Occupational therapy code of ethics (2015). *American Journal of Occupational Therapy, 69*(Suppl. 3), 6913410030. https://doi.org/10.5014/ajot.2015.696S03

Purtilo, R. B., & Doherty, R. F. (2011). *Ethical dimensions in the health professions* (5th ed.). St. Louis: Elsevier/Saunders.

Slater, D. Y. (Ed.). (2016). Glossary of ethics terms. In *Reference guide to the Occupational Therapy Code of Ethics* (2015 ed., pp. 291–292). Bethesda, MD: AOTA Press.

Veatch, R. M., Haddad, A. M., & English, D. C. (2010). *Case studies in biomedical ethics*. New York: Oxford University Press.

Wilcock, A. A. (2006). *An occupational perspective of health* (2nd ed.). Thorofare, NJ: Slack.

Part III.

APPLICATIONS

INTRODUCTION TO PART III

Janie B. Scott, MA, OT/L, FAOTA, and S. Maggie Reitz, PhD, OTR/L, FAOTA

The chapters in Part III each focus on a specific area of practice. Chapters 11–16 address the American Occupational Therapy Association's (AOTA's, 2016) primary practice areas:

- Mental health
- Productive aging
- Children and youth
- Health promotion and wellness
- Work and industry
- Participation, disability, and rehabilitation.

In addition to these primary practice areas, Chapter 17 addresses ethics in administration and management, Chapter 18 discusses ethics in higher education, Chapter 19 explores ethics in occupational therapy research, Chapter 20 discusses interprofessional ethics, and Chapter 21 addresses ethics and culture. Each chapter is aligned with the *Occupational Therapy Code of Ethics (2015)* (AOTA, 2015).

When reviewing the case studies and vignettes in Part III or addressing their own ethical dilemmas, readers are encouraged to remember and use their knowledge base as occupational therapy practitioners. Occupational therapy practitioners' and students' academic knowledge of activity analysis, human performance, and the other elements of competent practice provides them with the skills and ability to analyze and solve ethical dilemmas.

After examining the various situations and ways to approach dilemma resolution presented in Part III, readers can apply their knowledge of the topic area through reflective questions at the end of each chapter. The goal of this process is to increase readers' confidence in their own ability to personally take action, when necessary, for the good of clients and the profession.

References

American Occupational Therapy Association. (2015). Occupational therapy code of ethics (2015). *American Journal of Occupational Therapy, 69*(Suppl. 3), 6912310030. https://doi.org/10.5014/ajot.2015.696S03

American Occupational Therapy Association. (2016). *Practice.* https://www.aota.org/Practice.aspx

Chapter 11.

MENTAL HEALTH: ETHICS IN DIVERSE SETTINGS

Scott A. Trudeau, PhD, OTR/L, and Janie B. Scott, MA, OT/L, FAOTA

Learning Objectives

By the end of the chapter, readers will be able to

- Describe the unique ethical considerations for occupational practice in diverse mental health settings;
- Analyze the relationship of psychiatric symptoms and mental health considerations with ethical principles; and
- Apply the Principles and Related Standards of Conduct from the *Occupational Therapy Code of Ethics (2015)* to decisions that occupational therapy practitioners may encounter in mental health settings.

Key Terms and Concepts

- ✧ Assertive community treatment
- ✧ Comorbidity
- ✧ Delusions
- ✧ Integrated primary care practices
- ✧ Interprofessional team
- ✧ Partial hospital program
- ✧ Primary health care
- ✧ Psychosocial rehabilitation program
- ✧ Workforce development initiatives

The practice of occupational therapy with clients coping with mental illness poses specific ethical challenges that may be slightly different than those encountered with other populations. The basis of this difference is rooted in both the nature of the impairments associated with mental illness and the social context in which the illness occurs. Individuals with psychiatric morbidity deserve the same access to preventive and health care services as those without mental illness, yet disparities persist.

Socially, stigma and bias continue to run rampant—especially in the wake of events that associate horrific violent events with mental illness and draw major media coverage (Metzl & MacLeish, 2015). Therefore, the complexity of occupational therapy practice with individuals experiencing mental health challenges can present a multitude of ethical considerations for practitioners.

The intersection of legal and ethical considerations, which may at times be at odds with each other, is one of the most obvious areas of conflict for practitioners. The need to compromise an individual's basic right for self-determination by imposing unwanted treatment must never be taken lightly. Legally, that determination is typically made when an individual is assessed to be in imminent danger of significant harm to self or others (Brown, Beck, & Steer, 2000; Janofsky & Tamburello, 2006).

In spite of this legal determination, occupational therapy practitioners still need to develop a therapeutic relationship with each individual client. How does one support choice and motivation for engagement in occupational therapy interventions in this situation? This presents a significant challenge not only in the formulation of the interpersonal relationship but also in the development and client acceptance of the plan of care.

Further complicating the current provision of mental health services in the United States are the shifting priorities of the health care system and demands for ever-evolving service delivery models in response to health care reform legislation and the restructuring of reimbursement models. This relative uncertainty of demands in a variety of practice settings sets the stage for practitioners to experience unanticipated ethical challenges that must be recognized and systematically responded to by occupational therapy providers. This chapter reviews many of these issues and provides guidance for addressing ethical concerns that may arise when applying the *Occupational Therapy Code of Ethics (2015)* (referred to as the "Code"; American Occupational Therapy Association [AOTA], 2015b).

Comorbidity

People experiencing mental illness frequently have difficulty perceiving reality and thus may lack insight into their illness. ***Comorbidity*** is not infrequent among this population and is defined as "when two disorders or illnesses occur in the same person, simultaneously, or sequentially. Comorbidity also implies interactions between the disorder [or] illness that affect the course and prognosis of both" (National Institute on Drug Abuse, 2010, para. 1).

Comorbidity is often seen among the population seeking mental health or behavioral health services. Occupational therapy practitioners' knowledge of mental illnesses and substance use disorders is imperative when providing interventions to this population. According to the Substance Abuse Mental Health Services Administration (SAMHSA), "integrated treatment or treatment that addresses mental and substance use conditions at the same time is associated with lower costs and better outcomes" (2015, para. 20). The presence of comorbid conditions increases the complexity of the required care and treatment options. This can present ethical issues because decisions may need to be made about which issues are paramount at any given time.

Interprofessional Teams

Mental health practice has a long tradition of being interdisciplinary. The complex nature of cases with emotional burden that are seen in diverse mental health settings requires an experienced, synchronous, well-functioning interprofessional team to best serve clients. The varied contributions of each discipline can play an important role in addressing the individual needs of each client. This ***interprofessional team*** model meets the needs of clients while simultaneously providing a support system for staff.

Interprofessional teams in mental health practice include patients or clients and professionals (e.g., occupational therapy practitioners, psychiatrists, psychologists, nurses, pharmacists, students who work collaboratively in the best interest of the service recipient). This collaboration is especially important when lengths of stay could span months and therapeutic relationships need to be sustained across that period of time.

Interprofessional teams can serve as a source of support for practitioners as they strive to manage the inter- and intrapersonal demands of working with emotionally challenging cases. The team may serve as a resource in solving ethical dilemmas that are encountered during their transdisciplinary interventions, or are faced by a group member. Historically, people with mental illness were treated in institutional settings (see Chapter 2, "Historical Background of Ethics in Occupational Therapy"). Typically these institutions often were locked acute psychiatric units in general hospitals or, for people with more serious mental illness, a state hospital setting.

Changing Contexts of Mental Health Care

As early as the Mental Retardation Facilities and Community Mental Health Construction Act of 1963 (P. L. 88–164), legislators recognized that institutional care might not be the best model for the treatment of individuals with developmental or intellectual disabilities (Sheth, 2009). Since then, the U.S. health care system has attempted to shift focus from institutional care to new community-based models of care. This change has resulted in significantly decreased lengths of stay in acute inpatient contexts, which can have ethical implications (Ithman, Goplarkrishna, Beck, Das, & Petroski, 2014). Decreasing lengths of stay may result in individuals transitioning out of treatment sooner than desired by the interprofessional team.

Another issue resulting from this shift away from institutional care is that the threshold to be eligible for psychiatric hospitalization is much higher. This shift can be summarized by the colloquialism that mental health care is now "sicker and quicker." Service options now range from medical models to peer- or consumer-driven models of care. Models can range from locked acute psychiatric units to partial hospital programs to consumer-run clubhouse models.

Assertive Community Treatment

The shift to community models of care has generated the development of the concept of ***assertive community treatment,*** which is a "team-based care model to coordinate a client's care" (National Alliance on Mental Illness [NAMI], n.d., para. 6) and may involve mobile outreach treatment interventions. A clearly defined continuum of care no longer exists in mental health treatment. This fragmentation and variation in mental health service delivery make a clear definition of occupational therapy mental health practice difficult.

The movement of models of care, such as assertive community treatment, beyond the boundaries of traditional health care settings challenges care providers to think on their feet and often in isolation from other care providers. This context requires that occupational therapy practitioners know their ethical obligations so they can provide sound care to individuals with mental illness.

Settings where mental health services are delivered include but are not limited to

- Addiction recovery services (Mosaic, 2016),
- Behavioral health clinics (Mosaic, 2016; SAMHSA, 2015),
- Behavioral home health (Mosaic, 2016; SAMHSA, 2015),
- Hospital emergency rooms (Haiman & Slater, 2013; SAMHSA, 2015),
- Integrated primary care practices (SAMHSA, 2015),
- Jails and prisons (SAMHSA, 2015),
- Medical day care (Mosaic, 2016),
- Mobile treatment services (Mosaic, 2016; NAMI, n.d.),
- Mutual support groups and peer-run organizations (Haiman & Slater, 2013; NAMI, n.d.; SAMHSA, 2015),
- Psychiatric rehabilitation day programs (Haiman & Slater, 2013; Mosaic, 2016),
- Residential crisis programs (Mosaic, 2016; NAMI, n.d.),
- Residential rehabilitation services (Mosaic, 2016; NAMI, n.d.),
- Schools (SAMHSA, 2015),
- Substance abuse assessment and treatment services (Mosaic, 2016; NAMI, n.d.; SAMHSA, 2015), and
- Wrap-around services (Mosaic, 2016).

Integrating Health Care

New legislation may shift service delivery further. The Mental Health Reform Act of 2016 (S. 2680) and the Keeping Families on Mental Health Crises Act of 2016 (H.R. 2646) were folded into the 21st Century Cures Act (P. L. 114–255), which was signed into law December 2016. It seeks to address persistent health disparities by further integrating behavioral health (i.e., mental health) care into models of primary health care (American Psychological Association, 2016). ***Primary health care*** consists of integrated and accessible basic services, including programs aimed at promoting health, increasing early diagnosis of disease or disability, and preventing disease (AOTA, 2014). People with mental health disorders have higher rates of mortality than the average person. These higher mortality rates stem mostly from poor management of chronic illnesses coupled with poor health habits such as inadequate physical activity, poor nutrition, smoking, and substance abuse.

Barriers to primary care, coupled with difficulty maneuvering through the complex health care system, have contributed to limiting access to health maintenance activities for people with mental illness. These disparities raise concerns about the ethical Principle of Justice as it relates to accessing quality primary health care services. ***Integrated primary care practices*** embed traditional medically focused care with behavioral health care in the same clinical practice setting, thus providing a one-stop shop for clients (SAMHSA, 2016).

This integrated model seems to propose a holistic approach to wellness, embracing both physical and mental health needs, which is consistent with the occupational therapy philosophy of care. This legislation specifically identifies occupational therapy as a service necessary for workforce development initiatives to support integrated primary care practices. ***Workforce development initiatives*** include educational support and loan forgiveness programs funded by the government for practitioners from key disciplines. If enacted, this law could encourage future occupational therapy students/practitioners to consider working in behavioral health practice settings, ultimately increasing the presence of occupational therapy practitioners in mental health service delivery settings.

Shifting Role of Occupational Therapy

The profession of occupational therapy has its roots in working with soldiers with posttraumatic stress disorders and other mental illnesses, yet currently only a small percentage of occupational therapy practitioners identify their primary work setting as mental health (AOTA, 2015a). Further, one of the fundamental distinctions between occupational therapy and other rehabilitation professions is the training and emphasis on working with the emotional influences that may interfere with occupational performance.

According to AOTA (2015a), 5.2% of occupational therapists identified working in mental health in 2000, which declined to 2.4% in 2014. Similar trends were noted for occupational therapy assistants, with 5.4% reporting employment in mental health settings in 2000, decreasing to only 1.4% in 2014.

Moving away from working in mental health may represent an ethical dilemma for the occupational therapy profession. What is the possible cause for this shift in the workforce? Perhaps some of the complexity and variability of care settings may be part of the answer. We would be remiss, though, not to consider other factors. Is there a more malevolent force behind this issue? Are there perceived or real pay differences for work in mental health versus other settings? Could it relate to the stigma and bias that demonizes those with mental illness or mental health issues?

One might question whether bias has infiltrated our educational programs, leading to a lower priority being placed on preparation for mental health practice. For example, the Accreditation Council for Occupational Therapy Education® (ACOTE®) no longer requires that all entry-level students complete a mental health Level II Fieldwork (ACOTE, 2012). Without developing entry-level competencies through a Level II experience, how can a novice practitioner enter the complex work setting of mental health? As you can see, the answer to most ethical questions generates more questions. Weighing the multiple factors that influence situations to truly understand the core values through a process of ethical reasoning is rarely a purely linear path.

Ethical Considerations in Mental Health Occupational Therapy

The Code (AOTA, 2015b) is organized around six ethical Principles (i.e., Beneficence, Nonmaleficence, Autonomy, Justice, Veracity, Fidelity). In this section, each Principle is briefly presented, along with implications for occupational therapy mental health practice.

Principle 1. Beneficence

According to Principle 1, Beneficence, "occupational therapy personnel shall demonstrate a concern for the well-being and safety of the recipients of their services" (AOTA, 2015b, p. 2). This Principle speaks to the practitioner's imperative to make a positive impact on a client's life. In practice, this often centers on using our distinct skill set and practicing within the scope of our license to advance the occupational engagement of the clients we serve. Well-being and safety are always integral to the care of anyone with mental illness. However, as noted above, maintenance of safety often includes compromising self-determination and autonomy. Individuals whose safety is in question because of mental illness may lack insight into the gravity of their risk for harm. In this case, others must intercede to protect the individual

Case Study 11.1. Language Matters

Carlos was in a locked in-patient psychiatric unit with a diagnosis of schizophrenia, paranoid type, after reports that he threatened his mother with a butcher knife at home. His mother, **Rosa,** called 911, and the police transported Carlos to the emergency room for evaluation.

On intake, Carlos presented with limited English but readily conveyed basic needs. It was unclear, because of the language barrier and the presence of psychotic thinking, if he had been compliant with taking his prescribed medications recently. Because of Carlos's preference for speaking in his primary language, the team met to identify options to overcoming these language barriers.

The occupational therapist on the team explored the need for language interpreters and discovered in RSC 3J and Principle 4, Justice, the importance of reducing barriers for individuals to access services and providing services in a language that promotes their understanding. The team found an attending psychiatrist on staff who spoke fluent Spanish and also identified an interpreter service used by the hospital. The team also looked into another foreign language real-time translation service, MARTTI (My Accessible Real-Time Trusted Interpreter), used by behavioral health programs. The team reviewed these options and decided to use the hospital's interpreter service.

Carlos was injected with two doses of Haldol 10 mg, IM in the emergency room against his will. He had a history of 5 previous psychiatric admissions, each precipitated by similar aggressive behavior at home. Rosa reported that during this most recent incident, they were arguing over his taking medications.

Here, the desire to help Carlos regain his ability to process reality and limit his aggressive behavior superseded his right to refuse medication. Although the immediate threat of aggressive behavior would seem to justify this, a careful review of the details was required to ensure that other options that might not compromise his autonomy (Principle 3) were not overlooked.

Although this case did not seem to directly involve occupational therapy practitioners, this process set the stage for future occupational therapy involvement. Additionally, the occupational therapist was instrumental in advocating for Carlos during the team's conversation regarding the need and options for reducing language barriers to ensure that Carlos's need for involuntary medications was justified (RSC 3J).

or others from danger, at times without the client's consent. You can see that the process of ethical decision making is not always obvious, straightforward, or intuitive. Case Study 11.1 presents an ethical situation in which client consent, autonomy, and reducing language barriers are weighed.

Principle 2. Nonmaleficence

According to Principle 2, Nonmaleficence, "occupational therapy personnel shall refrain from actions that cause harm" (AOTA, 2015b, p. 3). Harm may be caused through a multitude of methods whereby practitioners provide undue influence on clients, students, individuals, supervised employees, research participants, and others. Occupational therapy practitioners are advised by the Code to avoid situations that may cause harm to others through direct action or inaction.

Several advisory opinions in the *Reference Guide to the Occupational Therapy Code of Ethics* (Slater, 2016) address circumstances where service recipients, colleagues, and others may be harmed if ethical practice is not followed. For example, Morris's (2016) advisory opinion on patient abandonment suggests that clients served through mental health systems can experience psychological abandonment from the interventionist when he or she separates him or herself to such a degree that the clients are abandoned. Personal awareness of one's reactions to clients can be a step toward forestalling this abandonment and upholding RSC 2B.

Occupational therapy practitioners are advised in RSC 2C to "recognize and take appropriate action to remedy personal problems and limitations that might cause harm to recipients of service, colleagues, students, research participants, and others" (AOTA, 2015b, p. 3). This harm can be through the imposition of undue influence (RSC 2D), conflicts of interest (RSC 2F), sexual exploitation (RSC 2G), or other forms of exploitation (RSC 2I).

Many of these situations can challenge occupational therapy practitioners engaged in mental health practice; practitioners must use their due diligence to avoid them. Active engagement in ongoing clinical supervision may be one strategy that affords occupational therapy practitioners with an objective forum for managing, reflecting on, and tracking their personal reactions to professional challenges. This structured supervision relationship with a trusted mentor is especially important for novice practitioners working in mental health settings to ensure that Principle 2 is not unintentionally or intentionally violated.

Principle 3. Autonomy

According to Principle 3, Autonomy, "occupational therapy personnel shall respect the right of the individual to self-determination, privacy, confidentiality, and consent" (AOTA, 2015b, p. 4). Individuals with serious mental illness may not recognize that their symptoms are part of an illness, which poses a challenge to the practitioner. By definition, an individual experiencing psychotic symptoms such as hallucinations or delusions is thought disordered, as evidenced by confusion, impaired judgment, a loss of contact with reality, or any combination of these. Thus, the Principle of Autonomy is, by nature of the psychotic illness, significantly jeopardized.

Superimpose on this ethical construct that the mental health care service delivery system and criminal/legal considerations often collide, and it is easy to appreciate how a person's autonomy could easily be compromised. For instance, an individual with bipolar disorder may have the grandiose delusional belief that he is the reincarnation of an historical figure and therefore resists treatment and medication interventions. Imposing treatment in this case challenges the individual's autonomy. Not imposing treatment may result in significant harm to this individual or others. Further, left unchecked, psychotic beliefs or behavior could escalate and result in criminal activity. Use of illicit substances in an effort to rid oneself of disturbing thoughts is one example of the intersection of the mental health and criminal justice systems.

In Vignette 11.1, Dekwan's situation exemplifies the balance of an individual with bipolar disorder desire for autonomy and the interprofessional team's efforts to ethically respect his preferences.

Principle 4. Justice

According to Principle 4, Justice, occupational therapy practitioners "shall promote fairness and objectivity in the provision of occupational therapy services" (AOTA, 2015b, p. 5). Individuals with mental illness face stigma, bias, and health disparities, which can compromise Principle 4. As a member of the interprofessional team, occupational therapy practitioners are obligated to challenge clinical decisions and facility policies that result in unequal access to services.

Occupational therapy practitioners are sometimes in a position to advocate for patients while educating members of interprofessional teams. The Principles of Justice and Fidelity are influential in the scenario described in Vignette 11.2.

What ethical Principles are at play in Vignette 11.2? One of the first areas to consider is how to advocate for this client's needs directly with the certified nursing assistant (CNA) and, potentially, with other team members. The ethical obligation for this advocacy is rooted in the Principles of Fidelity and

Vignette 11.1. Medication Compliance

Dekwan was a 30-year-old single African American male. He was diagnosed with bipolar disorder about 12 years ago. During the intake meeting with him upon admission to the ***psychosocial rehabilitation program*** (i.e., a community-based comprehensive mental health service), it was learned that he had more than 20 acute hospitalizations since his first psychotic break at age 18 years. He had not been hospitalized in the past 18 months because he had been maintained on Lithium and established a consistent relationship with his outpatient therapist and his psychopharmacologist.

Dekwan had a history of ambivalence about taking his medications as prescribed. Medication issues precipitated the majority of his previous acute admissions, which were necessary for stabilization and recompensation. At his intake, Dekwan expressed interest in community reintegration programs, especially the possibility of a supported work assignment, and the peer support program. The interprofessional team, including **Erin,** the occupational therapist, worked with Dekwan to identify strategies for goal achievement. The team was conflicted about the best plan of care and was at a crossroads to determine the course of action that would most benefit Dekwan.

Vignette 11.2. Insidious Bias

Oscar Charles Detwiler was admitted to the inpatient rehabilitation facility (IRF), a unit in a rehabilitation or other acute hospital for patients who can tolerate at least 3 hours of skilled therapy per day (Centers for Medicare and Medicaid Services, n.d.), where you were working as a staff occupational therapist. As you reviewed the chart in preparation for the initial evaluation, you learned that he was a 31-year-old divorced man and the father of 2 children for whom his wife had primary custody. He was admitted with bilateral ankle fractures, secondary to a mechanical fall. His ankle injuries were significant, and he was nonweight bearing at admission. You initiated your intervention plan, which focused on developing independence with self-care tasks at the wheelchair level and functional mobility. The first day of the intervention was limited by his complaints of pain and his report of dysregulation of his medication regime.

Just before your session on the second day, the CNA working with him pulled you aside and told you, "Your patient Oscar is crazy, you know. He told the nurse last night that he jumped out a third-floor window—that's how he fractured his ankles and that's why he's here. It just creeps me out!"

Justice. The belief that the CNA is acting from a position of bias or stigma is the first issue that needs to be addressed. Such bias has the potential to interrupt the quality of care that Oscar receives in this IRF.

Occupational therapy practitioners understand how physical and emotional factors can interfere with occupational performance and participation. Other members of the treatment team may see these issues as more dichotomous (i.e., they may think this unit is for physical rehabilitation and that psychiatric patients do not belong here). Advocating for Oscar while educating team members how his emotional needs affect his functional status will be necessary to effectively address and optimize his recovery.

Principle 5. Veracity

According to Principle 5, Veracity, occupational therapy practitioners are to "provide comprehensive, accurate, and objective information when representing the profession" (AOTA, 2015b, p. 6). Veracity is particularly challenging with individuals who may be psychotic and experiencing thought disorders. Although practitioners are obligated to provide accurate and complete information, this must be balanced with Principle 2, Nonmaleficence. For example, ***delusions*** are defined as fixed false beliefs, and the key word here is *fixed.* Therefore, confronting and challenging delusional thoughts with accurate information may be upsetting or agitating to the individual. Practitioners often must juggle Principles 2 and 5 in order to ethically meet the needs of clients with serious mental illness. This delicate balance is described in Vignette 11.3.

Occupational therapy practitioners often encounter individuals who have complex medical and psychiatric needs. It is imperative that practitioners serving these populations have demonstrated competence in their interventions. Multiple Principles are considered as the occupational therapist analyzes her options described in Case Study 11.2.

Principle 6. Fidelity

According to Principle 6, Fidelity, occupational therapy practitioners should "treat clients, colleagues, and other professionals with respect, fairness, discretion, and integrity" (AOTA, 2015b, p. 7). The Principle of Fidelity emphasizes that

Vignette 11.3. Visa Issues

Irina was a 32-year-old single woman. A Ukrainian geologist, she was in the United States on a work visa. She had been experiencing increasing stress at work because her company was reorganizing. She presented to the emergency room escorted by a coworker after she confided that she had not slept for the past 3 days. During her evaluation, Irina revealed that she has had increased energy and feelings of infallibility with plans to take over the multimillion-dollar company "to turn it around." She eluded to the fact that the Ukrainian government may be involved with the financial difficulties her employer was experiencing just so "they" could revoke her visa. In addition, last week she traded in her Honda Civic for a Mercedes C300. She was admitted for further assessment and treatment to the ***partial hospital program,*** which provides behavioral health interventions at an acute level of care that does not require that the individual be kept overnight as in an inpatient admission.

What Principles and core values could provide guidance to an occupational therapy plan of care?

Case Study 11.2. Eating Disorder

Maricelle weighed 71 pounds when she was evaluated for intake into the inpatient eating disorders program. She was at times so weak that her gait and standing tolerance were limited. At age 20 years and 5 feet 6 inches tall, her frame appeared emaciated.

Her weight loss began about 4 years ago when she began dieting to lose a few pounds. Receiving a favorable response from others, she continued to diet and increase her exercise, reaching an all-time low of 59 pounds. Her menses ceased about 3.5 years ago. She had a medical admission at her low weight and was treated for peptic ulcers. Within a month of her discharge from that hospitalization, she was admitted to an inpatient psychiatric ward. After 8 weeks in this program, she increased her weight to 78 pounds.

With outpatient support and treatment, she continued to do well and was approaching 100 pounds when she enrolled in college. With the increasing social and academic demands, she began dieting again, losing more than 20 pounds in the 6 weeks before this admission to the residential eating disorders program. This setting was chosen because of the high physical health risk caused by her eating disorder.

Maricelle's eating habits were ritualized, with meticulous cutting of food and moving it around her plate. She actively avoided, resisted, and refused foods that she considered to be high in fat or carbohydrate content. She experienced moderate hair loss. She was excessively anxious and preoccupied with her figure. She expressed concern that as she gains weight, her "womanhood" was evident to others.

Ceil, the occupational therapist assigned to the eating disorders program, was new to the unit and inexperienced with this patient population. She recognized the need for ethical and practice guidance that would help her develop effective intervention strategies. Because Ceil's supervisor was on vacation, she decided to use the Decision Table to help her determine the best course of action to take (Table 11.1).

Table 11.1. Decision Table for Case Study 11.2

Possible Action	Positive Outcomes	Negative Consequences
Take no action.	Ceil would uphold RSC 1E by not offering services beyond her level of competence.	Maricelle would not benefit from the therapeutic milieu, which potentially causes harm, a violation of RSCs 1A and 1C. RSC 3A would be upheld, however, placing Maricelle at greater risk of harm.
Meet with the covering supervisor.	Ceil would be mentored in the evidence-based interventions for Maricelle (upholding RSCs 1C, 6H, 6I). Interventions would not be delayed.	Ceil's supervisor might be disappointed to learn that Ceil didn't have the competencies needed to work with this patient population.
Conduct research about eating disorders to expand knowledge.	Ceil's knowledge base would improve as she learned about the complexity of providing interventions to this population. Seeking advice or consultation would be consistent with RSCs 1E, 1G, and 1I and with clinical practice standards established by the British Psychological Society and the Royal College of Psychiatrists (2004).	If Ceil delays providing services to Maricelle, her progress would potentially be thwarted (RSC 1A, 1C).
Refuse to provide services to this population until competency is established.	If Ceil thought that her supervisor expected her to provide services without demonstrated competencies, she might believe that she was upholding RSC 2H and that her supervisor had violated RSC 4H.	Ceil may jeopardize her position within the hospital and threaten her employment. Patients would not receive needed occupational therapy services. By not providing services, Ceil may avoid causing direct harm to patients (RSC 2A); however, she would abandon Maricelle and others and violate RSC 2B.

Note. RSC = Related Standard of Conduct.

occupational therapy practitioners hold true to their commitment to provide occupational therapy services within the scope of practice to the individuals they treat. Fidelity comes into play from the initiation of the therapeutic relationship and spans the course of the intervention.

In Case Study 11.2, one wonders if Ceil's supervisor was compliant with the Principle of Fidelity. Did the supervisor leave an untrained staff member in a position that would potentially harm clients? Was Ceil treated with fairness when her supervisor expected her to provide assessments and interventions without adequate experience? Were the clients and Ceil treated with integrity?

Summary

Individuals across the lifespan and in all living contexts may need mental health services at one or more points in time. Occupational therapy began as a focus of care for patients in mental institutions in the late 1800s. Today it has become an integral part of service to individuals with behavioral health and substance use disorders.

Occupational therapists and occupational therapy assistants receive academic preparation and clinical experiences that expose them to individuals of all ages in hospitals and com munity settings. These people can have emotional and biochemical disorders and other illnesses and disabilities, and they can benefit from occupational therapy's understanding of behavior and function. Occupational therapy services with each population and in each practice context present the potential for ethical dilemmas. The better the Code is understood by occupational therapy students, practitioners, researchers, and educators, the more likely those in the field will adhere to the profession's values and principles, and the profession's service to others will continue to be inspirational.

Reflective Questions

1. Refer to Vignette 11.1 and respond to the following questions: At least one of the peer counselors is quite anti-medication. Erin has been working closely with Dekwan on strengthening his work skills and believes that adherence to a medication management system will help his engagement in all life activities.
   - What are the issues?
   - What do you do?
   - Is it client centered to refuse his right to participate in the peer support program?
   - What Principles and RSCs from the Code support your position?
2. Refer to Case Study 11.2 and respond to the questions posted following Principle 6.
3. Considering the data reported from the *AOTA Salary and Workforce Survey* (2015a), identify strategies that would re-infuse occupational therapy into mental health practice contexts. How would this implicate ethical constructs and what barriers may interfere with these strategies?

References

21st Century Cures Act of 2016, P. L. 114–255.

Accreditation Council for Occupation Therapy Education. (2012). 2011 Accreditation Council for Occupational Therapy Education (ACOTE®) standards. *American Journal of Occupational Therapy, 66*(Suppl.6), S6–S74. https://doi.org/10.5014/ajot.2012.66S6

American Occupational Therapy Association. (2014). The role of occupational therapy in primary care. *American Journal of Occupational Therapy, 68*(Suppl. 3), S25–S33. https://doi.org/10.5014/ajot.2014.686S06

American Occupational Therapy Association. (2015a). *2015 AOTA salary and workforce survey.* Bethesda, MD: AOTA Press.

American Occupational Therapy Association. (2015b). Occupational therapy code of ethics (2015). *American Journal of Occupational Therapy, 69*(Suppl. 3), 6912310030. https://doi.org/10.5014/ajot.2015.696S03

American Psychological Association. (2016). *Mental Health Reform Act of 2016 moves forward in U.S. Senate.* Retrieved from http://www.apapracticecentral.org/update/2016/03-24/mental-health-reform.aspx

British Psychological Society, & Royal College of Psychiatrists. (2004). *Eating disorders: Core interventions in the treatment and management of anorexia nervosa, bulimia nervosa, and related eating disorders.* Retrieved from http://www.ncbi.nlm.nih.gov/books/NBK49301

Brown, G. K., Beck, A. T., & Steer, R. A. (2000). Risk factors for suicide in psychiatric outpatients: A 20-year prospective study. *Journal of Consulting and Clinical Psychology, 68*(3), 371–377. https://doi.org/10.1037/0022-006X.68.3.371

Centers for Medicare and Medicaid Services. (n.d.). *Inpatient rehabilitation facilities.* Retrieved from https://www.cms.gov

/Medicare/Provider-Enrollment-and-Certification /CertificationandComplianc/InpatientRehab.html

Haiman, S., & Slater D. Y. (2013). Ethics in diverse mental health settings. In J. B. Scott & S. M. Reitz (Eds.), *Practical applications to the Occupational Therapy Code of Ethics and Ethics Standards* (pp. 123–135). Bethesda, MD: AOTA Press.

Helping Families in Mental Health Crises Act of 2016, H.R. 2646, 114th Cong.

Ithman, M. H., Goplarkrishna, G., Beck, N. C., Das, J., & Petroski, G. (2014). Predictors of length of stay in an acute psychiatric hospital. *Journal of Biosafety and Health Education, 2*, 119. https://doi.org/10.4172/2332-0893.1000119

Janofsky, J. S., & Tamburello, A. C. (2006). Diversion to the mental health system: Emergency psychiatric evaluations. *Journal of the American Academy of Psychiatry and Law, 34*(3), 283–291.

Mental Health Reform Act of 2016, S. 2680, 114th Cong.

Mental Retardation Facilities and Community Mental Health Centers Construction Act of 1963, Pub. L. 88–164, 77 Stat. 282.

Metzl, J. M., & MacLeish, K. T. (2015). Mental illness, mass shootings, and the politics of American firearms. *American Journal of Public Health, 105*, 240–249. https://doi.org/10.2105 /AJPH.2014.302242

Morris, J. (2016). Patient abandonment. In D. Y. Slater (Ed.), *Reference guide to the Occupational Therapy Code of Ethics* (pp. 223–228). Bethesda, MD: AOTA Press.

Mosaic Community Services. (2016). *Programs and services.* Retrieved from http://www.mosaicinc.org/programs-services

National Alliance on Mental Illness. (n.d.). *Treatment settings.* Retrieved from https:// www.nami.org/Learn-More/Treatment /Treatment-Settings

National Institute on Drug Abuse. (2010). *Comorbidity: Addiction and other mental illness—What is comorbidity?* Retrieved from http://bit.ly/2jBgUDa

Sheth, H. C. (2009). Deinstitutionalization or disowning responsibility. *International Journal of Psychosocial Rehabilitation, 13*(2), 11–20. Retrieved from http://www.psychosocial .com/IJPR_13/Deinstitutionalization_Sheth.html

Slater, D. Y. (Ed.).(2016). *Reference guide to the Occupational Therapy Code of Ethics.* Bethesda, MD: AOTA Press.

Substance Abuse Mental Health Services Administration. (2015). *Behavioral health treatments and services.* Retrieved from http://www.samhsa.gov/treatment

Substance Abuse Mental Health Services Administration. (2016). *What is integrated care?* Retrieved from http://www .integration.samhsa.gov/about-us/what-is-integrated-care

Chapter 12.

PRODUCTIVE AGING: ETHICS FROM COMMUNITY TO SUPPORTIVE LIVING

Janie B. Scott, MA, OT/L, FAOTA

Learning Objectives

By the end of the chapter, readers will be able to

- Describe roles that occupational therapy practitioners may have in productive aging,
- Identify what Principles and Related Standards of Conduct apply to ethical dilemmas in productive aging practice, and
- Apply demographic projections and the Vision 2025 statement to the future of occupational therapy's ethical participation in productive aging.

Key Terms and Concepts

- ✧ Aging in place
- ✧ Cultural interfacing
- ✧ Discharge planning
- ✧ Livable communities
- ✧ Older adults
- ✧ Productive aging
- ✧ Vision 2025

People's engagement in their chosen occupations varies over time and is contingent on their health, interests, and abilities (see Figure 12.1). Occupational therapy practitioners consult for and intervene with the aging population by providing recommendations to improve energy conservation and community mobility and by identifying strategies for time management, work simplification, coping, and social and leisure participation in response to changing needs and interests (Scott, 2009). The *Occupational Therapy Code of Ethics (2015)* (hereinafter referred to as the "Code;" American Occupational Therapy Association [AOTA], 2015b) provides guidance for occupational therapy practitioners in ethical practice as they support older adults in aging productively.

Understanding Productive Aging

What is *productive aging?* Educator Ethel Percy Andrus first mentioned the construct in 1947 when advocating to insurance companies on behalf of older retired teachers. The organization, National

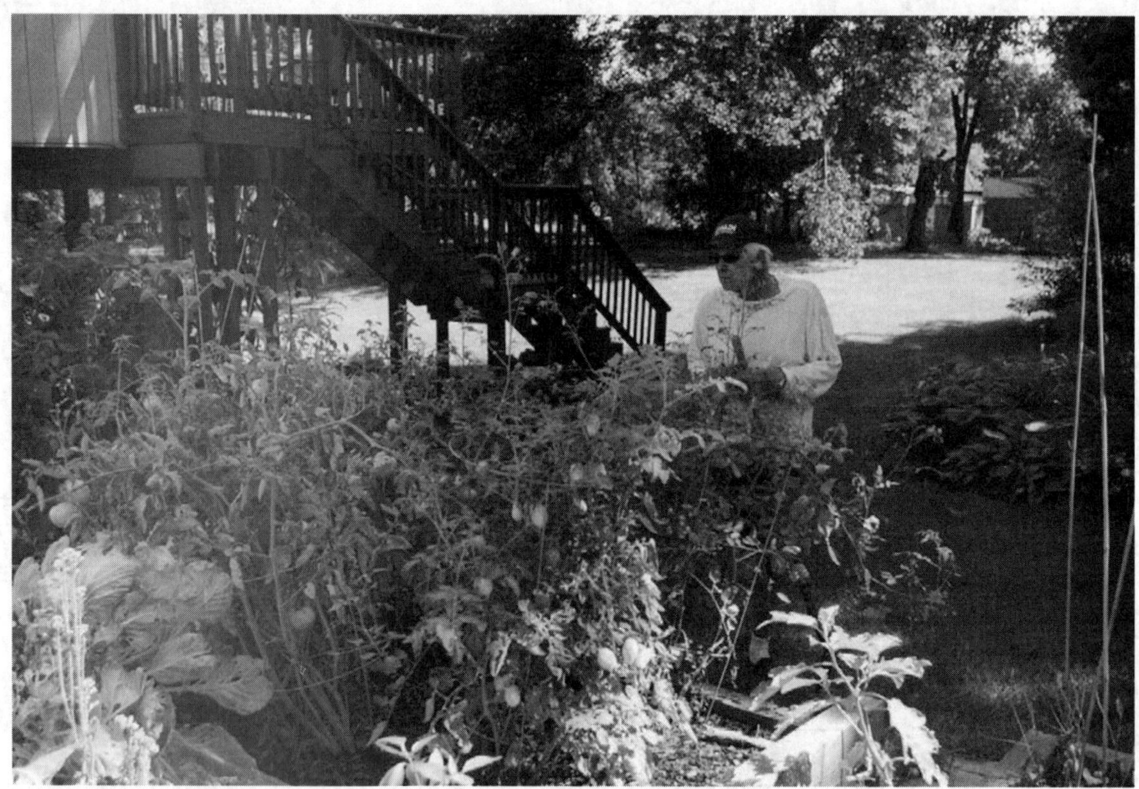

FIGURE 12.1

Occupational therapy practitioners provide interventions aimed at productive aging for clients with interests, such as continuing to work, resuming functional activities after a disability, gardening, and safely participating in home and community activities.
Source. J. Scott. Used with permission.

Retired Teachers Association, later became AARP (Jenkins, 2016). Dr. Robert N. Butler, the founding director of the National Institute on Aging, also used the term *productive aging* in his early work and throughout his career. He emphasized exercise, nutrition, social engagement, and naps as important to living a healthy and productive life (Agnvall, 2010).

Productive aging is the continued participation of older adults in self-care, work, volunteering, informal caregiving, civic participation, and engagement in leisure and social activities as they grow older. ***Older adults*** are categorized as individuals 65 or older (U.S. Department of Health and Human Services [DHHS], 2014; World Health Organization [WHO], 2016); however, when global and cultural factors are considered, the age demarcation may be lower. For example, WHO reported that the United Nations defines this population as 60-plus, with the exception of the classification of older adults in Africa, where the divide is age 50 (WHO, 2016.

Occupational Therapy's Role in Productive Aging

Productive aging applies to both older adults who are well and those who are living with illness or disabilities. Occupational therapy can help them achieve their goals through "the profession's core beliefs in the positive relationship between occupation and health and its view of people as occupational beings" (AOTA, 2014, p. S3). Occupational therapy's aim is to facilitate clients' ability to maintain balance between different areas of occupation (e.g., activities of daily living [ADLs], rest and sleep, leisure, social participation) so they can have a productive life (AOTA, 2014). Practitioners must consider the relationship of client factors (e.g., values, beliefs, spirituality) to a client's ability to maintain this balance in daily life, thereby achieving a productive and quality life. Through the occupational therapy process, practitioners can help facilitate the productive participation of older adults in life.

AOTA has recognized as a priority helping occupational therapy practitioners address the desire of older adults to remain productive. AOTA's Gerontology Special Interest Section and online forum are important sources of information and continuing education to help prepare the profession to meet this portion of society's needs. When 5,000 members of AOTA and its stakeholders participated in the development of ***Vision 2025,*** they generated the following statement to help guide the profession in coming years: "Occupational therapy maximizes health, well-being, and quality of life for all people, populations, and communities through effective solutions that facilitate participation in everyday living" (AOTA, 2016d, para. 1).

This statement and its guideposts, which include the terms *accessible, collaborative, effective,* and *leaders*, are inclusive of all areas of practice, including productive aging (AOTA, 2016d). The *Vision* serves as a tool for occupational therapy practitioners, consumers, policymakers, and others to appreciate the scope and benefits of occupational therapy interventions.

AOTA has solidified its focus on productive aging and gerontology. According to AOTA, "our society's rapidly aging population, increased longevity, the changing world of work, and Baby Boomers' focus on quality-of-life issues are some of the factors that will increase the need for services in this area" (AOTA, 2016c, para. 1). Occupational therapy practice areas in productive aging include

- Aging in place: home modifications, fall prevention, health promotion;
- Driving and community mobility;
- Primary care;
- Post-acute care and transition to home; and
- Palliative care (AOTA, 2016b, p. 4).

Demographic Trends in Productive Aging

The term *senior tsunami* has been used internationally by the popular press to describe the anticipated growth in the population of aging individuals, which will affect health care (including occupational therapy), housing, transportation, and social systems across the United States. The 2015 White House Conference on Aging (WHCOA) report declared that more than 10,000 Baby Boomers turn age 65 years every day. On the basis of these data and the fact that women older than age 85 years are the fastest growing demographic in the United States (WHCOA, 2015), occupational therapy practitioners must be prepared for the possibility of ethical dilemmas challenging conflicting values and ethical Principles of Autonomy and Justice within U.S. society.

Themes from the 2015 WHCOA included

- Need for collaboration between all parts of government, public and private sectors;
- Preparation to meet the needs of this growing population;
- Formal and informal support for caregivers;
- Breakdown of the silos among housing, transportation, health care, and long-term services and supports; and
- Increased access to and use of technologies (WHCOA, 2015).

Occupational therapy practitioners will have many opportunities to provide services to meet the needs of this increasingly diverse population in a culturally sensitive manner.

An emphasis on productive aging has implications both for housing and for the workforce. Many retirees want to age in place rather than move to warmer climates, retirement communities, or institutions (AARP, 2013). "Residing in one's preferred living arrangement and community mobility are two of the greatest challenges to maintaining occupational integrity" (Beitman, 2009, p. CE1). Unless these two conditions are met, opportunities for productive aging are severely compromised.

Changing demographics affect the current and future workforce. AARP projected a shortage of workers with experience to fill the gaps left by older, experienced workers; health care is an area where shortages are expected. At the same time, partly because of economic necessity and partly out of a desire for continuing productivity, older adults may choose to work part time or switch careers at traditional retirement age. "The continued increase in average retirement over the past decade is likely a reflection of various dynamics, both financial and non-financial. . . . Another factor that may be influencing the continued increase in the average retirement age is improved longevity" (AARP, 2015, p. 11). Changing expectations about retirement requires that people plan strategies for retirement in advance (e.g., Fuscaldo, 2012).

The Centers for Disease Control and Prevention (2013) projected that "by 2030, the percentage of older non-Hispanic white adults will make up 71.2% of the population, whereas Hispanics will make up 12%, non-Hispanic blacks nearly 10.3%, and Asians 5.4% (p. 1). Given the shift in demographics, employers may restructure their positions to use the skills of older workers, health care organizations and academic institutions may reframe their recruitment strategies toward people from more diverse backgrounds, and linguistic cultural competence and effectiveness may become a priority for all service providers.

Occupational therapy practitioners are dedicated to diversity and inclusion in their practice, and this emphasis will grow to meet society's needs (Wells, Black, & Gupta, 2016). As noted in the Code, "AOTA members are committed to promoting inclusion, participation, safety, and well-being for all recipients in various stages of life, health, and illness and to empowering all beneficiaries of service to meet their occupational needs" (AOTA, 2015b, p. 1).

Related Standard of Conduct (RSC) 3J of the Code obligates practitioners to "facilitate comprehension and address barriers to communication (e.g., aphasia; differences in language, literacy, culture) with the recipient of service (or responsible party), student, or research participant" (AOTA, 2015b, p. 5). Principle 4, Justice, guides the occupational therapy practitioner to "relate in a respectful, fair, and impartial manner to individuals and groups with whom they interact" (AOTA, 2015b, p. 5). Respect and impartiality is derived from the ability to understand how living conditions and life factors affect an individual's life. Further, RSC 4D introduces encouragement

---

Vignette 12.1. Facilitating Transition to Retirement With Cultural Competence

Camila, a 59-year-old Hispanic woman, was recently admitted to a community behavioral health program after a 28-day admission to the behavioral health unit of a local hospital. Camila's treatment for bipolar illness was complicated because of a recent diagnosis of diabetes secondary to obesity. Medication management, new meal preparation guidelines, and Camila's difficulty in adhering to schedules complicated her psychiatric, medical, and occupational therapy care. During the course of her hospitalization, Camila decided that the stress of her maintenance job was too much and that she would retire in 6 months at age 60.

Camila's occupational therapist, **Elaine,** had recently obtained her National Board for Certification in Occupational Therapy (NBCOT) certification. Elaine recognized that Camila had multiple occupational therapy needs (e.g., managing time, planning meals, expanding leisure interests, developing a retirement planning strategy). However, Elaine was uncomfortable working with Camila because of their cultural and language differences. Elaine discussed her feelings with **Nick,** her supervisor, who reminded her of her obligations under RSC 3J (facilitate open and collaborative dialogue with clients and their comprehension of services). This necessitated referral to another provider who had the linguistic skills necessary to serve Camila (RSC 1I).

This action, based on Elaine and Nick's concerns, underscores occupational therapy practitioners' obligation to take cultural orientation into account in service delivery. Cultural competence was important to Nick, in part because of the community outreach program to underserved populations. Practitioners were expected to locate translators when language barriers existed and to learn about sociocultural beliefs that could affect the therapeutic relationship with clients and their families. His commitment to this goal also supported the agency's imperative to review policies that limited clients' access to occupational therapy and other services (RSC 4D).

To that end, Elaine and Nick agreed to the following plan to support the evolution of Elaine's cultural sensitivity and competence. Elaine would

- Locate resources to facilitate her communication with Camila (e.g., Thrash, 2006);
- Identify a process to obtain real-time language translation services;
- Explore healthy and culturally sensitive food preferences that Camila could use;
- Assist Camila, if she was interested, in reconnecting with her religious community; and
- Pursue further knowledge about the cultural habits and preferences of Camila and Elaine's other clients and use that knowledge to increase her ***cultural interfacing,*** which includes the verbal and nonverbal communications used in interactions between people of different cultures and languages (Bloomfield, 1994).

to "advocate for changes to systems and policies that are discriminatory or unfairly limit or prevent access to occupational therapy services" (AOTA, 2015b, p. 5). A situation in which an occupational therapist is challenged to provide culturally appropriate practice is described in Vignette 12.1.

Ethical Dilemmas in Service Delivery to Older Adults

Occupational therapy practitioners who face ethical dilemmas in providing services to older adults need to consider whether to attempt to resolve the situation locally through direct communication with the supervisor or primary party involved, whether to file an ethical or legal complaint, or whether the best solution is to resign. Ethical situations practitioners encounter during the delivery of occupational therapy services to older adults will be explored in the next section.

Aging in Place

Many older adult occupational therapy clients live independently or with supports in the community, and they desire to continue aging in place. ***Aging in place*** reflects an individual's desire to remain in the living environment of their choosing with access to services that support their ability to live as independently as possible. Occupational therapy, with its focus on productive aging and aging in place, will be in high demand as such clients age.

Many practitioners in the area of aging in place primarily focus on making the home environment accessible to allow older adults and people with disabilities to continue living in their homes through home modifications.

On a broader scale, occupational therapy practitioners work to ensure ***livable communities;*** specifically, practitioners "evaluate barriers in the environment that contribute to health inequities and diminished quality of life; design and modify home and community environments; and create opportunities for engagement in meaningful physical, social, vocational, and cultural activities" (AOTA, 2016a, p. 1). "A livable community is one that has affordable and appropriate housing, supportive community features and services, and adequate mobility options, which together facilitate personal independence and the engagement of residents in civic and social life" (Kochera & Straight, 2005, p. 16).

Occupational therapy service delivery includes safety assessments of the home and community; recommendations and education with elderly clients and caregivers on environmental modifications; identification of resources that connect elders to community services; and consultations with builders, organizations, and agencies.

Occupational therapy practitioners also support clients' desires to age in place by providing driver screening and evaluations, training seniors in the use of public transportation, providing sensitivity training to drivers, and enabling the use of adaptive equipment for driving, ADL performance, and employment productivity. Beitman (2009) observed that "occupational therapy intervention for older adults living in the community is most beneficial when it is client-centered and focused on health maintenance and successful adaptation to challenges associated with the aging process" (p. CE6).

Entry-level education for occupational therapists addresses this area of practice through course content on universal design and environmental modifications. Practitioners can advance their knowledge in this practice area through AOTA continuing education and credentialing (e.g., Specialty Certification in Environmental Modification), the National Association of Home Builders Certified Aging-in-Place Specialist (CAPS) designation, and other academic and continuing education programs.

Public support for occupational therapy and other services to promote aging in place comes from legislation (see *Olmstead v. L.C.,* 1999) and initiatives through the Administration on Aging and aging advocacy organizations. DHHS's document *Healthy People 2020* details the nation's health objectives for the next decade, among them to "improve the health, function, and quality of life of older adults" (DHHS, 2014, para. 1). This document incorporates aging-in-place perspectives into many focus areas and objectives, such as fall prevention, engagement in leisure activities including exercise, and caregiver access to training and support—areas that are ideal for occupational therapy intervention (DHHS, 2014). As noted in *Healthy People 2020,*

> most older adults want to remain in their communities as long as possible. Unfortunately,

when they acquire disabilities, there is often not enough support available to help them. States that invest in such services show lower rates of growth in long-term care expenditures. (DHHS, 2014, para. 3)

In Case Study 12.1, an occupational therapist confronts competing priorities in her own efforts to age in place. Case Study 12.2 describes an occupational therapist's efforts to ethically ensure adequate care for her home care clients.

Case Study 12.1. Balancing Ethical Obligations to Enable Aging in Place

Marcie, a 61-year-old wife, mother, and grandmother, worked as an occupational therapist in a community-based senior center. Her duties included program evaluation and planning, group leadership, and client advocacy with community agencies. Her husband, **Stephen,** was age 66 years and became disabled after suffering a left-sided stroke while playing tennis. Marcie became the primary breadwinner for the family. Her position at the senior center required that she work a flexible schedule that included weekends when the center offered special events. Stephen began attending the center to be near his wife and to have mealtime supervision, opportunities for social engagement, and limited physical activity. The senior center context met both Marcie and Stephen's needs.

After a few months, Stephen's dependence on Marcie began to have a negative impact on her work performance. Stephen wanted Marcie to have lunch with him each day, go with him on center outings, and help him perform some of his ADLs. If Marcie were to attend to all of Stephen's needs, she would not have time to fulfill her job responsibilities. Marcie was torn between meeting the duties of her position at the senior center and to her husband. She identified the following dilemmas:

- Stephen wanted Marcie to eat lunch with him every day. Before he attended the senior center, Marcie used her lunch hour to interact with center members or contact community agencies on clients' behalf to arrange for services. Did Marcie have a greater duty to attend to Stephen's needs or to continue to function in her position as she had previously? Was Marcie obligated to work through her lunch, or was she entitled to alter her behavioral patterns and use her lunch hour to eat with her husband?
- Stephen wanted Marcie to go on center outings with him. Center staff often alternated in attending these events. If Marcie attended the ones that included Stephen, would she be able to attend to other members' needs? Would Marcie become more of a center member than staff? Did the center benefit from having Marcie so involved?
- Marcie was also conflicted about whether Stephen should be included in the groups she led. Would her attention be too directed to Stephen, to the detriment of the other group members' needs, presenting a conflict of interest?

Some questions for Marcie to consider include

- What are Marcie's duties and responsibilities in her position with the center? Has she discussed her dilemmas with her supervisor? If she acquiesces to Stephen's requests, will she still be meeting the essential requirements of her job?
- Should Marcie have a frank conversation with Stephen about her conflicted feelings? She doesn't want to hurt his feelings, but she feels compelled to share her thoughts with him. If Marcie's income is a major concern, they need to decide what to do so as not to jeopardize Marcie's job.
- Are current center members harmed by the diversion of Marcie's attention?

The responses to these questions will help Marcie analyze to whom she owes the greatest duty and how she decides between competing priorities. To more clearly understand the pros and cons of her dilemma, she used the Decision Table (Table 12.1) to help crystallize her thinking before making recommendations to her husband and employer.

(Continued)

Case Study 12.1. Balancing Ethical Obligations to Enable Aging in Place *(Cont.)*

Table 12.1. Decision Table for Case Study 12.1

Possible Actions	Positive Outcomes	Negative Consequences
Enroll Stephen in another senior center (RSCs 3B, 6C).	Marcie would be able to fulfill obligations to her employer and center participants (avoids violating RSC 2I).	Stephen might become depressed from reduced connection with Marcie (Principle 1). Marcie may worry about Stephen and become inefficient (RSCs 2C, 2D, 2F).
Schedule Stephen into groups and activities that don't involve Marcie (RSCs 3D, 6J).	Marcie would have fewer distractions and meet her employer's expectations. (RSC 6M). Marcie and Stephen would have greater autonomy (Principle 3). Stephen would increase his socialization and participation within the senior center.	Stephen may initially have difficulty transitioning to a new schedule.
Marcie and her supervisor realign her daily schedule so she regularly has lunch with Stephen (RSCs 3D, 6H, 6J, 6M).	Marcie would set work boundaries that satisfy her employer and Stephen (RSC 4L). Marcie would increase her ability to meet required job duties (RSCs 2F, 6E).	Marcie may have to realign her work duties, extending her workday.

Note. RSCs = Related Standards of Conduct.

Case Study 12.2. Addressing Client and Caregiver Needs in Home Care

Deidre, age 73 years, and her partner, **Alex,** age 82 years, were retired. Alex had had a mild stroke 12 years ago, and he had quadruple bypass surgery 1.5 years ago. Deidre maintained an active schedule, exercising daily, snow skiing a few times a year, reading journal articles, and maintaining an active social life.

Deidre was diagnosed with Parkinson's disease 3 years ago and was feeling the consequences of the disease physically, cognitively, and emotionally. Deidre devoted a significant amount of her time to maintaining her own wellness and trying to stay actively and socially engaged with Alex and their friends, but Deidre's acceptance of her diagnosis was difficult. Alex and their occupational therapist, **Regina,** were working with Deidre to encourage her to consider her current and future needs relative to her ability to age in place.

Although Deidre was the primary focus of the occupational therapy intervention, Regina believed it was imperative to consider Alex's needs and level of function so he could optimize his health and remain a supportive caregiver. Regina wanted to ensure that she would not be breaching the Code or Medicare policies by providing occupational therapy services to both Deidre and Alex. She reviewed several ethical decision-making models, the Code, and Medicare policies, specifically billing for caregiver education under Part A. She used the series of steps described in Chapter 4 to guide her decision making.

Regina sought first to gather the facts. Alex and Deidre could both benefit from occupational therapy intervention, but Medicare sets limits on reimbursement for people receiving home health services. Deidre needed evaluation and possible intervention regarding environmental adaptations, safety, energy conservation, and executive functions. Alex would benefit from stress management techniques, transfer and home safety strategies, and methods to provide Deidre with emotional support. The key people involved were

(Continued)

Case Study 12.2. Addressing Client and Caregiver Needs in Home Care *(Cont.)*

Deidre, Alex, Alex and Deidre's friends and family, and Medicare representatives. Deidre and Alex had a long-term relationship, and support was available from family and friends.

Regina was a licensed occupational therapist in good standing with the state regulatory board, AOTA, and within the local community, and she wanted to provide high-quality occupational therapy services to this couple. Deidre and Alex would do whatever was necessary, including privately pay for services, to enable them both to age in place.

Regina's dilemma was as follows: Could she ethically and legally provide occupational therapy services to both Alex and Deidre?

Regina listed the following possible courses of action:

- Evaluate and intervene only with Deidre and offer caregiver training to Alex under the Medicare rules.
- Accept private payment by the couple and evaluate and provide recommendations.
- Investigate and advocate for other sources of funding for the required services and environmental modifications.
- In light of Deidre's potential cognitive deficits, need to conserve energy, and manage her Parkinson's disease, Regina would review appropriate literature. From this review, Regina discovered a fact sheet, *Occupational Therapy's Role in Home Health* (AOTA, 2013) that had tips on managing daily activities and cognitive and behavioral health conditions that might be applicable to the situation.

Regina's actions needed to be consistent with the following Principles and RSCs of the Code: Principle 1, Beneficence; RSC 2C (avoid relationships that exploit the client); and Principle 4, Justice, especially RSCs 4E (uphold laws and maintain adherence to guidelines established in AOTA official documents) and 4B (advocate for clients to obtain needed services through available means). In her research, Regina checked with the Centers for Medicare and Medicaid Services (CMS) and found the *Medicare Benefit Policy Manual*. It noted that "If skilled therapy services by a qualified therapist are needed to instruct the patient or appropriate caregiver regarding the maintenance program, such instruction is covered" (CMS, 2016, p. 175). This information was related to outpatient therapy services and may not be helpful to Deidre and Alex. Regina also reviewed the original physician referral for occupational therapy evaluation and intervention, Medicare guidelines, Deidre's and Alex's priorities, and the Code.

Regina decided to set up a formal meeting with Deidre and Alex, during which she shared the results of her initial assessment and collaborated with them to develop an intervention plan. Regina agreed to provide the evaluation and services to Deidre in compliance with Medicare guidelines. At Regina's suggestion, Deidre agreed to contact the local Area Agency on Aging to see if grant funds or special programs were available to pay for environmental renovations and caregiver education. The three parties also agreed on a plan to re-evaluate Deidra and Alex's needs on a regular basis.

Institutional Care

In discussions on AOTA's *OTConnections,* an online discussion forum (e.g., gerontology, mental health), occupational therapy practitioners often discuss ethical dilemmas they face. Among those they typically encounter in institutional settings are requests by supervisors to modify the results of evaluations; offer interventions that lack evidence; provide services to clients, who in their professional opinion, don't need services; document a client's care at levels that aren't accurate; pad the minutes billed to Medicare to reflect the facility's productivity standards; and document services when none were delivered. (*Note.* Suspicions about Medicare fraud and abuse can be anonymously reported to the Medicare Hotline at 1-800-MEDICARE.)

Some participants consider leaving their employment rather than compromise their ethics, be in noncompliance with state regulations, or participate in billing fraud. An occupational therapist's efforts

Vignette 12.2. Promoting Client Well-Being in a Skilled Nursing Facility

Amrit was an occupational therapist with several years of experience in acute care who was now working in long-term care. He was assigned to evaluate and work with a 93-year-old woman, **Zelda,** who was frail and had multiple chronic illnesses, including dementia. Zelda was recovering from a recent hip fracture and needed rehabilitative care. Amrit was concerned that Zelda was too old and frail to benefit from occupational therapy. He expressed his concerns to his supervisor, who instructed him to fulfill the referral because no other occupational therapist was available to evaluate and intervene. Amrit's dilemma existed because of his concern that he would devote valuable time to a person who was unlikely (in his professional opinion) to benefit from occupational therapy interventions while other patients needing occupational therapy services were unserved.

After thoughtful reflection and review of the Code and the AOTA advisory opinion on patient abandonment (Morris, 2016), Amrit realized that occupational therapy values and principles encouraged the advancement of Zelda's well-being through the administration of occupational therapy services. He considered Zelda's comprehensive needs and decided to focus her intervention on working with nursing staff to reduce her risk of falling, promoting her cognitive engagement, assessing her ability to summon help using the call button, and increasing her participation in dressing and feeding.

to ensure that he is avoiding unethical practice in a skilled nursing facility are described in Vignette 12.2.

Discharge Planning

Discharge planning is a process that considers the needs of a client or resident prior to their transition from a care setting (CMS, n.d.). When a client's treatment in an institution comes to an end, occupational therapy practitioners have significant insights to contribute to the discharge planning process, and they need to embrace ethical principles to promote client safety and care. The Code obligates occupational therapy practitioners to terminate therapy in collaboration with the client when goals have been met (RSC 1H), to advocate for clients to obtain needed services through available means (RSC 4B), and to advocate for just and fair treatment for clients (RSC 4D).

Atwal and Caldwell (2003) examined occupational therapy's role and participation in discharge planning and determined that occupational therapy practitioners unintentionally fail to uphold Principles related to Autonomy and Confidentiality, Beneficence, Nonmaleficence, and Social Justice. Practitioners have an ethical obligation to contribute to the discharge planning process with interdisciplinary and multidisciplinary teams and to participate on such teams equally and assertively. In Vignette 12.3, an occupational therapy student and

Vignette 12.3. Advocating for Adequate Discharge Planning

Selena was an occupational therapy student on her Level II fieldwork assignment at a behavioral health inpatient unit of a community hospital. Her midterm evaluation was positive, with the comments focusing primarily on improving her communication skills, particularly her assertiveness during interactions with professional staff. Selena was reluctant to speak up at times (e.g., at team and discharge planning meetings). She was surprised to receive this feedback because her supervisor, **Marco,** rarely contributed in these settings.

Selena had been working with **Mrs. Boxer** following Marco's initial evaluation of her 2 weeks previously. Marco had identified several safety concerns in his assessment, and several of them remained unresolved, including short-term memory deficits, self-care, safety, and health. Selena voiced her concerns to Marco about Mrs. Boxer's plans to be discharged to her home. The day after their discussion, a discharge planning meeting was held involving the entire team, including family members. Team members mentioned some minor problems with short-term memory; however, all felt that Mrs. Boxer was safe to go home. Although Selena and Marco had information to the contrary, they were not asked for their input, and they did not offer their opinions.

Selena was distressed immediately after the meeting adjourned for a short break. She knew that the occupational therapy professionals had important information that should have been communicated to the team, and she expressed this to Marco. They realized that they had a duty to the patient and her family to share their knowledge and potentially protect Mrs. Boxer from a premature discharge that involved a high potential for injury. Although the team had moved on to the discussion of another patient, Selena and Marco returned to the subject of Mrs. Boxer and communicated their reports and recommendations.

Privately, they both recognized the dangers that could result from silence and failure to advocate for their patients, and they established personal goals to overcome their lack of assertiveness and to consistently speak up on behalf of their patients in all future meetings.

her fieldwork supervisor struggle with their ethical obligation to participate assertively on a client's discharge planning team.

Hospice and End-of-Life Care

Should conversations about productive aging include hospice and end-of-life care? Occupational therapists' ethical obligation to serve clients continues in the late stages of clients' lives. The Code reminds us that "*freedom* and personal choice are paramount in a profession in which the values and desires of the client guide our interventions" (AOTA, 2015a, p. 2). Support for clients' dignity, also a foundational value in occupational therapy, is critical in the end stages of life. Principle 1, Beneficence; Principle 3, Autonomy; and Principle 4, Justice, establish occupational therapy practitioners' responsibility to provide services to all clients, even those with a terminal condition, and to avoid an authoritative or paternalistic attitude toward clients by listening to their wishes and engaging them collaboratively in the therapeutic process.

Occupational therapy emphasizes occupational engagement for people throughout the lifespan, and preparing to die and dying are part of that process. The role of occupational therapy continues to support "quality of life by supporting their engagement in daily life occupations that clients find meaningful and purposeful" (AOTA, 2011, p. S67). Pizzi (2010) discussed the construct introduced in the palliative care literature of a "good death," which he believed could be achieved through the power of occupation: "Well-being and wellness can be goals for people with terminal illnesses" (p. 493).

Occupational therapy's role in hospice and end-of-life care includes strategies to enhance participation in meaningful occupations as well as specific ways to obtain reimbursement for these skilled services. Medicare, Medicaid, and other third-party payers supplement the cost of these needed services (AOTA, 2011). Practitioners use their knowledge and experience in task analysis, energy conservation, psychosocial conditions, and the aging process to introduce new strategies, including use of

Vignette 12.4. Addressing Lack of Vigilance in Hospice

Mandy was an occupational therapist and independent contractor with experience in the practice area of productive aging in a skilled nursing facility, a state behavioral health hospital unit, and an assisted living residence. She decided to expand her practice to include traditional home health services and hospice care to older adults living in their homes.

Mandy enjoyed working with clients in their homes. She felt that the care she delivered was more focused on each person's needs and priorities. Mandy developed close and rewarding relationships with some of her clients and their families. Occasionally her clients demonstrated their appreciation by taking her to lunch or giving her gift cards and other gifts. She enjoyed the attention and welcomed the gifts. Sometimes she used the gifts, and at other times she exchanged them for cash. Mandy found herself engaging in relationships with elderly clients at the end of their lives to deceptively attempt to obtain gifts and bequests, often by taking advantage of their diminished cognitive state. When a family member filed a complaint with the home health agency that contracted Mandy to provide occupational therapy services, the agency terminated her employment. The complaint alleged that Mandy exploited the complainant's parent by taking advantage of her poor judgment to obtain money and gifts from her.

David, the agency's vice president, filed a police report and reported Mandy to the state board regulating occupational therapy practice. He also filed a complaint with the AOTA Ethics Commission (see AOTA, 2015a) citing violation of RSC 2I (avoid relationships that exploit the client), RSC 2F (avoid situations in which one is unable to maintain clear professional boundaries), and RSC 4J (refrain from accepting gifts from clients and their families).

When a client or family member offers a gift to an occupational therapy practitioner, the practitioner should review the Code, the NBCOT *Candidate/Certificant Code of Conduct* (NBCOT, 2016), institutional policies, and federal regulations for relevant guidelines. The AOTA, NBCOT, and some state regulatory boards advise the occupational therapy practitioners they govern or regulate to avoid harming the person under their care. For example, Principles 1, 2, 3, and 4 of AOTA's Code (AOTA, 2015b); NBCOT Principle 4, 6 (NBCOT, 2016); and one board of occupational therapy practice (Maryland) advise against permitting one's desire for financial gain to interfere with decisions made about client care (Department of Health and Mental Hygiene, 2012). Harm may occur when a patient or client tries to express his or her appreciation to the therapist through gift giving when the gesture may cause financial or emotional harm.

Regulations established to govern the receipt of gifts for federal employees can be complex. Under some circumstances, employees may accept coffee, a doughnut, plaques, certificates, or other gifts of less than $20 (Office of the General Counsel, 2015). These guidelines help protect practitioners from engaging in relationships leading to conflicts of interest.

assistive and adaptive devices, to facilitate engagement in meaningful activities important to the client. Vignette 12.4 demonstrates a violation of the Code in end-of-life care.

Summary

Occupational therapy practitioners must have the knowledge, skills, and cultural competence to embrace AOTA's *Vision 2025:* "Occupational therapy maximizes health, well-being, and quality of life for all people, populations, and communities through effective solutions that facilitate participation in everyday living" (AOTA, 2016b). When working with older adults to maximize their productive aging, practitioners must incorporate evidence-based research into their practice and create effective solutions to life challenges, regardless of whether services are delivered in institutional settings or the community. Fulfilling *Vision 2025* will advance the profession and also build confidence and awareness among older adults who strive to age productively.

The construct of productive aging has been used for decades to emphasize occupational performance areas that are important to older adults. Occupational therapy has an important role in helping older adults develop, increase, or maintain ADLs and instrumental activities of daily living, work and volunteer roles, leisure pursuits, civic activities, and caregiving roles. The contexts for service provision include skilled nursing facilities, hospices, senior centers, private homes, employment settings, and community recreational programs. Occupational therapy practitioners also work with older adults as they transition from one phase of life to another (e.g., from full-time work to partial work to retirement). The Code and other resources can help occupational therapy practitioners examine and resolve ethical dilemmas during service delivery.

Reflective Questions

1. Review *Vision 2025* and the demographic projections presented in this chapter and create and describe at least 2 innovative directions for occupational therapy practitioners within the practice area of productive aging.
2. Refer to Vignette 12.2. Identify which Principles and RSCs support (or refute) Amrit's decision to provide occupational therapy interventions to Zelda.
3. Selena and Marco's continued silence in Vignette 12.3 would have led to violations of which Principles and RSCs of the Code?

References

AARP. (2013). *The future of home sweet home (Part 1): Housing.* Retrieved from http://www.aarp.org/home-family/your-home/info-06-2013/aging-in-place-inside-e-street.html

AARP. (2015). *The business case for workers age 50+: A look at the value of experience 2015.* Retrieved from http://www.aarp.org/content/dam/aarp/research/surveys_statistics/general/2015/A-Business-Case-Report-for-Workers%20Age%2050Plus-res-gen.pdf

Agnvall, E. (2010, June 8). How to live a longer, happier life. *AARP Bulletin.* Retrieved from http://www.aarp.org/health/longevity/info-06-2010/how_to_live_a_longer_happier_lifesubhed_longevity_expert_robert_butler_has_the_answers.html

American Occupational Therapy Association. (2011). The role of occupational therapy in end-of-life care. *American Journal of Occupational Therapy, 65*(Suppl.), S66–S75. https://doi.org/10.5014/ajot.2011.65S66

American Occupational Therapy Association. (2013). *Occupational therapy's role in home health* [Fact Sheet]. Retrieved from http://www.aota.org/-/media/Corporate/Files/AboutOT/Professionals/WhatIsOT/PA/Home-Health.pdf?la=en

American Occupational Therapy Association. (2014). Occupational therapy practice framework: Domain and process (3rd ed.). *American Journal of Occupational Therapy, 68*(Suppl. 1), S1–S48. http://dx.doi.org/10.5014/ajot.2014.682006

American Occupational Therapy Association. (2015a). Enforcement procedures for the Occupational Therapy Code of Ethics. *American Journal of Occupational Therapy, 69*(Suppl. 3), 1–13. http://dx.doi.org/10.5014/ajot.59.6.643

American Occupational Therapy Association. (2015b). Occupational therapy code of ethics (2015). *American Journal of Occupational Therapy, 69*(Suppl. 3), 691230030. http://dx.doi.org/10.5014/ajot.2015.696S03

American Occupational Therapy Association. (2016a). AOTA's societal statement on livable communities. *American Journal of Occupational Therapy, 70*(Suppl. 2), 7012410020. http://dx.doi.org/10.5014/ajot.2016.706S01

American Occupational Therapy Association. (2016b). *Occupational therapy's distinct value: Productive aging.* Retrieved from http://www.aota.org/-/media/Corporate/Files/Practice/Aging/Distinct-Value-Productive-Aging.pdf

American Occupational Therapy Association. (2016c). *Productive aging.* Retrieved from http://www.aota.org/Practice/Productive-Aging.aspx

American Occupational Therapy Association. (2016d). *Vision 2025.* http://www.aota.org/AboutAOTA/vision-2025.aspx

Atwal, A., & Caldwell, K. (2003). Ethics, occupational therapy and discharge planning: Four broken principles. *Australian Occupational Therapy Journal, 50,* 244–251. http://dx.doi.org/10.1046/j.1440-1630.2003.00374.x

Beitman, C. L. (2009). Wellness interventions in community living for older adults. *OT Practice, 14*(3), CE1–CE8.

Bloomfield, R. D. (1994). Cultural sensitivity and health care. *Journal of the National Medical Association, 86,* 819–820.

Centers for Disease Control and Prevention. (2013). *The state of aging and health in America 2013.* Retrieved from http://www.cdc.gov/aging/pdf/state-aging-health-in-America-2013.pdf

Centers for Medicare and Medicaid Services. (n. d.). *Discharge planning.* Retrieved from https://www.cms.gov/Outreach-and-Education/Medicare-Learning-Network-MLN/MLNProducts/Downloads/Discharge-Planning-Booklet-ICN908184.pdf

Centers for Medicare and Medicaid Services. (2016). *Medicare benefit policy manual (chapter 15).* Retrieved from https://www.cms.gov/Regulations-and-Guidance/Guidance/Manuals/Downloads/bp102c15.pdf

Department of Health and Mental Hygiene. (2012). Title 10, Subtitle 46. Board of Occupational Therapy Practice, Chapter 2, *Code of Ethics.* Retrieved from http://dhmh.maryland.gov/botp/docs/comar/10.46.02.00.pdf

Fuscaldo, D. (2012). *10 steps to get you ready for retirement.* Retrieved from http://www.aarp.org/work/social-security/info-05-2011/10-steps-to-retire-every-day.1.html

Jenkins, J. A. (2016, March, 22). *The many ways Ethel Percy Andrus made history* [Web log post]. Retrieved from http://blog.aarp.org/2016/03/22/the-many-ways-ethel-percy-andrus-made-history/

Kochera, A., & Straight, A. (2005). *Beyond 50.05. A report to the nation on livable communities: Creating environments for successful aging.* Retrieved from http://assets.aarp.org/rgcenter/il/beyond_50_communities.pdf

Morris, J. F. (2016). Patient abandonment. In D. Y. Slater (Ed.), *Reference guide to the Occupational Therapy Code of Ethics* (2015 ed., pp. 223–228). Bethesda, MD: AOTA Press.

National Board for Certification in Occupational Therapy. (2016). *NBCOT candidate/certificant code of conduct.* Retrieved from http://www.nbcot.org/code-of-conduct

Office of the General Counsel. (2015). *Ethics frequently asked questions.* Retrieved from https://www.nasa.gov/offices/ogc/general_law/ethicsfaq.html

Olmstead v. L. C., 527 U.S. 581 (1999).

Pizzi, M. A. (2010). Promoting wellness in end-of-life-care. In M. E. Scaffa, S. M. Reitz, & M. A. Pizzi (Eds.), *Occupational therapy in the promotion of health and wellness* (pp. 493–511). Philadelphia: F. A. Davis.

Scott, J. B. (2009). Consultation. In E. B. Crepeau, E. S. Cohn, & B. A. B. Schell (Eds.), *Willard and Spackman's occupational therapy* (11th ed., pp. 964–972). Philadelphia: Lippincott Williams & Wilkins.

Thrash, J. (2006). *Common phrase translation: Spanish for English speakers for occupational therapy, physical therapy, and speech therapy.* Burbank, CA: Author.

U.S. Department of Health and Human Services. (2014). *Healthy People 2020 topics and objectives: Older adults.* Retrieved from https://www.healthypeople.gov/2020/topics-objectives/topic/older-adults

Wells, S. A., Black, R. M., & Gupta, J. (Eds.). (2016). *Culture and occupation: A model for effectiveness in health care, research, and education* (3rd ed.). Bethesda, MD: AOTA Press.

White House Conference on Aging. (2015). *2015 White House Conference on Aging: Final report.* Retrieved from http://www.whitehouseconferenceonaging.gov/2015-WHCOA-Final-Report.pdf

World Health Organization. (2016). *Proposed working definition of an older person in Africa for the MDS Project.* Retrieved from http://www.who.int/healthinfo/survey/ageingdefnolder/en/

Chapter 13.

CHILDREN AND YOUTH: ETHICS IN SERVICE PROVISION ACROSS CONTEXTS

Susanne Smith Roley, OTD, OTR/L, FAOTA, and Mary Alice Singer, MS, OTR/L

Learning Objectives

By the end of the chapter, readers will be able to

- Identify the core values of occupational therapy as it relates to ethical practice with children, youth, and their caregivers;
- List 5 potential areas of ethical conflict with a client, employer, organization, or colleague when providing services to children, youth, and their caregivers;
- Differentiate between positive solutions during an ethical dilemma and those that violate the Principles and Related Standards of Conduct of an occupational therapy practitioner working with children and youth; and
- Recognize circumstances in the delivery of occupational therapy services to children and youth that require additional support from authorities, including the American Occupational Therapy Association, to ensure provision of ethical practice.

Key Term and Concept

✧ Co-occupations

Societies place a high value on protecting children and youth, one of the most vulnerable populations. This vulnerability is reflected in the laws and guidelines societies enact to protect children and youth, such as child protective services, child custody, and institutional review boards. The public outcry against those who exploit the vulnerability of children and youth and fail to protect them is echoed in the media. For example, *Time* published an article titled "FBI: Child Abuse 'Almost at an Epidemic Level' in U.S." that highlighted exploitation of impoverished and neglected children for pornography and sex trafficking (Johns, 2015).

Occupational therapy practitioners are obligated to provide services in compliance with laws and professional standards of practice (American Occupational Therapy Association [AOTA], 2015c). As such, practitioners are bound by the standards of care espoused by the occupational therapy profession to ensure that each client receives the services he or she needs to fully participate in society (AOTA, 2015a). Related Standard of Conduct (RSC) 4E of the *Occupational Therapy Code of Ethics (2015)* (hereinafter referred to as the "Code") obligates occupational therapy practitioners to "maintain awareness of current laws and AOTA policies and Official Documents that apply to the profession of occupational therapy" (AOTA, 2015a, p. 6).

In this chapter, the Code's six Principles are applied to occupational therapy practice with children and youth. It is trite, but true, that everybody makes mistakes. Table 13.1 provides examples of mistakes violating each of the six Principles in the Code. Ethical practitioners strive for best practice; recognize their mistakes; confront concerns affecting the lives of children, youth, and families; immediately take steps to report and repair errors; and make a firm commitment not to participate actively or passively in potentially harmful or dishonest situations.

Table 13.1. Vignettes Describing Breaches of the Code in the Practice Area of Children and Youth

Principle	Vignette
1. Beneficence	**Michelle,** an occupational therapist, provided a thorough community-based evaluation of **Todd,** an adolescent who was experiencing heightened anxiety and depression with suicidal thoughts. The evaluation provided an analysis of Todd's deficits but did not acknowledge his strengths. Michelle knew several immediate environmental modifications that would help Todd, but she did not share them with the family because she believed that this information involved remediation and wished to bill for the information. Michelle provided community-based suggestions over an 8-week period rather than as part of the evaluation report, consuming Todd's annual allotment of insurance coverage for occupational therapy. Besides breaching Principle 1, Beneficence, Michelle also violated Principle 2, Nonmaleficence; Principle 4, Justice; and Principle 5, Veracity.
2. Nonmaleficence	**Michael,** an occupational therapist, was working with **Juaquin,** who was macrocephalic because of hydrocephalus, was nonverbal, blind, and had cerebral palsy with contractures of the elbow and wrist. Michael decided that stretching the joints was necessary. The mother reported that Juaquin, who was typically good-natured and happy during therapy sessions, whined and cried throughout the stretching. Michael insisted that stretching was necessary and that Juaquin had to work through the pain. Later, a doctor discovered that Michael had torn Juaquin's biceps tendon. Michael violated RSC 2A, "Avoid inflicting harm or injury to recipients of occupational therapy services, students, research participants, or employees" (AOTA, 2015a, p. 4).
3. Autonomy	**Carla** was an occupational therapist working in a private practice serving a variety of children. Her desk was visible from the parent waiting room. She turned from working on a report to talk with a child. While she and the child were talking, a parent walked by, read portions of the report that was open on her computer screen, and proceeded to discuss this private information with another parent in the waiting room. The mother of the child discussed in the report overheard the conversation and was mortified and angry. Carla violated RSC 3H, "Maintain the confidentiality of all verbal, written, electronic, augmentative, and nonverbal communications in compliance with applicable laws, including all aspects of privacy laws and exceptions thereto" (AOTA, 2015a, p. 5).
4. Justice	A **5-year-old child** experiencing learning and behavior difficulties at school was referred to **Shawna,** an occupational therapist. Shawna informed the child's parents that there was a lengthy waiting list for evaluation and intervention. They were anxious for their child to receive services as quickly as possible, so the child's father offered to purchase and donate any piece of equipment needed for the practice, implying that he wanted his child to be moved to the top of the waiting list. Shawna rechecked the schedule and "found" an unexpected opening, ignoring the waiting list and removing a low-income, non-English speaking family from the roster. She scheduled the child and provided the parents her wish list of equipment for the gym, violating the Principle of Justice relative to the other families on her waiting list.

(Continued)

Table 13.1. Vignettes Describing Breaches of the Code in the Practice Area of Children and Youth (*Cont.*)

Principle	Vignette
5. Veracity	**Kenan,** an adolescent receiving inpatient intervention for cancer, was provided with occupational therapy services. The administrator insisted that the occupational therapist, **Akeia,** continue to see Kenan until discharge. Following reevaluation using the Canadian Occupational Performance Measure (Law et al., 2005) and other assessments, however, Akeia determined that Kenan had achieved all appropriate goals. The administrator also directed Akeia to use billing codes that did not reflect her intervention but had been preapproved by the insurance company, thereby violating the Principle of Veracity, or truthfulness, when billing.
6. Fidelity	A nonprofit organization providing specialized services for children invited **Cassandra,** an occupational therapist, to be a member of the board of directors. Cassandra accepted the position, even though her ownership of a for-profit business providing products and programs similar to those of the nonprofit organization constituted a conflict of interest. She intimidated affiliates of the organization, including past board members and current staff, by making slanderous statements about them in public. During the following year, she successfully lobbied for several of her business affiliates to fill vacant board positions; she intended to close two departments of the nonprofit and change key staff in the other departments and needed the additional votes to do so. With the new board members in place, Cassandra moved to the board chair position and proceeded to fire long-standing staff, replacing them with staff members loyal to her. Subsequently, their operations resulted in reduced services to members, poor quality educational opportunities, and inadequate intervention services for families. The community's confidence in occupational therapy services was diminished, therefore violating the Principle of Fidelity.

Note. AOTA = American Occupational Therapy Association; RSC = Related Standard of Conduct.

Occupational Therapy With Children and Youth

Occupational therapy practitioners' concern for children addresses children's need for food, love, and shelter (see Figure 13.1) but goes beyond these basic needs. Pediatric practices include children and families with a wide variety of presenting concerns and diagnoses (AOTA, 2014b). Occupational therapy practitioners work with individuals, organizations, and populations related to children and youth from prenatal care to age 21 years. Occupational therapy services are delivered in various contexts, including environments such as hospitals, communities, schools, homes, and clinics.

Depending on the area of pediatric practice, occupational therapy practitioners require different skill sets. Examples of types of practice that require distinct competencies include

- Counseling pregnant women;
- Providing identification of developmental risks in an Early Head Start program;
- Providing interventions to premature infants and their parents in a neonatal intensive care unit (NICU); and
- Working in prevocational training centers, juvenile detention facilities, women's shelters, and community mental health centers.

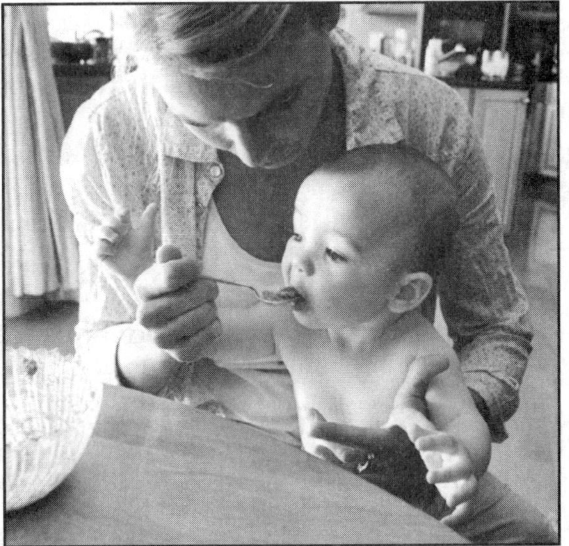

FIGURE 13.1

Practitioners often consult with parents on feeding techniques during a home visit.

Source. S. Smith Roley. Used with permission.

Occupational therapy practitioners who work with children and youth also work with their caregivers in various family constellations, cultural contexts, environments, and communities. Clients' concerns are central to the provision of occupational therapy; thus, family-centered care is imperative. Because caregivers spend the most time with their children, know them the best, and have the largest impact on their development, caregivers are the cornerstone of service provision to this population. Occupational therapy interventions often provide a critical source of support for development, remediation, education, and resilience in the lives of children who are at risk or who have disabilities, and their families.

To provide evidence-based, data-driven, and value-driven services, occupational therapy practitioners rely on high-quality occupational therapy education, research, administration, and innovations in practice and depend on the utmost integrity of the people, programs, and systems that provide them. Authorities and mentors often set the bar for what to do and what not to do; when this is not the case, situations arise that require practitioners to make tough choices. They base their practice on promoting clients' engagement in occupation to achieve health, well-being, and participation in life within the domain and process of occupational therapy (AOTA, 2014a). The value of engagement in activities drives what the practitioner will do; the values of altruism, equality, freedom, justice, dignity, truth, and prudence drive how the practitioner will do it (AOTA, 2015a).

Occupational therapy practitioners must be aware of potential conflicts of interest and must decline to engage in activities corrupted by motives of self-interest. Part of professional practice is ongoing vigilance for possible conflicts linked to personal gain such as salary, power, and position. In addition, practitioners need to act responsibly by discussing potential conflicts, requesting feedback from peers and authorities, and finding ways to approach conflicts so the outcome is in the best interest of the client and the profession.

Principle 1. Beneficence

According to Principle 1, Beneficence, RSC 1C, occupational therapy practitioners should "use, to the extent possible, evaluation, planning, intervention techniques, assessments, and therapeutic equipment that are evidence based, current, and within the recognized scope of occupational therapy practice" (AOTA, 2015a, p. 3).

Occupational therapy is a helping profession. Although multiple motivations bring someone to the profession, the desire to positively influence the lives of others is often the strongest driving force. Although they also may desire the other benefits, such as salaries, professional prestige,

Vignette 13.1. Promoting Beneficence in Services to Families

A **group of occupational therapy practitioners** provided services as part of an early intervention program focusing on children with autism and their families. Several families traveled more than 60 miles each way to attend the weekly program. The practitioners were aware that the program director took on clients who could be receiving services closer to their homes to prevent a competing program from receiving the business. The program director refrained from sharing information about geographically closer services with the families. The practitioners identified the following options to address this dilemma:

- Tell the families in private about other options for services.
- Meet with the director to discuss their discomfort with the situation.
- Solicit more clients within a reasonable geographic region.
- Set up meetings with similar agencies to discuss the referral process to better meet families' needs.
- Suggest providing unique and sophisticated intervention options that warrant the extra effort by families to attend that early intervention program.

After reviewing all of the possible plans of action, the practitioners developed a plan for soliciting more clients in the surrounding area. They also met with the therapy team at an agency closer to the families in question to create a referral plan to better serve the families. The final step was a meeting with the director of the program to update him on the networking and to suggest ways that the children and families would be better served. The proposal of a plan for attracting new clients allowed the meeting to go smoothly.

friendships, or standing in the local community, in the end occupational therapy practitioners working with children and youth should primarily wish to provide services that benefit this important segment of society. Clients in this area of practice necessarily include both children and youth and their primary caregivers (AOTA, 2014a). Therefore, it is essential to provide services that respect the values and beliefs of families and other caregivers.

Occupational therapy practitioners gather essential information from families and caregivers to better understand the child and improve the ***co-occupations*** they engage in—that is, activities that are intrinsically shared (e.g., parenting and being parented, family dining). Vignette 13.1 describes a situation in which occupational therapists promoted Beneficence in an early intervention setting.

Occupational therapy practitioners working with youth and children are responsible for maintaining the highest possible standards of practice (Figure 13.2). Therapists and assistants entering a new practice area must commit to updating their knowledge and skills. Entry-level skills and abilities are honed through practice and mentorship. Specialized knowledge and skills must be obtained, particularly in situations where the client is the most vulnerable, such as acute hospital care (e.g., NICU environments) and when children have difficulty with eating, feeding, and swallowing. When a client needs expertise beyond the level of a practitioner, the practitioner must find resources such as mentors or another practitioner to assist in the intervention (see Case Study 13.1).

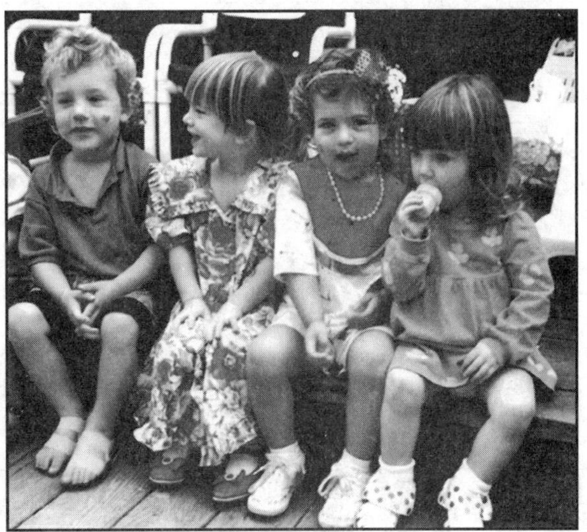

FIGURE 13.2

Occupational therapy practitioners working with youth and children are responsible for maintaining the highest possible standards of practice.
Source. S. Smith Roley. Used with permission.

Case Study 13.1. Maintaining Currency of Practice

Eva, a pediatric occupational therapist, was recently hired for a position in a busy hospital setting. Her responsibilities included NICU inpatient care and outpatient follow-up, including feeding interventions for babies who had graduated from the NICU and returned home.

Eva had some experience in a NICU setting but was not confident about her expertise in feeding. She was asked to feed a medically unstable infant with low-birth-weight born 25 weeks premature. Acutely aware that handling medically fragile infants requires constant physiological and cardiac monitoring specific to stress responses that may undermine their homeostasis and metabolic functions, she requested supervision by the occupational therapist with expertise in the NICU environment before handling the neonate. The therapist was aware that the nursing staff in the NICU was highly trained and quite protective of their precious charges. The experienced occupational therapist recommended that the treating therapist ask that a nurse be present during the feedings until the neonate was more stable.

Eva determined that she required additional skills for this new position before taking responsibility for working with the babies in the NICU, particularly after looking at documents outlining the knowledge and skills needed in this area of practice (AOTA, 2006). She considered the potential solutions identified in Table 13.2

(Continued)

Case Study 13.1. Maintaining Currency of Practice *(Cont.)*

Table 13.2. Decision Table for Case Study 13.1

Possible Action	Positive Outcomes	Negative Consequences or Costs
Take no action.	None.	Risk eroding other team members' opinions of the value of occupational therapy. Fail to provide the highest level of practice for the babies and their families.
Seek consultation and mentorship with an experienced therapist with postgraduate specialization in common feeding interventions for babies in the NICU.	Gain knowledge of techniques and evidence for providing feeding interventions for babies in the NICU. Complete CEU workshops dealing with NICU feeding intervention practice.	No negative effect on infant care. Requires investment of time and finances.
	Review literature such as AOTA Knowledge and Skills document specific to NICU practice (AOTA, 2006) and pediatric journals for evidence in neonatal care and feeding interventions.	Requires investment of time and finances.
Explore options for further education in this occupational therapy practice area.	Schedule meeting with nurses, primary caregivers, or both to determine procedures for inpatient care. Participate in team meeting for discharge planning, including creating a holistic plan for family life at home and in the community.	No negative effect on infant care.
Seek collaboration with other team members.	Collaborate with the parents specific to attachment, sensory sensitivities, motor development, feeding issues, and discharge planning.	May create unintended paternalistic relationship or result in culturally insensitive care.
Engage family in discharge planning for home follow-up.	Empowers and supports family with resources and options following hospital discharge.	Family may not be able to afford recommended care.

Note. AOTA = American Occupational Therapy Association; CEU = continuing education unit; NICU = neonatal intensive care unit.

Principle 2. Nonmaleficence

In Principle 2, Nonmaleficence, RSC 1C states, "occupational therapy personnel shall refrain from actions that cause harm" (AOTA, 2015a, p. 3). The phrase, *primum non nocere,* commonly used in medicine, means "First, do no harm." This Principle reminds practitioners to humbly consider whether intervening would be worse than doing nothing.

When working with vulnerable children and youth, occupational therapy practitioners must commit to updating their knowledge and skills to ensure that their clients are receiving the best possible services. This commitment is necessary both when entering practice with children and youth and when changing focus within this practice area. Practitioners must obtain specialized knowledge and skills, particularly in settings (e.g., NICU) or situations in which clients are the most vulnerable (e.g., difficulty with eating, feeding, and swallowing). Entry-level skills and abilities can be honed through practice and mentorship, but when the client needs expertise beyond the practitioner's skill level, the practitioner must find resources such as a mentor or a competent practitioner to assist in the intervention.

The more educated occupational therapy practitioners are, the more depth of knowledge they have when communicating with parents and professionals. Families rely on practitioners to provide expertise that supports their efforts to care for their children under stressful conditions. Caregivers are critical to a child's well-being; therefore, their input must be included in intervention planning, intervention, and follow-up programs. If practitioners educate parents and other caregivers regarding the purpose and methods used during intervention, parents and other caregivers are more likely to carry this learning over into the settings where children spend most of their time.

Parent education begins with evaluation results, which must be written in language that parents understand. Collaboration between practitioners and parents or caregivers is paramount in creating a support system for children at home and in the community. The supports must include transition opportunities when services are diminished or discontinued or when the adolescent transitions out of supports such as their educational environment (AOTA, 2015b). In Vignette 13.2, a practitioner confronts a dilemma involving the duty to do no harm.

Principle 3. Autonomy

Principle 3, Autonomy, states in RSC 1C that practitioners "shall respect the right of the individual to self-determination, privacy, confidentiality, and consent" (AOTA, 2015a, p. 4). Infants and children often do not have a voice in decision making related to their care, so the adults responsible for their well-being must be sensitive to their best interests. Occupational therapy practitioners require finesse to understand the primary needs of infants, children, and youth and then advocate for their best interests while traversing cultural differences in caregiving, parenting styles, and families' hopes and dreams as well as limitations in funding streams and service delivery models.

Occupational therapy practitioners often have access to sensitive information about their clients when providing services, including not only health and educational records but also family dynamics and financial status. The obligation to sustain confidentiality is expressly stated in laws such as the Health Insurance Portability and Accountability Act of 1996 (P. L. 104–191). Protecting the privacy of clients' written records is easy, however, compared with maintaining their privacy when collaborating with other parents or professionals and

Vignette 13.2. Avoiding Harm

While diapering a **child with Down syndrome** during an early intervention program, the occupational therapist noticed bruises on the child's legs. The nanny had mentioned to the therapist that she was frustrated with the child's hyperactivity and lack of compliance when told to do something. Both parents were away on a business trip. The therapist suspected that the nanny had used corporal punishment on the child.

The various responsibilities of the occupational therapist in this situation were as follows:

- Prevent further harm from happening to the child.
- Report suspected abuse to child protective services.
- Notify the child's parents about her suspicions and be aware of any future incidents.
- Inform the administration of the early intervention program about the suspected abuse.
- Consult with the nanny on positive behavioral approaches.
- Provide the nanny with contact information for the social worker on staff for assistance if needed.

The first step the occupational therapist took to prevent further harm to the child was to notify the child's parents and the program's administrator of her suspicions. The therapist provided the nanny with written information on positive behavioral approaches and opened a dialogue with the nanny about intervention strategies specific to the behavior she was finding difficult to manage. She gave the nanny a referral to a local respite program to add support. The child's parents returned home and, after meeting with the nanny, decided to hire additional help for the nanny when they were going to be out of town at the same time.

Vignette 13.3. Respecting Individual Determination

Trisha, a private practitioner, provided an independent occupational therapy evaluation to a family referred by a child advocacy group. On completing the evaluation, the father paid for the evaluation in cash, proudly stating that he had saved for 1 year to provide this evaluation for their child. Trisha knew that the father was a day laborer and did not have a bank account but understood that she had to respect the family's desire for services. She realized that her fees were a significant drain on the family's resources, but she had already committed to further services at a mutually agreed-on fee, including creating goals and objectives, consulting with the child's school district, and attending the individualized education program (IEP) meeting.

Trisha identified the following potential options to address this dilemma:

- Continue with the services as previously negotiated.
- Return the money for the evaluation to the father.
- Take the money and purchase something for the family.
- Provide the remainder of the agreed-on services with no further charge.

Trisha considered the ethical issues in this case and came to the following conclusions: She was providing a service to the family, and they needed to reimburse her, but the fees she charged should not put undue financial strain on a family already stressed by a child with serious health issues. Trisha decided to establish a sliding scale for her services and charged the family a reduced fee for the overall evaluation, recommendations, and attendance at the IEP meeting. This reduction in fees allowed the family to purchase equipment Trisha recommended to enhance the health and well-being of their child.

when addressing a history of child abuse or neglect. The occupational therapist in Vignette 13.3 faced a dilemma regarding a family's ability to pay for services.

Principle 4. Justice

Principle 4, Justice, states that RSC 1C, "Occupational therapy personnel shall promote fairness and objectivity in the provision of occupational therapy services" (AOTA, 2015a, p. 5). The occupations of children and youth may differ from those of other age groups, but the overarching goal of occupational therapy practice is still "achieving health, well-being, and participation in life through engagement in occupation" (AOTA, 2014a, p. S2), regardless of the age, disability, economic status, culture, or ethnicity of the client (see Figure 13.3). Access to and engagement in meaningful, needed, and desired activities are intrinsic to the health and well-being of children and youth and to their eventual participation as contributing members of society.

Provision of occupational therapy services allows children to be an active family and community member to the best of their ability. Practitioners strive to provide needed services to individuals, populations, and organizations without economic, ethnic, or cultural bias. Occupational therapy services are not limited by cultural or political boundaries and are provided with the aim of enhancing health, well-being, and

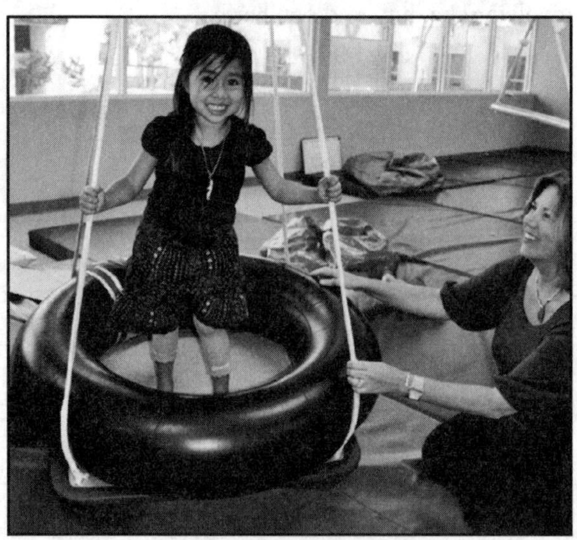

FIGURE 13.3

Practitioners should consider children's social needs within their communities to promote child development and well-being.

Source. S. Smith Roley. Used with permission

Vignette 13.4. Ensuring Adherence to Legal Obligations

Derek, a school-age child, attended a social skills training class led by **Bianca,** an occupational therapist, at a clinic. Derek's parents were in the process of a contentious divorce and custody settlement agreement, and each had independently requested that Bianca testify as a witness during Derek's custody hearing. In the meantime, the noncustodial parent under the current custody agreement tried to pick Derek up after therapy on days that were assigned to the custodial parent. No social workers or attorneys were available for consultation at the clinic.

Bianca identified the following options to address this dilemma:

- Consult with the AOTA Ethics Commission and the state regulatory board.
- Insist that the custodial parent be the only person transporting the child to and from therapy.
- Suggest that the parents go to mediation.
- Decline to provide testimony during the hearing.
- Meet with Derek's parents, and if they are unable to agree on who will transport Derek to and from therapy, discharge the child from the caseload.

Bianca scheduled a meeting with Derek's parents and explained that testifying in court for either parent compromised her neutrality and impaired her ability to provide child-centered therapy for Derek. She gave the parents a referral to a family therapist who was experienced in conflict resolution and suggested that to support Derek, both parents needed to focus on behavior that put his needs first. She explained that conflict over who was transporting Derek was impairing the therapeutic environment she was attempting to create for Derek, and she stated that she would not release him to the noncustodial parent. Bianca made it clear that these conditions were not negotiable and that the parents were free to choose another therapist if they could not agree to them. Derek's parents agreed to her stipulations and attended mediation to work out their issues.

participation in the lives of youth and children. Practitioners must provide appropriate supervision and mentoring for staff therapists, particularly those new to an area of practice. Regardless of whether the payer is a family, school district, employer, insurance company, or state or federal agency, fees for services should be fair and commensurate with the services provided. Vignette 13.4 presents a dilemma for the occupational therapist working with a child whose parents are in the midst of a contentious divorce.

Principle 5. Veracity

Principle 5, Veracity, states in RSC 1C that practitioners "shall provide comprehensive, accurate, and objective information when representing the profession" (AOTA, 2015a, p. 7). Accurate and reliable information provided to consumers of occupational therapy services and collaborators in the professional community is fundamental to the integrity of occupational therapy services. Occupational therapy practitioners are often the ones who work most closely with clients and their families to ameliorate challenges in carry out activities of daily living. Clients and their caregivers deserve the most accurate information in a format that enables them to best understand and apply that information. Practitioners must present information in a way that enhances understanding and avoids impairing family dynamics. In Vignette 13.5, an occupational therapist had to repair the damage caused by a colleague who violated the ethical Principle of Veracity. Case Study 13.2 describes a situation in which an occupational therapist intervened because a child's safety was at risk.

Principle 6. Fidelity

The Principle of Fidelity requires practitioners to practice reliably and faithfully and to make and keep commitments to others (AOTA, 2015a). Colleagues who are trusted implicitly are the ones who do what they say and say what they do; they are trustworthy and follow through on their commitments or responsibilities. Being reliable ensures that clients can trust the information and interventions provided. To ensure this level of reliability, practitioners must be honest about their knowledge base and the limitations of their expertise. They also

Vignette 13.5. Rectifying Breach of Veracity

The parents of **Eileen,** a 5-year-old child who was having difficulty in school, requested a second-opinion evaluation by **Tima,** an occupational therapist. Eileen had a history of developmental delays and extreme sensory sensitivities for which she had received intervention. Another occupational therapist from the same practice, **Robert,** had recently evaluated Eileen. The parents complained to Tima that they had spent a lot of money for a report that was confusing and did not address their concerns.

Robert had reported findings from prior assessments completed by other therapists but based his recommendations solely on observations in his office. Robert's evaluation report was written haphazardly, emphasized erroneous theories about neurology that lacked support in the literature, and claimed that with extensive intervention in his clinic, Eileen would be completely cured. Not only was the information incorrect, it was impossible to pick out the salient details that would be used to guide Eileen's intervention.

Tima communicated her concerns about Robert's report to her supervisor and set up a team meeting with the family. Tima also considered the following steps:

- Discuss her concerns with Eileen's parents regarding the need for additional testing and evidence-based review of information about Eileen's occupational performance and her needed and desired engagement in activities and, with the parents' permission, provide a complete evaluation and report on Eileen.
- Provide a suggested reading list for the parents.
- Write a concise and easily understood evaluation report with recommendations.
- Give the parents handouts that explain home and community activities that will benefit Eileen.
- Discuss the situation with the state regulatory board, the National Board for Certification in Occupational Therapy (if Robert is certified), and AOTA's Ethics Commission (if Robert is an AOTA member), supplying facts and documentation as necessary.
- If Eileen's parents provide consent, provide a copy of her current report and recommendations to Robert, the original therapist.
- Demonstrate intervention strategies within the sessions and explain how Eileen's parents can adapt them during the week to support her progress toward therapy goals.
- Provide Eileen's parents with a home program for follow-up to therapy; update the program periodically as Eileen progresses.

Tima scheduled a meeting with Eileen's parents and explained the need for further evaluation with standardized tests to determine her level of occupational performance in comparison to her same-age peers. Tima also described how services were provided and intervention decisions were made in their facility but avoided making disparaging remarks about Robert. After Eileen's parents agreed to further evaluation, Tima provided an evaluation with a clear explanation of Eileen's functional levels with recommendations for community and home activities that would help Eileen achieve her goals. Eileen's parents observed her therapy sessions and were provided with explanations of therapy approaches and ways to adapt them for home follow-up. Tima recommended reading for Eileen's parents about her challenges and ways to support her at home and school and in the community.

Tima determined that Robert was not a member of AOTA but was licensed. She reported him to the state regulatory board, which began an investigation into his practice.

Case Study 13.2. Ensuring Safety of Service Recipients

As part of a nonpublic agency (NPA) service, **Juanita,** an occupational therapist, provided twice-weekly one-on-one intervention to **Megan,** an elementary student, as indicated on Megan's IEP. On 3 out of 4 occasions over a 2-week period, on the day Juanita was to provide therapy, Megan had a grand mal seizure lasting about 20 minutes. The teacher told Juanita not to worry because she had managed the child during the seizures by wrapping her in a blanket in the corner of the classroom until the seizure subsided. On the fourth therapy day, Juanita happened to be at the school when Megan's mother picked her up. Juanita told the mother about the seizure activity and suggested that she call the physician to make an appointment to get Megan's blood checked for medication levels. The mother told her that because the physician did not expect to draw blood for another month, she hadn't thought to request it earlier.

The physician determined that because Megan had grown, the prescription was too weak. When

(Continued)

Case Study 13.2. Ensuring Safety of Recipients of Service *(Cont.)*

the prescription was modified, the seizure activity was eliminated. Later that week, Juanita received a call from the teacher reprimanding her for speaking directly to Megan's mother and undermining the teacher's authority. Juanita consulted the Code and found that Principle 5, Veracity, RSC 5D—"Identify and fully disclose to all appropriate persons errors or adverse events that compromise the safety of service recipients" (AOTA, 2015a, p. 7)—applied in this case.

She considered the following courses of action:

- Review the school district's policy related to health management specific to seizures.
- Request an emergency IEP team meeting, including the parents, and invite members of the child's medical team.
- Approach the district about the need to revise the line of supervision for NPA-related services.
- Cease providing services to this district because of the conflict between their policies and Juanita's legal and moral obligations.

After reviewing the school district's policy regarding seizures, Juanita determined that Megan's teacher had neglected to follow established procedures and alert both the school principal and Megan's parents of the increase in her seizure activity. She requested an emergency IEP team meeting, at which Megan's parents, teacher, and other therapy providers agreed on immediate notification of her parents regarding changes in the frequency of seizures or Megan's overall behavior. Juanita scheduled a meeting with the school principal to clarify the line of supervision for NPA-related services and arranged ongoing direct contact with the principal instead of the classroom teacher. Juanita established that consultation with the family and school staff was an essential part of the occupational therapy service included in the IEP. This resolution provided the confidence Juanita needed to continue to provide therapy services to this district in a manner that ensured Megan's health and safety along with the other students on her caseload.

Table 13.3. Decision Table for Case Study 13.2

Possible Action	Positive Outcomes	Negative Consequences or Costs
Take no action.	None.	Child does not receive necessary services because of the conflict between district policies and Juanita's legal and moral obligations.
Approach the district about the need to revise the line of supervision for NPA-related services. Review the school district's policy related to health management specific to seizures. Request an emergency IEP team meeting, including the parents, and invite members of the child's medical team.	Juanita continues to provide therapy services to this district in a manner that ensures Megan's health and safety along with the other students on her caseload.	By challenging the chain of command, Juanita risked her position in the organization. She believed it was more important to protect her occupational therapy license and reduce the possibility of malpractice. She therefore accepted the risk that she might have to change jobs.

Note. IEP = individualized education program; NPA = nonpublic agency.

Vignette 13.6. Ensuring Fidelity to Scope of Practice

Mariko, an occupational therapist providing rural home health services for homebound, medically fragile children, was asked by her employer to provide speech, nursing, and physical therapy to clients after being given cross-training in each of the other disciplines. Mariko saw that sufficient professionals were not available to meet the needs of these children. She knew the professional community in the area and wanted to maintain and develop her relationships with colleagues and organizations in the area. But she also knew that if she refused, she would lose her job, and this high-needs population might not be served.

Mariko considered the following courses of action:

- Seek consultation and mentorship with experienced home health therapists and administrators.
- Provide her employer with relevant sections from licensure laws and the Code.
- Attend as much continuing education as possible to cover the needs of these children and families.
- Review scope of practice documents (e.g., AOTA, 2014b).
- Consult frequently with other disciplines on issues relevant to the cases.
- Limit her caseload to force the agency to hire more therapists.
- Refuse to offer services outside of those covered by licensure laws.

Mariko decided to meet with the administrator and provide him with both the scope of practice standards and relevant sections of the licensure laws. She discussed the legal and ethical necessity not to provide therapeutic intervention outside of her area of expertise. The administrator agreed to provide her with continuing education for this population of clients. Mariko sought out mentorship from home health therapists in her area who understood the client population she was dealing with. She established monthly meetings with other therapists in her area for support and mentorship.

must avoid unnecessary disruptions to their personal and professional lives because of negligence, difficulty prioritizing, or lack of attention to essential duties and the needs of others. Vignette 13.6 describes the issues an occupational therapist faced in protecting her own competencies and those of other professionals.

Summary

When working with children and youth, their best interest is the ultimate goal of occupational therapy. This goal influences the ways in which occupational therapy practitioners decide what to do and how to do it. It is not enough to follow others' examples; practitioners must examine the ways in which actions or non-actions potentially influence others. Sometimes ethical practice requires going against the status quo. Practitioners who are uncertain about the right thing to do will benefit from seeking the advice of those who are knowledgeable about professional ethics and wise in their implementation.

Reflective Questions

1. How does an occupational therapy practitioner who is an employee of a large organization provide services to children and families according to his or her ethics and simultaneously meet the administration's dictates?
2. What actions can an occupational therapy practitioner take when providing services to children and youth with updated and evidence-based developmental methods that are challenged by their supervising therapist?
3. What potential responses can an occupational therapy practitioner give to a parent who is skeptical about the evaluation results and effectiveness of the proposed intervention and insists that the family is not going to provide suggested activities at home or in the community? What is the best course of action and why?
4. What are possible solutions when providing occupational therapy services to an adolescent client who is verbally and physically abusive to anyone perceived as an authority, including the practitioner?

References

American Occupational Therapy Association. (2006). Specialized knowledge and skills for occupational therapy practice in the neonatal intensive care unit. *American Journal of Occupational Therapy, 60*(6), 659–668. https://doi.org/10.5014/ajot.60.6.659

American Occupational Therapy Association. (2014a). Occupational therapy practice framework: Domain and process (3rd ed.). *American Journal of Occupational Therapy, 68*(Suppl. 1), S1–S48. https://doi.org/10.5014/ajot.2014.682006

American Occupational Therapy Association. (2014b). Scope of practice. *American Journal of Occupational Therapy, 68*(Suppl. 3), S34–S40. https://doi.org/10.5014/ajot.2014.686S04

American Occupational Therapy Association. (2015a). Occupational therapy code of ethics (2015). *American Journal of Occupational Therapy, 69*(Suppl. 3), 6912310030. https://doi.org/10.5014/ajot.2015.696S03

American Occupational Therapy Association. (2015b). Occupational therapy's perspective on the use of environments and contexts to facilitate health, well-being, and participation in occupations. *American Journal of Occupational Therapy, 69*(Suppl. 3), 6913410050. https://doi.org/10.5014/ajot.2015.696S05

American Occupational Therapy Association. (2015c). Standards of practice for occupational therapy. *American Journal of Occupational Therapy, 69*(Suppl.3), 6913410057. https://doi.org/10.5014/ajot.2010.64S106

Health Insurance Portability and Accountability Act of 1996, Pub. L. 104–191, 100 Stat. 2548.

Johns, T. (2015). *FBI: Child abuse "almost at an epidemic level."* Retrieved from http://time.com/3978236/american-children-sold-sex/

Law, M., Baptiste, S., Carswell, A., McColl, M. A., Polatajko, H., & Pollock, N. (2005). *The Canadian Occupational Performance Measure* (4th ed.). Ottawa, ON: CAOT Publications.

Chapter 14.

ETHICS IN HEALTH PROMOTION AND WELLNESS

S. Maggie Reitz, PhD, OTR/L, FAOTA

Learning Objectives

By the end of the chapter, readers will be able to

- Describe occupational therapy health promotion services,
- Determine when an ethical situation is present during the planning and implementation of a health promotion initiative, and
- Apply Principles and Related Standards of Conduct from the *Occupational Therapy Code of Ethics (2015)* to address ethical tensions during the provision of occupational therapy health promotion services.

Key Terms and Concepts

✧ Health promotion
✧ Occupational therapy health promotion services
✧ Pragmatism

Occupational therapy was born during a time of great social change in the United States. In the early 1900s, the lingering impact of the Civil War, the influx of immigrants, and innovations in mental health care all coincided with the emergence of pragmatism. Breines (1986) defines ***pragmatism*** as the belief that "human development proceeds through experience in life with objects and individuals in the environment. Knowledge and truth is constantly being revised, and interpretation of reality is influenced by individual and collective experience" (p. x). Pragmatism, a school of philosophy, was initially conceived in the United States in the late 1880s by William James, George Herbert Meade, and John Dewey. Dewey also was known as the leading education reformer of the time.

The profession of occupational therapy was established during this rich time of social activism. Both Dewey's Laboratory and Jane Addams's Hull House in Chicago, which emphasized active learning, became a hub for social activists. Social activists, using the philosophy of pragmatism, "asserted that active occupations was a means of promoting and restoring health" (Breines, 1986, p. x).

Each of the Principles in the *Occupational Therapy Code of Ethics (2015)* (hereinafter referred to as the "Code"; American Occupational Therapy Association [AOTA], 2015b) applies to occupational therapy practice that promotes health and well-being. The relationships between the six Principles of the Code and health promotion practice are discussed in this chapter. A recurring theme in the vignettes and case studies presented is the importance of obtaining current and relevant knowledge and competencies surrounding health promotion before engaging in this type of practice.

Health Promotion and Occupational Therapy

Health promotion includes efforts to ensure that members of the public have access to the knowledge, information, and strategies they need to minimize threats to health and maximize well-being. Health promotion activities should be available for all individuals regardless of their health or ability status. Occupational therapy practitioners have long been involved in the promotion of health and well-being among individuals and have the potential for greater involvement with communities and populations (Reitz, 2010; Reitz & Scaffa, 2010). The number of occupational therapy practitioners engaging in this type of practice has been small (AOTA, 2015a).

According to AOTA (2013), "Occupational therapy practitioners have three critical roles in health promotion and prevention:

1. To promote healthy lifestyles;
2. To emphasize occupation as an essential element of health promotion strategies; and
3. To provide interventions, not only with individuals but also with populations. It is important that occupational therapy practitioners promote a healthy lifestyle for all individuals and their families, including people with physical, mental, or cognitive impairments" (p. S50).

Although many of the same skill sets are used in this practice area as in other areas, practitioners may need to acquire additional skills, knowledge, and experience to provide interventions in an ethical manner.

Principle 1: Beneficence

Health promotion reflects Principle 1, Beneficence (i.e., doing good), because ***occupational therapy health promotion services*** are interventions designed to enhance the pursuit of wellness in individuals, families, institutions, and populations. The intended outcome of these efforts is the enablement of occupational engagement, health, and well-being (AOTA, 2013). Outcomes are facilitated through customized initiatives that facilitate clients' abilities to make positive, self-directed choices about occupational engagement in their pursuit of well-being.

Clients, whether individuals, families, or communities, determine their own definition of well-being on the basis of values shaped by culture, age, ethnicity, geography, and other unique factors. Occupational therapy practitioners support the Principle of Beneficence by ensuring that clients receive a benefit from services, that those services are based on best practices, and by respecting clients' values and their right to self-determination.

Educating for Health Promoting

Educating occupational therapy students in a manner that supports their development of knowledge and skills to provide occupational therapy health promotion services at various levels (e.g., individuals, groups, families, communities, populations) is supported by the Principle of Beneficence, as it clearly articulates the need for occupational therapy practitioners to only provide services for which they have been educated (see Related Standards of Conduct [RSCs] C, D, E, F, G). Preparation of occupational therapy students for this practice area is the subject of Case Study 14.1.

Disaster Preparedness and Recovery[1]

Many citizens, including occupational therapy practitioners, are moved by the Principle of Beneficence to assist in times of disaster. They can be prepared to help if a disaster occurs in their community, county, or state. Investigating local opportunities to volunteer and receive training as a responder before a disaster occurs gives people more options to serve if the circumstances arise.

[1]The material in this section is adapted from Reitz and Harcum (2010). Copyright © 2010 by American Occupational Therapy Association. Used with permission.

Case Study 14.1. Promoting Competency for Community Practice

Yael was hired as the third faculty member in a new occupational therapy department at a small liberal arts college that recently began offering graduate programs. She was excited to move from a health promotion–focused, community-based practice working with older adults, caregivers, and various agencies to an academic position. Yael had taught for 10 years before taking time off to care for her mother and then moving to community-based practice. She wanted to work in academia to help students become excited about working in community- and population-based programming because she saw the potential for the profession to influence a great many more lives.

However, once Yael took a closer look at the curriculum, she realized there was no coursework to prepare students for community-based practice. When she questioned **Martha,** the program director, she was told that the students were going to be well trained in the use of an occupational profile across diagnostic groups and that they would be able to easily generalize this process to the provision of health promotion services with families and communities.

Yael considered her next step. She remembered attending an ethics presentation at the state occupational therapy association's conference and reviewed her notes from the talk. She also identified relevant Principles from the Code. Yael was concerned that the students' ability to benefit from their occupational therapy education might be limited by the current curriculum design, and thus the program would be in violation of Principle 1, Beneficence. The students' preparedness to address issues surrounding Autonomy (i.e., Principle 3), Justice (i.e., Principle 4), and Veracity (i.e., Principle 5) in this practice area also could be limited.

Next, Yael reviewed the current accreditation standards for entry-level master's-degree programs (Accreditation Council for Occupational Therapy Education [ACOTE], 2012). She was simultaneously pleased and dismayed when she identified 10 ACOTE standards directly related to health promotion and community-based practice (see Table 14.1). Although she was pleased that this much attention was directed to a practice area she loved, she was dismayed because the proposed curriculum at her college could be out of compliance with many, if not all, of these standards.

Yael requested a formal meeting with Martha to review the curriculum, ACOTE standards, and official AOTA documents to formulate a plan to cover the material called for in the standards. The plan Yael developed included the addition of a community-based class, which she volunteered to develop and teach, as well as earlier infusion of additional content on family theory and community practice. Martha was embarrassed about her lack of knowledge about these standards and thanked Yael for her efforts to ensure that the program and curriculum would meet or exceed the standards.

Table 14.1. ACOTE Standards Related to Health Promotion and Community-Based Practice

No.	Standard
B.2.4	Articulate the importance of balancing areas of occupation with the achievement of health and wellness for the clients.
B.2.5	Explain the role of occupation in the promotion of health and the prevention of disease and disability for the individual, family, and society.
B.2.6	Analyze the effects of heritable diseases, genetic conditions, disability, trauma, and injury to the physical and mental health and occupational performance of the individual.
B.2.9	Express support for the quality of life, well-being, and occupation of the individual, group, or population to promote physical and mental health and prevention of injury and disease considering the context (e.g., cultural, personal, temporal, virtual) and environment.
B.5.17	Develop and promote the use of appropriate home and community programming to support performance in the client's natural environment and participation in all contexts relevant to the client.

(Continued)

Case Study 14.1. Promoting Competency for Community Practice *(Cont.)*

Table 14.1. ACOTE Standards Related to Health Promotion and Community-Based Practice (*Cont.*)

No.	Standard
B.5.18	Demonstrate an understanding of health literacy and the ability to educate and train the client, caregiver, family and significant others, and communities to facilitate skills in areas of occupation as well as prevention, health maintenance, health promotion, and safety.
B.5.19	Apply the principles of the teaching–learning process using educational methods to design experiences to address the needs of the client, family, significant others, communities, colleagues, other health providers, and the public.
B.5.26	Demonstrate use of the consultative process with groups, programs, organizations, or communities.
B.6.1	Evaluate and address the various contexts of health care, education, community, political, and social systems as they relate to the practice of occupational therapy.
B.6.5	Analyze the trends in models of service delivery, including, but not limited to, medical, educational, community, and social models, and their potential effect on the practice of occupational therapy.

Note. ACOTE = Accreditation Council for Occupational Therapy Education.
Adapted from "Accreditation Council for Occupational Therapy Education (ACOTE) Standards 2011," by Accreditation Council for Occupational Therapy Education, 2012, *American Journal of Occupational Therapy*, Vol. 66, Suppl. 6, pp. S6–S74. Copyright © 2012 by the American Occupational Therapy Association. Used with permission.

Readers are encouraged to locate the nearest Community Emergency Response Team (Federal Emergency Management Agency [FEMA], Department of Homeland Security, 2016; National Office of Citizen Corps, FEMA Individual and Community Preparedness Division, n.d.) training opportunity. Potential negative consequences of untrained attempts to provide aid in a disaster are described in Vignette 14.1, and a more successful example is detailed in Vignette 14.2.

Vignette 14.1. Gaining Competency Before Disaster[2]

Portia was saddened and concerned about the eastern rural portion of a neighboring state that had been hit that morning by a series of tornadoes. As an occupational therapist, she believed she could contribute to the disaster recovery efforts. She quickly packed some clothes and her dog into her car. As she drove east, a string of heavy thunderstorms resulted in flooded roads. She became lost in the darkness. The next day, she and her dog were rescued at taxpayers' expense.

Vignette 14.2. Promoting Well-Being After Disaster

After Hurricane Katrina struck in August 2005, **Frank Pascarelli** used his occupational therapy skills to combat lack of access to basic communication services in Pascagoula, Mississippi. Frank had greater ability to assist at a disaster site than most occupational therapy practitioners because of his unique dual roles as an Air Force reservist and employee of the Centers for Disease Control and Prevention.

Frank decided to facilitate a low-cost method for affected people to communicate and reconnect with family and friends. Many people had lost their mailboxes in the storm, so Frank acquired and distributed replacement mailboxes and provided a cordless drill. Residents used the drill to attach their new mailbox to some physical structure remaining on their property (e.g., tree, fence post). The same cordless drill was passed from neighbor to neighbor, thus rebuilding a sense of community along with the communication system.

Frank's next challenge was to assist in reclaiming a school playground to allow children to resume developmentally appropriate occupations (Hofmann, 2008).

[2]The vignettes in this chapter originally appeared in "Principle 4. Social Justice," by S. M. Reitz and S. Harcum. In J. B. Scott and S. M. Reitz (Eds.), *Practical Applications for the Occupational Therapy Code of Ethics and Ethics Standards*, pp. 65–76. Copyright © 2010 by the American Occupational Therapy Association. Reprinted with permission.

Upholding the Principle of Beneficence in times of disaster involves a unique set of ethical concerns. Occupational therapy practitioners must reflect on their motivations, pursue relevant training and ensure competence, and seek a position with an authorized disaster aid organization before embarking on disaster relief (AOTA, 2011). An example of disaster preparedness would be working with a community through authorized organizations to ensure that age-appropriate opportunities for occupational engagement are available at disaster shelters. Ensuring that communities have procedures for evacuating all members in a safe and orderly way supports both the Principle of Beneficence and Principle 4, Justice.

Principle 2: Nonmaleficence

Occupational therapy practitioners are reminded of the importance of preventing harm by Principle 2, Nonmaleficence. The potential to do harm is very real in health promotion practice (Reitz, Pizzi, & Scaffa, 2010). Examples of well-meaning health promotion interventions with the potential to result in physical or fiscal harm to a community include

- Using a boilerplate process to replicate a fitness program in all the senior centers in a county or local jurisdiction without customizing the program to meet the interests, health needs, and values of each center's membership.
- Replicating programs with no formal evaluation process in place, thereby failing to include a mechanism to uncover and address unforeseen negative effects.
- Supporting or assisting programs that use or promote fear to change behavior in adolescents and young adults without an understanding of the complex role of fear in health decision making. Research evidence has shown that fear is ineffective in changing the desired health behavior and in some cases can encourage unhealthy engagement in this age group (Prevention First, 2008).
- Establishing a health promotion program in an at-risk community with no plans to sustain the program once funding ends.

Failure to consider potential harm when developing health promotion programs or conducting research in this area can result in negative ripples of influence that travel through a community or population and compromise future efforts to gain access to the community.

Blatant abuse of a community's trust to meet personal needs or goals as a researcher or student or to collect data for a publication, grant, or course without concern for the long-term welfare of the community is unethical and in direct violation of Principle 1 and RSC 2A (avoid inflicting harm or injury to clients) and RSCs 2F and 2G (avoid relationships that exploit clients).

To ensure a win–win outcome in community-based health promotion programming and research, plans must address the sustainability of services or the program at the outset of negotiations. Failure to do so undermines access to the community by future students, researchers, or others seeking research participants. The Tuskegee experiment (1932–1972), in which researchers studied the long-term effects of syphilis among a group of African American men without notifying participants of their diagnosis or offering treatment for them or their partners, should be a warning to all who engage in public health or health promotion research without concern for the impact on the population. The legacy of this experiment is lingering mistrust of government public health officials and researchers (Jones, 1981; Thomas & Quinn, 1991).

Principle 3: Autonomy

The pursuit of wellness is a self-directed activity of individuals, communities, populations, or a society. One cannot impose wellness on a person or community; it must be initiated by the client. Although health promotion programs are developed to encourage health behavior change and the adoption of a wellness philosophy, deciding how to use the delivered information or experience rests solely with the client. When decisions are made regarding what programs are needed in a community, care should be taken to include community members and leaders in the needs assessment and decision-making process (Fazio, 2010).

Principle 3, Autonomy (i.e., client self-direction), should be upheld while assessing needs, developing programs, and evaluating outcomes with communities as well as individuals. As shown in Case Study 14.2, knowledge of health behavior

Case Study 14.2. Fostering Autonomy in Program Planning

Veranda enjoyed living and working in the city. She loved commuting to her job as an occupational therapist at the city hospital via mass transit. Having grown up in a quiet rural area on a farm, she thrived on the hustle and bustle of city life.

The hospital had recently received a grant to promote the health and well-being of families in the surrounding area. Staff could apply for funds to develop programs in support of the hospital's initiative. Veranda decided that the best way to improve the families' health and well-being was to provide basic parenting training. She was successful in obtaining funding to provide an evening parenting tips program. Because she had observed that the parents who brought their children for outpatient occupational therapy always seemed rushed, she decided that time management would be the focus of the first session; on the basis of the attention that the obesity epidemic was receiving in the media, she selected healthy eating habits as the second topic for the evening.

Veranda was in a hurry as she prepared for the parenting class. The night before, she remembered that 5 years earlier, a professor in her university health class had provided materials on the two topics she planned to discuss. Veranda located her class notebook, removed the professor's name and copied the material onto hospital letterhead, and made copies for the parenting class. Athough she momentarily considered that her actions constituted plagiarism, she brushed away those concerns. She was tired and wanted to get to sleep.

The night of the first session, she was happy to see 10 people in attendance. The program started off well; Veranda was a friendly, outgoing person who could put people at ease. Veranda sensed a growing tension as she distributed the materials on time management and healthy eating. Nevertheless, she proceeded to review the time management information, and when she sensed that the information was not being well received, she suggested a break. During the break, **Teddy,** a rehabilitation aide who was attending the class, told her that some people in the room could only read at about a 9th-grade level, and they were embarrassed and frustrated with the materials. Teddy further explained that he knew about the SMOG readability assessment (National Cancer Institute [NCI], 2001) from his health education graduate studies. Veranda thanked Teddy for the information.

After the break, Veranda switched to discuss the importance of serving fresh fruits and vegetables as part of a healthy diet. These materials contained more visuals and less text, so Veranda thought she was back on track. However, one attendee stood up and said, "Honey, I know you mean well, but where am I supposed to get fresh fruits and vegetables?" Veranda was speechless and said, "I don't understand." The person calmly explained that the closest grocery store was 10 miles away. Some convenience stores in the area carried fruits and vegetables, but the selection was limited, the quality was poor, and the cost was high. Veranda asked if there were any farmers markets in the area and was told there were none on this side of the river.

Veranda thought quickly; she needed to do something to reconnect with the group. She used her occupational therapy problem-solving skills and knowledge of occupational therapy theory, specifically the Ecology of Human Performance (Dunn, Brown, & McGuigan, 1994), to develop a potential plan for the next session. After thanking people for coming, she asked, "What do you think about spending next week's session having you introduce me to the local neighborhood and then brainstorm ideas to get a farmers market on this side of the river?" Teddy said, "Now that is much more like what we need!"

Teddy stayed after the others left. He gently asked Veranda if she had ever studied any health behavior frameworks or theories. She replied that she had not. Teddy suggested she start by reading two free sources that were available online. The first was Theory at a Glance (NCI, 2005), and the second was known in health education and behaviors circles as the "pink book" (NCI, 2001).

Veranda spent time the next weekend reviewing the materials. She became excited about blending health behavior theories with occupational therapy theories to support the development of a farmers market. She also asked Teddy if he would be co-facilitator for the project. Veranda was happy that the group's effort could be far more meaningful than she first imagined. Instead of merely affecting the 10 people who had attended the group, the group's combined efforts to obtain a farmers market could benefit the entire community.

literature and support from other disciplines can enhance occupational therapy practitioners' work and success as well as their adherence to the Code.

Principle 4: Justice

According to Plato, the "ideal" government was one that promoted the health of its citizens and prevented poverty (Lyons & Petrucelli, 1987, p. 219). Health promotion, especially at the community and population levels, can help address the disparities in health seen in the United States (U.S. Department of Health and Human Services, 2010). The presence of the Principle of Justice in the Code and the fact that health and wellness was one of the focus areas of AOTA's *Centennial Vision* (AOTA, 2007) support the need for continued focus on health promotion and community health in occupational therapy practice. In addition, the AOTA's *Vision 2025,* which states "Occupational therapy maximizes health, well-being, and quality of life for all people, populations, and communities through effective solutions that facilitate participation in everyday living" (AOTA, 2016, para. 1), also supports this focus.

Although the *Centennial Vision*, Vision 2025, and ACOTE standards (see Table 14.1) reflect an appreciation and acknowledgment of the important role of occupational therapy practitioners in health promotion, including population health (Braveman, 2015), the latest AOTA workforce survey (AOTA, 2015a) indicates that only 1.9%, slightly down from 2% in the previous study, of occupational therapy practitioners work in the community. Because this number includes practitioners who work in prevention or wellness programs as well as practitioners who work in adult day care, community residential care facilities, group homes, and other community settings, the proportion of practitioners who have health promotion as their primary work focus is very small indeed. Not included in these figures, however, are the health promotion efforts of occupational therapy practitioners working in other areas such as hospitals or schools; the professional literature provides little or no evidence of the impact of this work.

The profession as a whole has a shared responsibility to determine the next best steps to take to ensure that RSC 4D, "advocate for changes to systems and policies that are discriminatory or unfairly prevent access to occupational therapy services" (AOTA, 2015b, p. 5), is upheld. One strategy for the future is to educate the public and legislators about the value of occupational therapy in promoting health and wellness, which upholds RSC 4D.

RSC 4E, Justice, obligates occupational therapy practitioners to "maintain awareness of current laws and AOTA policies and Official Documents that apply to the profession of occupational therapy" (AOTA, 2015b, p. 5). In Case Study 14.2, Veranda failed to uphold this RSC in her parenting program because she was not aware of or had not referenced AOTA documents such as *Occupational Therapy's Perspective on the Use of Environments and Contexts to Facilitate Health, Well-Being, and Participation in Occupations* (AOTA, 2015c) and *Occupational Therapy in the Promotion of Health and Well-Being* (AOTA, 2013).

Veranda also had no knowledge of the health behavior change literature. She presented healthy eating information using the food pyramid (Figure 14.1; U.S. Department of Agriculture [USDA], 2005) instead of the updated "My Plate" tool (Figure 14.2; USDA, 2011), which is much easier to understand (Vastag, 2011). Furthermore, according to RSC 1E, occupational therapy practitioners must remain current on the available knowledge and evidence to deliver health promotion services ethically.

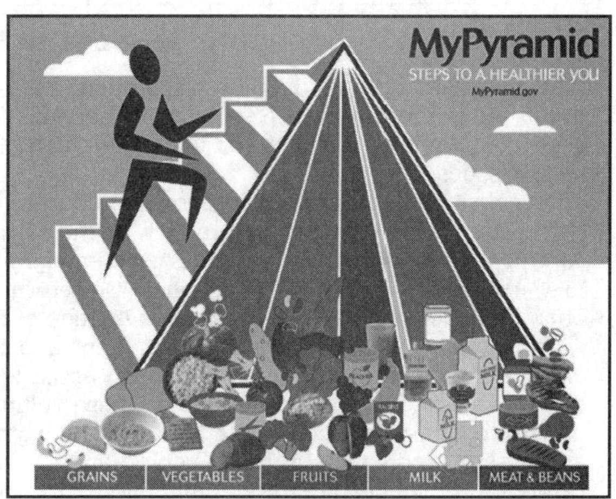

FIGURE 14.1

MyPyramid: Food guidance system recommended by the U.S. Department of Agriculture, 2005–2011.

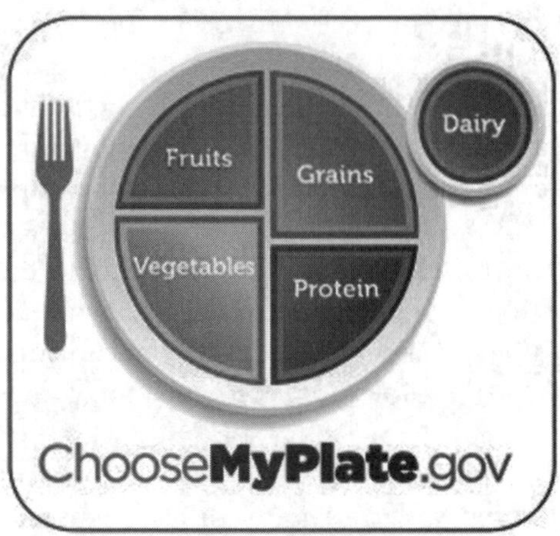

FIGURE 14.2

MyPlate: Food guidance system recommended by the U.S. Department of Agriculture since 2011.

Vignette 14.3 describes an occupational therapy practitioner's efforts to address justice for immigrants.

Principle 5: Veracity

Health promotion practice, like any other area of practice, requires practitioners to practice Principle 5, Veracity, and be truthful in their work. Examples of these behaviors include being honest about credentials, expertise, payment structures, and assessment data. In health promotion practice, as in other areas of practice, it is imperative to present one's expertise, training, and credentials in an honest fashion, including currency of all credentials.

In addition, all anticipated client payments, including charges for supplies or access to educational materials that supplement health promotion initiatives, must be clearly communicated before commencing care. If an additional resource is later identified, then this resource and the additional cost should be clearly communicated to the client in a timely manner. It should then be the client's decision as to whether this added cost is acceptable.

In Case Study 14.2, Veranda failed to uphold RSC 5B (be honest and accurate in all communication) and RSC 5H (do not plagiarize). As Teddy and Veranda talked about the source of the material she distributed, they realized she had plagiarized and failed to recognize her professor's work. At a minimum, Veranda needed to contact her professor to apologize and ask what actions she would like Veranda to take. She also needed to alert her supervisor to her mistake and follow supervisor and hospital guidance as long as the advice was in alignment with the Code.

Principle 6: Fidelity

Principle 6, Fidelity, requires occupational therapy practitioners to "treat colleagues and other

Vignette 14.3. Extending Services to Underserved Populations

Maria was an occupational therapist working as a consultant at a nonprofit women's health center in an urban area. The center offered all of its services for free or on a sliding-scale basis. In her role, Maria assisted in the development and implementation of educational programs and pamphlets about women's health issues.

Recently she had attended a continuing education course on the topic of cultural awareness and sensitivity. The course included an overview of the demographics in her city, which she learned had a significant population of relatively recent Asian immigrants, particularly from Southeast Asian nations such as Vietnam, Thailand, and the Philippines. On returning to work, Maria noticed that few or no Vietnamese, Thai, or Filipino women were taking advantage of the center's programs.

Maria was able to find several prominent and trusted members of the local Vietnamese, Thai, and Filipino communities who were willing to assist with recruitment of participants and the translation of marketing and educational materials. These volunteers also agreed to serve on a board of directors to assist the center in meeting the needs of the women in the community. This inexpensive strategy both addressed the disparity in those served and leveraged community stakeholders to assist in the identification of other needs of the community. This action upholds Principle 4, RSC 4B (help people access necessary services), RSC 4C (remove barriers to necessary services), RSC 4D (advocate for necessary services), as well as Principles 1 (Beneficence), 2 (Nonmaleficence), and RSC 3J (facilitation of meaningful communication).

professionals with respect, fairness, discretion, and integrity" (AOTA, 2015b, p. 7). As has been seen throughout this chapter, health promotion frequently intersects with other areas of practice, settings, and disciplines. For these initiatives to be successful, practitioners need to take care to nurture respectful and professional relationships. Positive partnerships both enhance client health promotion services and support the Principle of Fidelity. Failure to uphold this Principle can negatively affect service delivery, as shown in Vignettes 14.4 and 14.5, and can even place one's license or livelihood at risk.

Summary

Occupational therapy practitioners are trained to provide health promotion services to clients that directly relate to the completion of activities of daily living and instrumental activities of daily living with individuals. However, there is a need for occupational therapy practitioners to become involved in prevention and health promotion activities beyond the scope of the individual client.

Occupational therapy practitioners who want to provide services at the community or population

Vignette 14.4. Maintaining Fidelity in Program Development

Colleagues **Lilly** and **Irene** developed a fall prevention program while working for a private hospital. They both spent a lot of time working on the project and were proud of the program, including the title, TREAD (*T*rip *R*eduction *E*ducation, *A*nalysis, *D*emonstration). Irene left the facility to develop a private practice. While grocery shopping, Lilly noticed a set of flyers advertising a fall prevention program with Irene's picture. The title and program description were exactly the same as those they had developed at the hospital. Lilly was shocked that Irene had stolen and replicated the program because it belonged to the hospital.

Lilly, knowing that one should handle ethical issues locally before escalating to a complaint, contacted Irene and shared her concerns. At first, Irene shrugged it off, but when she saw how upset Lilly was, she offered to pay Lilly a percentage of the profit from the program. Lilly declined this solution and told Irene that she would contact the state regulations board to report Irene's unethical behaviors unless she cancelled the program, refunded any payments received, and ceased offering the program in the future. In addition, Lilly told Irene that she would inform her supervisor at the hospital of their actions to address the situation.

Table 14.2. Decision Table for Vignette 14.4

Possible Action	Positive Outcomes	Negative Consequences
No action.	Avoid uncomfortable situation.	Lilly would be in violation of Principle 2, Nonmaleficence; Principle 4, Justice; Principle 5, Veracity; and Principle 6, Fidelity, including RSCs 6A, 6B, 6C, and 6E.
Use social media to confront Irene.	Irene may refrain from her behavior.	Irene could feel betrayed. Lilly would be in violation of Principle 2, Nonmaleficence; Principle 3, Autonomy, including RSC 3I (inappropriate use of social media); Principle 4, Justice; and Principle 6, Fidelity, specifically RSC 6A.
Report Irene immediately to the hospital's legal counsel.	Hospital's interest would be protected.	Irene could feel betrayed. Lilly could be in violation of Principle 2, Nonmaleficence; Principle 4, Justice; and Principle 6, Fidelity, specifically RSC 6J.
Confront Irene	Hospital's interest would be protected. Irene would have the opportunity to resolve the issue. Lilly would uphold Principle 6, Fidelity, specifically RSC 6J.	Irene could feel betrayed.

Note. RSC = Related Standard of Conduct.

Vignette 14.5. Observing Fidelity in Assisting Colleagues

Dean had a background in private practice with children and youth in a bustling mid-Atlantic metropolitan area. He was hired as an assistant professor at a private faith-based university 45 miles east of the city in a rural farming community at the foot of the Appalachian Mountains. The chair of the occupational therapy department, **Kate,** met with Dean to share the university's mission and the guidelines for promotion and receipt of tenure. In the ensuing discussion, Kate encouraged Dean to become involved in health promotion service learning within the community to position himself for success at the university.

Being pragmatic, Dean thought he would provide an evaluation service embedded in a class he was scheduled to teach the following fall semester. Dean spent the next 9 months securing resources (e.g., a meeting place at the library) for a weekly evaluation clinic for young children. He anticipated community interest in the free evaluation service and expected the students to gain useful hands-on practice experience.

During the first 2 weeks, no one showed up for the free evaluation service. He was perplexed and concerned. Dean sought guidance from **Sam,** a health science faculty member who had been teaching at the university for 20 years. Sam asked questions about Dean's knowledge of health promotion and Appalachian culture. Dean acknowledged that he had very little. Sam provided him with resources about Appalachian culture and suggested he visit a local museum. Sam also suggested that he become familiar with health behavior models and frameworks, which would help him better plan and implement programs once he became known to and knowledgeable about the community he sought to assist.

levels should remain current on the literature on health behavior, health education, and public health and should consider partnering with experts in these areas to jointly provide services. A variety of publications are available from AOTA (e.g., AOTA, 2013, 2015c; Bailey, 2016; Braveman, 2015) to assist occupational therapy practitioners in providing guidance for best practice.

Reflective Questions

1. Review Vignettes 14.1 and 14.2.

- Which RSC related to the Principle of Beneficence could guide behavior during a disaster?
- What resources from AOTA and the World Federation of Occupational Therapists could inform Portia's future actions in disaster recovery?

2. Using the Four-Step Decision-Making Model, analyze the situation described in Vignette 14.5. Be sure to identify the ethical Principles and RSCs Dean violated. Consider Kate's responsibility in the situation.

- Did her behavior violate any of the principles?
- What should Dean do to address the situation in its totality?

3. Identify resources at AOTA and elsewhere that can help inform ethical occupational therapy health promotion services. How could these resources help?

References

Accreditation Council for Occupational Therapy Education. (2012). 2011 Accreditation Council for Occupational Therapy Education (ACOTE®) standards. *American Journal of Occupational Therapy, 66*(6 Suppl.), S6–S74. https://doi.org/10.5014/ajot.2012.66S6

American Occupational Therapy Association. (2007). AOTA's *Centennial Vision* and executive summary. *American Journal of Occupational Therapy, 61,* 613–614. https://doi.org/10.5014/ajot.61.6.613

American Occupational Therapy Association. (2011). The role of occupational therapy in disaster preparedness, response, and recovery. *American Journal of Occupational Therapy, 65*(6 Suppl.), S11–S25. https://doi.org/10.5014/ajot.2011.65S11

American Occupational Therapy Association. (2013). Occupational therapy in the promotion of health and well-being. *American Journal of Occupational Therapy, 67*(6 Suppl.), S47–S59. https://doi.org/10.5014/ajot.2013.67S47

American Occupational Therapy Association. (2015a). *2015 AOTA salary and workforce study.* Bethesda, MD: AOTA Press.

American Occupational Therapy Association. (2015b). Occupational therapy code of ethics (2015). *American Journal of Occupational Therapy, 69*(Suppl. 3), 6912310030. https://doi.org/10.5014/ajot.2015.696S03

American Occupational Therapy Association. (2015c). Occupational therapy's perspective on the use of environments and contexts to facilitate health, well-being, and participation in occupations. *American Journal of Occupational Therapy, 69*(Suppl. 3), 6913410050. https://doi.org/10.5014/ajot.2015.696S05

American Occupational Therapy Association. (2016). *Vision 2025*. Retrieved from https://www.aota.org/AboutAOTA/vision-2025.aspx

Bailey, R. R. (2016). Managing sedentary behavior to improve and enhance health. *OT Practice, 21*(6), 15–20.

Braveman, B. (2015). Population health and occupational therapy. *American Journal of Occupational Therapy, 70*(1), 1–6. https://doi.org/10.5014/ajot.2016.701002

Breines, E. (1986). *Origins and adaptation: A philosophy of practice*. Lebanon, NJ: Geri-Rehab.

Dunn, W., Brown, C., & McGuigan, A. (1994). The ecology of human performance: A framework for considering the effect of context. *American Journal of Occupational Therapy, 48*, 595–607. https://doi.org/10.5014/ajot.48.7.595

Fazio, L. S. (2010). Health promotion program development. In M. E. Scaffa, S. M. Reitz, & M. A. Pizzi (Eds.), *Occupational therapy in the promotion of health and wellness* (pp. 195–207). Philadelphia: F. A. Davis.

Federal Emergency Management Agency, Department of Homeland Security. (2016). *Community emergency response teams*. Retrieved from https://www.fema.gov/community-emergency-response-teams

Hofmann, A. O. (2008). *Rebuilding lives: Occupational therapy and disaster relief*. Retrieved July 13, 2008, from www.aota.org/News/Consumer/Rebuilding.aspx

Jones, J. H. (1981). *Bad blood: The Tuskegee syphilis experiment—A tragedy of race and medicine*. New York: Free Press.

Lyons, A., & Petrucelli, R. (1987). *Medicine: An illustrated history*. New York: Abradale Press.

National Cancer Institute. (2001). *Making health communication programs work: A planner's guide*. Bethesda, MD: National Institutes of Health.

National Cancer Institute. (2005). *Theory at a glance: A guide for health promotion practice* (2nd ed.). Bethesda, MD: National Institutes of Health.

National Office of Citizen Corps, FEMA Individual and Community Preparedness Division. (n.d.). *Search CERT programs by zip code*. Retrieved from http://www.citizencorps.fema.gov/cc/searchCert.do?submitByZip

Prevention First. (2008). *Ineffectiveness of fear appeals in youth alcohol, tobacco and other drug (ATOD) prevention*. Springfield, IL: Author.

Reitz, S. M. (2010). Historical and philosophical perspectives of occupational therapy's role in health promotion. In M. E. Scaffa, S. M. Reitz, & M. A. Pizzi (Eds.), *Occupational therapy in the promotion of health and wellness* (pp. 1–21). Philadelphia: F. A. Davis.

Reitz, S. M., & Harcum, S. (2010). Principle 4; Social justice. In T. B. Scott & S. M. Reitz (Eds.), *Practical applications for the occupational therapy code of ethics and ethics standards* (pp. 65–76). Bethesda, MD: AOTA Press.

Reitz, S. M., & Scaffa, M. E. (2010). Public health principles, approaches, and initiatives. In M. E. Scaffa, S. M. Reitz, & M. A. Pizzi (Eds.), *Occupational therapy in the promotion of health and wellness* (pp. 70–95). Philadelphia: F. A. Davis.

Reitz, S. M., Pizzi, M. A., & Scaffa, M. E. (2010). *Evaluation principles in health promotion*. In M. E. Scaffa, S. M. Reitz, & M. A. Pizzi (Eds.), *Occupational therapy in the promotion of health and wellness* (pp. 157–172). Philadelphia: F. A. Davis.

Thomas, S. B., & Quinn, S. C. (1991). The Tuskegee syphilis study, 1932 to 1972: Implications for HIV education and AIDS risk education programs in the Black community. *American Journal of Public Health, 81*, 1498–1505. http://dx.doi.org/10.2105/AJPH.81.11.1498

U.S. Department of Agriculture. (2005). *My Pyramid tracker*. Retrieved from https://www.cnpp.usda.gov/sites/default/files/archived_projects/MiniPoster.pdf

U.S. Department of Agriculture. (2011). *My Plate*. Retrieved from https://www.choosemyplate.gov/MyPlate

U.S. Department of Health and Human Services. (2010). *Healthy People 2020* [Brochure]. Retrieved from https://www.healthypeople.gov/sites/default/files/HP2020_brochure_with_LHI_508_FNL.pdf

Vastag, B. (2011, June 3). Moving from pyramid to plate. *The Washington Post*, p. A4.

Chapter 15.

WORK AND INDUSTRY: ETHICAL CONSIDERATIONS FOR OCCUPATIONAL THERAPY PRACTITIONERS

Jeff Snodgrass, PhD, MPH, OTR/L, FAOTA

Learning Objectives

By the end of the chapter, readers will be able to

- Describe ethical dilemmas related to the practice area of work and industry,
- Identify and analyze potential ethical dilemmas in a variety of work-related practice settings, and
- Apply ethical Principles and Related Standards of Conduct to vignettes and case studies representing real-world ethical dilemmas in work and industry.

Key Terms and Concepts

- ✧ Americans With Disabilities Act of 1990
- ✧ Americans With Disabilities Act Amendments Act of 2008
- ✧ Ergonomics
- ✧ Functional capacity evaluation
- ✧ Occupational and Safety Health Act of 1970
- ✧ Occupational Safety and Health Administration
- ✧ OSHA Form 300 logs
- ✧ Person with a disability
- ✧ Pre-employment examination
- ✧ U.S. Equal Employment Opportunity Commission
- ✧ Work reconditioning

Work and industry is a well-established area of practice for occupational therapy practitioners. Because the profession has always been strongly grounded in work as a central occupation, occupational therapy practitioners are found in various settings with diverse client populations, including people with developmental disabilities, adolescents and younger workers, older workers, and people with mental health illness. Traditional venues include outpatient settings, either hospital based or freestanding, and inpatient rehabilitation centers as well as clients' homes and work sites (Kaskutas & Snodgrass, 2009).

Work and industry interventions may include application of ergonomics to prevent injury and work reconditioning programs to prepare employees to return to work. ***Ergonomics*** is the scientific discipline concerned with understanding the interactions among humans and other elements of a system. Ergonomics is also the profession that applies theoretical principles, data, and methods to design in order to optimize human well-being and overall system performance (International Ergonomics Association [IEA], 2016, para. 1). ***Work reconditioning*** is a generalized approached to rehabilitation focused on physical conditioning, including strength, endurance, cardiopulmonary fitness, range of motion and flexibility, and coordination (Haruka, Page, & Wietlisbach, 2013).

In addition to understanding and adhering to the *Occupational Therapy Code of Ethics (2015)* (hereinafter referred to as the "Code"; American Occupational Therapy Association [AOTA], 2015), occupational therapy practitioners must be aware of and understand the workplace regulatory and policy environment in which they provide services to effectively serve their clients. Regulatory and policy issues provide an important contextual component of ethical decision making in the workplace (Snodgrass & Gupta, 2014).

Workplace Policy, Regulations, and Programming

Numerous types of work-related legislation have been enacted since the early 20th century. In the United States, legislation and programming have been enacted and implemented over the last several decades to protect employers and employees, to ensure that hiring practices are fair, and to promote safe working conditions. This section describes some of the relevant legislation that influences the ethical practice of occupational therapy. Although the intent of this chapter is to focus on professional ethical issues, the reader should keep in mind that the regulations presented in this section must be considered as part of the ethical decision-making process.

Americans With Disabilities Act of 1990

The ***Americans With Disabilities Act of 1990*** (ADA; P. L. 101–336) was "the most comprehensive legislation for people with disabilities ever passed in the United States" (Karger & Rose, 2010, p. 74). The intent of the broad and inclusive legislation was to socially integrate people with disabilities. The ADA defines a ***person with a disability*** as someone with a recorded physical or mental impairment that substantially limits his or her participation in one or more life activities, such as work. ADA prohibited discrimination in employment on the basis of disability and required accessibility of state and federal government programs and services, specifically in public accommodations, transportation, and telecommunications. Employers are prohibited from discriminating against workers with a disability who qualify for employment as long as they can meet the essential job functions with or without reasonable accommodations in the workplace.

Americans With Disabilities Act Amendments Act of 2008

The ***Americans With Disabilities Act Amendments Act of 2008*** (ADAAA; P. L. 110–325) was enacted to explicitly reject the narrowing of the definition of disability by the courts and to clarify the language so courts can consistently apply the broad intent and purpose of the act. In essence, the ADAAA focuses on discrimination of individuals with disabilities rather than on their disability (Snodgrass & Gupta, 2014).

U.S. Equal Employment Opportunity Commission

Created in 1965, the ***U.S. Equal Employment Opportunity Commission*** (EEOC) is a federal agency that enforces antidiscrimination laws and provides oversight to protect workers from being discriminated against on the basis of their race, color, religion, sex (including pregnancy, gender identity, and sexual orientation), national origin, age (40 years or older), disability, or genetic information (EEOC, 2015).

ADA is enforced in the workplace by the EEOC. When the ADAAA was enacted in 2008, the EEOC was directed to make the necessary changes to the Title I ADA regulations and the interpretive guidance documents (EEOC, 2015).

Occupational Safety and Health Administration

The federal agency responsible for oversight of safe and healthy workplaces is the ***Occupational Safety and Health Administration*** (OSHA), which operates under the U.S. Department of Labor. When the ***Occupational and Safety Health Act of 1970*** (OSH Act; P. L. 91–596) was passed, it had a two-fold charge: (1) assure safe and healthful workplaces by setting and enforcing standards and (2) provide training, outreach, education, and assistance to employers and employees.

Employers are required to comply with all applicable OSHA standards and also must comply with the General Duty Clause of the OSH Act, which requires employers to maintain a safe workplace free any of known and serious hazards. The OSH Act encourages states to develop and administer their own job safety and health programs, although OSHA must approve and monitor all state plans (OSHA, 2015). OSHA's jurisdiction covers private-sector employers but excludes self-employed individuals, family farm workers, and government workers, except in states with approved state plans.

The OSH Act requires employers to record and report work-related fatalities, injuries, and illnesses. Although OSHA states that it cannot inspect all 7 million workplaces it covers each year, the agency does focus its inspection efforts on the most hazardous workplaces (Jung & Makowsky, 2012).

Workplace Ethical Dilemmas

It is imperative that occupational therapy practitioners adhere to standards of ethical behavior in work and industry. Ethical conduct by practitioners requires understanding and application of the Code (AOTA, 2015). This section provides two case studies that pose several ethical dilemmas requiring examination of ethical conduct and application of the Code, one in an industrial work site setting and the other in a hospital setting. The occupational therapist in Case Study 15.1 works as an independent contractor providing on-site services, including work reconditioning, preplacement examinations, job simulation for return to work, ergonomics consultation, and injury prevention programs, in various work settings.

Ethical Decision Making

Ethical decision making is akin to decision making with a client; it includes evaluation, development of an intervention plan, and assessment of outcomes (AOTA, 2014). Most ethical decision-making frameworks or models follow similar steps (see Chapter 4, "Solving Ethical Dilemmas").

The process for analyzing ethical problems used in this chapter combines ethical decision frameworks by Purtilo and Doherty (2011) and Jennings, Kahn, Mastroianni, and Parker (2003) into the following six-step process:

1. Gather relevant information, and identify key issues.
2. Identify the type of ethical problem, and clarify the facts.
3. Analyze the problems, and identify the stakeholders.
4. Explore the practical alternatives and possible courses of action.
5. Select and complete the best course of action.
6. Evaluate the process and outcomes.

To adequately and appropriately address the ethical tensions described in Case Study 15.1, Susan applied this six-step process to help her remain objective and exercise sound judgment.

Gather relevant information, and identify key issues

In Case Study 15.1, Susan faced several possible issues that she felt compelled to address before moving forward with her program. Susan reflected on the situation and identified three essential issues.

First, Susan determined that failing to inform the company's senior administration about the risk factors she identified was a problem. She recalled the human resources (HR) director's instruction to report all findings directly to him instead of sharing them with the president and other managers. She now wondered if this process of reporting was typical procedure or reflected a culture of silence and lack of transparency. She believed that the Safety and Healthy for Injury Prevention (SHIP) committee was the place to address and discuss her findings, which, in turn, were reported to the president via meeting minutes and reports.

Second, Susan considered the company's history of OSHA violations that had gone unresolved. Susan recognized her responsibility to confront the company's key stakeholders because of her belief that the company had a duty and legal obligation to address OSHA citations. Susan also knew that this discussion might be unpleasant and could have negative consequences.

Case Study 15.1. Confronting Ethical Dilemmas in a Work Site Program

Susan, an occupational therapist working as an independent contractor, established a limited liability corporation (LLC) 5 years ago when she decided to leave her long-time employer to provide occupational therapy services at work sites in her region. Her contracting service was called Occupational Rehabilitation Consulting Services, LLC.

Susan enjoyed relative success with several companies by establishing comprehensive injury prevention and ergonomic programs. She presented her positive outcomes at a regional occupational safety and health symposium that was well attended by local and state health safety officials, plant managers and supervisors, and health care providers. After her presentation, she was approached by the HR direc tor of a midsize company in the area that produced small engine parts for a large automobile manufacturer. The HR director was interested in discussing Susan's recent successes with designing and implementing injury prevention programs, and he invited her to visit the company's facility to meet with management and safety professionals.

On her arrival at the facility, Susan was given a tour and saw firsthand the operations and production areas. After the walkthrough of the facility, Susan sat down with the company's president, HR director, safety and health manager, and senior production supervisor. The president expressed his concern about the company's rising work-related injury rates and resultant increase in workers' compensation claims and costs. The HR director went on to explain that over the past several years, their workers' compensation costs had skyrocketed because of coverage of medical treatment and benefits paid while their injured workers were recuperating away from work. Through their discussions, Susan determined that this company was committed to reducing injuries and improving the overall quality of the work environment.

At the conclusion of the first meeting, Susan was asked if she would be willing to work with the company to design and implement a comprehensive injury prevention program. Susan replied that she would certainly consider the opportunity, but she would first need to conduct a preliminary needs assessment to determine the magnitude of the problem. Both parties, Susan and the company, agreed to draw up an initial letter of agreement to establish a working relationship.

After the letter of agreement was signed, Susan began her work in earnest as a consultant. She requested access to their OSHA Log of Work-Related Injuries and Illnesses (Form 300) for the past 3 years and overall workers' compensation costs for the same period. ***OSHA Form 300 logs*** are used to classify work-related injuries and illnesses and to note the extent and severity of each case (OSHA, 2004a). The company president initially expressed concern about revealing this information, but Susan reassured him that all information would be treated with strict confidentiality. The HR director suggested that she sign a nondisclosure statement to protect the company's private and sensitive information and any proprietary information she might be privy to during her needs assessment. Susan signed the nondisclosure statement and began reviewing the company's OSHA Form 300 logs.

Before presenting her final needs assessment analysis, Susan reviewed the latest U.S. Bureau of Labor Statistics (BLS, 2015) data for cases requiring days away from work for musculoskeletal disorders by nature of injury and part of body. Susan used the national data as a means for benchmarking and comparing the company's rate of injury to the national standard.

On the basis of the preliminary needs assessment, Susan concluded that the company had indeed had a significant number of OSHA-recordable work-related injuries over the past 3 years. In fact, she had been provided with 5 years of data from the company's workers' compensation insurance carrier, and she discovered that the company's OSHA-recordable work-related injuries amounted to hundreds of thousands of dollars in compensable workers' compensation claims. Susan compared the company's injury rates to the national data from BLS (2015). Of particular concern was the fact that the company's average days away from work because of musculoskeletal injuries was 8 days longer than the national average. Most of the company's OSHA-recordable injuries were related to overexertion and repetitive work. The most common injuries were to the low

(Continued)

Case Study 15.1. Confronting Ethical Dilemmas in a Work Site Program *(Cont.)*

back (e.g., low-back strains, sciatica) and upper extremities (UE; e.g., rotator cuff tears, lateral epicondylitis, carpal tunnel syndrome). From a thorough review of records, Susan found that the company had received several OSHA citations under the OSHA General Duty Clause (OSHA, 2004b) related to poor work station design, excessive exposure to awkward postures and forceful exertions (e.g., lifting, pushing, pulling, carrying), and repetitive motions.

The HR director scheduled a meeting with Susan and the safety and health manager to discuss the results of her preliminary needs assessment. This meeting revealed that the company had not addressed most of the OSHA citations. The HR director pulled Susan aside after the meeting and informed her, "You need to report all of your findings directly to me rather than sharing them with the president and other managers." He explained that it was important to first report the findings to him to create a "proper flow of information."

Susan began to design a comprehensive injury management and prevention program. She conducted a series of roundtable discussions and focus interviews with senior administration, middle management, frontline supervisors, and rank-and-file employees. From these roundtable discussions, Susan noted several emerging themes, including an organizational culture that lacked transparency and a general distrust of management among the rank-and-file employees. However, these discussions also revealed the acknowledgment that the status quo was no longer acceptable and assurance by all stakeholders that they were willing to reimagine their company as a leader in workplace safety and as an employee-supportive work environment.

After the roundtable discussions and focus interviews, Susan formed a SHIP committee. All levels of the organization were represented on the SHIP committee, and Susan was chair.

The program's initial rollout phase involved management and select employees, as agreed on by the SHIP committee. The committee targeted one part of the manufacturing area, which included 2 shift supervisors and 12 employees. Working directly with the supervisors and employees, Susan conducted ergonomic evaluations on each of the four small-parts assembly workstations. After the evaluations, she first presented the findings to the HR director. Although he expressed concern regarding her findings, he agreed that she should present her findings to the SHIP committee, discuss issues and concerns, and then begin problem solving and implementing solutions with the employees.

The full phase-in of the program began after the initial phase was successfully completed. At this stage, Susan started experiencing significant resistance from the HR director and safety and health manager, both of whom were members of the SHIP committee. The HR director and safety and health manager were concerned that Susan's findings were too critical of the company's current work practices and that her findings would create potential OSHA violations that could lead to citations. At first, Susan believed the resistance she encountered was merely the typical resistance to change she had seen in many other companies where she implemented similar programs. Susan had learned that change does not come easily in most instances, and part of her job was to cultivate and facilitate a culture of change to enable her programs to be successful.

One day, however, Susan was invited to a meeting with the HR director and safety and health manager to "discuss progress to date." They informed Susan that the company was concerned because her program had identified several deficiencies (e.g., excessive repetitive motions, forceful exertions, awkward postures involving UE) on their small-parts assembly line that might be red flags to OSHA and the state's occupational and safety health administration. In addition, since the initial implementation of the program, the company had experienced a significant increase in employees reporting musculoskeletal discomfort and other OSHA-recordable injuries, and they worried that this increase would trigger an inspection by a state health compliance officer to investigate the increase. The HR director and safety and health manager asked Susan to refocus her program to encourage employees to "work through the pain and discomfort" rather than report their injuries so the company could meet the production schedule and minimize the number of recordable injuries while implementing the program.

(Continued)

Case Study 15.1. Confronting Ethical Dilemmas in a Work Site Program *(Cont.)*

Table 15.1. Decision Table for Case Study 15.1

Possible Action	Positive Outcomes	Negative Consequences
Take no action; simply continue to implement the program and keep her concerns to herself.	The program is implemented. Susan is able to work with the employees to address ongoing work design issues.	Federal and state regulations are potentially violated. Internal policies and procedures are not revised to address the issues.
Meet with the HR director about his insistence on keeping information from the president.	The HR director agrees to allow the flow of information directly to the president.	The HR director continues to serve as a communication barrier, and the underlying problems Susan identified persist.
Raise her concerns and identified issues in a SHIP committee meeting and devise a plan of action to deal with the issues at hand.	Plan of action is formulated and approved.	The HR director influences the SHIP committee's decision, and the plan of action is opposed.
Meet with the president and share her concerns about the suppression of information and lack of support for the program.	President agrees to work with HR director and SHIP committee to revise policy and procedures.	President disagrees and terminates Susan's contract.

Note. HR = human resources; SHIP = Safety and Health for Injury Prevention.

Finally, Susan was concerned about the HR director's request that she refocus her program to encourage employees to "work through pain and discomfort" instead of reporting their injuries in order to maintain the production schedule and minimize reports of recordable injuries. Susan understood from her educational background and practice experience that workers in labor-intensive jobs sometimes experience a certain amount of pain and discomfort. However, she also understood that workers who experience significant pain and discomfort are at much greater risk for developing a work-related musculoskeletal disorder (Zuccarello, 2010). In fact, she knew that epidemiological studies have found a strong correlation between exposures to work-related risk factors (e.g., forceful exertions, repetitive motions) and musculoskeletal injuries (Kaskutas & Snodgrass, 2009).

Identify the type of ethical problem, and clarify the facts

As an AOTA member, Susan was bound by the Code, which had been adopted by her state regulatory board. She used the Code as a resource and guide to help identify the ethical problems she had encountered. Susan determined that the following ethical Principles had been or might be violated: Principle 1, Beneficence; Principle 4, Justice; and Principle 5, Veracity.

Principle 1. Beneficence, and Principle 4. Justice. Susan was especially concerned that the company had received numerous citations from OSHA and the state's occupational safety and health administration that had gone unresolved. Thus, she believed that segments of the company were acting unethically. Susan was obligated to consider the reporting process because of Principle 4, Related Standard of Conduct (RSC) K, which states the need to "report to appropriate authorities any acts in practice, education, and research that appear unethical or illegal" (AOTA, 2015, p. 5). The HR director's request that she advise workers to work through pain and discomfort would violate Principle 1, RSC A, which obligates practitioners to "provide appropriate evaluation and a plan of intervention for recipients of occupational therapy services specific to their needs" (AOTA, 2015, p. 2).

Susan feared that asking employees to work through their pain was similar to asking them to ignore what could be a sign of a significant problem, especially in light of the evidence of a connection between exposure to work-related risk factors, reported discomfort, and the development of musculoskeletal injuries.

Susan's conversations with the HR director and the safety and health manager led her to fear that the company was failing to follow state and federal rules. In addition, she believed that not reporting her concerns to the company's president compromised her integrity and the ethical Principle of Justice. After reviewing the Code, Susan believed she risked violating Principle 4, RSC L, "collaborate with employers to formulate policies and procedures in compliance with legal, regulatory, and ethical standards and work to resolve any conflicts or inconsistencies" (AOTA, 2015, p. 5), and Principle 4, RSC N, "ensure compliance with relevant laws, and promote transparency when participating in a business arrangement as owner, stockholder, partner, or employee" (AOTA, 2015, p. 6). Therefore, Susan felt compelled to highlight to senior administration where the potential violation of rules existed and encourage the formulation of appropriate policies and procedures to ameliorate the violations.

Principle 5. Veracity. Lack of truthfulness was a significant concern for Susan. She believed that she had been asked on several occasions to hide her findings by sharing them with only a select few individuals and to discourage employees from reporting problems. Susan realized that she would violate Principle 5, RSC B, if she complied with these requests; this RSC obligates practitioners to "refrain from using or participating in the use of any form of communication that contains false, fraudulent, deceptive, misleading, or unfair statements or claims" (AOTA, 2015, p. 6).

Analyze the problems, and identify the stakeholders

Susan identified the key stakeholders in this situation as herself, the HR director, the safety and health manager, members of the SHIP committee, frontline supervisors, rank-and-file employees, and the president. Susan used two perspectives on ethics—human rights and utilitarianism—to provide insight into the situation and help resolve her ethical tension (Thomas, 2005). Weighing these two perspectives helped Susan gain a clearer picture of the situation and decide on her best course of action.

From the human rights perspective, Susan recognized the importance of maintaining the dignity of all of those involved and her obligation to protect those most vulnerable to work-related injuries (e.g., rank-and-file workers) if it all possible. Susan believed that being asked to "work through the pain" compromised the rank-and-file workers' dignity by discouraging them from reporting their symptoms and discomfort.

Using the utilitarian perspective, Susan looked at the potential consequences of her action, and inaction, and how each action would affect the entire company. She determined that the overall benefits of implementing her program far outweighed the potential costs of ignoring workers' reported symptoms and withholding her findings from the president. In fact, Susan had presented this cost–benefit analysis to the key stakeholders when she initially presented her program.

Susan also considered the laws, rules, and regulations that govern workplace safety. Susan was familiar with the federal OSH Act, which requires that employers provide their employees with working conditions that are free of known dangers (OSHA, 2004a). Workers have the right to a safe work environment that is free from conditions that pose a risk of serious harm. Thus, Susan knew that the company was bound by federal law to provide workers with a safe work environment and address any known issues.

In addition to incorporating ethical perspectives and considering issues of jurisprudence, Susan also found it helpful to draw on prior experiences from her own work and trusted colleagues' work in the field. This action is a recommended strategy when facing ethical challenges (Thomas, 2005). After doing some background investigation and networking with several colleagues and recognized experts in the field of industrial rehabilitation, Susan found an emerging theme when others were faced with similar dilemmas (i.e., resistance from employers to acknowledge and address identified risk factors).

Explore the practical alternatives and possible courses of action

After much critical thought and deliberation, Susan developed a list of possible courses of action she could take to address the identified ethical issues (see Table 15.1).

Select and complete the best course of action

Susan spent the better part of a weekend considering the key issues, identifying and analyzing the ethical problems, and detailing possible courses of action. She decided to schedule a one-on-one meeting with the company president to share her concerns. During the meeting, Susan objectively presented the key issues, identified ethical issues, and outlined what she believed were the best strategies to address her concerns to continue with implementation of the program. The president expressed concern about the suppression of findings and lack of transparency in the organization. He informed Susan that he wanted to meet with her and the SHIP committee to establish an open and honest dialogue regarding the issues and solutions.

After meeting with the president, Susan called a meeting of the SHIP committee and president. The meeting was difficult for Susan to lead and facilitate, but in the end she was able to establish an open and honest dialogue between the key stakeholders concerning the ongoing implementation of the program. After this meeting, SHIP committee members reached a consensus, and Susan felt confident that implementation of her program would proceed as planned.

Evaluate the process and outcomes

Susan spent time reflecting on and evaluating the process she took to resolve her ethical dilemma. Susan compared and contrasted the ethical issues with this company with her past experience in similar situations. Susan scheduled a lunch meeting with her mentor to further discuss and consider how she handled the situation and what, if anything, she should have done differently. She and her mentor agreed that Susan handled the situation appropriately by addressing the issue directly with the company's president.

However, her mentor provided one suggestion for consideration should she be faced with this type of ethical dilemma in the future. Susan's mentor suggested that Susan always include in her initial meetings with prospective clients the need for transparency and veracity of reporting when discussing any and all ergonomic assessment findings and recommendations. Her mentor noted that the potential for ethical dilemmas is always present, but using strong communication skills is critical to successful resolution of dilemmas.

Susan arrived at a satisfactory conclusion by following a formal process of ethical decision making. The process involved gathering relevant information, identifying the ethical problem, applying ethical perspectives to analyze the problems, identifying stakeholders, exploring alternatives, selecting the best course of action, and evaluating the outcomes. This systematic process for ethical problem solving can help occupational therapy practitioners practicing at work sites and in other settings address and resolve ethical issues.

In Case Study 15.2, the occupational therapist struggles to maintain objectivity when providing a functional capacity evaluation (FCE). Three vignettes (Vignette 15.1–15.3) follow to provide opportunity to reflect and consider the best course of action to take in the context of ethical principles.

Summary

Practice in work and industry requires occupational therapy practitioners to navigate a variety of potential ethical concerns in the context of the Code and

Case Study 15.2. Functional Capacity Evaluation

Darrell, an occupational therapist, received a referral to conduct a FCE on a client, **Carter,** who was male, age 38 years, and married with children. An ***FCE*** is an "evaluation of capacity of activities that is used to make recommendations for participation in work while considering the person's body functions and structures, environmental factors, personal factors and health status" (Soer, van der Schans, Groothoof, Geertzen, & Reneman, 2008, p. 394).

An external case manager, **Trudy,** coordinated Carter's referral. After receiving the written physician's order and Carter's past medical and vocational history, Darrell called Trudy the day before the scheduled FCE. Trudy indicated that Carter had been "very difficult" in terms of lack of progress with rehabilitation efforts. Trudy indicated that Carter had been moody and, at times, angry during her interaction with him. As Darrell was asking Trudy about Carter's course of medical, pharmacological, and rehabilitation treatment thus far, he asked her what questions needed to be answered based on the results of the FCE. Trudy indicated that ultimately the FCE needed to assist

(Continued)

Case Study 15.2. Functional Capacity Evaluation *(Cont.)*

her and the physician in deciding whether Carter was capable of returning to his pre-injury job. If not, was he capable of competitive employment in another line of work?

However, she noted at the end of their phone conversation, "Between you and me, I don't think Carter has any plans or desire to return to work. I think he is malingering and just trying to work the system to get on Social Security Disability, or he is at least trying to obtain reasonable accommodations for an easier job." Darrell responded to Trudy by thanking her for the background information but informed her of his concern about her biased remarks regarding Carter.

Ethical Decision Making

To reconcile what Darrell believed was an obvious ethical dilemma, he referred to the Code, state licensure law (i.e., practice act), and his training as an FCE evaluator. Darrell had received extensive training to conduct objective, reliable, and valid FCEs. He had been performing FCEs for more than 10 years and estimated he had performed at least 300 FCEs.

As an experienced evaluator, Darrell knew and understood that an FCE must be approached from an objective and unbiased viewpoint. In fact, he was a highly sought-after FCE evaluator in his community on the basis of his professional reputation for his ability to conduct a thorough and unbiased FCE without pressure or influence from payer sources, employers, referral sources, or any combination of these.

Type of Ethical Problem

Darrell quickly identified the potential ethical issues. He determined that the following Principles had been or might be violated: Principle 2, Nonmaleficence, and Principle 6, Fidelity.

Principle 2. Nonmaleficence

Darrell perceived the conversation that he had with the case manager to lack adequate objectivity and inappropriately biased against the client. He believed that had he engaged Trudy further in her assertions that the client was malingering, he would have violated Principle 2, RSC F, "avoid dual relationships, conflicts of interest, and situations in which a practitioner, educator, student, researcher, or employer is unable to maintain clear professional boundaries or objectivity" (AOTA, 2015, p. 3).

Principle 6. Fidelity

Similar to the potential to violate Principle 2, RSC F, Darrell also knew that engaging in communication that was not based on facts, and ultimately, not germane to the client's care, would potentially violate Principle 6, RSC G, which states that occupational therapy practitioners should "refrain from communication that is derogatory, intimidating, or disrespectful and that unduly discourages others from participating in professional dialogue" (AOTA, 2015, p. 7).

Course of Action

Ultimately, Darrell knew from his extensive experience as an occupational therapist conducting FCEs that he should always refrain from engaging other professionals in communications about clients that lacked objectivity, were unnecessarily biased, and ultimately would serve as a barrier for professional dialogue. After analyzing the ethical dilemmas, Darrel conducted the FCE from an objective and unbiased perspective and submitted the report and results to the case manager and physician.

Evaluate the Process and Outcome

After Darrell submitted his FCE report, he received a follow-up call from Trudy. She thanked Darrell for his thorough assessment and recommendations to facilitate the client's return to work. She indicated that she was surprised by his findings with respect to the lack of "malingering" issues in the report. Darrell stated that Trudy's initial suggestion that the client was malingering was not based on objective facts. He explained to her that he is bound by his professional code of ethics and he could not engage in any communications that were biased and might potentially serve as a barrier to professional dialogue.

Vignette 15.1. Developing Pre-Employment Examination, Post-Offer Screening Program

Shelly, an occupational therapist, worked in the Department of Employee and Occupational Health as the coordinator of health promotion and injury prevention at a midsized suburban medical center. Because of a significant amount of work-related musculoskeletal injuries (e.g., low-back strains, shoulder sprains) among the CNAs at the hospital, the director of employee and occupational health, **Tamara,** charged Shelly with developing a pre-employment examination, post-offer screening program for all candidates applying for a CNA position at the medical center. The aim of a ***pre-employment examination*** is to screen job applicants who may have an increased risk for occupational disease or injury while on the job (Mahmud et al., 2010). Tamara and Shelly had been investigating options for the best testing packages for the screening program.

After reviewing and discussing several options, Tamara recommended purchasing a screening program offered by a well-known company. The screening program included a screening protocol, evaluation equipment, and software for analysis and documentation of results. Although the program was cost-effective, Shelly had concerns about the validity and reliability of the program, especially as it applied to the population of clients to which it would be applied, CNAs. In fact, the program had no published results on this population; its results were only for manufacturing and construction industries. Shelly was concerned that if they purchased this particular program, she would face potential ethical issues related to the Code.

Note. CNAs = certified nursing assistants.

Vignette 15.2. Zero-Lift Policy in a Skilled Nursing Facility

The administrators at a 200-bed SNF decided to institute a zero-lift policy for all direct care staff, (i.e., nurses, physical therapists, occupational therapists, speech–language pathologists). This was in response to an increasing number of OSHA-recordable injuries. **Humphrey,** the director of rehabilitation at this SNF, was responsible for developing and implementing the zero-lift policy. Humphrey used OSHA's (2009) *Guidelines for Nursing Homes* to guide his program design and implementation.

In addition, Humphrey referenced the latest evidence-based practice research to further inform and support his approach to developing the facility's policy by using databases such as OT Seeker and ProQuest. He knew, for instance, that Principle 1, RSC C, states that "occupational therapy personnel shall use, to the extent possible, evaluation, planning, intervention techniques, assessments, and therapeutic equipment that are evidence based, current, and within the recognized scope of occupational therapy practice" (AOTA, 2015, p. 2).

Note. RSCs = Related standards of Conduct; SNF = skilled nursing facility.

Vignette 15.3. State Workers' Compensation Policy Reform

An ad hoc commission was formed by the governor of one of the largest states in the United States. The governor asked the commission to review the state's current workers' compensation statutes and regulations and submit recommendations to the governor to "reform and transform our current workers' compensation system."

Lisa, an occupational therapist and owner of a large, work-focused outpatient rehabilitation clinic, was appointed to serve on this commission. Other members included a physician, nurse, lawyer, physical therapist, hospital administrator, chief executive officer of a private corporation, and a human resources director.

The first charge from the governor to the commission was to recommend a set of evidence-based clinical guidelines that all clinicians must follow when providing services under the state's workers' compensation system. During the commission's discussion, the physician appointee, **Judy,** was adamant that the only clinical guidelines that should be followed were those published by the American College of Occupational and Environmental Medicine (ACOEM). She argued that the guidelines were comprehensive, updated on a regular basis, and had already been adopted by other states for their workers' compensation clinical guidelines.

The majority of the commission members quickly acquiesced to Judy's recommendation, except Lisa. Lisa raised the issue of whether the ACOEM's guidelines were sufficiently comprehensive and inclusive to be appropriate and applicable to the practice of allied health professions. Specifically, Lisa indicated that the ACOEM's guidelines were developed with the express intent of guiding the practice of physicians, not necessarily the practice of other allied health professions.

various work-related policies and laws as presented in this chapter. The case studies and vignettes presented provide the context for practitioners to anticipate some of the more common ethical dilemmas in work and industry. For example, an occupational therapist performing a work-site assessment of an injured employee and the possibility of the client returning to work must balance the need to exercise sound ethical judgment, clinical reasoning, and knowledge of applicable work-related regulations. Often, this balancing act comes with tensions that the practitioner must resolve. This resolution only comes with a sound knowledge and understanding of the Code within the context of the practice setting.

Reflective Questions

1. Review Vignette 15.1, "Developing a Pre-Employment, Post-Offer Screening Program."
   - What potential ethical issues would you anticipate in this scenario? *Hint:* Review Under Principle 4, Justice, RSC F.
   - Think about potential work-related policies and laws that would need to be considered in the development of a pre-employment examination, post-offer screening program. If you were Shelly, what would you recommend as the best course of action?
2. Review Vignette 15.2, "Zero-Lift Policy in a Skilled Nursing Facility." As Humphrey develops the program and associated policies for the SNF, he is concerned about whether instituting a zero-lift policy is feasible, evidence-based, safe for the patients and staff, and cost-effective. Using the six-step process described in this chapter, analyze the key ethical issues that Humphrey should consider.
   - What specific ethical Principles and RSCs should be considered?
   - How would you address the potential conflict between RSCs and the need to develop and implement a zero-lift policy?
   - Think about what work-related regulations should be considered.
3. Review Vignette 15.3, "State Workers' Compensation Policy Reform." Lisa was placed in an unenviable position of being the lone voice of dissent. With the majority of the commission members in agreement with a recommendation to adopt the ACOEM's guidelines, Lisa must carefully consider how to approach this situation. Before the commission's next scheduled meeting, Lisa must grapple with the potential ethical dilemmas that she believes are present with the possible adoption of the ACOEM's guidelines.
   - What are the potential ethical dilemmas, real or perceived, from the perspective of occupational therapy?
   - What documents should Lisa review to help inform and support her recommendations to the commission?

References

Americans With Disabilities Act of 1990, Pub. L. 101–336, U.S.C. 42 § 12101.

Americans With Disabilities Act Amendments Act of 2008, Pub. L. 110–325, 122 Stat. 3553.

American Occupational Therapy Association. (2014). Occupational therapy practice framework: Domain and process (3rd ed.). *American Journal of Occupational Therapy, 68*(Suppl. 1), S1–S48. https://doi.org/10.5014/ajot.2014.682006

American Occupational Therapy Association. (2015). Occupational therapy code of ethics (2015). *American Journal of Occupational Therapy, 69*(Suppl. 3), 6912310030. https://doi.org/10.5014/ajot.2015.696S03

Haruka, D., Page, J., & Wietlisbach, C. (2013). Work evaluation and work programs. In H. Pendleton & W. Shultz-Krohn (Eds.), *Pedretti's occupational therapy practice skills for physical dysfunction* (pp. 337–380). St. Louis: Elsevier.

International Ergonomics Association. (2016, January 08). *Definition of ergonomics*. Retrieved from http://www.iea.cc/whats/

Jennings, B., Kahn, J., Mastroianni, A., & Parker, L. S. (Eds.). (2003). *Ethics and public health: Model curriculum.* Retrieved from http://www.aspph.org/app/uploads/2014/02/EthicsCurriculum.pdf

Jung, J., & Makowsky, M. D. (2012). *Regulatory enforcement, politics, and institutional distance: OSHA inspections 1990–2010.* Retrieved from http://webapps.towson.edu/cbe/economics/workingpapers/2012-02.pdf

Karger, H., & Rose, S. R. (2010). Revisiting the Americans with Disabilities Act after two decades. *Journal of Social Work in Disability and Rehabilitation, 9,* 73–86. https://doi.org/10.1080/1536710X.2010.493468

Kaskutas, V., & Snodgrass, J. (2009). *Occupational therapy practice guidelines for individuals with work-related injuries and illnesses.* Bethesda: AOTA Press.

Mahmud, N., Schonstein, E., Schaafsma, F., Lehtola, M. M., Fassier, J. B., Reneman, M. F., &, Verbeek, J. H. (2010).

Pre-employment examinations for preventing occupational injury and disease in workers. *Cochrane Database of Systematic Reviews 2010*, 12. Art. No.: CD008881. https://doi.org/10.1002/14651858.CD008881

Occupational Safety and Health Act of 1970, Pub. L. 91–596, 84 Stat 1590.

Occupational Safety and Health Administration. (2004a). *Injury and illness recordkeeping forms—300, 300A, 301.* Retrieved from https://www.osha.gov/recordkeeping/RK-forms.html

Occupational Safety and Health Administration. (2004b). *Sec. 5, Duties.* Retrieved from http://www.osha.gov/pls/oshaweb/owadisp.show_document?p_table=OSHACT&p_id=3359

Occupational Safety and Health Administration. (2009). *Guidelines for nursing homes.* Retrieved from https://www.osha.gov/ergonomics/guidelines/nursinghome/final_nh_guidelines.html

Occupational Safety and Health Administration. (2015). *State plans: Office of State Programs.* Retrieved from https://www.osha.gov/dcsp/osp/index.html

Purtilo, R., & Doherty, R. (2011). *Ethical dimensions in the health professions* (5th ed.). Philadelphia: Elsevier/Saunders.

Snodgrass, J., & Gupta, J. (2014). Work occupations. In J. Hinosjosa & M. L. Blount (Eds.), *Texture of life: occupations and related activities (*4th ed., pp. 317–336). Bethesda, MD: AOTA Press.

Soer, R., van der Schans, C., Groothoof, J., Geertzen, J., & Reneman, M. (2008). Towards consensus in operational definitions in functional capacity evaluation: A Delphi Survey. *Journal of Occupational Rehabilitation, 18*, 389–400. https://doi.org/10.1007/s10926-008-9155-y#page-1

Thomas, J. C. (2005). Skills for the ethical practice of public health. *Journal of Public Health Management and Practice, 11*(3), 260–261.

U.S. Bureau of Labor Statistics. (2015). *Nonfatal occupational injuries and illnesses requiring days away from work, 2014.* Retrieved from http://www.bls.gov/iif/oshcdnew.htm

U.S. Equal Employment Opportunity Commission, (2015). *About EEOC.* Retrieved from http://www.eeoc.gov/eeoc/index.cfm

Zuccarello, V. (2010). The use of ergonomic analysis in medical causation cases to support or debunk compensability claims for musculoskeletal disorders. *Work and Industry Special Interest Section Quarterly, 24*(3), 1–4.

Chapter 16.

PARTICIPATION, DISABILITY, AND REHABILITATION: ETHICAL CHALLENGES

Timothy Holmes, OTD, OTR/L, COMS

Learning Objectives

By the end of the chapter, readers will be able to

- Understand how decisions made by clients or their families may conflict with clinical judgment, causing ethical dilemmas;
- Develop an awareness of how ethical dilemmas arise in a variety of rehabilitation settings; and
- Identify resources and methods to resolve ethical dilemmas to facilitate optimal clients' participation in valued occupations.

Key Terms and Concepts

- ✧ Background knowledge
- ✧ Case analysis
- ✧ Disability
- ✧ Ethical dilemmas
- ✧ Occupational therapy process
- ✧ Participation
- ✧ Participation restrictions
- ✧ Patient-Centered Care Ethics Analysis Model for Rehabilitation
- ✧ Process model
- ✧ Self-assessment

Occupational therapy practitioners working in the practice area of rehabilitation services may be faced with many ethical challenges. The occupational therapy profession has a long history of ethics-based practice. Ties to ethics can be seen as early as the Moral Treatment era in the late 1800s, in which pioneers of the profession such as Philip Pinel and Samuel Tuke began replacing physical restraints with work and leisure activities (Quiroga, 1995).

This tradition of providing rehabilitation services in an ethical manner remains an important tenet for the profession of occupational therapy. The current trend of length-of-stay reduction combined with medical and technological advances has the potential to lead to conflicts that occupational therapy practitioners may struggle to resolve.

Ethical conflict resolution is important for many reasons. Atwal and Caldwell (2003) go so far as to suggest that ethical issues that are not managed successfully not only lead to poor client interactions but may also contribute to burnout and an occupational therapy practitioner leaving clinical practice.

This chapter explores potential ethical challenges that occupational therapy practitioners may face as individual practitioners or as part of organizational systems. Case studies and vignettes cover various rehabilitation practice settings such as acute care, inpatient rehabilitation, and outpatient services. This chapter is meant to stimulate personal reflection and professional dialogue regarding potential rehabilitation situations that address disability and participation in chosen occupations.

Ethical vs. Legal

Occupational therapy practitioners must be able to distinguish between issues related to ethical professional practice and those that fall under legal jurisdiction. Ethical issues involve situations that present a moral dilemma but do not have a clear answer or solution (Scott, 1998). ***Ethical dilemmas*** may involve attempting to solve a conflict in which each "solution of the conflict may contain undesirable outcomes for one or more parties involved" (Kassberg & Skär, 2008, p. 204). Ethical issues related to occupational therapy practice may be manifested during assessment of client performance, in direct clinical intervention, or during supervision of students or occupational therapy practitioners.

Legal statutes related to professional practice are parameters that constitute action that is binding by state or federal law. Occupational therapy practitioners must comply with legal statutes or risk consequences that could range from written reprimand to suspension or revocation of professional license to incarceration. Examples of legal noncompliance or violation might include providing clinical services without a license or billing for services not rendered.

Practitioners facing ethical dilemmas should seek resources to assist with conflict resolution. These resources may include the *Occupational Therapy Code of Ethics (2015)* (hereinafter referred to as "the Code;" American Occupational Therapy Association [AOTA], 2015); AOTA's Ethics Commission or its ethics program manager; in-house ethics committees; state licensure boards; and Chapter 4, "Solving Ethical Dilemmas."

In some instances, practitioners may be unsure if a situation presents significant ethical challenges to warrant action. Occupational therapy practitioners should become familiar with the Code to guide one's ethical practice. In addition to the Code, the *Occupational Therapy Practice Framework* (hereinafter referred to as the *Framework;* AOTA, 2014), offers guidance in providing services that are based on the client–practitioner relationship. These services may be delivered through direct intervention, advocacy, and consultation.

Through the *Framework,* AOTA (2014) defines the ***occupational therapy process*** as the provision of services that is client-centered:

> The process includes evaluation and intervention to achieve targeted outcomes, occurs within the purview of the occupational therapy domain, and is facilitated by the distinct perspective of occupational therapy practitioners when engaging in clinical reasoning, analyzing activities and occupations, and collaborating with clients. (p. S10)

By infusing practice guidelines as described in the *Framework* with the profession's core values reflected in the Code, practitioners can feel confident they are providing services that are both meaningful to the client and ethically sound.

Disability and Participation

In AOTA's *Vision 2025,* the practice area of rehabilitation, disability, and participation was identified as important to occupational therapy service delivery in the 21st century (AOTA, 2016). The constructs of disability and participation used within the process rehabilitation (or habilitation) are included in the *Framework* and the *International Classification of Functioning, Disability and Health* (World Health Organization [WHO], 2001).

WHO (2001) defines ***disability*** as a general term for impairments, activity limitations, and restrictions in participation. Under the Americans With

Disabilities Act of 1990, *disability* is a legal term as opposed to a medical term, defined as

> a person who has a physical or mental impairment that substantially limits one or more major life activity. This includes people who have a record of such an impairment, even if they do not currently have a disability. It also includes individuals who do not have a disability but are regarded as having a disability. (Americans With Disabilities Act National Network, n.d.)

The *Framework* does not provide a specific definition for *disability* but rather provides guidance in developing an intervention plan based on client factors, performance skills and patterns, context and environment, and activity demands that have the potential to disrupt occupational performance and participation in life (AOTA, 2014).

WHO defines ***participation*** as "involvement in a life situation" (WHO, 2002, p. 10). Thus, ***participation restrictions*** are difficulties one may experience in the attempt to engage in life situations. According to the *Framework,* the domain and process of occupational therapy services are designed to enable client participation in health, well-being, and engagement in daily life activities. Active engagement in occupations by those who may be at risk for participation restriction is viewed as the key to fulfilling these aspirations (AOTA, 2014).

Ethical dilemmas faced by occupational therapy practitioners can affect client participation in desired occupations and anticipated outcomes. These dilemmas may occur directly during clinical interventions or indirectly through personal conflicts, professional conflicts, or both. Vignette 16.1 explores a personal and professional ethical conflict where the client is unable to communicate personal care choices to his family and the occupational therapy practitioner.

Case Study 16.1 considers when client preferences, client safety, and legal and ethical obligations collide. Vignette 16.2 provides an opportunity to reflect upon how a client's autonomy may conflict with

---

Vignette 16.1. Demonstrating Concern for Service Recipients While Respecting Individuals' Rights

Thomas, an occupational therapist who provides occupational therapy interventions for a neurosurgical ICU, received a referral to fabricate bilateral hand splints to prevent joint deformity. Upon review of the medical record, subsequent evaluation of the client, and discussion with the charge nurse of the day, Thomas learned the client had severe brain damage, was comatose, and had a poor prognosis. Additionally, the client had no spasticity that would indicate potential contracture development. Thomas decided, based on clinical reasoning, not to fabricate the splints as ordered by the neurosurgeon.

After he made his decision, Thomas contacted the neurosurgeon to report that he did not believe that splint fabrication and wear was indicated and offered his rationale for the decision. The next day, the neurosurgeon sent a second referral and, in addition, paged Thomas and stated that the client's family was demanding "everything be done" for the client and wanted the splints fabricated. Thomas continued to believe the splints were not indicated and the time and resources should be allocated elsewhere.

Later in the day, the surgeon contacted the manager of rehabilitation services and reported that Thomas refused to complete the referral for splint fabrication. Although the surgeon acknowledged the splints would not be particularly beneficial for the client, they would potentially help calm the traumatized family. The manager then contacted Thomas to discuss the situation. Thomas felt conflicted because he had made his decision based on the client's specific need and as supported by the Code's RSC 1A, which states, "occupational personnel shall provide appropriate evaluation and a plan of intervention" (AOTA, 2015, p. 2). However, Thomas felt pressured by the neurosurgeon and his manager to fulfill the referral.

Thomas identified the following ethical conflicts and references in the Code that directed his decision making:

- Concern for the well-being of his client, including his family, while concurrently providing services that meet reasonable expectations for clinical improvement on the basis current evidenced-based practice (RSCs 1A, 1C, 6E).
- Respecting the client's wishes while being a good steward of the hospital's resources (RSCs 3A, 6E).

Upon further reflection of his clinical reasoning and the family's expressed concerns and desires, Thomas decided to fabricate the splints. Because of his comatose state, the client was not able to participate in care-related decisions, and the family was the surrogate decision maker. Thomas determined that honoring the family's rights held greater value than deferring an intervention that may have been of marginal value.

Note. ICU = intensive care unit; RSC = Related Standard of Conduct.

Case Study 16.1. Client Well-Being, Autonomy, and Right to Privacy

Jesse, age 85 years, was admitted to an inpatient rehabilitation unit after becoming severely debilitated following surgery for esophageal cancer. One surgical procedures involved the insertion of a percutaneous epigastric tube. The medical team informed Jesse and his spouse that no food was to be taken by mouth and that any food taken by mouth would lead to aspiration, which, in turn, would cause pneumonia and possible death. Jesse demonstrated the cognitive capacity to understand the information presented by the physicians.

During an occupational therapy session, Jesse mentioned that one of his goals was to make enough progress to be discharged home and attend a family reunion. He informed **Evan,** the occupational therapy assistant, that he was well aware of the consequences of eating a regular diet; however, given his advanced age and wanting to "enjoy my time left" (implying quality of life), he planned to enjoy the reunion by eating some of his favorite dishes that family members would bring. He appeared excited about attending the reunion and asked Evan not to disclose his intentions of eating food at the reunion to his wife and the rehabilitation team. Evan felt compelled to inform the team but also recognized the trust Jesse placed in him during the conversation. He believed he should share Jesse's comments with his wife, so she would be aware of his intentions and potentially prevent Jesse from eating regular-consistency foods.

Evan felt a strong conflict as he considered whether Jesse's right to confidentiality and self-determination with regard to making decisions based on personal values (RSCs 3A, 3E, 3F) outweighed the obligation to report behavior that might affect the client's quality care and safety (see RSC 6H). Evan believed that when Jesse was discharged home he would eat food by mouth and likely experience consequences that could lead to readmission to the hospital and potential death. At the same time, Evan was empathic to what might be considered end-of-life wishes.

To resolve this conflict, Evan referred to the Code (AOTA, 2015) as the initial step. He thus followed "a systematic process that includes analyzing the complex dynamics of the situations, weighing consequences, making reasoned decisions, taking action, and reflecting on outcomes" (AOTA, 2015, p. 1).

Evan identified the major dilemma along with situational dynamics: Does Jesse's right to self-determination and confidentiality (RSCs 3A, 3E, 3F) outweigh the professional obligation to report behavior that may be deemed self-injurious (RSC 6H)? Evan had a deep belief and respect for a client's desire to live life as meaningfully as possible, especially during the end of one's life, so he believed he should maintain Jesse's wish for confidentiality. However, he felt uneasy keeping this to himself as he pondered the repercussions of Jesse's potential post-discharge behavior. In addition to the ethical issue, Evan also considered whether he would face any legal consequences (e.g., patient neglect) if Jesse followed through with his intent to eat a regular-consistency diet that could result in serious secondary medical conditions.

Evan proceeded to the next phase and considered various courses of action. He wrote down possible actions:

- Maintain complete confidentiality and not discuss the situation with anyone.
- Discuss the situation only with Jesse's spouse.
- Discuss the situation with his clinical supervisor.
- Discuss the situation with members of the treatment team (e.g., nurse, attending physician).
- Contact the in-house ethics committee for suggestions.
- Refer to the state licensure board of occupational therapy.
- Contact the AOTA ethics program manager.

Evan considered the potential consequences of each action and then decided on what he believed was a reasonable course of action. His first conclusion was that the issue contained enough complexity for him to seek guidance not just from professional reference material but also from additional team members.

Evan's first action was to inform his clinical supervisor of the situation along with the resources he used as a basis for his decision. Both Evan and his

(Continued)

Case Study 16.1. Client Well-Being, Autonomy, and Right to Privacy *(Cont.)*

supervisor collaboratively proceeded to consult with the attending physician, because she was ultimately responsible for Jesse's comprehensive rehabilitation plan of care. The three of them decided to contact the in-house ethics committee and determine the best method to approach both Jesse and his spouse.

Finally, Evan reflected on the outcome of his decision. He concluded this course of action was for his client's greater good, and any possible conflicts in future intervention sessions with Jesse could be resolved by his disclosing his rationale and concern for Jesse's well-being.

the clinical judgment of an occupational therapy practitioner.

Models for Ethical Decision Making

Occupational therapy intervention is often guided by the practitioner's personal and professional values and beliefs (Kassberg & Skar, 2008) and may "influence the process of making evidence-based practice decisions" (Wright-St. Clair & Newcombe, 2014, p. 156). To resolve ethical challenges, practitioners may first begin by using various strategies or models. This section provides a brief overview of some of these resources that might serve as a guide to helping occupational therapy practitioners.

Patient-Centered Care Ethics Analysis Model for Rehabilitation

Hunt and Ellis (2013) developed the ***Patient-Centered Care Ethics Analysis Model for Rehabilitation*** (PCEAM–R) to address the specific needs of an inpatient rehabilitation unit. They suggest these types of units often have distinctive features of care as compared to acute care, where more life-and-death decisions are made. Ethical issues on a rehabilitation unit may arise from "negotiation of expectations; goals and roles between clinicians, patients, and families; and issues related to risk and capacity" (Hunt & Ellis, 2013, p. 819). The authors chose to ground their model in patient-centered care because of the expectation of active patient participation and because of the focus on optimizing function.

The PCEAM–R has six steps:

1. Identify the ethical issues to address.
2. Collect information.
3. Review and analyze.
4. Identify and weigh options.
5. Make decisions.
6. Evaluate and follow up.

Each step contains multiple questions and prompts designed to "stimulate reflection, discussion, and careful deliberation among those involved in an ethically challenging situation" (Hunt & Ellis, 2013, p. 822). This model is not a detailed algorithm but rather a method to support systematic assessment of important features and options in an effort to make ethical decisions in rehabilitation care.

Process Model

Gervasis (2005) developed a ***process model*** that health care professionals may use to make ethically informed decisions. The intent behind this model was to not only take into account individual client encounters and clinical alternatives to decisions (as is the basis for more traditional bioethics models) but to also consider institutional and societal features. It proposes three types of preparation for making an ethical decision: (1) background knowledge, (2) case analysis, and (3) self-assessment.

Background knowledge

Background knowledge draws on facts of the situation and also on societal and health system characteristics and the realities of a particular health care system. The moral compass of the health care provider is also necessary when using professional ethics codes for decision making. Advocacy is considered a cornerstone of this approach.

Case analysis

Case analysis requires review of the facts along with consideration of professional and instructional contexts and identification of problems and options. These elements are not new to traditional

Vignette 16.2. Concern for Well-Being, Right to Self-Determination, and Objectivity

Alice, an occupational therapist, received a referral for evaluation and intervention for a client who was admitted to an observation unit within a Level I trauma hospital. The client, **Roberta,** was a 65-year-old woman with a history of numerous medical co-morbidities, including significant alcohol use.

Roberta had fallen and sustained a left nondisplaced hip fracture. The consulting orthopedist determined that surgical intervention was not indicated. However, Roberta would need to adhere to left lower extremity non–weight bearing precautions for several weeks. She would need to use a rolling walker during functional mobility tasks and IADLs. She would also need to temporarily discontinue many IADLs, such as driving, shopping, and heavy home management tasks.

Upon initial evaluation, Alice determined that Roberta was able to verbalize accurate details of the accident, her living situation, and her typical daily routine. When asked about the circumstances of the fall, Roberta admitted to having several alcoholic drinks while on her porch and then falling as she ascended the short threshold into her house. Roberta lived alone and was independent in all basic personal care and IADLs (including taking care of her small dog, medication management, and driving) before the fall. She did have friends who visited and with whom she socialized. From Alice's observations, it appeared that Roberta was able to verbalize accurate details about her living situation and was able to coherently verbalize her goals and desires.

During the mobilization aspect of the occupational therapy evaluation, Alice observed that Roberta was unable to adhere to her weight-bearing precautions. Alice observed Roberta's difficulty ambulating and transferring to various surfaces (e.g., toilet). Alice discussed her findings with the physical therapist. When this was brought to her attention, Roberta stated she realized the challenge; however, she desired to be discharged back home given that she needed no further medical or surgical management. Roberta also stated that while she would have periods of time throughout the day in which she would be alone, she could call on individuals within her social support system for many tasks she would initially be unable to perform.

After documenting the results of the evaluation, which included a recommendation for discharge to a subacute rehabilitation facility, the team members met with Alice to discuss the results and her documented recommendations. Alice reported she believed Roberta was unsafe to return home given her high fall risk and her unpredictable access for assistance. Alice was informed the client did not meet the criteria for a three-day qualifying stay in the hospital and subsequently would not have Medicare funding for admission to a subacute facility. Team members asked Alice to change her documentation to support discharge home because discharge to a subacute facility was not financially realistic. Alice was uneasy about discharging Roberta home because of the high likelihood for additional injury. She believed she faced an ethical dilemma in being asked to change her recommendations.

In this situation, Alice considered the many factors that would have an impact in developing an appropriate discharge plan:

- The client has many risk factors (e.g., difficulty maintaining the weight-bearing restrictions, history of heavy alcohol use) that led Alice to believe discharge to Roberta's home without constant supervision would be unsafe.
- The client does not have the financial resources to stay at any type of facility supported by caregiving staff.
- The client has the capacity to make her own decisions.
- The client has explicitly expressed a desire to return home.

Although Alice was not completely comfortable with the plan to discharge Roberta home, she acknowledged that Roberta had the right to make her own decisions regarding her care and her expressed wishes should be respected (RSCs 3A, 3B, 3D). Alice decided to provide Roberta with fall prevention education, recommendations for home safety techniques and appropriate home medical equipment, and follow-up home health occupational therapy. Alice also discussed the potential to obtain a medical alert device and suggested Roberta develop a schedule in which people in her support system would assist her with IADL tasks, such as laundry and shopping.

When it appeared that Roberta would go home, Alice contemplated whether she should change her documentation recommendations because she believed there was a conflict between her recommendations and the actual discharge plan. Alice also felt pressured from team members to change her documentation. However, Alice decided that to change previously documented information would violate RSCs 5B, 5C, and 4O that pertain to the Principles of Veracity and Justice.

Note. IADLs = instrumental activities of daily living; RSCs = Related Standards of Conduct.

Case Study 16.2. Concern for Well-Being, Respect of Privacy, and Objective Services Provision

Monique was one of two occupational therapists in an outpatient clinic that provided services for clients with neurological impairments, such as stroke, TBI, and Parkinson's disease. One of the services offered in the clinic was driving evaluation and intervention.

Monique had several years' experience as an occupational therapist; however, she was new to the outpatient setting and had not received formal training in driving evaluation and rehabilitation. The other occupational therapist in the clinic was a CDRS; however, she was on vacation when Monique received a referral for evaluation of treatment for **Marcus,** a 65-year-old man who had sustained a stroke.

Upon chart review and evaluation, Monique determined that Marcus had a complete left homonymous hemianopia from a posterior circulating artery stroke. Although the stroke resulted in a visual field deficit, the client did not demonstrate any concurrent physical or cognitive impairment. Marcus was going to receive only occupational therapy outpatient services.

Marcus was retired, and before the stroke, he had been independent in all basic self-care and home management tasks. He also performed all shopping and community mobility tasks independently and regularly attended church services. He lived alone in a rural area where public transportation was limited.

As part of the evaluation, Monique asked Marcus his reason for pursuing occupational therapy and the goals he would like to achieve. Marcus began by mentioning difficulty reading books and engaging in computer tasks. However, he reported the most meaningful issue to address was his need to return to driving to various locations to perform his desired occupations.

Monique discovered that although the client did have some support from family and friends, they were not available to provide transportation for all of his needs and activities on a regular basis.

Monique began to discuss some of the potential improvements that may occur with reading and computer tasks. Marcus shifted the conversation to driving. The state's Division of Motor Vehicles did not allow an individual to drive if the person had less than 140 degrees of visual field. When Monique informed Marcus of this law, he became frustrated and questioned the accuracy of the information. After further discussion, Marcus informed Monique that, regardless of the state law, "I plan on driving anyway."

Marcus left after setting up follow-up appointments. His niece drove him to the initial occupational therapy appointment, and Monique assumed she or other family members would continue to provide transportation. Monique decided not to report Marcus's remarks to any team members or authorities because she believed his remarks were made out of frustration of being told he could not drive; she did not think he actually intended to do so. Although she did not report Marcus's remarks to anyone, she did document them in the medical record.

Marcus was making good progress toward improving his performance on computer-related tasks and various reading materials. Several sessions later, Monique noticed some facial and upper-extremity bruising on Marcus. When she inquired about the source of the injury, Marcus acknowledged that he had driven and caused an accident in which another person was injured. At this point, Monique was unsure what, if anything, to report or document.

Monique was faced with the following ethical dilemmas at two crucial times. The first conflict occurred at the end of the initial evaluation when Marcus stated he planned on driving regardless of

(Continued)

Case Study 16.2. Concern for Well-Being, Respect of Privacy, and Objective Services Provision *(Cont.)*

state regulations. Monique had to weigh Marcus's right to privacy and self-determination (RSCs 3A, 3B, 3F, 3H) with her obligation to report issues that may affect client safety (RSCs 5C, 5D, 6H). The second major conflict was when Marcus informed Monique that he was the responsible party in causing an accident.

When Monique found out that Marcus was involved in an accident, she wondered whether she was obligated to report the objective findings of the initial evaluation along with his remarks. She decided to use a decision table to guide her next step (see Table 16.1).

After reviewing the potential outcomes and consequences, Monique decided the best course of action was to immediately discuss the situation with the therapy services manager. This allowed her to obtain immediate feedback and plan subsequent actions. Although there was the potential for serious consequences, Monique felt she needed to accept responsibility to prevent the potential for further injury.

Table 16.1. Decision Table for Case Study 16.2

Possible Action	Positive Outcomes	Negative Consequences
Take no action.	Avoid any potential consequences. Maintain positive relationship with Marcus.	Potentially unsettled subjective feeling of responsibility and guilt. Potential legal consequences if Marcus is involved in legal action and medical records are obtained and reviewed.
Wait to discuss the situation with the other OT/CDRS when she returns from vacation.	Can discuss with someone who has much more experience.	Possibility that Marcus will continue to drive and be a risk to himself and others.
Discuss the situation immediately with the manager of therapy services.	Can get immediate feedback and suggestions regarding potential subsequent actions. May prevent further injury. May have less internal stress regarding the situation.	May be at risk of disciplinary action. May be at risk of legal consequences.
Review available references and guidelines that list recommendations.	Will assist in building knowledge base for future reference. Can immediately use information learned to inform clients regarding laws and regulations.	Review may reveal actual violation of legal statutes.

Note. CDRS = certified driving rehabilitation specialist; OT = occupational therapist; RSCs = Related Standards of Conduct; TBI = traumatic brain injury.

ethics models. The process model suggests further analysis of and attention to the "embeddedness" (Gervasis, 2005, p. 187) of a health care professional when considering their role in solving clinical problems. Factors that often contribute to ethical problems may include professional arrangements and relationships as well as institutional structure and policies.

Self-assessment

Self-assessment is introspective evaluation of oneself and consists of four elements: (1) adequacy of background knowledge, (2) personal capacity for determining and then doing the right thing, (3) personal moral convictions, and (4) moral courage to advocate for a potentially

Vignette 16.3. Fairness and Objectivity in Services Provision, Accurate Representation of Profession, and Intervening With Integrity

Sierra provided occupational therapy services in an outpatient, low vision clinic. She received referrals from several local hospitals and from an optometrist who specialized in low vision evaluation. She recently received a referral to evaluate and provide low vision occupational therapy services for a client, **Josh,** who had recently lost his vision and now had no light perception (i.e., completely blind). The client was otherwise physically healthy and did not exhibit any cognitive impairment.

Josh's main goal was to be able to walk to a fitness center and take public transportation to the local library. Josh expressed much anxiety regarding mobility tasks because accomplishing his goals would necessitate walking down sidewalks and crossing several traffic intersections. Josh also stated he had never taken public transportation and was unfamiliar with how to proceed. Although Sierra had much experience in working with clients with moderate to severe low vision, she did not have any experience providing intervention to clients with complete blindness.

Sierra was aware that the state in which she lived provided support and intervention without charge through the state DSB. She had been told in CE workshops that these services were very limited because the agency's budget had recently been reduced. Because community mobility is a billable service, she felt her plan of care would be covered by Josh's medical insurance. She felt confident she could review mobility techniques she had observed in CE seminars and could teach him how to use the long white cane to navigate the short distance to the fitness center and take public transportation to the library.

Questions to consider:

- Does this fall under the scope of occupational therapy? (RSC 1E)
- Is Sierra competent to provide these services? (RSCs 5A, 6I)
- Would her attempt to provide these services reduce the public trust in or have a negative impact on the profession of occupational therapy? (RSCs 6K, 6L)
- What other options does Sierra have?

Sierra believed Josh's needs would not fully be met through the state DSB. The dilemma occurred when Sierra was considering offering services she was not fully qualified to perform. Upon reflection of the potential risk for Josh, Sierra investigated additional resources to assist Josh and referred him to the most appropriate professionals in the most appropriate manner (RSCs 6H, 6I, 6L, 6M).

Note. CE = continuing education; DSB = Division of Services for the Blind; RSCs = Related Standards of Conduct.

difficult decision. A potential outcome of the self-assessment step may be to seek specialized guidance or study.

The final steps to the process model are to make a decision, act and then evaluate the entire process. The individual must weigh options to reach a decision that is congruent with one's moral compass. If conflicts are identified, one must inquire into and use available resources. Case Study 16.2 is an example of the safety of a client and his community being at odds with client confidentiality.

Vignette 16.3 emphasizes appropriate services provision by those with appropriate qualifications.

Summary

Occupational therapy practitioners working in the practice area of physical disability, rehabilitation, and participation can be faced with significant ethical challenges as the complexity of the health care environment grows. Resolving ethical dilemmas involves balancing the client's abilities, needs, and rights while adhering to professional ethical guidelines (Kassenberg & Skär, 2008). Occupational therapy students and practitioners are encouraged to use the resources identified in this chapter and book to assist them in resolving the ethical dilemmas encountered in this practice area.

Reflective Questions

1. You are working in an outpatient rehabilitation clinic with a client who sustained a traumatic brain injury. She is making progress toward her goal of returning to work at a local restaurant. Per your plan of care, you anticipate another 3 to 4 weeks of intervention; however, her insurance has denied further reimbursement. You

believe she will not reach optimal potential if she is unable to complete her course of occupational therapy.

- Given your ethical obligation of concern for client well-being and promoting fairness in provision of services, what might your next steps be?

2. A client on your caseload in an acute inpatient rehabilitation unit has had a stroke. He was admitted with mild motor deficits but significant cognitive impairment. He has progressed to a level that a client might typically be discharged home, although he still has cognitive impairments that preclude independence with various IADLs and he cannot return to work as a physician. He and his spouse have a newborn infant, and she is overwhelmed by the current circumstances. She asks you to continue to advocate for extension of his stay on the rehabilitation unit.
   - How do you balance the concern for client and family with your duty to be a good steward of appropriate resources?
3. You observe a colleague frequently providing interventions that have no evidence to support effectiveness.
   - What potential strategies could you approach your colleague with to discuss your ethical concern of what you view as ineffective practice?

References

American Occupational Therapy Association. (2014). Occupational therapy practice framework: Domain and process (3rd ed.). *American Journal of Occupational Therapy, 68*(Suppl. 1), S1–S48. https://doi.org/10.5014/ajot.2014.682006

American Occupational Therapy Association. (2015). Occupational therapy code of ethics (2015). *American Journal of Occupational Therapy, 69*(Suppl. 3), 6912310030. https://doi.org/10.5014/ajot.2015.696S03

American Occupational Therapy Association. (2016). *Vision 2025.* Retrieved from http://www.aota.org/AboutAOTA/Get-Involved/ASD/npp.aspx

Americans With Disabilities Act of 1990, Pub. L. 101–336, 42 U.S.C. § 12101–12213.

Americans With Disabilities Act National Network. (n.d.). In *What is the definition of disabilities under the ADA?* Retrieved from https://adata.org/faq/what-definition-disability-under-ada

Atwal, A., & Caldwell, K. (2003). Ethics, occupational therapy and discharge planning: four broken principles. *Australian Occupational Therapy Journal, 50*(4), 244–251. https://doi.org/10.1046/j.1440-1630.2003.00374.x

Gervasis, K. G. (2005). A model for decision making to inform the ethics education of future health care professionals. In R. B. Purtilo, G. M. Jensen, & C. B. Royeen (Eds.), *Educating for moral action: A sourcebook in health and rehabilitation ethics* (pp. 185–190). Philadelphia: F. A. Davis.

Hunt, M. R., & Ellis, C. (2013). A patient-centered care ethics analysis model for rehabilitation. *American Journal of Physical Medicine and Rehabilitation, 92*(9), 818–827. https://doi.org/10.1097/PMH.0b013e318292309b

Kassenberg, A., & Skär, L. (2008). Experiences of ethical dilemmas in rehabilitation: Swedish occupational therapists' perspectives. *Scandinavian Journal of Occupational Therapy, 15*(4), 204–211. https://doi.org/10.1080/11038120802087618

Quiroga, V. (1995). *Occupational therapy: The first 30 years.* Bethesda, MD: American Occupational Therapy Association.

Scott, R. (1998). *Professional ethics: A guide for rehabilitation professionals.* St. Louis: Mosby.

World Health Organization. (2001). *International classification of functioning, disability and health.* Geneva: Author.

World Health Organization. (2002). *Towards a common language for functioning, disability and health.* Retrieved from http://www.who.int/classifications/icf/training/icfbeginnersguide.pdf

Wright-St. Clair, V. A., & Newcombe, D. B. (2014). Values and ethics in practice-based decision making. *Canadian Journal of Occupational Therapy, 8*(3), 154–62. https://doi.org/10.1177/0008417414535083

Chapter 17.

ADMINISTRATION AND MANAGEMENT: ETHICAL CHALLENGES

Missi Zahoransky, MSHS, OTR/L

Learning Objectives

By the end of the chapter, readers will be able to

- Understand the ethical dilemmas facing managers and administrators in the delivery of occupational therapy services within a variety of settings,
- Describe key components in the development of a culture of integrity and an ethically sound workplace,
- Understand major ethical issues faced in the current health care market, and
- Describe how the Patient Protection and Affordable Care Act of 2010 has affected ethics in health care delivery.

Key Terms and Concepts

- ✧ Bullet directive
- ✧ Client-centered approach
- ✧ Codes of ethics
- ✧ Ethical purity
- ✧ Ethical standards
- ✧ Improving Medicare Post-Acute Care Transformation Act of 2014
- ✧ Patient Protection and Affordable Care Act of 2010
- ✧ Social media

When most occupational therapy students start their education, they are usually focused on making a difference in direct patient care. Over time and as they gain experience, some develop an interest in administration and management as a way to help more people; others are tapped to fill roles at these levels because of a leadership void.

Occupational therapy practitioners often start positions in management with little preparation. Successful leaders must use a multitude of skills and knowledge bases to garner respect, loyalty, and confidence from peers, staff, and other team members.

Ethical considerations are not a "might-happen" situation; they are now part of the everyday health care arena, and practitioners must be prepared and understand how to navigate and lead in the model of care they are managing.

Our current health care system is rapidly changing, and the emergence of new regulations and payment models lends itself to potential ethical challenges and concerns. Our modern-day health care system and the emphasis on outcomes have directed the focus of care and management toward meeting the needs of a complex medical community and have made ethical challenges and concerns common.

Common areas of ethical challenges faced by occupational therapy managers and administrators are explored in this chapter. The purpose of this chapter is to provide a road map for administrators and managers to follow to assist them in developing, successfully managing, and refining a culture of ethical integrity.

Overview of Ethics in Management and Administration

What are some major ethical issues occupational therapy managers and administrators face? If this question were asked to a large group of managers and administrators, the predominant theme would likely be balancing high-quality care with expected efficiency. An ethical dilemma arises when occupational therapy practitioners, managers, and administrators begin to question the priorities of patient care and safety when driven by efficiency.

According to the World Health Organization (WHO; 2008), people

> expect their families and communities to be protected from risks and dangers to health. They want health care that deals with people as individuals with rights and not as mere targets for programs or beneficiaries of charity. They are willing to respect health professionals but want to be respected in turn, in a climate of mutual trust. (p. 14)

This tenet of mutual trust requires health care practitioners to be proactive and reactive when faced with ethical dilemmas.

Management's Role

Managers and administrators ensure that care is provided safely, effectively, and efficiently to meet the needs of the health care organization while protecting the client and ensuring the highest caliber of care. Although most organizations have an ethics committee to address ethical concerns within the facility, managers and administrators could institute the practice of having an ethical component within the department's meeting structure. To do this, managers and administrators must first understand the *Occupational Therapy Code of Ethics (2015)* (hereinafter referred to as the "Code"; American Occupational Therapy Association [AOTA], 2015) as well as the facility's or agency's ethical policies and procedures. This knowledge allows for managerial competence when addressing and discussing ethical dilemmas common to the area of practice.

Managers and administrators can discuss ethical concerns at all staff meetings or during individual meetings with staff. This process allows for the development of an ethical culture and advocacy. It can enable a department or group to reach a fair consensus on how an ethical dilemma should be resolved.

Codes of Ethics

Codes of ethics generally guide a profession's conduct in providing care. Managers and administrators in health care must consider client safety and accept that additional institutional values must be addressed as well. Managers and administrators must consider a variety of professional codes of ethics. Practitioners might focus on the codes of ethics that drive the profession, but leaders must be aware of the codes of ethics that drive, support, and surround the arena of practice.

Understanding how ethical considerations are part of daily management is a hallmark of successful leaders. Peter Drucker (2014) once said, "Management is doing things right; leadership is doing the right things" (para. 5). Each manager may have his or her own style, but when dealing with ethics, a manager or administrators must display ethical leadership and serve as a role model who follows the practice's codes of ethics. Is safety important? Of course it is, but as an administrative representative, a manager must look at all of the competing values and understand that one action may affect other departments and can have far-reaching positive or negative consequences that need to be addressed within the system.

Policy change, ethical dilemma interpretation, and overall facility or agency enhancement as a health care provider are a few examples of positive consequences. Ignoring concerns, avoiding censure of employees, declining to take corrective action, or turning a blind eye to situations are negative consequences that will not lead to a successful workplace.

Occupational therapy practitioners, managers, and administrators must understand the role of codes of ethics and the implication and application of such codes. They then must understand, follow, educate, and promote the Code within all areas of practice.

Patient Protection and Affordable Care Act

> The issue of health care reform brings important ethical issues of justice to the forefront, as individuals, communities, and the legislature struggle with how to provide quality health care for the many without sacrificing the basic rights of even the few. (Sorrell, 2012, p.1)

The ***Patient Protection and Affordable Care Act*** (ACA: P. L. 111–148, 2010) addresses comprehensive health insurance reforms. Health care professionals need to understand the primary tenet of the ACA (i.e., allowing for affordable health care for more individuals in a cost-effective manner), how this tenet affects health care delivery practices, and the ethical dilemmas it can engender (Lachman, 2012).

Although the ACA is intended to address injustices in the access to health care, confusion about the fundamentals of the law and its enforcement can result in ethical quandaries when efforts to implement the mandates are attempted. This confusion occurs when providers or payers do not fully understand the law and misinterpret the ACA guidelines and policy directives.

For example, a hospital system might institute policies and procedures regarding the exchange of patient information between providers of care that are more restrictive and cumbersome than the law mandates. If team members are restricted in sharing pertinent patient information that would facilitate better care, the overly restrictive policies can prevent optimal care. In addition, when a facility or agency "overinterprets" policy, others may also mandate increasingly complex systems into an already complex arena of care, potentially increasing costs. This adds layers of work to health care providers, which is unnecessary and time-consuming.

The ACA was considered by most to be the biggest change to the Medicare and Medicaid programs since their inception in 1965. Although current analysis of the effectiveness of the ACA shows more patients receive health care coverage, occupational therapy managers and practitioners continue to face many challenges. "Although the ACA does much to expand access to health insurance coverage, it falls short of the goals espoused by the right to health movement" (Christopher & Caruso, 2015, p. 958). The ACA addresses insurance coverage and availability of this coverage to a portion of individuals who were previously uninsured. This approach continues to be based on financing health care and not on the philosophy of the basic human right to health care, which would ensure coverage for everyone in the United States (Christopher & Caruso, 2015).

This right-to-health movement is inclusive to all providers of health care, which affects occupational therapy practitioners. As more people receive health care coverage, the number of potential clients receiving occupational therapy services increases, and occupational therapy practitioners should be involved in discussions about how to meet the needs and manage the increased demands and the ethical challenges that can occur. Therefore, practitioners, managers, and administrators must develop sound ethical standards within their work environment.

Upholding Ethical Standards of Practice

WHO established strict parameters and guidelines addressing health-related research with the development of Research Ethics Committees (RECs) internationally, nationally, and locally. Successful managers and administrators incorporate a variety of knowledge and skills to help guide them through the process of ethical decision making.

Health care is a human-driven process, and as such, the philosophical discussion of ***ethical purity,*** or the ability to act ethically with integrity and consistency, can be confusing. Reviewing established guidelines and blending them with current managerial skills advance an ethical leader's effectiveness. Through the RECs, a manager or administrator can address an ethical dilemma by applying knowledge and working within the Decision Table (Appendix G).

In the following paragraph from WHO, interpret "approval or disapproval" as Decision Table outcomes and replace "research" with "client intervention"; you can see a pattern that mirrors the ACA, the Code, and many health care organizational standards addressing ethics.

> Approval or disapproval is based on the *ethical acceptability* of the research, including its social value and scientific validity, an acceptable ratio of potential benefits to risks of harm, the minimization of risks, adequate informed consent procedures (including cultural appropriateness and mechanisms to ensure voluntariness), measures to ensure protection of vulnerable populations, fair procedures for selection of participants, and attention to the impact of research on the communities from which participants will be drawn, both during the research and after it is complete. The review takes into account any prior scientific reviews and applicable laws. (WHO, 2011, p. 12)

Vague Language and Bullet Directives

One challenge many administrators and managers face is that, in interpreting a professional code of ethics, the language to guide one through the process is sometimes vague. Many administrators and managers are frustrated by the lack of finite examples. Vague language can lead to misinterpretation of the law as well as implementation of policy by leadership that may impact a department's operations and, subsequently, affect patient care.

As with ACA interpretation, many managers are issued bullet point–style directives to ensure ethical practice; the manager or administrator is then left to define and develop processes to manage whatever dilemmas may arise in the provision of care. As with code of ethics interpretation, vague and unproven policy can affect the overall successful functioning of practice patterns and ultimately impede quality patient care.

One example of vague guidance arises in regard to reimbursement and productivity. Managers often receive a ***bullet directive,*** a short, decisive statement, to focus on productivity and reimbursement of services. These directives from administration often demand specific targets for both of these aspects of patient care. These targets may make financial sense on paper but can infringe on areas such as clinical competency.

This issue is so important that the three national therapy associations (i.e., AOTA, American Physical Therapy Association, & American Speech–Language–Hearing Association, 2014) joined forces to develop the *Consensus Statement on Clinical Judgment in Health Care Settings.* This document clearly supports the codes of ethics for all three disciplines when it states, "Clinicians are ethically obligated to deliver services that they believe are medically necessary and in the client/patient's best interest, based upon their independent clinical reasoning and judgment as well as objective data" (p. 1). An illustration of this ethical obligation would be in a skilled nursing facility when a practitioner feels pressure to treat a patient for a specific amount of minutes, regardless of human components (see Vignette 17.1).

Administrators and managers need a comprehensive approach to identify, analyze, and address complex ethical issues. ***Ethical standards*** are generally developed to provide a moral compass to help guide practitioners, managers, and administrators through challenges encountered in the current health care climate. These standards allow administrators, managers, and practitioners to operate in an honest and trustworthy environment.

Ethical practice is an ongoing concern and affects every area of occupational therapy practice, regardless of setting, population, or practitioner. According to Jonsen, Siegler, and Winslade (2006), "to understand the ethical issues in a case, it is necessary to consider the clinical situation of the patient, that is, the nature of the disease, the treatment proposed, and the goals of the intervention" (p. 15). Jonsen and colleagues cite that a clear understanding of these factors is paramount to resolving an

Vignette 17.1. Skilled Nursing Facility

Mr. Davis was recently diagnosed with pneumonia. Upon the occupational therapy practitioner's arrival to the patient's room to transport him to therapy, Mr. Davis requested deferral until the next day when he hoped to feel better. The practitioner agreed that therapy would not be productive, but upon return to the department, the manager reiterated the need for the minutes to be completed that day to avoid reimbursement issues. The manager felt the pressure to enforce a blanket policy that had not been clearly defined, and the practitioner felt the need to avoid treating a patient who would not benefit in that moment in time. Both the manager and the clinician faced an ethical dilemma.

Vignette 17.2. Ethical Teamwork

Margie was admitted to the hospital after having an episode of right-sided weakness and loss of speech. A physician diagnosed her with TIA and ordered occupational therapy, physical therapy, and speech–language pathology evaluations. Upon evaluating the client's level of function the following morning, **Yolanda,** the occupational therapist, discussed recommendations with Margie. Based on information Margie shared, they developed an intervention plan together. Yolanda coordinated care with the other team members, and the overall plan of care was developed and documented per hospital policy adhering to HIPAA guidelines (P. L. 104–191). Yolanda discussed the plan with the assigned occupational therapy assistant and maintained communication on Margie's progress. Margie completed the stipulated number of evidence-based occupational therapy sessions, achieved the anticipated outcomes, and returned home. The discharge recommendations included occupational therapy services through home health care and use of DME.

Note. DME = durable medical equipment; HIPAA = Health Insurance Portability and Accountability Act; TIA = transient ischemic attack.

ethical dilemma. Vignette 17.2 is an example of an ethically sound case because the client, physician, occupational therapist, occupational therapy assistant, and other team members share the same values and core principles to achieve success and agree with an acceptable course of care.

Many of the Code's Principles are reflected throughout the care process in Vignette 17.2:

- *Principle 1, Beneficence (Related Standards of Conduct [RSCs] A, D, E, H, I):* Completing a comprehensive evaluation and formulating a plan specific to the client's needs; referring to appropriate providers (home health care) upon discharge; care is driven by evidence and coordinated with team (Principle of Fidelity is also evident).
- *Principle 3, Autonomy (RSCs A, B, D, H):* Discussion with the client regarding wishes and expectations as well as development of the care plan; collaboration with all team members; documentation per policy and HIPAA.
- *Principle 4, Justice (RSCs A, B, H, M, O):* Response in a timely manner; billing accordingly for services and reflected in documentation; providing appropriate supervision of personnel.

Social Media

One component of modern-day health care that can cause considerable ethical dilemmas for managers and administrators is social media. ***Social media*** is an information technology for information sharing and interaction with a broad or targeted community.

> Social media represents a brave new world for health care. It offers a venue for communicating with consumers quickly and inexpensively, such as promoting new wellness programs, marketing new services, and announcing the latest achievements in patient care. It also presents challenges, including risks to information accuracy, organizational reputation, and individual privacy. (Backman et al., 2011, p. 20)

Although many venues for social media are harmless in nature, staff must be educated on the dangers and unintended consequences of using social media. The unfortunate reality of social media is its instantaneous and binding nature; it is also essentially uncontrolled by management when done at the employee level.

Many areas of social media engagement might be perceived as no or low risk, when the opposite can be true. Consider the use of professional blogs and discussion forums available to occupational therapists. A patient's condition and other pertinent information may be discussed openly with a large audience, and because other examples are shared and discussed, this is seen as helpful and ethical. Shared information, regardless of a patient's name being redacted, can still violate a patient's privacy rights.

Furthermore, social media lacks the intangibles that face-to-face conversation holds. "One incorrect or flippant remark can become indelible, reaching audiences who lack the ability to read facial expressions or hear intonation. They may not be able to discern something said in jest from something said in earnest" (Backman et al., 2011, p. 12). A simple ethical concern can be exacerbated into a grievous concern, regardless of validity, because of the ability to share information

Case Study 17.1. Confidentiality Breach Via Social Media

Ashley, a manager in a hospital, had a general rule not to be active with staff on social media outlets. **Lily,** one of the staff therapists, asked to speak to Ashley in confidence. During the discussion, Lily shared that **Fred,** another staff therapist, was sharing a patient scenario on social media. Lily was clearly upset and concerned regarding this incident. She also was hesitant to give details and did not want "to get anyone in trouble."

As a manager, Ashley recognized that more information had to be obtained before any action could occur. She assured Lily that the meeting was confidential to allow for an environment of trust. Ashley also clearly defined that the conversation would remain "on point" and address only this particular instance. This was done to ensure no additional personal feelings or concerns would cloud the issue being discussed. Ashley knew that, as a manager, she had to remain neutral and focused on this investigation to determine if Lily's concern was valid. She began to collect data with basic questions such as, What was the incident that occurred? When did the incident occur? What was the social media outlet? Were specific names mentioned? She also asked to see the posting.

Lily informed Ashley that she could show her the postings on the computer. First, Ashley ensured that the postings were viewed without violating any polices. Upon viewing, Ashley saw that Fred had posted information regarding a patient. The posting posed a question regarding treatment for specific deficits. No names were used, but Fred's profile included his place of employment. Second, because most social media is in the public domain, Ashley felt comfortable making a copy of the posting. This decision was a managerial one, and multiple considerations were taken into account, including the nature of the complaint, the possibility of a HIPAA violation, and the fact that social media can be manipulated (e.g., postings can be removed). Before continuing, Ashley told Lily that she would look into the situation to determine whether any violations occurred.

In analyzing the data, Ashley first went to the hospital's Policy and Procedure Manual for guidance on HIPAA regulations and social media use. She found that the facility had no specific policy about social media, but HIPAA guidelines are very specific. Ashley decided not to go to others to corroborate the information she received because that would lead to unnecessary complexities. As a manager, Ashley's biggest concern was potential HIPAA violation. If a client's name had been used, an ethical and legal breach may have been made with consequences that could be far-reaching for the hospital. Because a client's name was not mentioned, Ashley needed to handle this situation according to policy and established standards. However, Ashley discovered that the facility did not have a distinct policy on social media.

Using the Code, Fred potentially violated Principle 1, Beneficence (RSC F); Principle 3, Autonomy (RSC H); Principle 4, Justice (RSC E); and Principle 6, Fidelity (RSCs A, K, L; see Table 17.1).

By completing the last two options in the Decision Table, Ashley would not only have supported the Code in a vast number of Principles and RSCs but also would have advanced the ethical conduct promoted by the hospital. An advantage to using the Decision Table is the inherent processing that occurs with its use. As scenarios are developed and options noted, a clear picture begins to emerge as to the best course of action. Using the Decision Table also may lead to several options that jointly evolve into a successful plan.

Following up with Lily was a choice Ashley had to make. In no instance should the details or discussion with Fred be disclosed. Ashley could choose to inform Lily it was handled, which also would be apparent when the new policy was addressed at a staff meeting. It also would allow Lily to know she was heard and a fair approach was taken. Most therapists would appreciate that the manager wanted to keep everything confidential because they would want the same respect if they were in a situation of concern.

Another approach would be to handle the situation without discussion of the resolution. Every manager knows his or her staff and the dynamics within, as well as the personalities. Consideration of this is part of the overall managerial style developed. A manager must take into account the

(Text continued on p. 200)

Case Study 17.1. Confidentially Breach Via Social Media *(Cont.)*

Table 17.1. Decision Table for Case Study 17.1

Possible Action	Positive Outcomes	Negative Consequences
No action.	None.	Further postings could occur, and additional information could come out, which could compromise the client's privacy and well-being (Principle 2, Nonmaleficence, RSC E). The facility could then be at risk. Lack of policy is unreported (Principle 4, Justice, RSCs F, K, L). Lily might go to Ashley's supervisor if no action is taken.
Inform Fred that he will be written up for unprofessional conduct. Explain to Fred that he cannot post information regarding a patient on social media, and when asked, explain that another staff reported the incident.	Lily feels validated and believes Ashley is a successful manager and has upheld the Code with emphasis on Nonmaleficence and Justice.	Without personally verifying that the incident occurred as reported, Ashley may, in turn, violate the Code herself (RSCs 1F, 2C, 4F, 5D, 5G). This approach could result in unjust disciplinary action. Other staff members may view Ashley as unfair and unjust and not respect her authority or decision-making process as a supervisor.
Ashley reports the incident to the hospital's ethics board and HIPAA compliance officer, asks them to determine if there are violations, and if so, have them address the issue with Fred.	Promotes transparency within the organization regarding potential concerns about ethical behavior and client privacy.	This action could result in the administration perceiving that Ashley is an ineffective manager, and she would be in violation of the Code (RSCs 1F, 1G, 4H, 4L, 6J).
Consult with the HIPAA compliance officer regarding the issue to determine if any follow-up is required at the HIPAA level. Work with the organization to establish new policies regarding social media posts directly related to client care and the organization as a whole.	Avoids a "passing the buck" mentality and applies managerial responsibilities with well-informed actions. Advances the organization in regard to social media, a growing concern within the health care arena. Supports the Code's Principle 4, Justice (RSCs L, N).	None foreseen.
Educate Fred regarding proper social media outlets for information sharing and ways to handle. Have Fred review the Code and discuss the areas that had potential consequences, specifically HIPAA. At a later staff meeting, introduce new social media policies. Follow up with Lily, reporting that the situation was handled, without discussing details. Based on facts, Fred could receive a verbal or written warning, according to other policies within the organization.	Establishes clear ethical and legal standards in policies and procedures regarding social media that will benefit the entire facility. This supports adherence to Principle 3, Autonomy (RSCs H, I) and Principle 4, Justice (RSCs E, F, H, K, L). Early investigation and intervention also support Principle 5, Veracity (RSCs D, G).	None foreseen.

Note. HIPAA = Health Insurance Portability and Accountability Act; RSCs = Related Standards of Conduct.

(Continued)

Case Study 17.1. Confidentially Breach Via Social Media *(Cont.)*

message being sent. If it is clear the situation was handled, silence may be the correct course. Keep in mind that the staff members need to know there was a resolution, regardless of the course of action, or they may begin to view the manager with less respect or trust. There is no right or wrong answer to this dilemma, and it exemplifies another tough decision that a manager must be prepared to make.

In regard to the potential HIPAA violation, a manager must discuss it with the HIPAA officer (which is required by law) and determine if a breach occurred. If the HIPAA officer determines the posting on social media did not violate the HIPAA statute, it would no longer be pursued at that level and the issue returns to the internal department management for resolution.

with a large group of people at the push of a button. Case Study 17.1 illustrates ethical challenges related to social media.

Client-Centered Care

Occupational therapy uses a ***client-centered approach*** with the client as the ultimate decision maker. AOTA, through the *Occupational Therapy Practice Framework* states,

> the occupational therapy process is the client-centered delivery of occupational therapy services. The process includes evaluation and intervention to achieve targeted outcomes, occurs within the purview of the occupational therapy domain, and is facilitated by the distinct perspective of occupational therapy practitioners when engaging in clinical reasoning, analyzing activities and occupations, and collaborating with clients. (AOTA, 2014, p. S10)

The client, as a member of the care team, identifies his or her needs, priorities, and the focus of the intervention process. The clinician and client must be able to communicate realistically and responsibly to develop a true client-centered course of care. Discussions regarding goals and outcomes are a large part of the process, but under the current model of health care in the United States, conversations about coverage and resources also play a key role in care planning.

When a client needs a tub seat for safety but it is not a covered DME under Medicare and the client does not have the funds, what is the ethical responsibility of the occupational therapy practitioner? The simple answer is to provide it free of charge to make sure the client is safe. The realistic answer is that a practitioner can research additional areas of funding or resource allocation and still not be able to make this a feasible option. Is the clinician ethically irresponsible? No. Although the system may be perceived as flawed and these situations are not uncommon, the professional standards were met during care.

Another challenge facing clinicians and managers alike was discussed in a 2015 Global Health Ethics report by WHO. In the key findings, WHO (2015) stated, "Health practitioners seeking to provide the best possible care to their patients in the most ethical manner may find it difficult to balance the right to information with the need to avoid information overload" (p. 17).

How much information is enough, and what can the client absorb and retain? Is the client competent to make decisions, and conversely, is the family or caregiver legally privy to the information? Although some aspects may have legal guidance (i.e., HIPAA), many of these occurrences must rely on a practitioner's sound clinical reasoning skills.

Although the client is at the core of the process, many challenges can affect care. Practitioners sometimes encounter a situation in which a client identifies goals that might be unrealistic regarding anticipated outcomes. What is the practitioner's ethical or moral responsibility? For example, a client is receiving care in the occupational therapy department in a SNF and wants to take a break every 10 minutes to go outside to smoke. After a discussion on how frequent breaks affect goal attainment, the client demands that he has the right to smoke. What do you do?

Balancing a patient's desire for autonomy and his or her long-term safety can be a dilemma for even an experienced occupational therapy practitioner, who could benefit from using the Decision Table in

Vignette 17.3. Home Health Care

A home health occupational therapist, **Acacia,** approached **Kaley,** her supervisor, regarding a concern that her client, **Bruno,** was not following her recommendations. Bruno lived alone in a ranch-style home with a basement. He was a widower of many years and did not have much involvement with his children. His laundry was in the basement as was a walk-in shower he installed years ago. Acacia evaluated Bruno, and the results indicated that he was cognitively intact; however, he was a fall risk because of unsteady gait and impulsive decision making. Acacia made safety recommendations for ADL, and IADLS, specifically to use the first-floor shower. She took sample DMEs (i.e., grab bar, tub seat, and hand-held showerhead) to demonstrate their uses to Bruno to increase his safety. Bruno politely refused all recommendations and told Acacia he "will keep doing it my way."

Acacia was concerned that if she went along with Bruno's wishes, she would violate Principle 1, Beneficence, of the Code because Bruno would be at risk. Under the Decision Table model, Kaley assessed the situation and shared with Acacia that although the safety of a client is paramount, Bruno had the right to choose unsafe behavior because he was deemed competent. In fact, if Acacia tried to "coerce" Bruno's compliance, she would violate the principle of Autonomy, particularly with respect to Bruno's wishes (see RSC A) and the right to refuse occupational therapy services regardless of potential poor outcomes (see RSC E).

Note. ADLs = activities of daily living; DME = durable medical equipment; IADLs = instrumental activities of daily living; RSCs = Related Standards of Conduct.

concert with a consultation with a manager or supervisor. Very few arenas in health care delve into safety and patients' desires and values as practicing in the patient's home environment does (see Vignette 17.3).

Impact Act

The ***Improving Medicare Post-Acute Care Transformation Act of 2014*** (IMPACT Act; P. L. 113–185) requires the submission of standardized data by long-term care hospitals, SNFs, home health agencies, and inpatient rehabilitation facilities (Centers for Medicare and Medicaid Services [CMS], 2015). These data allow transparency in regard to outcomes, resource utilization, and best practices by being able to be compared across different post-acute care settings. The IMPACT Act also meets a key aim of the National Quality Strategy of providing health care that is affordable, reliable, accessible, and safe (CMS, 2015). The IMPACT Act shifts occupational therapy practitioners' focus to outcomes and management of chronic diseases, thereby making sure practitioners are knowledgeable and competent to provide care and participate in a culture of integrity.

This act resonates with the Code, specifically in regard to Principle 1, Beneficence, and Principle 2, Nonmaleficence. Effective managers and administrators must understand specific policy and how it affects practice within the setting to ensure ethical integrity and staff education meet the needs of the facility or agency. Ensuring staff members have the opportunity to advance their skills and engage in educational advancement is necessary to build a culture of ethics and excellence.

As discussed above, the ACA was mandated to give all individuals the right to health care (Lachman, 2012). As health care coverage expands, occupational therapy practitioners have greater access to clients. Although this can positively affect the profession and personal careers, growth carries inherent risk, particularly regarding ethical behavior. Although the ACA mandated increased coverage, individual freedom of choice is still a concern in an environment where the law's mandates are developed and carried out by states, insurance companies, and private health care providers.

Occupational therapy practitioners must be engaged in developing and monitoring processes to ensure inclusion in the burgeoning health care delivery system. Practitioners need to deliver evidence-based care that is ethically sound to help guide the occupational therapy profession into becoming a major stakeholder in future health care models. According to the Code, practitioners have a responsibility to use evidence in their interventions (RSC 1C) and be competent in the services they deliver (RSC 1G) as they strive to address and reduce barriers to care (RSCs 4C, 4D).

Developing a Culture of Ethical Integrity

In the world of insurance and audits, health care entities are cautious in their provision of care, and occupational therapy practitioners face the ongoing ethical dilemma of access to care. Throughout health care, systems are in place to manage access to care and determine care needs based on data collected at the beginning of care. Because practitioners are in the business of human care, they understand that needs can change daily, and they are faced with ethical and moral value concerns. Possessing a clear understanding of ethical standards will help in conversations and add clarity and rationale to approaches taken in meeting care needs.

Clear Communication

Open dialogue with staff as well as clients boosts the ethical culture of integrity. Ensuring a transparent atmosphere for information sharing as well as encouraging forthright and understandable dialogue regarding ethics and ethical integrity allows the culture to become a foundation for the future. Clients, staff, and management flourish in an environment of care that is soundly and fairly structured in regard to ethics.

> People obviously want effective health care when they are sick or injured. They want it to come from providers with the integrity to act in their best interests, equitably and honestly, with knowledge and competence. The demand for competence is not trivial: it fuels the health economy with steadily increased demand for professional care (doctors, nurses and other non-physician clinicians) who play an increasing role in both industrialized and developing countries. (WHO, 2008, p. 16)

Consistency

One quality of ethical consciousness is consistency. An ethics rubric is essential because it allows the manager or administrator to use a consistent tool to collect and analyze the necessary data to reach a decision. The Code and state regulatory boards all play key roles in this process by providing the road map that a manager or administrator can follow for fair and consistent resolution.

Promotion of an Environment of Integrity

Ethical leadership also consciously promotes an environment that supports a culture of "high-quality, value-driven healthcare but promotes the ethical behavior and practices of individuals throughout the organization" (American College of Healthcare Executives, 2015, para. 2). Managers and administrators promote an environment of ethical integrity through role modeling and educating staff about the values, ethical standards, and policies and procedures of the department and facility. Managers and administrators establish and communicate processes and systems for addressing ethical concerns.

Although creating a culture of integrity is paramount, the challenge comes in maintaining this culture, which ultimately leads to an environment of integrity and compliance. As occupational therapy practitioners advance their knowledge of an ethical culture, they move toward an aspirational rather than punitive way of consistently incorporating ethical standards into health care environments. This new culture promotes learning from mistakes so they do not occur again.

Differentiation Between Legal and Ethical Issues

When ethical conflicts occur in health care, legal rules may sometimes set limits to ethical options or even create ethical conflicts (Jonsen et al., 2006). Although managers and administrators need not have extensive knowledge of law, they must have an understanding of what constitutes legal issues and actions. Jonsen et al. further reiterate the importance of not allowing the legal context to override the ethical issue. The solution for either may be different and must be handled by concepts and reasoning specific to each area.

Just because something is legal does not make it ethical. For example, although no law prohibits investing vast amounts of taxpayer dollars into researching the effects of a rare, nontoxic parasite, is this an ethical use of funds? Another example is that, although you have a constitutional right to freedom of speech, is it ethical to demean or make derogatory statements to a team member or patient?

When administrators and managers establish and maintains a culture of ethical integrity and competence, overall client care and staff satisfaction improves. The challenge for many in management is not in having the "right staff" for change but in understanding how to implement or make the change to the culture.

The following strategies are essential for managers and administrators who want to develop and maintain a culture of ethical integrity:

- Serve as a role model by quoting policy and ethical standards. Sending the message that these rules are for others is a quick descent into a negative culture.
- Be clear regarding the values and ethical standards expected by all. Everyone should understand that these standards are held in high regard and inform daily decisions.
- Make sure the facility or agency and department standards are evident to all and discussed routinely. Let everyone know that there are consequences to unethical behavior and that no one is exempt from these consequences, regardless of position or role.
- Create an avenue for reporting concerns. This is one of the hardest endeavors but is also one of the soundest. Managers and administrators must create an environment where others can discuss or report concerns without retribution.
- Consider developing a culture and values statement to complement your vision statement. In our current world of technology, mistrust, and constant change, prominently displaying your ethical culture and values can go a long way in calming any worries in clients and eliciting loyalty in staff.
- Understand the environment you manage. Many health care organizations have ethics committees or legal representation to review concerns and provide guidance. Understand and educate the staff you manage on the policy and procedures of these committees or representatives.

If a manager had used the strategies identified above, she may have been able to prevent the issues detailed in Case Study 17.2.

Appropriate communication is a powerful preventive tool to avoid potential harm to clients and colleagues. Vignette 17.4 describes a situation in which there is a need to confront both unethical verbal communication and written documentation.

Summary

The constructs of ethical behavior and integrity are not new. However, because of an ever-changing health care system, the frequency of ethical challenges and misbehaviors are compounded and of growing

Case Study 17.2. While I Am Away

Adina supervised staff in an outpatient clinic. **Danielle,** an occupational therapist under Adina's supervision, reported that while she was on vacation, **Heather,** another occupational therapist, covered her patients. Danielle was concerned about what transpired. She reported that when a client came in for her scheduled visit with Heather, the client reported issues regarding part of her care.

The client reported she felt "concerned" about some of the care she received under the covering therapist. The client reported that Heather told her they "would try some new things to get the wrist moving better" and that "some things work and some things don't." The client reported that Heather also attempted to "hook her up" to the transcutaneous electrical nerve stimulation unit but could not turn it on correctly and then said Heather told her she "wasn't comfortable using it." Upon further discussion, the client stated "she tried it once or twice, and it kept jolting me, so she stopped." Upon questioning Danielle further, Adina found that Danielle had left very detailed instructions for Heather in regard to specific modalities, exercises, and expected outcomes. Danielle also expressed concern that there was no documentation in Heather's notes of the procedures performed.

Upon further fact finding, Adina found that Heather did not share any concerns regarding treatment or modalities with Danielle before agreeing to provide vacation coverage. Adina determined that under RSC 1E, "Provide occupational therapy services, including education and training, that are within each practitioner's level of competence and scope of practice" (AOTA, 2015, p. 3), there was sufficient data to require action regarding a violation of ethics standards by Heather. Furthermore, Adina also reflected on her need to assess whether she had been out of compliance with RSCs 1D and 1E when assigning cases to Heather.

Vignette 17.4. Did He Really Just Say That?

Team members are discussing clients and their status at a meeting. Upon discussing **Mrs. Jones,** one of the physical therapists, **Calvin,** states that Mrs. Jones wanted him to pray with her to get better. Before any further conversation could occur, one of the occupational therapist, **Gary,** makes derogatory remarks about Mrs. Jones and says the SNF does not treat with "the laying on of hands." He goes on to state that Mrs. Jones was a "frequent flyer" and "you just need to treat her, tell her you are praying with her and it is working, and discharge her home." After the meeting, Calvin comes to you and shares additional concern regarding Gary. Calvin reports, "He came in and did his evaluation at the same time and asked me to change times so we didn't overlap."

You need to address multiple serious concerns. The derogatory statements violate Principle 3, Autonomy, by implied deception to a patient (RSCs B, F) as well as a lack of collaborative effort (RSC D). Gary's actions further violate Principle 4, Justice, by not only being disrespectful to the client but to other staff as well. Depending on the facility's policies and procedures and Gary's prior behavior, a written warning would be completed and reviewed with Gary, at a minimum. Of greater concern is the request to change times on legal documentation. Although this is clearly an ethical compromise of Principle 2, Nonmaleficence, RSCs F and H, it also violates Principle 4, Justice, which states occupational therapy personnel should relate in a respectful and fair manner and respect professional standards and laws. In this instance RSCs 4E, 4M, and 4O are clearly compromised, but more important, this situation could have entered the world of fraudulent billing.

Note. RSCs = Related Standards of Conduct; SNF = skilled nursing facilities.

concern. The ethical challenges facing administrators and managers today are inherently complex because the health care arena is rapidly changing and is driven by outcomes, technological advances, and payment. Understanding the policies and procedures of a department and organization regarding ethics is a small part of the process. By educating and surrounding oneself with guidance and standards, such as the Code, the practitioner becomes part of the solution.

Effective administrators and managers must incorporate the Code's Principles and RSCs, together with practice laws (state and national), as well as facility or agency policies and procedures. The Code further delineates the need for mindful reflection when addressing ethical challenges.

Successful managers and administrators must understand the need to systematically address ethical challenges when defining outcomes. By consistently using a matrix or Decision Table, each case, although different in nature, is dealt with in a fair and professional manner. This approach leads to a culture of ethical integrity and allows for professional growth and development for the entire health care team.

Reflective Questions

1. How can administrators and managers foster a culture of integrity and ethical responsibility that will create a powerful environment for client care?
2. How have occupational therapy practitioners been affected by the implementation of the ACA?
3. What factors in the rapidly advancing health care system have directly affected our profession and ethical integrity?
4. Based on the future of promoting ethics in the U.S. health care system, what knowledge and skills will you, as a manager or administrator, need to be successful?

References

American College of Healthcare Executives. (2015). *Creating an ethical culture within the healthcare organization.* Retrieved from https://www.ache.org/policy/environ.cfm

American Occupational Therapy Association. (2014). Occupational therapy practice framework: Domain and process (3rd ed.). *American Journal of Occupational Therapy, 68*(Suppl. 3), S1–S48. https://doi.org/10.5014/ajot.2014.682006

American Occupational Therapy Association. (2015). Occupational therapy code of ethics (2015). *American Journal of Occupational Therapy, 69*(Suppl. 3), 6912310030. https://doi.org/10.5014/ajot.2015.696S03

American Occupational Therapy Association, American Physical Therapy Association, & American Speech–Language–Hearing Association. (2014). *Consensus statement on clinical judgment in health care settings AOTA,*

APTA, ASHA. Retrieved from http://www.aota.org/~/media/Corporate/Files/Practice/Ethics/APTA-AOTA-ASHA-Concensus-Statement.pdf

Backman, C., Dolack, S., Dunyak, D., Lutz, L. Tegen, A., Warner, D. & Wieland, L. (2011). Social media + healthcare. *Journal of AHIMA, 82*(3), 20–25. Retrieved from http://library.ahima.org/doc?oid=103686#.WDYZ1E0VDEY

Centers for Medicare and Medicaid Services. (2015). *IMPACT Act of 2014 and cross–setting measures.* Retrieved from https://www.cms.gov/Medicare/Quality-Initiatives-Patient-Assessment-Instruments/Post-Acute-Care-Quality-Initiatives/IMPACT-Act-of-2014-and-Cross-Setting-Measures.html

Christopher, A. S., & Caruso, D. (2015). Promoting health as a human right in the post-ACA United States. *AMA Journal of Ethics, 17*(10), 958–965. https://doi.org/10.1001/journalofethics.2015.17.10.msoc1-1510

Drucker, P. (2014). These 10 Peter Drucker quotes may change your world. *Entrepreneur.* Retrieved from https://assets.entrepreneur.com/article/1411582563-10-peter-drucker-quotes.jpg?_ga=1.57666722.942625902.1467249445

Health Insurance Portability and Accountability Act of 1996, Pub. L. 104–191, 42 U.S.C. § 300gg, 29 U.S.C § 1181–1183, and 42 USC 1320d-1320d9.

Improving Medicare Post-Acute Care Transformation Act of 2014, Pub. L. 113–185, 128 Stat. 1952.

Jonsen, A. R., Siegler, M., & Winslade, W. J. (2006). *Clinical ethics: A practical approach to ethical decisions in clinical medicine* (6th ed.). New York: McGraw-Hill.

Lachman, V. (2012). Ethical challenges in the era of health care reform. *MedSurg Nursing, 21*(4), 248–251. Retrieved from http://www.nursingworld.org/MainMenuCategories/EthicsStandards/Resources/Ethical-Challenges-in-the-Era-of-Health-Care-Reform.pdf

Patient Protection and Affordable Care Act, Pub. L. 111–148, 42 U.S.C. §§ 18001–18121 (2010).

Sorrell, J., (2012). Ethics: The Patient Protection and Affordable Care Act: Ethical perspectives in 21st century health care. *OJIN: The Online Journal of Issues in Nursing, 18*(1). Retrieved from https://doi.org/10.3912/OJIN.Vol18No02EthCol01

World Health Organization. (2008). *The World Health Report 2008—Primary health care (now more than ever).* Retrieved from http://www.who.int/whr/2008/en/

World Health Organization. (2011). *Standards and operational guidance for ethics review of health-related research with human participants.* Retrieved from http://apps.who.int/iris/bitstream/10665/44783/1/9789241502948_eng.pdf?ua=1&ua=1

World Health Organization. (2015). *Global health ethics: Key issues.* Retrieved from http://apps.who.int/iris/bitstream/10665/164576/1/9789240694033_eng.pdf?ua=1

Chapter 18.

APPLICATION OF ETHICS IN HIGHER EDUCATION

Linda S. Gabriel, PhD, OTR/L

Learning Objectives

By the end of the chapter, readers will be able to

- Describe ethical issues facing students in occupational therapy education programs and the impact of responding to these issues on students' professional development,
- Describe ethical issues facing faculty in occupational therapy education programs and the impact of responding to these issues on faculty development and the ability to provide competent education to future practitioners, and
- Analyze a case study and vignettes regarding student and faculty behavior using the American Occupational Therapy Association's *Occupational Therapy Code of Ethics (2015)*.

Key Terms and Concepts

- ✧ Cheating
- ✧ Collaboration
- ✧ Collusion
- ✧ Explicit curriculum
- ✧ Faculty incivility
- ✧ Fair use
- ✧ Implicit curriculum
- ✧ Plagiarism
- ✧ Workplace or social bullying

No one wants an unethical practitioner, least of all the client or the client's family. No one wants a member of his or her profession to behave in a way that reduces the public's trust in that profession.

Acquiring ethical and virtuous habits does not begin when graduates sign their first contract to work as occupational therapy practitioners. Habits need to be established early in the professional education process and maintained through repetition in a supportive environment. One predictor of future unethical practice is unethical behaviors in the academic setting (Aaron, Webb, & Simmons, 2013; Lovett-Hooper, Komarraju, Weston, & Dollinger, 2007; Papadakis et al., 2005), which underscores the importance of making every effort to ensure students learn ethical behaviors through the explicit and implicit curricula.

The ***explicit curriculum*** describes how a program is designed and implemented and focuses on what is taught and is approved by external bodies and publicly shared with stakeholders. However, programs also have an ***implicit curriculum*** that focuses on how to teach the core knowledge (Crigger & Godfrey, 2014; Gallagher & Tschudin, 2010; Goulet & Owen-Smith, 2005; Hooper, 2008; Shepard & Jensen, 1990).

The implicit curriculum "encompasses the desired ways of being that are communicated through the culture of the program, its customs, its rituals, and its patterns of relating" (Hooper, 2008, p. 229). The implicit curriculum may be intentional or unintentional, visible or invisible, and it may have the greatest impact on the learning of ethical reasoning (Crigger & Godfrey, 2014; Shepard & Jensen, 1990).

This chapter explores how faculty and administrator behavior affects the implicit curriculum and the working environment in higher education. Student behavior, and how it affects students' professional formation and ability to become ethical practitioners, is also discussed. The *Occupational Therapy Code of Ethics (2015)* (hereinafter referred to as the "Code;" American Occupational Therapy Association [AOTA], 2015) is applied through case studies and vignettes featuring the behavior of students, faculty, and administrators in higher education. The Code contains Principles and Related Standards of Conduct (RSCs).

Ethical Problem Behaviors of Students

Cheating

One of the most basic ethical decisions confronting college students is whether "to cheat or not to cheat on their academic work" (McCabe, Treviño, & Butterfield, 2001, p. 220). ***Cheating*** is engaging in deceptive practices regarding one's academic work or the work of another student or actions taken to try to gain an unfair advantage. The data are not encouraging; cheating, also referred to as *academic dishonesty,* is prevalent in college, and some forms of cheating, such as unpermitted collaboration, have increased dramatically in the past 30 years (Krueger, 2014; McCabe et al., 2001).

Personal and contextual factors contribute to academic dishonesty or cheating (McCabe et al., 2001). Examples of personal factors include pressure from family, society, and self; inadequate preparation; lack of understanding of what constitutes academic dishonesty; and values and beliefs. Contextual factors include the climate in the institution, program, and classroom and shared attitudes in peer relationships (McCabe et al., 2001).

It would be comforting to think that the incidence of cheating among upper-level students in the health professions is lower than that among the total college population. In describing nursing programs, however, Fontana (2009) noted that "this does not appear to be the case. Not only are violations increasing, but methods of cheating are also becoming increasingly sophisticated" (p. 181). McCabe (2009) reached the same conclusion after analyzing surveys from 2,100 nursing students from 12 nursing schools and approximately 21,000 students majoring in other disciplines: "Approximately half of the graduate nursing students, in both the longitudinal survey and the nursing survey, self-reported one or more classroom cheating behaviors" (p. 622).

The rate of academic dishonesty does not appear to be decreasing; a recently published literature review of academic dishonesty in schools of nursing reported similar results (Klocko, 2014). Furthermore, the anonymity of online learning environments may pose unique challenges to academic integrity (Chertok, Barnes, & Gilleland, 2014). Student cheating is specifically addressed in Principle 4, Justice, RSC P: "Refrain from . . . unauthorized access to educational content or exams (including . . . sharing test questions, unauthorized use of or access to content or codes" (AOTA, 2015, p. 6).

Acts of omission can result in unethical behavior, just as acts of commission as illustrated in Vignette 18.1 in which a student is academically dishonest.

Plagiarism

Plagiarism continues to be problematic on campuses and "is the use of published or unpublished work or specific ideas of another person without giving proper credit to that person. It also includes submitting, as one's own work, materials that have been prepared by another person" (Gaberson, 1997, p. 14). A contributing factor is that not all students understand the breadth of what plagiarism involves (Kiehl, 2006; Kolanko et al., 2006; Savin-Baden, 2005). However, students must understand that

Vignette 18.1. Looking the Other Way

Dr. Robinson has been teaching at a large state university for 12 years. During that time, her class sizes have increased, and students seem less prepared and less mature than when she started. She is knowledgeable in her area of occupational therapy and, for the most part, is a good teacher. However, Dr. Robinson has grown tired of dealing with what she considers rude behavior on the part of students. Confronting students about their behavior often led to counter-accusations, paperwork, and meetings that took time away from her other work.

Students take their examinations on laptop computers issued by the program, using testing software. They are not allowed to have any other materials with them during exams. During a recent kinesiology exam, a student, **Mia,** approached Dr. Robinson and said that she had observed another student, **Sarah,** looking at answers she had written in several places on her clothing and body. Dr. Robinson stood and walked around the room, occasionally looking in Sarah's direction. She saw Sarah push up her sleeves and then pull them down but was not close enough to see writing. Dr. Robinson did not want to deal with the hassle that would ensue if Sarah was caught cheating. After the exam, the students left the room, and Dr. Robinson headed back to her office. She knew she should have asked to see Sarah's forearms, but she really did not want to get involved.

As Lovett-Hooper et al. (2007) noted, "Teachers who are reluctant to take measures to address academic dishonesty in the classroom may be persuaded to do so when they realize that this behavior is likely to continue" (p. 332). If faculty does not model and take positive actions to promote academic integrity, it is more likely that students will exhibit incivility and misconduct (Clark & Springer, 2007; Hutton, 2006). Dr. Robinson's decision to look the other way could be seen as an act of implicit collusion. Ethical issues presented in this vignette are identified (see Table 18.1).

Dr. Robinson's actions were a violation of the Code in her role as educator, just as not reporting unethical practice in a hospital would be a violation for a direct service provider. Frequently, ethical violations occur, not because occupational therapy practitioners fail to recognize an ethical problem, but because they choose not to take action. If students observe this type of behavior in the classroom, they may be less likely to demonstrate the moral courage necessary to address ethical issues in practice.

Table 18.1. Identification of Ethical Issues in Vignette 18.1

Ethical Issue	*AOTA Code of Ethics (2015)*
Allowing cheating to occur	Principle 2, Nonmaleficence, RSC 2A: "Avoid inflicting harm" (p. 3).
	Principle 4, Justice, RSC 4K: "Report . . . any acts in . . . education . . . that are unethical" (p. 5).
	Principle 5, Veracity, RSC 5G: "Be honest . . . in gathering and reporting fact-based information" about "student performance" (p. 6).

Note. AOTA = American Occupational Therapy Association; RSC = Related Standard of Conduct.

plagiarism constitutes theft of ideas and goes beyond forgetting to put quotation marks on a passage. Plagiarism "involves the taking of another's ideas, thoughts, and concepts from any source" (Kornblau & Ashe, 2015, p. 229). Sources can include workshops, videos, and the Internet, as well as traditional printed material. Plagiarism also includes omitting quotation marks (even if the source is cited), citing the source inaccurately, or citing the incorrect source altogether.

Almost every college or university has a writing center, and most occupational therapy programs are in divisions or schools that offer advice to students (and faculty) on how to prevent plagiarism. In addition, a plethora of Internet sites provides excellent guidance in this area. Many educational programs also provide students with assistance for poor time management, which can contribute to a temptation to plagiarize or otherwise cheat. In the midst of all these readily accessible resources, no one studying occupational therapy should engage in theft of another's ideas, intentionally or unintentionally. However, faculty needs to ensure that students know about the resources that are available and include these resources in course syllabi and on course sites supported by instructional technology.

Generational Issues

Faculty should make every effort to consider the characteristics of current students. Many current students are from the Millennial Generation, or Generation Y. This cohort of students was born between 1980 and the early 1990s and many are the children of Baby Boomers. Millennials, as a group, grew up in a busy world with a lot of structure (Twenge, 2009). Twenge discussed the impact of what she called "Generation Me" on medical education. She noted that the generational changes that are likely to have the greatest impact on medical education include "higher expectations, higher levels of narcissism and entitlement, increases in anxiety and mental problems, and a decline in the desire to read long texts" (p. 400).

Arhin (2009) examined the Generation Y perspective on academic dishonesty among nursing students. As they grew up, Generation Y students were taught to be resourceful, and they value social networks (Arhin, 2009). From their perspective, collaboration may be considered ordinary or morally acceptable in any situation, including one in which individual work is required. The classroom culture must actively identify and encourage academic integrity. According to Hutton (2006), faculty should recognize the importance of social networks and become a part of these networks by building relationships with students: "Creating and strengthening vertical connections between students and instructor is critical for maintaining the instructor's power base" (p. 175).

Generation Z (or "net gen") students are just now entering (or approaching the age of entry) into occupational therapy education programs. They are the cohort born in the early 1990s, extending to the late 2010s (Smith-Trudeau, 2016; Turner, 2015). Because they have not experienced life before the Internet, they are the first generation to be digital natives (Turner, 2015). Other global characteristics of this cohort are that they are diverse, came of age during difficult financial times, and were reared during a time of war (the oldest were age 7 or 8 years on September 11, 2001).

From the standpoint of professional education, these students' communication with each other and educators may be influenced by a preference for talking online rather than in real life (Turner, 2015). Communicating online reduces practice in reading social cues and the social negotiation involved in face-to-face communication. Online resources and social networking are thought to contribute to continuous partial attention or absent presence, meaning that the person may be physically present but his or her social attention and communication focus is elsewhere (Turner, 2015).

Teaching Generation Z students will require occupational therapy educators to increase their awareness of this generation's frame of reference to build relationships that foster the learning of ethical reasoning. According to Turner (2015),

> The explosion of technology is neither good nor bad; it is simply reality. When adults focus on the strengths of technology while also emphasizing continuing the traditions of personal connection, the results can only enhance the social interest for all. (p. 111)

Student Work

Occupational therapy students are commonly divided into small groups to work together on assignments. At other times, however, individual work is assigned to allow faculty members to evaluate each student's competence in the subject matter. Sometimes the lines between collaboration, collusion, cheating, and plagiarism can be blurry (Savin-Baden, 2005). According to Savin-Baden (2005), ***collaboration*** is "working together in some form of intellectual activity," whereas ***collusion*** is "more usually associated with copying work from a fellow student or the passing off of work done jointly as your own," and cheating is "trying to gain an unfair advantage or breaking a regulation" (p. 12). A more subtle form of collusion occurs when one student does not do his or her share of the work on a group project. Appropriate collaboration occurs when students work together to achieve learning outcomes and follow the instructions provided for the assignment.

Faculty needs to make sure that expectations for assignments are clear and that students understand the differences among collaboration, collusion, and plagiarism. Savin-Baden (2005) suggested asking groups of students to look at assignments, exams, and other assessments of their performance at the beginning of a course and to find all the ways in which they could plagiarize or collude. Then students could "be encouraged to contract with each other to collaborate rather than collude so that they all become stakeholders in both the agreement and the assessment" (p. 15).

Chertok and colleagues (2014) emphasized the importance of deliberately teaching health science students about academic integrity. They created the Survey of Online Knowledge and Attitudes (SOLKA) to measure outcomes of an online tutorial about academic integrity and plagiarism in an intervention group of 194 students (the control group contained 161 students). Although the SOLKA scores of both groups improved over the course of a semester, the intervention group's improvement was significantly higher than the control group. The authors "suggest that education is crucial in increasing students' knowledge of academic integrity which may lead to improving their attitudes and reducing their engagement in academic dishonesty" (p. 1329) and that "institutional policy and academic integrity statements should be communicated consistently and persistently to students throughout their programs of study" (p. 1329).

Case Study 18.1 illustrates the application of ethical reasoning to a case involving students working collaboratively in a group in a research course.

Case Study 18.1. Unequal Work in Student Groups

A professional doctorate program requires students to plan and implement a research project in small groups. The project is spread out over 3 semesters and, in addition to the instructor of record, each group has a faculty mentor. **Emma, Chloe,** and **Robert** are a research group comparing 2 handwriting programs in a first-grade classroom. Chloe and Robert are very interested in learning about the research process, are high achievers, and want to submit the finished manuscript for possible publication. Emma is more interested in the courses that have direct application to practice and is involved in several student organizations and outside activities. All assignments are turned in as a group. Even though students have bachelor's degrees before entering the program, they receive instruction on best practices when doing group projects.

During the first research course, Emma notices that Chloe and Robert are much more gung ho than she is and that if she does not have her part done they will likely assist her. This causes some strife within the group, but Chloe and Robert are more interested in a quality product than in arguing with Emma. During the second course, however, Robert decides the unequal work is a problem that needs to be addressed. After failing to resolve the problem of Emma's lack of (or substandard) contributions within the group, he seeks assistance from the instructor of record, **Dr. Wood.** Dr. Wood is sympathetic but does not want to spend time being a referee. Her suggestion is to leave Emma's name off the manuscript when it is submitted for publication. Dr. Wood goes one step further by telling Robert that she should be the first author because she is a faculty member. Ethical issues present in this case are identified in Table 18.2 and possible actions in Table 18.3.

Table 18.2. Identifying Ethical Issues in Case Study 18.1

Ethical Issue	AOTA *Code of Ethics (2015)*
Putting Emma's name on work that she did not do is a form of deception.	Principle 5, Veracity, RSC B: "Refrain from using . . . communication" that is deceptive, false, or misleading (p. 6).
Emma's actions are a form of exploitation of the other members of the group.	Principle 2, Nonmaleficence, RSC I: "Avoid exploiting any relationship" (p. 4).
Authorship should be in order of work contributed; if all persons contributed equally, alphabetical order is acceptable. A faculty member who advises the group but does not contribute to the research should not be first author, and doing so harms the students who are in a subordinate position.	Principle 6, Fidelity, RSC D: Avoid actions based on one's position that could lead to "real or perceived conflict of interest" (p. 7)

Note. AOTA = American Occupational Therapy Association; RSC = Related Standard of Conduct.

(Continued)

Case Study 18.1. Unequal Work in Student Groups *(Cont.)*

Table 18.3. Decision Table for Case Study 18.1

Possible Actions	Positive Outcomes	Negative Consequences
Take no action.	The path of least resistance may prevent escalating conflict with Emma and Dr. Wood.	Exploitation of Robert and Chloe continues by Emma (failing to do her fair share) and by Dr. Wood (claiming an authorship position that does not reflect her contribution). Emma graduates without meeting minimal competencies for research and its application to practice.
Robert and Chloe talk to the chair of the department. (Assume the chair resolves the situation in a fair and professional manner.)	Workload is more fairly distributed among the students. The ethical way to resolve a conflict of this type is modeled for the students and faculty. Robert and Chloe gain experience in moral courage (we become brave by doing brave acts) by reporting an unethical situation.	Dr. Wood may become angry and deny that she made the authorship request and then judge Robert's and Chloe's work harshly. Emma may be disciplined, resulting in negative social consequences to Robert and Chloe for being snitches.
Robert and Chloe complain about Emma to their classmates.	Complaining may relieve some of the internal frustration Robert and Chloe are feeling. Peer pressure might make Emma carry her share of the workload.	Robert and Chloe violate Principle 6, Fidelity, RSC 6J, of the Code by not trying to resolve interpersonal conflicts.

Note. RSC = Related Standard of Conduct.

Ethical Problem Behaviors of Faculty and Administrators

Faculty, administrators, and staff are powerful role models for students; therefore, their behavior can greatly affect students' academic integrity (Couch & Dodd, 2005; DiBartolo & Walsh, 2010; Malaski & Tarvydas, 2002; Tippitt et al., 2009). In addition to role-modeling ethical behavior, faculty members must act when they witness academic misconduct by students. McCabe and colleagues (2001) reported that faculty members often overlook student transgressions because they "do not want to become involved in what they perceive as the bureaucratic procedures designed to adjudicate allegations of academic dishonesty on their campus" (p. 220).

Faculty Incivility and Bullying

An issue with ethical implications that is receiving increased scrutiny in higher education is incivility and bullying. "Although much research has been done on workplace aggression and bullying over the past two decades, academics have paid relatively little attention to bullying in their own institutions" (Keashly & Neuman, 2010, p. 48). ***Faculty incivility*** describes rude, discourteous, or disruptive behaviors that often result in psychological or physiological distress for target faculty (Clark, Olender, Kenski, & Cardoni, 2013; Von Bergen, Zavaletta, & Soper, 2006).

In contrast, ***workplace or social bullying*** is defined as persistent and demeaning words or actions that occur over time and damage the physical or emotional health of the targeted faculty member (Goldberg, Beitz, Wieland, & Levine, 2013; Twale & De Luca, 2008). It is defined by its effect on the recipient rather than the intent of the bully (Dentith, Wright, & Coryell, 2015; Goldberg et al., 2013; Keashly & Neuman, 2010).

Bullying in academia includes "intimidation, persistent criticism, inaccurate accusations, ignoring or exclusion, public humiliation, malicious rumor, setting one up to fail, and work overload" (Dentith et al., 2015, p. 28). Other behaviors may include ignoring positive contributions while highlighting reported negative outcomes; not correcting false information; discounting another's accomplishments; eye rolling, glaring, or whispering when a targeted faculty member speaks; giving the silent treatment; or failing to give needed information or feedback (Cassell, 2011; Fogg, 2008; Twale & De Luca, 2008).

Bullying has a negative physical or psychological effect on the recipient (i.e., it causes harm). "Research has found evidence that bullying leads to emotional issues, health disorders, extreme stress, and feelings of worthlessness and shame" (Dentith et al., 2015, p. 29). Bullying by faculty and administrators affects all stakeholders in higher education and is a serious problem (Clark & Springer, 2007; Clark et al., 2013; Dentith et al., 2015; Keashly & Neuman, 2010; Kolanko et al., 2006; Twale & De Luca, 2008).

Although some might assume that people with advanced degrees in academic settings might be less likely than other professionals to engaging in bullying, it is actually more frequent in academia than in other corporate workplaces (Hollis, 2012; Keashly & Neuman, 2010). Hollis found that close to 62% of respondents reported "that they had been bullied or witnessed bullying in their higher education positions in the last 18 months" (p. 36) and that this frequency is about 60% higher than has been reported among corporate employees. Clark et al. (2013) found that 68% of a sample of 588 nursing faculty found faculty-to-faculty incivility to be a moderate or serious problem.

In fact, some of the very characteristics of academia may make it a breeding ground for bullies (Olwell & Gunsalus, 2006; Twale & DeLuca, 2008).

Vignette 18.2. Don't Outshine Me

Dr. Scott has been teaching in an occupational therapy program for about 4 years. She is creative, energetic, and popular among the students. Students' level of achievement is also high in the practice area in which she teaches. She makes extensive use of technology and sometimes records lectures that students view online before coming to class so that more class time can be devoted to discussion. Dr. Scott submitted a research proposal to the university's institutional review board on the effectiveness of CIMT in collaboration with a local occupational therapy practitioner.

Dr. Bergen has been teaching in the program for a number of years and submitted an article on CIMT to a journal several years ago, but it was not accepted. Dr. Bergen and another faculty member began griping to each other about Dr. Scott and her popularity. Dr. Bergen began to complain to others, first in the halls and other common areas, and then in the curriculum committee. Her complaints included that Dr. Scott took unfair advantage of her work on CIMT, uses unconventional and questionable teaching methods, and is damaging the collegiality of the department with her ambitious and selfish personality. Dr. Bergen is a member of the school's promotion and tenure committee and has let it be known that she would have a problem supporting Dr. Scott for promotion and tenure when the time comes. The chair of the department met with Dr. Bergen and told her to stop badmouthing her colleague. However, Dr. Bergen's behavior only escalated. The chair is now on a leave of absence, and the climate in the department is becoming toxic. Ethical issues present in this vignette are identified in Table 18.4.

Table 18.4. Identification of Ethical Issues in Vignette 18.2

Ethical Issue	*AOTA Code of Ethics (2015)*
This pattern of behavior by Dr. Bergen exemplifies bullying.	Principle 2, Nonmaleficence, RSC 2A: "Avoid inflicting harm" on others (p. 3).
	Principle 2, Nonmaleficence, RSC D: "Avoid" behavior "that may . . . compromise the ability to competently provide . . . education" (p. 3).
	Principle 5, Veracity, RSC 5B: "Refrain from . . . any form of communication that contains false, . . . deceptive, . . . or unfair statements or claims" (p. 6).
	Principle 6, Fidelity, RSC 6F: "Refrain from verbal . . . or emotional harassment of peers or colleagues" (p. 7).
	Principle 6, Fidelity, RSC 6G: "Refrain from communication that is derogatory . . . or disrespectful and that unduly discourages others from participating in professional dialogue" (p. 7).

Note. AOTA = American Occupational Therapy Association; CIMT = constraint-induced movement therapy; RSC = Related Standard of Conduct.

These characteristics include the decentralized structure of many universities, long-term employment (i.e., tenure), manipulation of concepts of academic freedom, big egos, and tolerance of behaviors not accepted elsewhere (Fogg, 2008; Olwell & Gunsalus, 2006; Twale & DeLuca, 2008). As a result of decentralized structure, the majority of management is left to the department chairpersons, who often lack management training and may not know how to respond effectively to bullying (Fogg, 2008). The promotion and tenure processes add unique stresses to those working in academia and may contribute to bullying, as well as to the reluctance to report bullying for fear of retaliation (Clark et al., 2013; Hollis, 2012; Twale & DeLuca, 2008). Although not all competition is destructive, when a faculty member uses destructive means to win a competitive advantage, it is considered bullying.

Who is most likely to be the target of bullying in higher education? Faculty members who are younger, women, adjunct or not yet tenured, and those who excel in their work (Cleary, Walter, Horsfall, & Jackson, 2013; Dentith et al., 2015; Twale & DeLuca, 2008). "According to the literature, outspoken women in particular are commonly targeted as they are often prepared to speak up about unjust matters—their competence and success is perceived to be a threat by those engaging in the bullying behaviors" (Cleary et al., 2013, p. 266).

The harm caused by bullying can extend beyond the recipient of bullying to include others who witness the bullying and the overall functioning of the department (Dentith et al., 2015; Luparell, 2008). Coworkers who witness bullying may also experience stress and guilt because they do not have the courage to try to stop it. It is not surprising that low productivity and higher-than-average turnover can be the result of bullying in an academic setting (Dentith et al., 2015; Keashly & Neuman, 2010; Twale & DeLuca, 2008). Vignette 18.2 illustrates social bullying of a faculty member.

Environmental Pressure

Pressures surrounding costs in the academic environment can foster unethical behavior. Ethical distress for faculty members can occur when students are treated as customers and the administration acts to keep customers satisfied at the expense of faculty integrity, as illustrated in Vignette 18.3. Use of adjunct faculty can help address the shortage of

Vignette 18.3. Customer Is Always Right

Dentith and colleagues (2015) described a story of a student (called **Trevor** in this vignette) who was unhappy with his grade and complained to the dean that the faculty member who assigned the grade (called **Kathy**) was unprepared for classes and incompetent. The dean notified the chair of the department, who notified Kathy that she was a problem. Kathy produced evidence to dispute the student's accusations and was supported by one senior member of the faculty, but neither the chair nor the dean was willing to listen. The dean wanted it handled by the chair, and the chair was currying favor with the dean and did not want to rock the boat. In addition, as rumors of the incident spread, several other faculty members started making snide comments and providing Kathy with unsolicited helpful advice about how to improve her course. Borrowing from a similar case described by Twale and De Luca (2008), other faculty members supported Trevor, who "they said was a very bright and a good student" (p. 12). Kathy was unable to dispute the rumor of her incompetence because no one was willing to openly talk about it. Ethical issues present in this vignette are identified in Table 18.5.

Table 18.5. Identification of Ethical Issues in Vignette 18.3

Ethical Issue	*AOTA Code of Ethics (2015)*
The dean, chair, and other faculty members made assumptions without ensuring the accuracy of the information.	Principle 2, Nonmaleficence, RSC 2A: "Avoid inflicting harm" (p. 3).
	Principle 5, Veracity, RSC 5B: "Refrain from communication . . . that is false . . . deceptive, misleading" (p. 6).
Derogatory information was communicated, and professional dialogue was discouraged.	Principle 6, Fidelity, RSC 6G: "Refrain from communication that is derogatory . . . or disrespectful and that unduly discourages others from participating in professional dialogue" (p. 7).

Note. AOTA = American Occupational Therapy Association; RSC = Related Standard of Conduct.

Vignette 18.4. Adjunct Faculty

Excellent University is a large private university. Over the past 10 years, the university has shifted from one of faculty governance to a more corporate culture. Universities are competing for increasingly scarce financial resources. One cost-cutting strategy has been to increase the number of part-time adjunct faculty in proportion to full-time tenure-track faculty.

The occupational therapy department has 2 vacant tenure-track faculty positions. The vice president for health sciences, **Dr. Kilgore,** directs the department to leave those positions vacant and to use existing faculty and hire adjunct (i.e., part-time) faculty to teach the necessary courses. He even offers to pay the existing faculty a bonus for each course they teach above the normal courseload. Several faculty members, as well as alumni, of the program raise concerns about how this will affect student learning in both the short term and the long term. Dr. Kilgore addresses the concerns at a faculty meeting, stating that adjunct faculty brings fresh perspectives and real-world experience to the students. He reminds faculty that the strong demand for admission to the occupational therapy program provides them with job security and that he is paying extra to those who take on a heavier load. Ethical issues present in this vignette are identified in Table 18.6.

Table 18.6. Identifying Ethical Issues in Vignette 18.4

Ethical Issue	*AOTA Code of Ethics (2015)*
Continuity of curriculum and impact on student learning. Typically, adjunct faculty is not as knowledgeable about the implicit and explicit curriculum as full-time faculty. This may compromise its ability to provide necessary vertical and horizontal integration of content across courses.	Principle 2, Nonmaleficence, RSC 2D: "Avoid any undue influences that may . . . compromise the ability to . . . provide occupational therapy education" (p. 3).
Although some faculty will get a modest financial bonus for teaching extra courses, the workload is increased not only by courses but also by the need to mentor new adjunct faculty who may also be new to academia. Faculty workload is also increased by having fewer faculty to hold positions on school and department committees. There is an increased risk of faculty burnout.	Principle 1, Beneficence: "Examples of beneficence include protecting and defending the rights of others, preventing harm from occurring to others, removing conditions that will cause harm to others" (Beauchamp & Childress, 2013, as cited in AOTA, 2015, p. 2). Principle 2, Nonmaleficence, RSC 2D: "Avoid any undue influences that may . . . compromise the ability to . . . provide occupational therapy education" (p. 3).
Adjunct faculty is more vulnerable than tenure-track faculty, making it less likely to complain and easier to manipulate.	Principle 2, Nonmaleficence, RSC 2I: "Avoid exploiting any relationship established as an occupational therapy . . . educator . . . to further one's own . . . interests" (p. 4).
Scholarship and research productivity for the department will likely decrease, jeopardizing faculty's promotion and tenure and its ability to contribute to the occupational therapy body of knowledge.	Principle 2, Nonmaleficence, RSC 2D: "Avoid any undue influences that may . . . compromise the ability to . . . provide occupational therapy education" (p. 3).

Note. AOTA = American Occupational Therapy Association; RSC = Related Standard of Conduct.

faculty or bring specialized expertise. However, if multiple adjunct faculty are used as a less expensive alternative to hiring a full-time, tenure-track faculty member, harm may result to the curriculum and the students as illustrated in Vignette 18.4.

Modeling Unethical Behavior

Faculty sometimes makes copies (paper or digital) of book chapters or other copyrighted products for student learning. However well intended this may be, it can violate copyright law (and is also plagiarism, if not attributed). ***Fair use*** allows distribution of some copied materials but with restrictions. Requesting permission takes time and faculty may be tempted to copy anyway because others do it without consequences (Metcalfe, Diaz, & Wagoner, 2003).

It is unethical for faculty members to make unauthorized copies, and it sends the wrong message to students. How can students be expected to refrain from plagiarism or copyright infringement if faculty models it when teaching, either directly or indirectly, by asking students to use material that has violated copyright protection? As Reed (2011) puts it, "We need to be more diligent about honoring the work of colleagues in our field. And if we choose to remain silent in the face of blatant copyright violations among our peers, we have to recognize our tacit complicity in the act" (p. 48). When using material without the permission of the author and/or publisher, faculty is infringing on the rights of publishers and authors alike.

Faculty needs to be familiar with laws for fair use and copyright and know how to access this information. University libraries frequently have resources to assist faculty to avoid violating copyright laws. A good online resource is the Copyright and Fair Use website of Stanford University Libraries (http://fairuse.standford.edu).

Summary

Occupational therapy educators have a special responsibility and opportunity to shape the ethical behavior of future occupational therapy practitioners. In addition to teaching about codes of conduct, honor, ethics, and other didactic content, faculty must find ways to promote academic integrity and ethical and civil behavior in the classroom. This content is especially important given the nature of the profession and the potential consequences of unethical practice for future clients.

Although dealing with student misconduct can be bothersome and time consuming, educators should keep in mind that both action and inaction can affect client safety in the future (Danielson, Simon, & Pavlick, 2006; Fontana, 2009; Malaski & Tarvydas, 2002) and that unethical conduct among students must be directly addressed at every opportunity.

Faculty attitudes, behaviors, and actions include how faculty members relate to each other, in addition to how they relate to students. Social and workplace bullying in higher education occurs and has negative and harmful consequences. "There is little peace in academia: warfare is common and no less deadly because it is polite" (Baldridge, 1971, p. 107). The harmful consequences can affect the target, the bully, peers, students, departments, and educational institutions (Dentith et al., 2015; Goldberg et al., 2013; Hollis, 2012; Keashly & Neuman, 2010; Twale & De Luca, 2008). The Code applies to all occupational therapy personnel, including practitioners, researchers, administrators, educators, and students. Mistreatment of colleagues is harmful and unethical in both clinical and academic settings. In academic settings, the harm caused by one or two individuals can directly or indirectly affect the preparation of untold future practitioners.

Reflective Questions

1. Do you intentionally promote integrity and civility with your students and colleagues? If yes, describe your methods. If no, why not?
2. Compare and contrast acts of commission and acts of omission when you notice an ethical issue in higher education. How often do you take action when you notice an ethical issue, and how often do you not take action? How might this affect the quality of services provided by future occupational therapists?
3. Reflect on instances in which you have witnessed incivility or bullying of another faculty member. How did witnessing this behavior affect your job satisfaction or morale?

References

Aaron, L., Webb, D. G., & Simmons, P. (2013). The influence of academic dishonesty on professionalism. *Radiologic Science and Education, 18,* 25–30.

American Occupational Therapy Association. (2015). Occupational therapy code of ethics 2015. *American Journal of Occupational Therapy, 69*(Suppl. 3), 6913410030. https://doi.org/10.5014/ajot.2015.696S03

Arhin, A. O. (2009). A pilot study of nursing students' perceptions of academic dishonesty: A Generation Y perspective. *Association of Black Nursing Faculty in Higher Education Journal, 20,* 17–21.

Baldridge, J. V. (1971). *Power and conflict in the university: Research in the sociology of complex organizations.* Hoboken, NJ: Wiley.

Cassell, M. A. (2011). Bullying in academe: Prevalent, significant, and incessant. *Contemporary Issues in Education Research, 4,* 33–44. https://doi.org/10.19030/cier.v4i5.4236

Chertok, I. R. A., Barnes, E. R., & Gilleland, D. (2014). Academic integrity in the online learning environment for health sciences students. *Nurse Education Today, 34,* 1324–1329. https://doi.org/10.1016/j.nedt.2013.06.002

Clark, C. M., Olender, L., Kenski, D., & Cardoni, C. (2013). Exploring and addressing faculty-to-faculty incivility: A national perspective and literature review. *Journal of Nursing Education, 52,* 211–218. https://doi.org/10.3928/01484834-20130319-01

Clark, C. M., & Springer, P. J. (2007). Incivility in nursing education: A descriptive study of definitions and prevalence. *Journal of Nursing Education, 46,* 7–14.

Cleary, M., Walter, G., Horsfall, J., & Jackson, D. (2013). Promoting integrity in the workplace: A priority for all academic health professionals. *Contemporary Nurse, 45,* 264–268. https://doi.org/10.5172/conu.2013.45.2.264

Couch, S., & Dodd, S. (2005). Doing the right thing: Ethical issues in higher education. *Journal of Family and Consumer Sciences, 97,* 20–27.

Crigger, N., & Godfrey, N. (2014). From the inside out: A new approach to teaching professional identity formation and professional ethics. *Journal of Professional Nursing, 30,* 376–382. https://doi.org/10.1016/j.profnurs.2014.03.004

Danielson, R. D., Simon, A. F., & Pavlick, R. (2006). The culture of cheating: From the classroom to the exam room. *Journal of Physician Assistant Education, 17,* 23–29.

Dentith, A. M., Wright, R. R., & Coryell, J. (2015). Those mean girls and their friends: Bullying and mob rule in the academy. *Adult Learning, 26,* 28–34. https://doi.org/10.1177/1045159514558409

DiBartolo, M. C., & Walsh, C. M. (2010). Desperate times call for desperate measures: Where are we in addressing academic dishonesty? *Journal of Nursing Education, 49,* 543–544. https://doi.org/10.3928/01484834-20100921-01

Fogg, P. (2008, Sept. 12). Academic bullies. *Chronicle of Higher Education, 55,* B10.

Fontana, J. S. (2009). Nursing faculty experiences of students' academic dishonesty. *Journal of Nursing Education, 48,* 181–185. http://dx.doi.org/10.3928/01484834-20090401-05

Gaberson, K. B. (1997). Academic dishonesty among nursing students. *Nursing Forum, 32,* 14–20. https://doi.org/10.1111/j.1744-6198.1997.tb00205.x

Gallagher, A., & Tschudin, V. (2010). Educating for ethical leadership. *Nurse Education Today, 30,* 224–227.

Goldberg, E., Beitz, J., Wieland, D., & Levine, C. (2013). Social bullying in nursing academia. *Nurse Educator, 38,* 191–197. https://doi.org/10.1097/NNE.0b013e3182a0e5a0

Goulet, C., & Owen-Smith, P. (2005). Cognitive–affective learning in physical therapy education: From implicit to explicit. *Journal of Physical Therapy Education, 19,* 67–72.

Hollis, L. P. (2012). *Bully in the ivory tower: How aggression and incivility erode American higher education.* Wilmington, DE: Patricia Berkly.

Hooper, B. (2008). Stories we teach by: Intersections among faculty biography, student formation, and instructional processes. *American Journal of Occupational Therapy, 62,* 228–241. https://doi.org/10.5014/ajot.62.2.228

Hutton, P. A. (2006). Understanding student cheating and what educators can do about it. *College Teaching, 54,* 171–176. https://doi.org/10.3200/CTCH.54.1.171-176

Keashly, L., & Neuman, J. H. (2010). Faculty experiences with bullying in higher education: Causes, consequences, and management. *Administrative Theory and Praxis, 32,* 48–70. https://doi.org/10.2753/ATP1084-1806320103

Kiehl, E. M. (2006). Using an ethical decision-making model to determine consequences for student plagiarism. *Journal of Nursing Education, 45,* 199–203.

Klocko, M. N. (2014). Academic dishonesty in schools of nursing: A literature review. *Journal of Nursing Education, 53,* 121–125. https://doi.org/10.3928/01484834-20140205-01

Kolanko, K. M., Clark, C., Heinrich, K. T., Olive, D., Serembus, J. F., & Sifford, K. S. (2006). Academic dishonesty, bullying, incivility, and violence: Difficult challenges facing nurse educators. *Nursing Education Perspectives, 27,* 34–42.

Kornblau, B. L., & Ashe, A. M. (2015). Avoiding plagiarism. In D. Y. Slater (Ed.), *Reference guide to the occupational therapy code of ethics* (2015 ed., pp. 229–234) Bethesda, MD: AOTA Press.

Krueger, L. (2014). Academic dishonesty among nursing students. *Journal of Nursing Education, 53,* 77–87. https://doi.org/10.3928/01484834-20140122-06

Lovett-Hooper, G., Komarraju, M., Weston, R., & Dollinger, S. J. (2007). Is plagiarism a forerunner of other deviance? Imagined futures of academically dishonest students. *Ethics and Behavior, 17,* 323–336. https://doi.org/10.1080/10508420701519387

Luparell, S. (2008, April/May). Incivility in nursing education: Let's put an end to it. *National Student Nurses Association Imprint,* pp. 42–46.

Malaski, C., & Tarvydas, V. M. (2002). Teaching ethics and the ethics of teaching: Challenges for rehabilitation counselor educators. *Rehabilitation Education, 16,* 1–13.

McCabe, D. L. (2009). Academic dishonesty in nursing schools: An empirical investigation. *Journal of Nursing Education, 48,* 614–623. https://doi.org/10.3928/01484834-20090716-07

McCabe, D. L., Treviño, L. K., & Butterfield, K. D. (2001). Cheating in academic institutions: A decade of research. *Ethics and Behavior, 11,* 219–232. https://doi.org/10.1207/S15327019EB1103_2

Metcalfe, A., Diaz, V., & Wagoner, R. (2003). Academe, technology, society, and the market: Four frames of reference for copyright and fair use. *Libraries and the Academy, 3,* 191–206. https://doi.org/10.1353/pla.2003.0043

Olwell, R., & Gunsalus, C. K. (2006). Dealing with bullies. *Inside Higher Education.* Retrieved from https://www.insidehighered.com/views/2006/11/30/gunsalus

Papadakis, M. A., Teherani, A., Banach, M. A., Knettler, T. R., Rattner, S. L., Stern, D. T., & Hodgson, C. S. (2005). Disciplinary action by medical boards and prior behavior in medical school. *New England Journal of Medicine, 353,* 2673–2682. https://doi.org/10.1056/NEJMsa052596

Reed, D. K. (2011). Plagiarism isn't just an issue for students. *Journal of Staff Development, 32,* 47–49.

Savin-Baden, M. (2005). Why collaborate when you can cheat? Understanding plagiarism in OT education. *British Journal of Occupational Therapy, 68,* 11–16. https://doi.org/10.1177/030802260506800103

Shepard, K. F., & Jensen, G. M. (1990). Physical therapist curricula for the 1990s: Educating the reflective practitioner. *Physical Therapy, 70,* 556–573.

Smith-Trudeau, P. (2016, January–February–March). Generation Z nurses have arrived. Are you ready? *Vermont Nurse Connection,* pp. 3–4.

Tippitt, M. P., Nell, A., Kline, J. R., Tilghman, J., Chamberlain, B., & Meagher, P. G. (2009). Creating environments that foster academic integrity. *Nursing Education Perspectives, 30,* 239–244.

Turner, A. (2015). Generation Z: Technology and social interest. *Journal of Individual Psychology, 71,* 103–113. https://doi.org/10.1353/jip.2015.0021

Twale, D. J., & DeLuca, B. M. (2008). *Faculty incivility: The rise of the academic bully culture and what to do about it.* San Francisco: Jossey-Bass.

Twenge, J. M. (2009). Generational changes and their impact in the classroom: Teaching generation me. *Medical Education, 43,* 398–405. https://doi.org/10.1111/j.1365-2923.2009.03310.x

Von Bergen, C. W., Zavaletta, J. A., & Soper, B. (2006). Legal remedies for workplace bullying. *Employee Relations Law Journal, 32,* 14–40.

Chapter 19.

ETHICS IN OCCUPATIONAL THERAPY RESEARCH

Elizabeth Larson, PhD, OTR, FAOTA

Learning Objectives

By the end of the chapter, readers will be able to

- Articulate the ethics of producing, critically evaluating, and using research in service of occupational therapy intervention;
- Explain and contrast the influence of the profession's theoretical foundations and current sociocultural forces in driving the profession's research agenda; and
- Describe the hallmarks of ethically conducted research.

Key Terms and Concepts

- ✧ Epistemic culture
- ✧ Epistemology
- ✧ Evidence-based medicine
- ✧ Habitus
- ✧ Impact factor
- ✧ Impact ratings
- ✧ Informed consent
- ✧ Institutional review board
- ✧ Ongoing consent
- ✧ Qualitative methods
- ✧ Randomized controlled trial
- ✧ Research question
- ✧ Written consent

Before beginning to examine the ethics of conducting research, it is important to consider the ethics of using research in everyday occupational therapy practice. There is a strong impetus to use evidence to inform and guide decision making in daily practice, but some have argued that not all interventions with demonstrable research support are congruent with the profession's occupation-focused philosophy (Gustafsson, Molineux, & Bennett, 2014), nor can group data be easily applied to individual cases.

Occupational therapy's holistic perspective and agentic values invite a collaborative teaming with clients that may be counter to using prescriptive pathways of interventions. Thus, it is important to discern which evidence to use and how to use it when serving clients. Key to doing this is evaluating what evidence we have access to or choose to generate as a profession. These choices of the creation and application of evidence are ethically driven. The occupational therapy profession must respond ethically to the political and social forces that direct policy and funding for research while embracing our core professional values.

This chapter begins by unpacking the habitus and epistemic culture of occupational therapy's knowledge generation and is followed by discussing the need to remain focused on occupation and participation. This is followed by a consideration of what is valuable as evidence for practice, which, in turn, influences the research methods used by occupational therapy researchers. To provide a context for ethics in research design and methods, a brief historical review outlines the missteps that led to the development of current standards for ethical research. This is followed by an exploration of ethical considerations and challenges in designing, conducting, and reporting research. Often overlooked but essential issues in the ethical conduct of research are highlighted as well as emerging ethical issues in research using technology-based or web-based data collection.

Research in Occupational Therapy

Research is often viewed in U.S. culture as an objective way of discovering or validating knowledge. The popular belief is that immutable facts are revealed through carefully designed research that is executed and analyzed in precise and systematic ways. Although excellent research displays these hallmarks, designing and conducting high-quality research also requires a series of carefully considered ethical decisions. In addition, social scientists have pointed out that scientific inquiry is not a value-free activity but is shaped by cultural context and, at times, even political pursuits (Albert, Laberge, & Hodges, 2009).

Researchers' choices regarding the framing of questions and method selection are influenced by their current theoretical framework, their disciplinary and scholarly values, their methodological training, and the sociopolitical and historical contexts surrounding research. Scientific practices are formed by the disciplinary ***habitus*** (i.e., way of doing) and ***epistemic culture*** (i.e., valued way of knowing) of the discipline (Becher & Trowler, 2001; Bordieu, 2004). Schools of thought that embrace specific theoretical orientations are often centered in different universities or research centers, each with its own cultural values and historic traditions. Through graduate training, new generations of researchers are enculturated into specific research values, roles, and approaches (Albert et al., 2009).

The health care climate, the needs of occupational therapy consumers, and occupational therapy practitioners' professional values and beliefs shape how occupational therapy research is produced and used within occupational therapy practice. Occupational therapists now enter the profession with graduate degrees in part because of the necessity for therapists to be competent in evaluating and using research evidence for best practice (Accreditation Council for Occupational Therapy Education [ACOTE], 2012). Three core ethical issues affect research in occupational therapy:

1. The centrality of research to professionalism and professional power, reflected in the identification and selection of specific research topics that produce knowledge of value to the profession and the general public (i.e., occupational therapy's epistemic culture).
2. The design and conduct of studies (i.e., disciplinary habitus) in beneficent and principled ways, including in emerging areas of research in which fewer guidelines exist.
3. Publication of this knowledge to inform occupational therapy practice.

Ethical practice in research requires more than simply following a prescribed set of behaviors or professional principles. Often situations arise that include competing interests among research stakeholders (e.g., funders, researchers, and participants) or conflicts in the application of ethical principles. In these circumstances, occupational therapy practitioners and researchers must carefully evaluate their own and others' interests and consider the balance among ethical principles to choose the most ethical response.

Research's Role in Professionalism and Professional Power

Science was the cornerstone of the American Occupational Therapy Association's ([AOTA], 2007)

Centennial Vision for occupational therapy: "We envision that occupational therapy is a powerful, widely recognized, science-driven, and evidence-based profession with a globally connected and diverse workforce meeting society's occupational needs" (p. 613). Generating a substantive knowledge base is viewed as critical to supporting best practice, increasing and broadening occupational therapy's reach to serve all those who can benefit from occupational therapy services, and allowing the profession to flourish within current and future health care climates. AOTA's (2016) *Vision 2025* states, "Occupational therapy maximizes health, well-being, and quality of life for all people, populations, and communities through effective solutions that facilitate participation in everyday living" (para. 1). *Vision 2025* builds on the *Centennial Vision* and advances it by emphasizing the need for effective solutions supported by evidence. The *Occupational Therapy Code of Ethics (2015)* (hereinafter referred to as the "Code") binds therapists not only to provide client-centered evidence-based services but also efficient, cost-effective services (AOTA, 2015b).

Occupation and Participation

Although occupational therapy has long claimed participation in occupation as the foundation of health and well-being, the focus on examining the relationship of health and participation has spread to other health professions across the world. For example, scientists in the fields of epidemiology, psychology, and other social sciences have developed participation measures (e.g., Brown et al., 2004; Van Brakel et al., 2006). How occupational therapy practitioners conduct their scholarship in occupation influences how the profession is viewed and positioned within the larger realms of science and society. Whether occupational therapy practitioners are recognized as the experts in participation and health depends upon how well researchers and clinicians continue to generate relevant and high-quality evidence, promote public awareness of this research, and apply it for effective service delivery.

A recent systematic review of interventions aimed at improving the participation of children with disabilities suggested that occupational therapy is making major inroads in participation research (Adair, Ullenhag, Keen, Grandlund, & Imms, 2015). A combination of tools used or developed by occupational therapists was used in key studies cited in this particular review.

Occupational therapy practitioners hold a common belief in the power of occupation to foster health. In pursuing a core phenomenon, a profession may have competing paradigms that promote different theoretical approaches and research methods (Christiansen, 1981; Kuhn, 1962). Tensions between influences inside and outside the profession, as well as pragmatic considerations, also influence the profession's research agenda. Outside the profession, the agendas set by funders of research and their review panels control the available resources for research and historically have often promoted certain methodologies and research foci that are more likely to get support. In addition, funders of occupational therapy services and legislators are demanding evidence of the efficacy of occupational therapy practice (Bernstein, Collette, & Pederson, 2010).

Levels of Evidence

Leaders of the profession have waged a strong response to calls for data on the efficacy of services. This response has been incorporated into the Code in Related Standard of Conduct (RSC) 1C: "Use, to the extent possible, evaluation, planning, intervention techniques, assessments, and therapeutic equipment that are evidence based, current, and within the recognized scope of occupational therapy practice" (AOTA, 2015b, p. 2). Indeed, demonstrating that occupational therapy services promote improved functioning and well-being is an ethical imperative (Christiansen & Lou, 2001). Likewise, it is important that occupational therapy services do no harm. Christiansen and Lou pointed out that ineffective intervention has psychological, financial, and other costs to clients. These costs may present in the form of reduced opportunities, diminished self-efficacy, and wasted personal and health care resources. AOTA's leaders have forged a plan to promote the development and publication of certain kinds of research to target specific goals. The publication priorities of the *American Journal of Occupational Therapy's* editorial board are aligned with the *Centennial Vision* (Table 19.1).

These priorities emphasize producing the highest levels of evidence (Sackett, Richardson, Rosenberg, & Haynes, 1997; Sackett, Straus, Richardson, Rosenberg, & Haynes, 2000). A pyramid of evidence showing what is considered increasing quality is displayed in Figure 19.1 (Dartmouth Biomedical

Table 19.1. Publication Topics and Goals of the *American Journal of Occupational Therapy*

Publication Topics	Goals
Occupational therapy interventions (clinical trials)	Effectiveness studies or outcome studies, systematic reviews, meta-analyses
Occupational therapy–relevant health services research Occupational therapy–relevant health policy research	Efficiency studies assessing interventions in areas such as patient satisfaction and cost or time efficiency
Relationship of mechanisms (physiological and psychological) and ability to participate, incidence and prevalence of client factors related to participation, and various populations' patterns of occupational engagement, activity participation, and quality of life	Studies linking occupational engagement to participation and health
Occupation-focused or -based assessments	Studies establishing reliability and validity of occupational therapy instruments
Pedagogy relating to occupational therapy education and interprofessional collaborations	

Source. From "Guidelines for Contributors to *AJOT*," by American Occupational Therapy Association, 2015a, *American Journal of Occupational Therapy, 69*(Suppl. 3), 6913430010. Copyright © 2015 by the American Occupational Therapy Association. Adapted with permission.

Laboratories, 2008). The highest levels are critical analyses of compilations of studies. Systematic reviews, evidence syntheses, and critical appraisals of studies are judged the most powerful evidence. The best "unfiltered" evidence (in order of decreasing quality) are the ***randomized controlled trial*** (RCT), the cohort study, and the case–control study. At the bottom of the pyramid is expert opinion. Proponents of evidence-based practice have suggested that, in some instances, the best possible evidence for a particular question may not be an RCT; rather, the research question should always direct the selection of study design (Sackett, Rosenberg, Gray, Haynes, & Richardson, 1996). In addition,

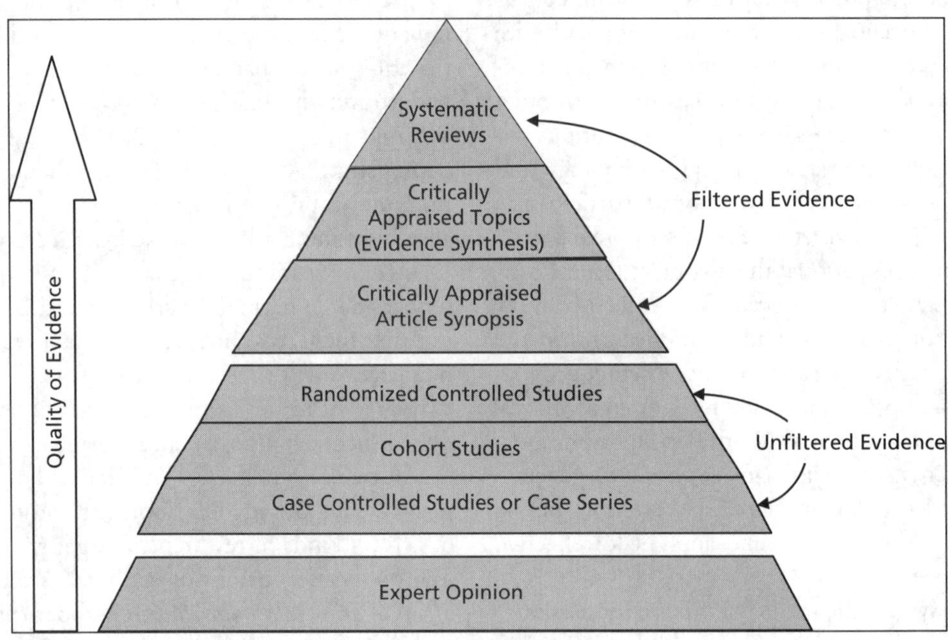

FIGURE 19.1

Quality of evidence in evidence-based medicine.
Source. From EBM Pyramid and EBM Page Generator. Copyright © 2008, Trustees of Dartmouth College and Yale University. All rights reserved. Produced by Jan Glover, David Izzo, Karen Odato, and Lei Wang. Adapted with permission.

they believe that the evidence must be considered in relation to client preferences and integrated with clinical expertise.

Heralded as a significant step forward for the health professions, the ***evidence-based medicine*** (EBM) model is not without critics. Critiques have focused on questions of *epistemology* and application of EBM in practice professions. Cohen, Stavri, and Hersch (2004) suggested a problematic imbalance in focusing on the empirical "purity" of studies (specifically, RCT methodologies) to the detriment of development of a core understanding of mechanisms and processes underlying health. They outlined three major points of concern:

1. Lack of evidence that RCTs and meta-analyses are more reliable than other research methods for answering clinical questions (which would entail research demonstrating better outcomes for clients of practitioners who apply evidence in practice).
2. Limited questions EBM is suited to answer.
3. Lack of integration of EBM with "other, non-statistical, forms of medical information, such as professional experience and patient-specific factors" (p. 39).

Cohen and colleagues (2004) believed that defining evidence in this way limits the questions that may be answered and leaves unanswered many questions essential to a practice profession:

> Questions specific to small patient populations, or those that require subjective evaluation (such as improvement in the quality of life) . . . cannot be studied by the methods that EBM deems "best." Furthermore, since the methods of EBM are epidemiological and statistical, clinically important details may be hidden, overlooked, or simply "averaged out" by the methods of the study. . . . Upshur describes a taxonomy that includes four types of evidence: qualitative–personal, qualitative–general, quantitative–personal, and quantitative–general. . . . Upshur's categorization conceptualizes the essential qualities of evidence as being the context of its use and its means of production, and does not rank one combination as inherently better than another. Of these four categories, EBM only specifically deals with the quantitative–general form of evidence. . . . Perhaps EBM should be renamed "methods of incorporating epidemiologic evidence into clinical practice." (p. 39)

Cohen and colleagues' (2004) insights suggest that, when generating evidence for practice, the means of best answering that question, and the context in which the resulting evidence will be used, all need to be considered in the study's design. In prioritizing RCTs and meta-analyses as research designs for the profession, an emphasis is being placed on developing key evidence to demonstrate the efficacy of occupational therapy services in populations. This first step in generating population-based evidence of the efficacy of an intervention needs to be followed by other types of research that focus on client-centered implementation or cost-effectiveness of that intervention.

Cochrane (2004, cited in Hope, 1997), the grandfather of the EBM movement, recognized that some questions essential to health care practice do not lend themselves to statistical manipulations. His book took a critical view of the efficiency and effectiveness of the British national health care system, noting that some common practices continued despite inefficiency or even possible patient harm. He noted that practitioners both care for and make efforts to cure their clients and that both the process of and the methods for intervention were important to health care services. The diagram in Figure 19.2 illustrates the scope of information important to the client (Circle C) that is not believed to be evidence based (Cochrane, cited in Hope, 1997).

In her Eleanor Clarke Slagle Lecture, Rogers (1983), like Cochrane (2004, cited in Hope, 1997), recognized this integrative interplay in the application of practice knowledge ("cure") and care for our clients as necessary for effective service delivery, which must include consideration of the dynamics of human relationships, an understanding of clients' preferences and capacities, and a process through which therapeutic change may occur. She noted that reflective, individualized practice results in ethical decisions about the approach and course of intervention. In her words, "without science, clinical inquiry is not systematic; without ethics, it is not responsible; without art, it is not convincing" (Rogers, 1983, p. 616).

Epistemology and Ethics

Epistemology is an examination of the origin, nature, methods, and suppositions of knowledge. Garnering and focusing the available resources,

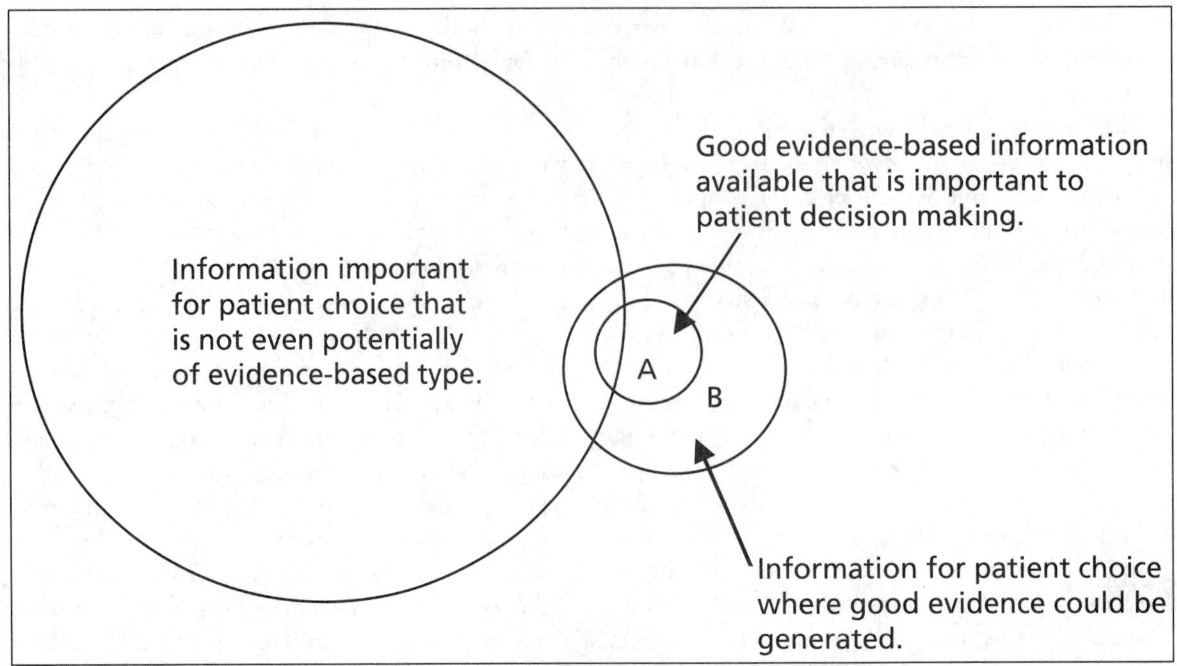

FIGURE 19.2

Availability of evidence-based information important to patient choice.
Source. From "Random Reflections on Health Services" by T. Hope, in *Effectiveness and Efficiency: Random Reflections on Health Services* (p. xxv), and by A. J. Cochrane, 1972, London: Nuffield Provincial Hospitals Trust. (Reprinted in 2004 for Nuffield Trust by the Royal Society of Medicine Press, London.) Adapted with permission.

occupational therapy researchers need to carefully consider what knowledge is needed and useful to professional practice and to society. The following epistemic questions must be addressed:

- What is worth knowing? Specifically, which theories, ideas, or models should be investigated?
- How should this knowledge be generated? What methods and designs (qualitative, quantitative, or mixed methods) should be used?
- How should this knowledge be applied in practice?

These are all ethical questions. The first question addresses the unique niche occupational therapy practitioners inhabit within health care and community-based practice. The decision as to what studies to pursue not only demonstrates what is valued but also shapes the way information is filtered in professional and nonprofessional groups. Occupational therapy practitioners think occupationally about their clients, in terms of doing. Hooper (2006), citing Palmer (1983), pointed out that values become a lens for viewing the world that influences what is seen, what rises to awareness, and what motivates actions. In turn, this "way of knowing" the world then shapes interactions such that "our epistemology is quietly transformed into our ethic" (Palmer, 1983, cited in Hooper, 2006, p. 21).

Occupational therapy scholars have debated what knowledge is useful and essential to the profession (Abreu, Peloquin, & Ottenbacher, 1998; Carlson & Clark, 1991; Spencer, 1993; Yerxa, 1992). In a seminal article on ethics and epistemology, Yerxa (1992) advocated that to be ethical, occupational therapy science must be commensurate with practitioners' view of occupation. She outlined the following guidelines for knowledge generation in occupational therapy:

- Elucidate client capacities rather than limitations.
- Study people in context.
- Focus at the person level.
- Consider developmental and lifespan processes of occupation.

- Focus on the person's experience of occupation.
- Examine the organization and balance of occupation in daily life.
- Synthesize knowledge across disciplines to address occupational complexity.

Research that follows these guidelines requires a contextualized approach to examine the person's experience while he or she is engaged in the world of everyday life activities. In this way, the research produced would be both beneficent and socially just, providing knowledge about clients' occupational needs that is rooted in their unique personal, social, and cultural influences. In Yerxa's (1992) view, only qualitative methods have the breadth and depth to study occupation without losing its core essence.

Similarly, Spencer (1993) advocated for the need to study meaning, context, and change processes within intervention. She advocated for efforts to enhance a practical understanding of how physical and cultural contexts influence recovery and daily functioning for people with disabilities. Research that fosters an understanding of consumers' perspectives is crucial to promote effective life change.

Qualitative methods

Qualitative methods are naturalistic approaches that use systematic methods (e.g., participant observation, in-depth interviews, focus groups) to define a focus, gather, and analyze data. These methods are generative, allowing the pursuit of emerging novel findings, and more complex understandings of culture and context. These methods have an important role to play in occupational therapy's epistemic culture.

Qualitative research can be both generative, producing new insights, and grounded in the participant's perspective rather than the researcher's perspective or previous theory (Gutman, 2008, 2009). As Yerxa (1992) and Spencer (1993) enjoined, these methods can increase practitioners' understanding of clients and their occupational choices and of what matters to them, how their experience evolves over time during the course of intervention, and what bolsters their healthy participation within their particular contexts.

Qualitative methods can help practitioners understand why clients refuse to use or do not use strategies or adaptive equipment, even after these interventions have been demonstrated to be effective through various research methods. The rich descriptions generated through qualitative approaches provide sufficiently detailed information to allow occupational therapy practitioners to make case-by-case decisions about which clients may benefit from specific interventions and under what circumstances. These methods can be used in tandem with experimental designs or alone to better identify the critical person and process features that are vital to optimal outcomes.

Research design and methodology

Many research designs and methodologies can generate data for practice on occupational participation both in context and in relation to individual client factors. Hinojosa (2013) argued that occupational therapy practitioners should thoughtfully and critically consider whether and how the evidence hierarchy they adopt aligns with their professional values and supports practice. Tomlin and Borgetto (2011) propose this alternative evidence hierarchy (see Figure 19.3).

Several exemplars of occupational therapy research have used designs aligned with occupational therapy practitioners' professional values and focused on occupation and have also produced high-level evidence. Several RCT trials have examined occupational therapy interventions using personally tailored and contextualized intervention programs (e.g., Clark et al., 1997; Gitlin et al., 2009). This kind of approach has, in some cases, been associated with better outcomes (Adair et al., 2015). Studies using rigorous RCT designs with large populations, assessing standardized intervention protocols that were personalized to each client's interests and desires, are in line with occupational therapy's epistemology, professional values, and need for evidence.

The application of RCT findings is described in Case Study 19.1. This case reflects not only the tensions in translation of evidence from groups to individuals but also the tailoring of evidence to apply it to the whole family unit.

Ethically, practitioners owe it to the forces outside the profession demanding evidence of efficacy to provide evidence that occupational therapy services are effective and socially useful. Current and accepted methods for demonstrating efficacy need to be used in ways that align with the profession's epistemic culture. Unlike drug or other

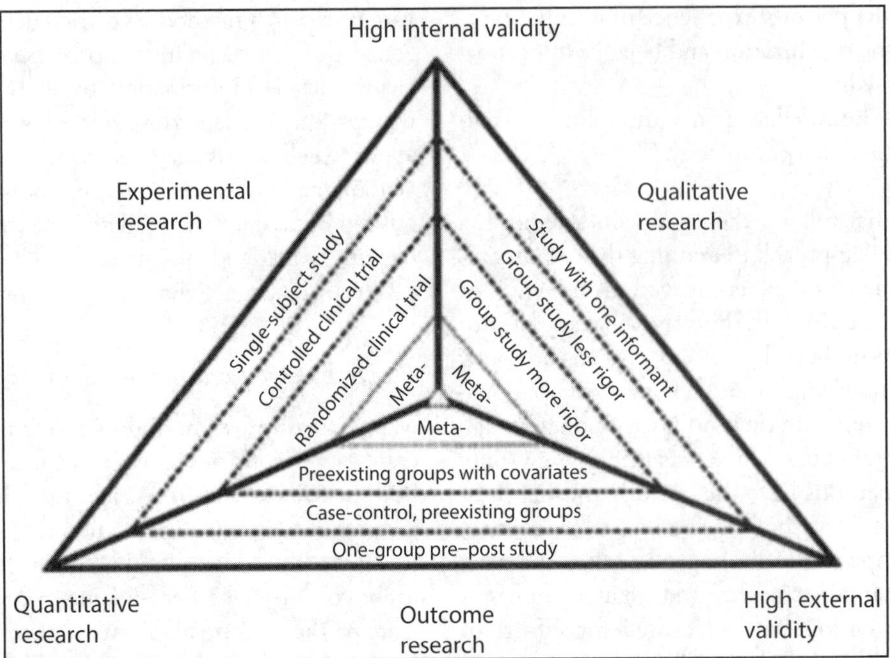

FIGURE 19.3

Alternative research pyramid.
Source. From "Research Pyramid: A New Evidence-Based Practice Model for Occupational Therapy," by G. Tomlin and B. Borgetto, 2011, *American Journal of Occupational Therapy, 65,* p. 191. Copyright © 2011 by the American Occupational Therapy Association. Used with permission.

single treatments, occupational therapy is a complex, person-centered practice. When choosing the direction and methods of the profession's research agenda, it is important to consider the usefulness, limitations, and applicability of any approach used to generate evidence. Designs need to consider the person factors and the therapeutic relationship.

In addition, practitioners should not ignore critiques leveled in medicine that research intended to generate evidence for practice cannot be atheoretical in conceptualization or design. For occupational therapy, these considerations mean that practice evidence should contribute to an understanding of the processes underlying achievement of health and well-being through occupational participation. Theoretical development and generation of evidence need to go hand in hand.

Ethical Design and Conduct of Research

Research has become increasingly regulated to ensure researchers follow the Principles of Beneficence, Nonmaleficence, Justice, and Veracity (AOTA, 2015b, p. 2). Researchers must carefully consider the balance between potentially beneficial research outcomes and the costs to research participants when making decisions about the design, conduct, and publication of their research. In addition, to redress past limitations, current guidelines encourage more socially just approaches, such as encouraging the study of previously understudied or vulnerable groups. Throughout the process, following the established guidelines—Justice—is essential to ensure the protection of human participants' rights. Finally, the Principle of Veracity also permeates the entire research process and is essential to producing knowledge that in the end is useful, accurate, and ethical.

Historical Foundations of Research Ethics

Historically, public outcry surrounding unethical studies led to the development of guidelines for recruitment and treatment of research participants (National Institutes of Health [NIH], 2004). In several infamous 20th-century studies, researchers embraced a utilitarian ethical principle. They believed that despite the high costs to a few participants, the

Case Study 19.1. Application of Randomized Controlled Trial Findings

You are a senior occupational therapist considering the possibility of developing a more effective intervention program for children with cerebral palsy in your clinic. In preparation, you have reviewed the available evidence, including one recent meta-analysis and systematic review of constraint-induced movement therapy (CIMT; Tinderholt Myrhaug Østensjø, Larun, Odgaard-Jensen, & Jahnsen, 2014). You hope to design a program that uses clinic resources effectively, that works well for families, and whose frequency and intervention strategies can be substantiated to insurance providers. The authors of the meta-analysis conclude,

> The present and other recently published systematic reviews have demonstrated the extensive and increasing evidence regarding CIMT. Studies on hand function had lower risks of bias compared with studies of gross motor function. Moreover, studies on gross motor function were typically characterised by a lower number of training sessions and longer training periods without home programs compared with studies that targeted hand function, which were characterised by higher number of training sessions and shorter training periods including home programs. These findings might suggest that more intensive training for a shorter period including practicing in the child's natural environment may be more effective for learning functional skills. Home training appears to play an important role in increasing the intensity of training. How to implement home training without disturbing the family's daily life in a negative manner remains to be resolved. Equal improvements in motor function and functional skills were reported for intensive interventions and conventional therapy or between two different intensive interventions in a majority of the included studies. The identification of the optimal intensity of interventions that target motor function and functional skills, as well as the possible harmful effects of intensive training, requires further investigation. (Tinderholt Myrhaug et al., 2014, p. 17)

How does this evidence shape your design of the program? What approach will you take in regard to home programs? What are the ethics of an imposed home program on families, even if the evidence suggests it is an essential element? After you have considered responses to these questions, review Table 19.2.

Table 19.2. Decision Table for Case Study 19.1

Possible Action	Positive Outcomes	Negative Consequences
Take no action.	Does not detract time from delivery of current strategies for children with CP and their families. Reduces family burden for those who cannot manage a home program in addition to child's daily care.	There is a failure to explore and offer best practice to children and their families. Clients may potentially have slower progress with greater treatment costs for families.
Continue to review evidence of RCT and pilot CIMT with a few children.	Findings applied on a case-by-case basis may benefit some.	Some children who could benefit will not receive CIMT treatment and may incur higher therapy costs because of the greater number of treatment sessions. Parents and children may be discouraged with the children's skill acquisition and progress.
Implement current RCT findings.	There is potential for greater improvements in fine motor skills with fewer sessions for a larger number of clients.	There is no clear evidence for frequency of therapy or home sessions to guide program development. Families may face an increased burden as a result of the home program component's further unbalancing family dynamics.

Note. CIMT = constraint-induced movement therapy; CP = cerebral palsy; RCT = randomized controlled trial.

studies' findings would benefit the many, outweighing the consideration of their participants' health and well-being.

For example, some medical researchers intentionally induced disease or failed to treat disease in their studies' participants (Corbie-Smith, 1999; Hornblum, 1997). These researchers sought readily available or easily influenced populations such as prisoners, institutionalized people with mental retardation, debilitated older adults in institutions, or illiterate or poor members of minority populations (Hornblum, 1997). Prisoners and residents of treatment centers were considered especially convenient and desirable research participants because they lived in controlled settings.

The first worldwide code for research was generated after the Nuremberg trials of Nazi physicians (see Appendix 19.A). The Nuremberg Code (1949) laid the foundation for core ethical principles in use today and included key provisions to protect participants and to ensure that studies were reasonable, necessary, and likely to produce humanitarian benefits. This code required studies to be rooted in prior scholarship, to be conducted by qualified researchers, to have a potential humanitarian benefit that exceeded potential risks to participants, to be conducted only if a priori evidence suggested that participation would not result in potential death or disability, and to be terminated at any time if continuation was believed to be harmful.

Unfortunately, after World War II, some U.S. physicians did not believe the Nuremberg Code applied to their research. These researchers encouraged prisoners' participation by offering early release or other privileges in exchange for participation in studies that involved intentional exposure to deadly disease, cancer, or radiation or unnecessary surgery (Hornblum, 1997). They reasoned that prisoners' research participation was moral, allowing them to right a wrong (their crime) or to contribute (during World War II) to the war effort by being human guinea pigs for studies, including radiation studies. Historical evidence has suggested that prison participants were not typically informed of the potential risks and that their participation was not voluntary by Nuremberg Code standards.

Likewise, psychological studies using deception have evoked concern. For example, Milgram's (1968) study examined the conditions under which and the likelihood that people would follow an authority figure's punitive demands for punishment. He found that when an authority figure wearing a white coat stood nearby, 65% of participants provided increasing and even deadly levels of electrical current to an actor they believed was a coparticipant making learning mistakes. After the study, participants were not debriefed on the study's deception. They were left to deal with altered self-perceptions of their capacity to do or not do harm to another person when influenced by a person in power.

In response to highly publicized abuses in the 1960s and 1970s, global and U.S. scientific councils outlined additional ethical standards for conducting research. The Declaration of Helsinki (World Medical Association, 2008), the Belmont Report (NIH, 2004), and the Office for Human Research Protections of the U.S. Department of Health and Human Services' (DHHS, 2005) rules for the protection of human participants provided additional research guidelines and requirements. The first Declaration of Helsinki was the first effort to regulate medical and clinical research worldwide. The Belmont Report emphasized three core ethics: respect for persons, beneficence, and justice (NIH, 2004). Carefully balancing the needs of a vulnerable population with the importance of studying their health, the DHHS rules specifically address the manner of and method for inclusion of vulnerable and under-researched populations in research (see Appendix 19.B; Office for Human Research Protections, DHHS, 2009).

These guidelines address the ethical treatment of participants through all steps of the research, beginning with the study's conceptualization and continuing through the steps of design, consent, conduct, conclusion, analysis, and publication. These codes are meant to assist researchers in designing studies that ensure that "serious efforts have been made to protect the rights and welfare of research subjects" (NIH, 2004, p. 4).

Ethics in Design

The study design and methods selected to address a ***research question*** must also be scientifically rigorous. Poorly designed or shoddy research violates basic ethical guidelines (Gilliam, Guillemin, Bolitho, & Rosenthal, 2009).

Research question

Study design begins with the identification of a significant and socially valuable question. The question

Vignette 19.1. Costs and Contributions—Is the Study Ethical?

As part of coursework, your group is assigned to develop a research question and study design and to collect initial data. Your group decides to investigate the training of occupational therapy students in interprofessional practice by surveying occupational therapy program faculty using an electronic survey that you develop. The response rate is low, around 9%; the findings are documented in a group paper you submit to your instructor but are not published. Is this a significant question? Is it important enough to justify the participants' time? Are the methods sufficiently rigorous? Given the lack of publication of the findings in a peer-reviewed journal, is the effort and time of the student researchers and participants ethical?

must be of sufficient importance to justify the participants' time and exposure to risks (Gilliam et al., 2009). Vignette 19.1 explores the need to balance gaining knowledge with costs to research participants.

Questions for research are often rooted in current social concerns. Presently, investigating and explaining the underlying roots of health disparities among ethnic groups is a key priority in U.S. health research (DHHS, 2011). This priority has spurred funding of studies inclusive across age, gender, ethnicity, sexual orientation, socioeconomic status, and educational attainment. Equitable inclusion of diverse people requires study designs that address a more complex heterogeneous participant selection.

In the past, medical researchers excluded female participants in an effort to control for variability attributable to hormone cycles. This practice led to the current problem of limited and insufficient understanding of women's responses to different medical treatments, including those for leading causes of mortality and disability. Efforts to control variability must be balanced against the need to produce research that benefits people of all groups, especially those most likely to have the specific conditions under study.

Vulnerable populations

Researchers must weigh choices to study vulnerable groups (defined as children; individuals with cognitive impairments; individuals with AIDS/HIV; prisoners; economically or educationally disadvantaged; pregnant women, neonates, or fetuses; students or employees) against the benefits likely to accrue to those group members and others from their participation and f rom the potential outcomes of the proposed studies. Concerns about past exploitation have led to strict guidelines for the participation of vulnerable people in research.

An ***institutional review board*** (IRB) is the local governing body that reviews research proposals to assure compliance with human subjects protection standards. In applications to the IRB, investigators must document whether a vulnerable population will be included and require evidence that the study safeguards and procedures address the specific needs of the vulnerable population. Measures may include specially designed recruitment material, simplified language in the informed consent form if needed, alternative procedures for low or nonliterate participants, and justification of the use of incentives to recruit or reward participants after study completion.

Informed consent

Planning and designing procedures for informed consent are a critical part of the research process. ***Informed consent*** is a process in which people, with a clear understanding of the study expectations, benefits, and risks and their individual rights, agree to participate in a research study. Many online resources are available to assist in developing informed consent forms that include all of the essential components and in assessing the grade level of language used, such as the SMOG readability formula and the Fry Readability Graph (Centers for Disease Control and Prevention, 2009). A common guideline is that the informed consent should be written at a 6th- to 8th-grade reading level. In cases in which participants' literacy is known to be more limited, the consent form should be at a reading level appropriate to the group's comprehension of language.

For example, when working with a group of Native American caregivers, research suggested that the literacy of some could be at the 4th-grade reading level; therefore, the consent form needed simpler vocabulary and paragraph structure and more active language. Consents for non–English-speaking participants may also need to be translated and back-translated (i.e., translated to the participants' first language and translated again to English to check the accuracy of the translation) to ensure that participants understand the expectations and procedures of the study.

In the case of research with children, minors are generally not legally able to consent to research participation, so their parents must consent on their behalf. Still, assent procedures are highly recommended for children ages 10 years or older. To obtain assent, researchers describe the study to a child in language he or she can understand and then give the child the option to note his or her agreement or refusal to participate.

In all studies, ***written consent,*** or the signing of the consent form, is only one part of the consent process. The research team is also obligated to discuss and explain study procedures to participants. Both the oral presentation, either in person or by phone, and the signing of the consent are important steps in ensuring that participants understand and agree to participate in the study. In addition, a review of recruitment materials and processes is part of the IRB requirements for approval of the study. The advertising scripts used to recruit participants must explain the study in a clear and accurate way, and wording of the risks and benefits must carefully parallel the wording used in the informed consent.

Progressive researchers are now also assessing participants' understanding of the informed consent process and obtaining ***ongoing consent.*** An additional step of surveying participants' understanding of the study's aims, the activities expected of them, and their rights helps to ensure and verify that vulnerable study participants truly understand the import of their consent (Buccini, 2009; Dunn, 2006). After such a survey, researchers can then provide further education in areas the participant did not understand well. This step is particularly useful in adult populations in which people's medical or health conditions are believed to potentially impair their capacity for autonomous decision making. Gauging a person's continuing willingness to share personal information has also been advocated, especially when a highly intense or emotionally charged topic is being investigated (Schelbe et al., 2015).

Impact of Research on Participants

Even with well-designed consents, surveys of consent comprehension, and considerable forethought in addressing the expected consequences of participation, research may have unintended effects on participants. For this reason, researchers must continue to monitor participants throughout the study for any ill effects, which must be reported to the IRB in yearly reviews. Intervention studies must provide participants with information about viable alternatives to those offered in the study, and researchers may need to offer treatment if undesired outcomes occur. In treatment studies in which the intervention results in positive outcomes, ethical researchers typically offer the same intervention to control group participants. This offer requires advance planning to ensure that the research budget includes control group treatment. Vignette 19.2 describes a situation when a research study was terminated early due to unintended consequences.

Little research has been done to examine the effects of study participation, even effects whose risks are typically considered minimal. In a follow-up of research on occupational therapy practitioners' ethical dilemmas in practice, Barnitt and Partridge (1999) interviewed therapists about their experience participating in the ethics study. Two therapists provided very different accounts of the experience of participating in this study:

> [I was asked] asked to describe an ethical problem I had encountered at work. I had had notice of this and had decided which one to report on. She just left me to talk, and I found that I was getting out of my depth, revealing things I didn't want exposed. (p. 256)

The second participant said, "My colleagues are nervous of discussing the dilemma [discharge of a confused elderly patient] because we can never agree. It was nice to talk about it without being judged" (p. 257). Although the first therapist felt vulnerable and overexposed, the second felt the study provided an open, affirming forum. In both cases, participating in research was neither objective nor neutral from the therapists' perspectives. Researchers need to recognize that participation can have life-altering effects on participants, and more study is warranted in this area.

Issues in Innovative Methodology and Confidentiality of Data

Several advances in research methods have highlighted the need for additional safeguards and study to determine how to ethically manage research participants' confidential information. For example, genetics researchers are currently concerned about third-party consent. People who consent to genetics

Vignette 19.2. Confronting Research Risks for Participants

While in graduate school in California, I received a call telling me that my mother had been hospitalized. I flew home to find her in a hospital bed, her left side black and blue from head to toe and a baseball-sized hematoma over her left eye, looking as if she'd survived a bad car wreck. Because of a "shower" of pulmonary embolisms, she'd passed out and fallen from midstair onto the concrete basement floor at home. Doctors said she'd beaten the odds; they had given her only a 30% chance of survival upon arrival in the ER. Using a textbook to guide them, they administered what was then a new "clot-busting" drug that saved her life.

My mom was a volunteer in the longitudinal Women's Health Initiative (WHI) study that was examining the effects of hormone replacement therapy (HRT) and other supplements on the incidence of heart disease and stroke. We suspected her life-threatening event was related to study-provided medications. The WHI study coordinator refused to provide us with any information; only after my mother's physician contacted the research team did they break the double-blind group assignments to reveal that she was indeed receiving HRT.

My mother's and others' experiences led to the early termination of the HRT part of the study in 2002, although she continues today to participate in the study's long-term follow-up. Despite practitioners' intuition that HRT was beneficial to women's health, this RCT demonstrated that HRT was not beneficial for many and caused harm for some (National Heart, Lung, and Blood Institute, 2002).

Do you agree with the research team's response to my family? Was the team's behavior consistent with the Principles of the Code? How and when should a negative event such as the one my mother experienced lead to an alteration in study procedures? How should my mother's and other participants' consent to this study have been reevaluated after this aversive reaction?

studies, by nature of the information analyzed, provide information about their family members. Incidental identification of conditions may be a risk the participant chooses to assume, but what of the family members who do not choose to participate in the study? The immediate or extended family may experience both the information sharing and the evaluation results as both unwelcome and life changing.

Another arena provoking discussion is online and app-based data collection. Online surveys have the benefits of being easily administered across wide geographic areas and of enabling simultaneous data compilation. Researchers typically promise anonymity to participants in web surveys. Yet with increasingly sophisticated software, some people are able to mine web interactions, or researchers may lack the technological sophistication to anonymize the responses.

In a recent online survey of university faculty on a highly controversial topic, the invitation to the study offered anonymity, but after receiving angry queries about biased questions the researcher offered participants the option to withdraw their data. To withdraw, the author of the survey would need an identifier that allowed him to delete an individual's data. Both statements to participants could not be true. Likewise, there is concern about app-based tools and surveys and the encryption of data at all points of transmission and storage; this work requires a team member with a high level of technological expertise.

These issues must be resolved to ensure participants' confidentiality and protection of their medical and other personal information. New technologies bring both opportunities and challenges for research methods.

Ethics in Publishing Research

Publishing, the last step in the process of research, is nonetheless an essential one. When an article is published, the researcher's choices throughout the process, as well as the findings, are documented and distributed for public consumption. Publication is vitally important because the dissemination of research efforts to a wider audience can create major shifts in practice or policy and provide evidence for practice.

Research findings are often presented in neat and tidy ways in publications, yet behind-the-scenes accounts of research processes are informative about the many dilemmas that exist in describing the design, its implementation, and findings published in research. Choices in how to describe the methods, which analyses to perform, what visual displays to use, and which findings to publish are all shaped by ethical decisions.

Typically, multiple articles may be published from a given study, with each focused on a specific aspect. Thus, researchers may limit descriptions of methods or refer readers to earlier published descriptions of methods to save space. This balance between providing depth of description of methods and dedicating more space to findings is one that researchers consider in publications.

The analyses that are selected need to be guided by scientific traditions and ethics. It is problematic for researchers to run multiple analyses in a fishing expedition for statistically significant findings. Analyses should be based on the theoretical assumptions about the relationships between variables guiding the study. In addition, null findings are often not published, despite the contribution they make to the knowledge base. In many instances, null findings are important to patient care—for example, in studies of the efficacy of specific treatments or medications. Knowing that a specific approach is not effective is important knowledge for practice.

False or Misleading Research

Many times, the focus at the publication stage is solely on considerations of the originality and veracity of the publication. Although in rare cases researchers have intentionally published false or misleading research (Farthing, 1998), these instances can have a widespread impact.

One recent infamous case includes the retraction of a *Lancet* article that suggested an association between the emergence of regressive autism and administration of a childhood vaccination (Deer, 2010). This discredited study has been responsible for worldwide decreases in the number of children being immunized and for increases in preventable diseases and deaths (e.g., measles, mumps, rubella) that previously were rarely seen.

Plagiarism

Similarly, plagiarism or duplicate data publications, also considered to be research misconduct, are rare but problematic. Errami et al. (2008) used a text analysis to identify an incidence of 0.04% potential plagiarism and 1.35%, or 117,550, duplicate publications in articles in the Medline database. Martinson, Anderson, and de Vries (2005) surveyed 3,247 NIH-funded scientists who reported engaging in plagiarism and duplicate data publications, as well as keeping inadequate records, dropping observations or data outliers on the basis of gut instincts, changing study design because of external pressures (e.g., funding sources), or ignoring human participant provisions. These problematic actions reflect inadequate attention to procedures and veracity, violating Principles 4, Justice, and 5, Veracity, of the Code (AOTA, 2015b). In a most egregious example, one occupational therapy professor's work was closely copied by a nursing colleague in publications, not once but twice (Erdley, 2011).

It is the function of peer review to carefully consider the quality of manuscripts submitted to journals, judge originality, and identify unintended errors in analyses or misleading narrative. Still, peer reviewers may miss self-plagiarism, use of large sections of a prior publication in a new one, inaccurate citations of others' work, or missing citations of foundational work. Using a complex analysis program, Simkin and Roychowdhury (2003) tracked inaccurate duplicate citations through generations of publications. They argued that these persistent errors represented researchers' repeated use of others' analyses of the literature without returning to the original sources and that only a paltry 20% of citers read the original source. This, too, is problematic because persistent errors can be transmitted through the literature.

Other Ethical Issues

Several other ethical considerations exist in publication, including timely dissemination of findings, selection of publication venue and audience for the information, and choices in reporting the data (e.g., how to visually display data in figures, whether to report null results, how to fairly represent the importance of the findings). For example, in occupational therapy, the researcher's choice of journal to submit to may be driven by a variety of inside and outside pressures.

The journal that represents the ideal audience for an article may not have a sufficiently high impact rating to support the researcher's progress in an academic career at a high-productivity university. ***Impact ratings*** are calculated by averaging the number of citations of all the published articles for a given period; this average of how often a publication's articles are cited gives an idea of the breadth of its impact. This consideration has been a challenge in occupational therapy and occupational science, although more of our professional journals are being rated for impact and what had been relatively low ***impact factor*** ratings are rising. A researcher may be torn between reaching occupational therapy practitioners, the ideal consumers of the research, and succeeding in academia by seeking out journals with higher distributions and impact factors.

Summary

Leaders and policymakers advocate that translation of research into practice is a high priority for occupational therapy practitioners. Because of this priority, entire courses in occupational therapy curricula are dedicated to the evaluation of the quality and use of research in practice. The implementation of knowledge in service of clients is being viewed both within and outside the profession as a moral imperative.

Occupational therapy practitioners must make a lifelong professional commitment to keep abreast of and use new knowledge in practice. Recognizing the appropriate uses and limits of knowledge translation, not merely its addition to practice, and addressing the gaps and needs in the knowledge base are essential to moving the profession forward.

Reflective Questions

1. What evidence do you believe is needed now to bolster the quality of and evidence for occupational therapy practice? What should our first priority be, and where should we put our resources?
2. How can we invite people with disabilities to participate in research, in order to produce knowledge that will serve people like them, in a manner that is respectful and fully informed?
3. Consider the impact of historic studies, such as those investigating genetically based differences in intelligence, on policies governing education and health care. This research has been viewed by some as misused (Gray & Thompson, 2004) to support policies that provide differential opportunities to people on the basis of race. What current policies that impact our clients' service options attempt to redress past inequities in education and health care?
4. Identify the relevant Principles and RSCs from Case Study 19.1 and its Decision Table (Table 19.2).

References

Abreu, B. C., Peloquin, S. M., & Ottenbacher, K. (1998). Competence in scientific inquiry and research. *American Journal of Occupational Therapy, 52,* 751–759. https://doi.org/10.5014/ajot.52.9.751

Accreditation Council for Occupational Therapy Education. (2012). 2011 Accreditation Council for Occupational Therapy Education (ACOTE®) standards. *American Journal of Occupational Therapy, 66*(6, Suppl.), S6–S74. https://doi.org/10.5014/ajot.2012.66S6

Adair, B., Ullenhag, A., Keen, D., Granlund, M., & Imms, C. (2015). The effect of interventions aimed at improving participation outcomes for children with disabilities: A systematic review. *Developmental Medicine and Child Neurology, 57,* 1–12. https://doi.org/10.1111/dmcn.12809

Albert, M., Laberge, S., & Hodges, B. D. (2009). Boundary-work in the health research field: Biomedical and clinician scientists' perceptions of social science research. *Minerva, 47,* 171–194. http://dx.doi.org/10.1007/s11024-009-9120-8

American Occupational Therapy Association. (2007). AOTA's *Centennial Vision* and executive summary. *American Journal of Occupational Therapy, 61,* 613–614. https://doi.org/10.5014/ajot.61.6.613

American Occupational Therapy Association. (2015a). Guidelines for contributors to *AJOT. American Journal of Occupational Therapy, 69*(Suppl. 3), 6913430010. https://doi.org/10.5014/ajot.2015.696S13

American Occupational Therapy Association. (2015b). Occupational therapy code of ethics (2015). *American Journal of Occupational Therapy, 69*(Suppl. 3), 6912310030. https://doi.org/10.5014/ajot.2015.696S03

American Occupational Therapy Association. (2016). *Vision 2025.* Retrieved from http://www.aota.org/aboutaota/vision-2025.aspx

Barnitt, R., & Partridge, C. (1999). The legacy of being a research subject: Follow-up studies of participants in therapy research. *Physiotherapy Research International, 4,* 250–261. https://doi.org/10.1002/pri.172

Becher, T., & Trowler, P. R. (2001). *Academic tribes and territories: Intellectual enquiry and the culture of disciplines* (2nd ed.). Philadelphia: Society for Research Into Higher Education/Open University Press.

Bernstein, J., Collette, D., & Pederson, S. (2010). Basing healthcare on empirical evidence. *Mathematica, 3,* 1–4.

Bordieu, P. (2004). *Science of science and reflexivity.* Cambridge, England: Polity Press.

Brown, M., Dijkers, M. P., Gordon, W. A., Ashman, T., Charatz, H., & Chen, Z. (2004). Participation objective, participation subjective: A measure of participation combining outsider and insider perspectives. *Journal of Head Trauma Rehabilitation, 19,* 459–481. https://doi.org/10.1097/00001199-200411000-00004

Buccini, L. D. (2009). *Developing an instrument to measure informed consent in non-cognitively impaired adults* (Doctoral thesis). University of Wollongong, Wollongong, New South Wales, Australia.

Carlson, M. E., & Clark, F. A. (1991). The search for useful methodologies in occupational science. *American Journal of Occupational Therapy, 45,* 235–241. https://doi.org/10.5014/ajot.45.3.235

Centers for Disease Control and Prevention. (2009). *Simply put: A guide for creating easy-to-understand materials* (3rd ed.). Atlanta: Author.

Christiansen, C. (1981). Toward the resolution of crisis: Research requisites in occupational therapy. *Occupational Therapy Journal of Research, 1,* 115–124. https://doi.org/10.1177/153944928100100201

Christiansen, C., & Lou, J. Q. (2001). Ethical considerations related to evidence-based practice. *American Journal of Occupational Therapy, 55,* 345–349. https://doi.org/10.5014/ajot.55.3.345

Clark, F., Azen, S. P., Zemke, R., Jackson J., Carlson, M., Mandel D., . . . Lipson, L. (1997). Occupational therapy for independent-living older adults: A randomized controlled trial. *JAMA, 278,* 1321–1326. https://doi.org/10.1001/jama.1997.03550160041036

Cochrane, A. J. (2004). *Effectiveness and efficiency: Random reflections on health services.* London, England: Royal Society of Medicine Press. (Original work published 1972)

Cohen, A. M., Stavri, P. Z., & Hersch, W. R. (2004). A categorization and analysis of the criticisms of evidence-based medicine. *International Journal of Medical Informatics, 73,* 35–43. https://doi.org/10.1016/j.ijmedinf.2003.11.002

Corbie-Smith, G. (1999). The continuing legacy of the Tuskegee syphilis study: Considerations for clinical investigation. *American Journal of Medical Science, 317,* 5–8. https://doi.org/10.1016/S0002-9629(15)40464-1

Dartmouth Biomedical Libraries. (2008). *Evidence-based medicine (EBM) resources.* Retrieved from http://www.dartmouth.edu/~biomed/resources.htmld/guides/ebm_resources.shtml

Deer, B. (2010). Secrets of the MMR scare: How the case against the MMR vaccine was fixed. *BMJ, 342,* c5347. https://doi.org/10.1136/bmj.c5347

Dunn, L. (2006). Capacity to consent to research in schizophrenia: The expanding evidence base. *Behavioral Sciences and the Law, 24,* 431–445. https://doi.org/10.1002/bsl.698

Erdley, D. (2011, Nov. 7). Repeat of plagiarism shocks professor. *Trib Live.* Retrieved from http://triblive.com/x/pittsburghtrib/news/s_765943.html

Errami, M., Hicks, J. M., Fisher, W., Trusty, D., Wren, J. D., Long, T. C., & Garner, H. R. (2008). Déjà vu: A study of duplicate citations in Medline. *Bio-informatics, 24,* 243–249. http://dx.doi.org/10.1093/bioinformatics/btm574

Farthing, M. (1998). The COPE report: Coping with fraud. *Lancet, 352,* 10–11.

Gilliam, L., Guillemin, M., Bolitho, A., & Rosenthal, D. (2009). Human research ethics in practice: Deliberative strategies, process and perceptions. *Monash Bioethics Review, 28,* 7.1–7.17.

Gitlin, L. N., Winter, L., Earland, T. V., Herge, E. A., Chernett, N. L., Piersol, C. V., & Burke, J. P. (2009). The Tailored Activity Program to reduce behavioral symptoms in individuals with dementia: Feasibility, acceptability, and replication potential. *Gerontologist, 49,* 428–439. https://doi.org/10.1093/geront/gnp087

Gray, J. R., & Thompson, P. M. (2004). Neurobiology of intelligence: Science and ethics. *Nature Reviews Neuroscience, 5,* 471–482. https://doi.org/10.1038/nrn1405

Gustafsson, L., Molineux, M., & Bennett, S. (2014). Contemporary occupational therapy practice: The challenges of being evidence-based and philosophically congruent. *Australian Occupational Therapy Journal, 61,* 121–123. https://doi.org/10.1111/1440-1630.12110

Gutman, S. (2008). From the Desk of the Editor—Research priorities of the profession. *American Journal of Occupational Therapy, 62,* 619–622. https://doi.org/10.5014/ajot.62.5.499

Gutman, S. (2009). From the Desk of the Editor—State of the journal, 2009. *American Journal of Occupational Therapy, 63,* 667–673. https://doi.org/10.5014/ajot.63.6.667

Hinojosa, J. (2013). The Issue Is—The evidence-based paradox. *American Journal of Occupational Therapy, 67,* e18–e23. https://doi.org/10.5014/ajot.2013.005587

Hooper, B. (2006). Epistemological transformation in occupational therapy: Educational implications and challenges. *OTJR: Occupation, Participation and Health, 26,* 15–24.

Hope, T. (1997). Evidence-based patient choice and the doctor-patient relationship. In M. Dunning & G. Needham (Eds.), *But will it work, doctor?* (pp. 20–24). London: Kings Fund.

Hornblum, A. M. (1997). They were cheap and available: Prisoners as research subjects in twentieth-century America. *BMJ, 315,* 1437–1341. https://doi.org/10.1136/bmj.315.7120.1437

Kuhn, T. S. (1962). *The structure of scientific revolutions* (3rd ed.). Chicago: University of Chicago Press.

Martinson, B. C., Anderson, M. S., & de Vries, R. (2005). Scientists behaving badly. *Nature, 435,* 737–738. https://doi.org/10.1038/435737a

Milgram, S. (1968). Some conditions of obedience and disobedience to authority. *International Journal of Psychiatry, 6,* 259–76. https://doi.org/10.1177/001872676501800105

National Heart, Lung, and Blood Institute. (2002, July 9). *NHLBI stops trial of estrogen plus progestin due to increased breast cancer risk, lack of overall benefit* [Press release]. Retrieved from https://www.nhlbi.nih.gov/news/press-releases

/2002/nhlbi-stops-trial-of-estrogen-plus-progestin-due-to-increased-breast-cancer-risk-lack-of-overall-benefit

National Institutes of Health. (2004). *Guidelines for the conduct of research using human subjects at the National Institutes of Health* (Publication No. ADM 00-4783). Washington, DC: U.S. Government Printing Office. Retrieved from http://sourcebook.od.nih.gov/ethic-conduct/Conduct%20Research%206-11-07.pdf

Nuremberg Code. (1949). In *Trials of war criminals before the Nuremberg military tribunals under Control Council Law No. 10* (Vol. 2, pp. 181–182). Washington, DC: U.S. Government Printing Office. Retrieved from http://history.nih.gov/research/downloads/nuremberg.pdf

Office for Human Research Protections, U.S. Department of Health and Human Services. (2009). *45 C.F.R. §46.111. Protection of human subjects.* Retrieved from http://www.hhs.gov/ohrp/humansubjects/guidance/45cfr46.html/

Palmer, P. (1983). *To know as we are known.* San Francisco: Harper.

Rogers, J. C. (1983). Clinical reasoning: The ethics, science, and art (Eleanor Clarke Slagle lecture). *American Journal of Occupational Therapy, 37,* 601–616. https://doi.org/10.5014/ajot.37.9.601

Sackett, D. L., Richardson, W. S., Rosenberg, W., & Haynes, R. B. (1997). *Evidence-based medicine: How to practice and teach EBM.* London: Churchill Livingstone.

Sackett, D. L., Rosenberg, W. M. C., Gray, J. A., Haynes, R. B., & Richardson, W. S. (1996). Evidence based medicine: What it is and what it isn't. *BMJ, 312,* 71. https://doi.org/10.1136/bmj.312.7023.71

Sackett, D. L., Straus, S. E., Richardson, W. S., Rosenberg, W., & Haynes, B. (2000). *Evidence-based medicine: How to practice and teach EBM* (2nd ed.). Edinburgh, Scotland: Churchill Livingstone.

Schelbe, L., Chanmugam, A., Moses, T., Saltzburg, S., Williams, L., & Letendre, J. (2015). Youth participation in qualitative research: Challenges and possibilities. *Qualitative Social Work, 14,* 504–521. https://doi.org/10.1177/1473325014556792

Simkin, M. V., & Roychowdhury, V. P. (2003). Read before you cite! *Complex Systems, 14,* 269.

Spencer, J. C. (1993). The usefulness of qualitative methods in rehabilitation: Issues of meaning, of context, and of change. *Archives of Physical Medicine and Rehabilitation, 74,* 119–126.

Tinderholt Myrhaug, H., Østensjø, S., Larun, L., Odgaard-Jensen, J., & Jahnsen, R. (2014). Intensive training of motor function and functional skills among young children with cerebral palsy: A systematic review and meta-analysis. *BMC Pediatrics, 14,* 292. https://doi.org/10.1186/s12887-014-0292-5

Tomlin, G., & Borgetto, B. (2011). Research pyramid: A new evidence-based practice model for occupational therapy. *American Journal of Occupational Therapy, 69,* 189–196. https://doi.org/10.5014/ajot.2011.000828

U.S. Department of Health and Human Services (2011). *DHHS action plan to reduce racial and ethnic disparities: A nation free of disparities in health and health care.* Retrieved from http://minorityhealth.hhs.gov/omh/browse.aspx?lvl=2&lvlid=10

Van Brakel, W. H., Anderson, A. M., Mutatakar, R. K., Bakirtzief, Z., Nicholls, P. J., Raju, M. S., & Das-Pattanayak, R. K. (2006). The Participation Scale: A key concept in public health. *Disability and Society, 28,* 193–203. https://doi.org/10.1080/09638280500192785

World Medical Association. (2008). *WMA Declaration of Helsinki—Ethical principles for medical research involving human subjects.* Retrieved from http://www.wma.net/en/30publications/10policies/b3/17c.pdf

Yerxa, E. J. (1992). Some implications of occupational therapy's history for its epistemology, values, and relation to medicine. *American Journal of Occupational Therapy, 46,* 79–83. https://doi.org/10.5014/ajot.46.1.79

Appendix 19.A. Nuremberg Code (1947)

1. The voluntary consent of the human subject is absolutely essential.

   This means that the person involved should have legal capacity to give consent; should be so situated as to be able to exercise free power of choice, without the intervention of any element of force, fraud, deceit, duress, overreaching, or other ulterior form of constraint or coercion; and should have sufficient knowledge and comprehension of the elements of the subject matter involved as to enable him to make an understanding and enlightened decision. This latter element requires that before the acceptance of an affirmative decision by the experimental subject there should be made known to him the nature, duration, and purpose of the experiment; the method and means by which it is to be conducted; all inconveniences and hazards reasonably to be expected; and the effects upon his health or person which may possibly come from his participation in the experiment.

   The duty and responsibility for ascertaining the quality of the consent rests upon each individual who initiates, directs, or engages in the experiment. It is a personal duty and responsibility which may not be delegated to another with impunity.
2. The experiment should be such as to yield fruitful results for the good of society, unprocurable by other methods or means of study, and not random and unnecessary in nature.
3. The experiment should be so designed and based on the results of animal experimentation and knowledge of the natural history of the disease or other problem under study that the anticipated results justify the performance of the experiment.
4. The experiment should be so conducted as to avoid all unnecessary physical and mental suffering and injury.
5. No experiment should be conducted where there is an a priori reason to believe that death or disabling injury will occur; except, perhaps, in those experiments where the experimental physicians also serve as subjects.
6. The degree of risk to be taken should never exceed that determined by the humanitarian importance of the problem to be solved by the experiment.
7. Proper preparations should be made and adequate facilities provided to protect the experimental subject against even remote possibilities of injury, disability or death.
8. The experiment should be conducted only by scientifically qualified persons. The highest degree of skill and care should be required through all stages of the experiment of those who conduct or engage in the experiment.
9. During the course of the experiment the human subject should be at liberty to bring the experiment to an end if he has reached the physical or mental state where continuation of the experiment seems to him to be impossible.
10. During the course of the experiment, the scientist in charge must be prepared to terminate the experiment at any stage, if he has probable cause to believe, in the exercise of good faith, superior skill and careful judgment required of him that a continuation of the experiment is likely to result in injury, disability or death to the experimental subject.

Note. From "Nuremberg Code," in *Trials of war criminals before the Nuremberg military tribunals under Control Council Law No. 10* (Vol. 2, pp. 181–182), 1949, Washington, DC: U.S. Government Printing Office.

Appendix 19.B. Criteria for Institutional Review Board Approval of Research From the Code of Federal Regulations

§46.111 Criteria for Institutional Review Board (IRB) approval of research.

(a) In order to approve research covered by this policy the IRB shall determine that all of the following requirements are satisfied:

1. Risks to subjects are minimized: (i) By using procedures which are consistent with sound research design and which do not unnecessarily expose subjects to risk, and (ii) whenever appropriate, by using procedures already being performed on the subjects for diagnostic or treatment purposes.
2. Risks to subjects are reasonable in relation to anticipated benefits, if any, to subjects, and the importance of the knowledge that may reasonably be expected to result. In evaluating risks and benefits, the IRB should consider only those risks and benefits that may result from the research (as distinguished from risks and benefits of therapies subjects would receive even if not participating in the research). The IRB should not consider possible long-range effects of applying knowledge gained in the research (for example, the possible effects of the research on public policy) as among those research risks that fall within the purview of its responsibility.
3. Selection of subjects is equitable. In making this assessment the IRB should take into account the purposes of the research and the setting in which the research will be conducted and should be particularly cognizant of the special problems of research involving vulnerable populations, such as children, prisoners, pregnant women, mentally disabled persons, or economically or educationally disadvantaged persons.
4. ***Informed consent*** will be sought from each prospective subject or the subject's legally authorized representative, in accordance with, and to the extent required by §46.116.
5. ***Informed consent*** will be appropriately documented, in accordance with, and to the extent required by §46.117.
6. When appropriate, the research plan makes adequate provision for monitoring the data collected to ensure the safety of subjects.
7. When appropriate, there are adequate provisions to protect the privacy of subjects and to maintain the confidentiality of data.

(b) When some or all of the subjects are likely to be vulnerable to coercion or undue influence, such as children, prisoners, pregnant women, mentally disabled persons, or economically or educationally disadvantaged persons, additional safeguards have been included in the study to protect the rights and welfare of these subjects.

Source. From *45 C.F.R. §46.111. Protection of Human Subjects,* by Office for Human Research Protections, U.S. Department of Health and Human Services, 2005. Retrieved from http://www.hhs.gov/ohrp/humansubjects/guidance/45cfr46.html/

Chapter 20.

INTERPROFESSIONAL ETHICS WITH INTERNAL AND EXTERNAL COMMUNITIES

Janie B. Scott, MA, OT/L, FAOTA, and S. Maggie Reitz, PhD, OTR/L, FAOTA

Learning Objectives

By the end of the chapter, readers will be able to

- Describe ethical dilemmas encountered in internal and external communities,
- Identify potential interprofessional partners across continuums of care, and
- Apply Principles from the *Occupational Therapy Code of Ethics (2015)* to potential ethical dilemmas in interprofessional communities.

Key Terms and Concepts

- ✧ Conflict of interest
- ✧ Ethical tension
- ✧ External organizations and bodies
- ✧ Groupthink
- ✧ Institutional rules
- ✧ Interprofessional collaboration
- ✧ Interprofessional teams
- ✧ Interprofessionality
- ✧ Lateral attack
- ✧ Mobbing
- ✧ Verbal abuse
- ✧ Workplace bullying
- ✧ Workplace sabotage

Most occupational therapy practitioners in the United States work in either the health care or education industries within interprofessional teams (American Occupational Therapy Association [AOTA], 2015a). ***Interprofessional teams*** are composed of the patient or client and involve some or all of the following professionals: occupational therapy practitioners, architects, contractors, nurses, physical therapists, speech–language pathologists, educators, physicians, psychiatrists, social workers, engineers, driver evaluators, volunteers, and others. The term *interprofessional* is interchangeable with *colleague* and *peer*.

Since 2013 AOTA has increased its attention on interprofessional collaboration within and outside of the profession (AOTA, 2013). ***Interprofessional collaboration*** is "a partnership between a team of health providers and a client in a participatory, collaborative and coordinated approach to shared decision-making around health and social issues" (Canadian Interprofessional Health Collaborative, 2010, p. 24). Occupational therapy practitioners engage with other professionals in a process of ***interprofessionality,*** which reflects the exchange of ideas and strategies that will benefit clients without the intrusion of professional conflicts of interest.

The U.S. health care industry has evolved into a complex system of for-profit and not-for-profit agencies and organizations that attempt to meet the health care needs of the public. More than 25% of occupational therapy practitioners are employed in the education system (AOTA, 2015a), which provides early intervention services and education to children and youth from kindergarten through 12th grade as well as to students in higher education. Occupational therapy practitioners employed in higher education work in occupational therapy academic programs as educators or researchers, or in a combination of these two roles, and in administrative positions such as department chairperson or dean.

This chapter first discusses how occupational therapy practitioners work in such systems within their immediate work setting, with institutional professionals, paraprofessionals, staff, and consumers. Occupational therapy practitioners also interact with a variety of ***external organizations and bodies,*** defined as those outside the specific settings where occupational therapy practice and education directly occur. Ethical issues related to interactions with external communities are the focus of the second half of this chapter.

Ethical Tension Within Institutions

Ethical issues can arise in any institution, so all institutions should take steps to minimize their occurrence. Administrators of an organization or leaders of an association should lead by example in this regard; the *Occupational Therapy Code of Ethics (2015)* (referred to as the "Code"; AOTA, 2015c), together with other resources (AOTA, 2011, 2014, 2015b; Glennon & Van Oss, 2010; Slater, 2016), can help guide ethical behavior within institutions.

Ethical tension occurs when there are conflicting values among team members, including patients and their families. "Primary ethical tensions seen in the literature are broadly categorized as systemic constraints, value conflicts, witnessing questionable behaviors, and failure to speak up" (Kinsella, Park, Appiagyei, Chang, & Chow, 2008, p. 181). Ethical tension within institutions can result from behaviors that include

- Ensuring respect for institutional rules (see Vignette 20.1)
- Discriminatory behavior (see Case Study 20.1)
- Sabotaging and mobbing (see Case Study 20.2)
- Workplace bullying.

Preventive strategies to avoid ethical tension in the workplace include transparency in decision making, disclosure of potential conflicts of interest, self-monitoring of motivations and possible conflicts of commitment, respect for colleagues and others, and use of a framework for analysis of ethical

Vignette 20.1. Ensuring Respect for Institutional Rules

Virginia, an occupational therapy student, was enrolled in an evening kinesiology lab section. She chose that particular section because she wanted to have a class with an instructor who was "in the trenches" as a currently employed full-time practitioner. Virginia was excited to meet **Leneida,** the course instructor, who came to class in scrubs and looked like the vision that Virginia imagined for herself. Virginia did not mind that Leneida let the first class out early because Virginia wanted to get to a friend's birthday celebration. However, when Leneida let the next two classes out early, Virginia became concerned that she was not receiving the same educational experience as the students in the daytime lab section, which had been meeting for the entire designated time period.

Before Virginia could decide what to do, **Bart,** a full-time professor, came to observe the class as part of the department's regular peer evaluation process. Bart saw that Leneida was behind on the course content timetable, so during a break, he inquired as to why Leneida was behind. She responded that the students needed more time to absorb the material. A half-hour after the break, Bart saw that many of the students were packing up their materials and looking at the clock. Leneida, seeing Bart's concern, announced that the students should be prepared to stay the entire class time that night and in the future and that they might need to take shorter breaks to catch up on the required material.

Virginia was glad she did not need to take action that time but made a commitment to herself that in the future she would take action if a teacher was not following departmental procedures and policies.

dilemmas when an issue arises (AOTA Ethics Commission, 2011).

Respect for Institutional Rules

Institutional rules are the values, policies, and procedures established by institutions that guide the actions of staff, volunteers, and students. These reference guides and materials serve as resources in orientation, ongoing training, and daily performance to facilitate adherence to organizational standards. Institutional rules establish standards that are clear and enforceable.

It is commonly accepted that there is greater strength in numbers, as when people come

Case Study 20.1. Combating Discriminatory and Noninclusive Behavior in a Volunteer Role

Nancy and **Philip,** who worked together at a skilled nursing facility, decided they would like to be more active in their state occupational therapy association. Nancy shared an e-mail notice soliciting volunteers to join the conference committee to support the planning of an upcoming state association conference. She and Philip reviewed the commitments and timing of the conference, and they concluded the work was manageable. Nancy and Philip were excited about the opportunity to contribute to the profession. Together they approached their supervisor, **Reina,** to see if they could modify their work schedule so they could travel to the planning committee meetings.

As they drove to the committee's first scheduled meeting, Nancy and Philip talked about how excited they were to meet other occupational therapy practitioners around the state and become involved. They arrived and were scanning the room for familiar faces when someone yelled out, "Oh look, great! We have a guy. Now we have someone to fetch the coffee and carry the boxes." The comment was received with giggles and whispered comments. Both Nancy and Philip were taken aback, but they started introducing themselves to the other people present.

After the meeting, Nancy and Philip discussed the comment and hoped it was simply an isolated event and someone's poor attempt at humor after a long workday. At the next meeting, however, additional male-bashing comments were made. Both Nancy and Philip believed that their technology and social media skills could benefit the group's planning and ultimately the success of the state conference. However, they were uncomfortable with the group's repeated disparaging and discriminatory remarks about men. They decided to consult with their work supervisor, Reina, regarding possible responses to this unprofessional behavior.

Together with Reina, they identified the potential actions outlined in Table 20.1. They decided that the best approach was to suggest that the conference committee offer an educative program, such as the Speak Up! program developed by the Southern Poverty Law Center (2005), both at a conference committee meeting and at the conference. Nancy and Philip had received Speak Up! training when they were student leaders at the university where they received their occupational therapy education, so they were able to lead the training. At the presentation to the conference committee, group members initially were defensive and then became embarrassed about the impact of their behavior; however, they accepted that their behavior needed to change. A well-attended Speak Up! session was conducted at the conference, and its success was evident from conference evaluation data. To their delight, Nancy and Philip were asked to co-chair the following year's conference committee.

There are many models for considering ethical dilemmas. The process depicted in Table 20.1 simply asks the person with the dilemma to consider the situation from three different perspectives. First, what are the possible courses of action that the individual can take? After that is determined, the person considers the positive outcomes and negative consequences for each action. By weighing the major issues; consulting the Code, regulations, and institutional policies and procedures; and then considering the roles or scopes of practice for other team members, individuals should be able to make a more informed decision.

(Continued)

Case Study 20.1. Combating Discriminatory and Noninclusive Behavior in a Volunteer Role *(Cont.)*

Table 20.1. Decision Table for Case Study 20.1

Possible Action	Positive Outcomes	Negative Consequences
Quit the conference planning committee.	Nancy and Philip avoid an uncomfortable situation and the potential conflict resulting from addressing their concerns with the group.	This action does not confront the discriminatory behaviors and thus fails to uphold RSCs 4D and 6J and Principle 6. The committee loses the benefit of Nancy's and Philip's technology skills without knowing the true reason behind their decision to quit. Committee members are likely to continue their unethical behaviors.
No action; continue to participate on the committee.	Nancy and Philip avoid an uncomfortable situation and the potential conflict resulting from addressing their concerns with the group. Nancy and Philip continue to contribute their technology expertise to planning the state conference.	Philip may continue to be subjected to an uncomfortable environment. This action does not confront the discriminatory behaviors and thus fails to uphold RSCs 4D and 6J and Principle 6.
Contact committee chairperson to discuss their concerns and ask for support in addressing behaviors.	Nancy and Philip attempt to uphold RSCs 4D and 6J, Principle 6. This action is transparent with the committee chair and minimizes meeting disruption.	The committee chairperson might dismiss their concerns. Committee members may become defensive.
Offer to provide an educative program, such as the Speak Up! program developed by the Southern Poverty Law Center (2005), for the committee and at the conference to help people develop skills to address discrimination in a nonconfrontational manner.	This action upholds RSCs 4D and 6J and Principle 6.	Committee members may become defensive.

Note. RSCs = Related Standards of Conduct.

together to solve a complex problem or situation. However, even a group of competent, usually ethical people can make poor choices (AOTA Ethics Commission, 2011). ***Groupthink*** occurs when group members feel pressure to conform at the expense of logical thinking, thereby negatively influencing the group's effectiveness. This diminished level of function can damage individuals and groups inside the institution and even the institution itself (Engleberg & Wynn, 2007). Most important, groupthink can bring harm to the clients or students the institution is designed to serve.

Discrimination and Lack of Inclusion

One hallmark of the occupational therapy profession is its commitment to nondiscrimination and inclusion. This commitment is supported by the Code and detailed in the AOTA (2014) position paper, *Occupational Therapy's Commitment to Nondiscrimination and Inclusion.* This commitment not only extends to clients but also guides relationships among and opportunities within the occupational therapy professional community: "Inclusion requires that we ensure not only that everyone is treated fairly and equitably but also that all individuals have the same opportunities to participate in the naturally occurring activities of society, such as . . . participating in professional organizations" (AOTA, 2014, p. S23). When individuals are excluded from participation in the occupational therapy professional community as practitioners, clients, or professional colleagues, ethical tensions may exist. Understanding and sharing values creates communities of inclusion (see Case Study 20.1).

Workplace Bullying

Bullying at school and in the workplace is getting increased attention (American Medical Association, 2011; Briles, 1994; Seeley, Tombari, Bennett, & Dunkle, 2011; U.S. Department of Health and Human Services, n.d.; Workplace Bullying Institute [WBI], 2014).

Workplace bullying is "repeated, health-harming mistreatment of one or more persons (the targets) by one or more perpetrators. It is abusive conduct that is

- Threatening, humiliating, or intimidating, or
- Work interference—sabotage—which prevents work from getting done, or
- Verbal abuse (WBI, 2014, para. 1).

Briles (1994), in her studies of workplace abuse among female health care workers, reported unprofessional gossiping, sabotaging, and other abusive behaviors. In this research and in previous research across other professions, Briles consistently found that women reported being mistreated at work more by other women than by men. This finding is consistent with WBI's research, which revealed that women tend to bully women more than they do men. In addition, people with college educations reported being bullied more often than those with less education (WBI, 2010).

Given that the majority of occupational therapy practitioners are college-educated women (AOTA, 2015a), institutions need to take measures to prevent and confront bullying. Occupational therapy practitioners are not immune from experiencing moments of lack of judgment and unprofessional behavior with students, each other, colleagues from other disciplines, or clients. This type of behavior becomes increasingly troublesome when the behaviors turn into a pattern or the behavior escalates.

Sabotaging and Mobbing

Sabotaging and mobbing are abusive behaviors and are forms of bullying. Florence Clark, while AOTA Vice President, observed that the use of lateral attacks is one of the obstacles to women-dominated health professions securing power and using their expertise to enhance quality of life and save health care dollars (Clark, 2009). A ***lateral attack,*** also known as *lateral or horizontal violence or abuse,* "is the disruptive, disrespectful or antagonistic behavior of others on the same hierarchical level within an organization" (Fuimano-Donley, 2011, p. 5).

Bullying, launching lateral attacks, and mobbing are examples of ***workplace sabotage,*** in which an employee or group distracts energy and attention from tasks that could move a department, unit, team, task force, commission, professional organization, or profession ahead. According to Briles (1994), "In healthcare, women's sabotaging behavior will definitely be directed toward other women" (p. 57). Examples from Briles's research included "lying, spreading rumors about personal matters and professional abilities," ganging up on someone before a meeting, or making them a target of gossiping or backstabbing, among other behaviors (pp. 57–58).

Mobbing, or bullying or sabotaging by a group, has been described as "emotional abuse in the workplace" through "malicious, nonsexual, nonracial, general harassment" (Mobbing-USA, 2010, para. 1). Like other forms of bullying, mobbing disrupts productivity and harms the target's health and well-being (Lovell & Lee, 2011; Niedhammer et al., 2011) and professional reputation. Mobbing perpetrators can include supervisors and subordinates, as well as coworkers at the same level in the organization, and is usually done to force the target to leave the place of employment (Mobbing-USA, 2010). Occupational therapy practitioners are susceptible to engaging in this behavior; Case Study 20.2 discusses how mobbing or sabotaging can negatively affect the work environment and employees.

Verbal Abuse

Verbal abuse is a pattern of derogatory utterances that seek to disempower an individual or a group.

Case Study 20.2. Confronting Mobbing in the Workplace

An occupational therapy department with 24 employees within a large county hospital had undergone a series of staff changes over the previous 3 years. Two recent graduates, **Keira** and **Teri,** who had been classmates, were hired to replace the latest two employees who had abruptly resigned. Keira and Teri were invited to have lunch with three of the current staff, **Rosalyn, Ursula,** and **Desdemona.** They were excited to be asked to join what seemed to be the popular group. During lunch, Keira and Teri were told to steer clear of **Inga** because she "never carried her weight" and was the physical therapy director's "pet." This information was followed by smirks and other innuendos.

After the first week, Keira was assigned to the stroke care team and Teri to the orthopedic team; these two teams had different lunchtimes, so the women did not get to see as much of each other as they thought they would when they accepted the positions.

Keira was assigned to the same unit as Inga. At first, Keira was deeply suspicious of Inga and avoided her; however, one day she was having a difficult time with a complex patient, and Inga came over and offered her assistance. Later that day, after Inga had left for the day, Rosalyn, Ursula, and Desdemona started imitating her accent and insinuating that Inga had left to "hook up" with the physical therapy director. Keira became upset because she had believed Inga when she told Keira that she had to leave to pick up her sick child from school. Keira thought she had been duped by Inga, as the others had warned her. As she prepared to leave, Keira said to the others, "I wish I had listened to your advice. I can't believe I fell for her ruse!"

As Keira was leaving the hospital, she walked by the pharmacy, where she saw Inga with a young child at the prescription pickup counter. Inga was trying to manage her wallet and purse while holding the child, who obviously was not feeling well. Keira went in and asked if she could help and walked with Inga to her car, carrying the prescriptions and a humidifier, while Inga carried the child. After Keira got home, she reflected on how she had so quickly jumped to the wrong conclusion and had readily joined a mob that was spreading malicious rumors without merit. The following week, Keira started to have lunch with Inga and found her to be an excellent mentor and, as a single mother of three children, too busy to be having an affair with anyone.

Teri routinely went to lunch with Rosalyn, Ursula, and Desdemona and was shocked to hear them criticizing Keira for becoming friends with Inga and saying how they were going to give a negative report of Keira's first-month performance to the occupational therapy director. They further shared that they were angry with Keira because before Keira came, they had almost "broken" Inga and gotten her to leave. Teri sat stunned, but not as stunned as she was by the next information they shared: Ursula said, "We know that Keira and Inga are having a joint affair with the physical therapy director." Teri tried not to laugh out loud. Teri had roomed with Keira, a self-proclaimed prude, for more than 4 years before Keira married, and she was confident that Keira was still madly in love with her spouse, who was currently deployed for combat duty.

Ursula saw a slight grin on Teri's face and misread the reason. She stated, "That's right, Teri, we have your back. We will get rid of Inga and Keira. We are experts at weeding out those who don't listen or work too hard. With Inga and Keira gone, you will gain more seniority when we hire the next crop in a couple of months. Stick with us; you will be safe, and we can get coworkers who speak English and work to the rule!" Teri realized that Rosalyn, Ursula, and Desdemona were targeting Inga and Keira out of fear and prejudice, but she was terrified and did not know what to do.

After work, Teri texted Keira and asked if they could get together and discuss their new jobs. After they shared their experiences interacting with Rosalyn, Ursula, and Desdemona, they sat back and pondered what to do. They decided that they should first let Inga know of the plot. Inga was mortified when she heard. As a single mother, Inga did not want to risk being unemployed or receiving a bad reference. As the three of them talked, they determined that the best form of employment security and the most ethical step to take was to request a meeting with the occupational therapy and physical therapy directors.

(Continued)

Case Study 20.2. Confronting Mobbing in the Workplace *(Cont.)*

The meeting was scheduled for the following week. The next day, as Keira was changing into her scrubs, Ursula slammed Keira's locker closed and yelled, "I heard about your meeting. Who do you think you are? You'd better get in line, or the next time, I will slam that locker door on your fingers. Then see how much longer you will be working!" Two of the other occupational therapists who had been working at the hospital for a while were changing clothes on the other side of the lockers. They heard the exchange and approached Keira, who was now shaking and sobbing. One of them, **Priscilla,** said "OK; this has gone too far. We, and I mean *we,* cannot wait a week to have this meeting. We are going to human resources now!" An immediate meeting was called, and Rosalyn, Ursula, and Desdemona were placed on paid leave pending an investigation. Priscilla lamented that she wished she had spoken up sooner. Keira responded, "At least you had the guts to do so when I really needed you. I was ready to quit the minute she slammed my locker door, and I would have if you had not supported me."

As part of the investigation, the occupational therapy staff was interviewed. A culture of fear was uncovered. All of the occupational therapy staff, including Rosalyn and Desdemona, shared that they were fearful of Ursula and either participated in the mobbing or ignored it because of this fear. Although Ursula resigned before the investigation was completed, the occupational therapy director reported Ursula's behavior to the State Regulatory Board (SRB), AOTA, and National Board of Certification in Occupational Therapy (NBCOT). Keira, Teri, and Inga secured restraining orders against Ursula. Rosalyn and Desdemona received a reprimand and were placed on probation for a year for sharing privileged information inappropriately (i.e., gossiping), and the rehabilitation executive secretary who had informed Ursula of the meeting also was placed on probation. The executive secretary and the rest of the occupational therapy staff were encouraged to seek counseling if they found that they had difficulty coping with the outcomes of their actions or inactions. The hospital hired a consultant in workplace violence who recommended that all current and newly hired staff receive in-service training on bullying and mobbing prevention and that policies on workplace bullying be implemented and monitored.

The actions taken by Keira, Teri, Inga, Priscilla, and the occupational therapy director were supported by the Code, specifically Principle 2 (Non maleficence), Principle 4 (Justice), RSC 4D (advocate for fair treatment for all), RSC 5B (refrain from participating in false communication), Principle 6 (Fidelity), and RSC 6J (attempt to resolve violations internally). Failure to report Ursula's behavior earlier by Rosalyn, Desdemona, and the other occupational therapy staff put them all in violation of Principles 2, Nonmaleficence; 5, Veracity; and 6, Fidelity. However, whether they were either coconspirators or unwitting bystanders in fear of intimidation should be weighed against their failure to report Ursula's actions.

In addition, the occupational therapy director's actions were supported by RSC 2A (avoid inflicting harm) and RSCs 2F and 2I (avoid exploitative relationships). The director chose not to report the failure to report of Rosalyn, Desdemona, and the other occupational therapy staff because of their dual roles as offenders and victims. Although RSC 6J directs occupational therapy practitioners to "use conflict resolution and internal and alternative dispute resolution resources as needed to resolve organizational and interpersonal conflicts, as well as perceived institutional ethics violations (AOTA, 2015c, p. 7), the director reported Ursula to the SRB, AOTA, and NBCOT because of the egregiousness of her actions.

Verbal abuse can be directed at students, colleagues, clients, and clients' families. Most people have said something disrespectful to another person at some point out of frustration, fatigue, or stress. When this happens, an apology often follows with an explanation. Verbal abuse is different; the perpetrator seeks to use language as a tool to hurt and control another person or persons as shown in Case Study 20.2.

The nursing profession continues to build on the work done by Briles (1994) by investigating various types of workplace bullying, including verbal abuse. A recent study of nurses in

Florida found that 83% of male nurses and 85% of female nurses reported being a victim of verbal abuse (Small, Porterfield, & Gordon, 2015). *Verbal abuse* was defined by the researchers as spoken "behavior that creates emotional pain and mental anguish" (p. 69). Behaviors such as accusing, blaming, trivializing, harassing, berating, disguising as a joke, discounting, name calling, yelling, gossiping, and other behaviors were included in the study. The top three verbally abusive behaviors reported by the study respondents were (1) gossiping, (2) blaming, and (3) accusing. Nurses with less education and experience more frequently reported being victims of bullying. The most frequent perpetrators were supervisors and coworkers. Male victims of verbal abuse were less likely to report incidents than female victims.

It is important that occupational therapy practitioners, especially supervisors, be cognizant of this phenomena in health care and be proactive. Proactive measures to prevent abuse among employees are supported by Principle 2, Nonmaleficence, and RSCs 2A, 2C, and 2I. Efforts to prevent verbal abuse of clients also is supported by this Principle and these RSCs as well as the Principle 3, Autonomy, and RSCs 3A and 3F. Clients and their families are best served in an environment in which coworkers partner collegially to facilitate optimal occupational therapy outcomes.

Ethical Guidelines and External Organizations

Most institutions have principles and standards that govern and determine ethical parameters for the institution. These may be expressed in a code of conduct for employees, contractors, consultants, volunteers, and boards of directors (The Joint Commission, 2009). Organizations also have policies and procedures that direct the structure, format, and content of activities conducted in health care or educational institutions. The principles, standards, policies, and procedures may originate in ethical principles governing professional behavior in a certain culture (e.g., health care, school system, higher education).

Accrediting bodies also may impose standards and requirements with which an organization must comply to attain the accreditation or certification. Often accreditation is required to receive funds (e.g., a hospital must be accredited by Medicare to receive Medicare funding for patient services delivered in that hospital). Through an arrangement with the Centers for Medicare and Medicaid Services (CMS), the Joint Commission has "deemed status" to conduct the accreditation process for certain health care organizations. Standards for such accreditation include compliance with federal and state laws and regulations and other standards set by CMS. The Joint Commission may go above and beyond these standards—for example, in promoting higher quality of services—but organizations must be compliant at least with the required and relevant laws, regulations, and standards.

In addition, professionals working within the institution may have their own professional code of ethics or conduct that governs their practice in the setting. Institutions and organizations that represent professionals and nonprofessionals often have specific procedures for enforcing their code of conduct. For example, AOTA has the *Enforcement Procedures for the Occupational Therapy Code of Ethics* (AOTA, 2015b) to inform members and the public about steps that can be taken to address breaches of the Code. In the sections that follow, we discuss institutional and professional standards and ethical principles within the context of case examples of interactions with external bodies and organizations. Each case study is preceded by a short introduction to provide context and a foundation for decision making. Readers are encouraged to use one of the ethical decision-making models presented in Chapter 4 to analyze each case.

Legal Compliance

Organizational activities and employee conduct are to be in compliance with all applicable laws and regulations. Principle 4, Justice, of the Code states, "occupational therapy personnel shall promote fairness and objectivity in the provision of occupational therapy services" (AOTA, 2015c, p. 5). Under regulations governing grants given by the U.S. Department of Health and Human Services (DHHS), the DHHS is required to ensure that recipients of service be citizens or have legal status in the United States (U.S. Code of Federal Regulations, 1999). To provide services to people who do not have legal status is in violation of these regulations and may be considered fraudulent and an abuse of the system. In Case Study 20.3, an occupational therapist weighs consideration of the legal status of a client against the Principle of Justice.

Case Study 20.3. Ensuring Legal Compliance With Funder Requirements

Jane, an occupational therapist, provided services part-time to an early intervention program for developmentally challenged infants and toddlers. The program billed Medicaid for screening of the infants and toddlers and private insurance for screenings and intervention when possible. The program also received federal funds to pay for other program services and for clients who did not have Medicaid or other insurance, including consultation by the occupational therapist.

Jane received a referral to see **Kiku,** a 2-year-old girl whom a neighbor referred to the clinic's doctor because she was not crawling and failed to make eye contact with the parents or the neighbor. Kiku's parents did not have insurance; her father worked as a day laborer. Kiku had two school-age siblings who attended a local elementary school. Her mother was a full-time homemaker and used a cane because she had lost a limb after a guerrilla attack.

As part of her assessment, Jane learned that Kiku's parents, **Mr. and Mrs. San,** were Somalian and had been in the United States for 6 years. They fled Somalia when militant gangs threatened their city and attacked the mother. Kiku's father and mother had been interviewed at intake, and they both spoke limited English. **Sondra** was the team member who provided social work services, and she approached Jane to ask about the parents. She had been unable to get Mr. San to bring in his pay stub or give her sufficient information about his or his wife's background to enable her to assist the family in applying for government benefits (i.e., food stamps, special supplemental nutrition program for Women, Infants, and Children) and explore whether they might be eligible for Medicaid because of Mrs. San's disability. Sondra suspected that Mr. and Mrs. San did not have legal status but knew Jane had an upcoming home visit. She wanted Jane to see what more she could find out to determine if Mr. and Mrs. San were illegal immigrants.

The program administrator program indicated that funding was "tight" because many people in the community were losing their jobs and seeking care at the clinic. Jane even feared that her job as a contractor might be in jeopardy if funding were lost. She was unsure whether her program was legally permitted to provide services to illegal immigrants under their funding contract. Jane reviewed the Code in an effort to understand her ethical responsibilities to the child, the family, and her employer. In particular, she wondered if she had any ethical responsibility as an occupational therapist under the ethical Principle 4, Justice.

The questions about the family's legal status made Jane and the agency cautious. According to RSC 3A, "Occupational therapy personnel shall respect and honor the expressed wishes of recipients of service" (AOTA, 2015c, p. 4). Jane recognized her obligation to respect the family's right to privacy and to avoid placing them or the agency she worked for in legal jeopardy. Jane and the family needed to make sure they understood each other as well as the process. In addition, Principle 4, Justice, states "occupational therapy personnel shall promote fairness and objectivity in the provision of occupational therapy services" (p. 5; see also RSCs 4C and 4D). Jane had a duty to advocate for the services that might be legally available to Kiku.

Principle 4, Justice, also presents the expectation that occupational therapy practitioners, "should also respect the applicable laws and standards related to their area of practice" (AOTA, 2015c, p. 5; see also RSCs 4C, 4D, 4E, and 4N). Thus Jane had a legal and ethical obligation to comply with current laws, regulations, AOTA association policies, and her employer's organizational guidelines. Jane, and possibly the agency, was obligated to learn or seek consultation with experts regarding Kiku's legal entitlement to services. Jane also had a responsibility to inform the agency of her obligations under the Code, particularly if her compliance with her employer's policies placed her activities in conflict with the Code. The Code, which emphasize values, would support Jane's efforts to seek alternative avenues to providing Kiku's care if traditional means were unavailable.

Conflict or Duality of Interest

Conflict of interest is a "conflict between the private interests and the official responsibilities of a person in a position of trust" (Merriam-Webster, n.d.). These conflicts may concern real or perceived interests. The ethical principle of avoiding conflict or duality of interest requires that occupational therapy practitioners be loyal to their institution and employer. It prohibits practitioners from using their position to profit personally or to help others profit via their connection with the institution: "Having a financial interest in a business venture such as product sales related to occupational therapy, while providing occupational therapy services to the client may be perceived as a conflict of interest" (Austin, 2016, p. 161).

Conflict of interest is mentioned in Principle 2, Nonmaleficence, and Principle 6, Fidelity. According to Principle 2, "Occupational therapy personnel shall refrain from actions that cause harm" (AOTA, 2015c, p. 3); RSCs 2F, 2I, and 2J provide more detail as does RSC 6D, "Avoid using one's position (employee or volunteer) or knowledge gained from that position in such a manner as to give rise to real or perceived conflict of interest among the person, the employer, other AOTA members, or other organizations" (AOTA, 2015c p. 7). In addition, RSC 6C is relevant to discussions of conflict of interest. In Case Study 20.4, an occupational therapy assistant weighs an opportunity for advancement against his obligations to his employer.

Case Study 20.4. Examining Duality of Interest

Gaines Rehabilitation Services was a freestanding rehabilitation company that provided physical and occupational therapy services in a suburban community. A husband–wife team who were physical therapists owned the company. *Ed* managed the business, and his wife, *Leora,* supervised the day-to-day operations and provided physical therapy evaluation and intervention to patients. Staff included *Calvin,* an occupational therapist; two other physical therapists; *Lloyd,* an occupational therapy assistant; and two physical therapy aides. The company's clients included patients recovering from neurological conditions, including brain trauma; orthopedic injuries, surgeries, and disorders; and acute and chronic pain syndromes.

Lloyd, the occupational therapy assistant, had worked for the practice for 6 months. He liked Calvin and enjoyed the clients served by the program. In addition to direct intervention, Calvin and Lloyd ran a work tolerance program designed to help injured workers return to work after injury or surgery. Many of these clients were being seen in the practice under workers' compensation insurance, and others were referred by a managed health care company with which the practice had a contract to provide return-to-work services for injured workers. Ed sometimes encouraged the therapy staff to "keep the patients on program" for extended periods, even when the therapists believed the clients were ready for discharge from the work therapy or tolerance program.

Lloyd was uncomfortable with this situation and planned to discuss it with Calvin. In the meantime, **Harold,** a client case manager from the managed care company and old school friend of Lloyd's, stopped by to check on his patients' progress and to have dinner with Lloyd afterward. At dinner, Harold mentioned that the company's patients seemed to be having trouble when they returned to work and that it would be good if a service could be provided to assist the workers on the job. Lloyd said he would talk to his employer about this, but Harold said the managed care company was not very satisfied with Gaines Rehabilitation Services but might be interested in contracting independently with Lloyd to assist workers when they returned to their jobs.

This seemed like an opportunity for Lloyd to advance himself, although he was concerned about whether he could take Harold up on his offer without the supervision of an occupational therapist. He also was concerned about being disloyal to Gaines Rehabilitation Services and wondered

(Continued)

Case Study 20.4. Examining Duality of Interest *(Cont.)*

if he had any legal obligation to the company. Lloyd knew he should review his contract with the company and, if he had any questions, seek the services of an attorney. (FindLaw.com could help him identify attorneys in his area and with the skill set he needed.)

Was Lloyd obligated to tell his employer about his conversation with Harold (e.g., negative feedback about Gaines Rehabilitation Services and his potential job offer with the managed care company), even though he had not specifically signed anything that bound him to the company? Unless the contract or work agreement included restrictive covenants or noncompete clauses, employees may resign at will. However, they should abide by previously agreed on resignation notification time frames. Although no specific ethical principle required Lloyd to inform Ed of the other company's dissatisfaction with their services, reporting this information would be supported by the Code, specifically Principle 6, Fidelity: "Occupational therapy personnel shall treat clients, colleagues and other professionals with respect, fairness, discretion, and integrity" (AOTA, 2015c, p. 7). Specifically, RSC 6C ("avoid conflicts of interest . . . in employment"; p. 7) and RSC 6D ("avoid using one's position . . . or knowledge gained from that position in such a manner that gives rise to real or perceived conflict of interest among the person, the employer"; p. 7) provide guidance regarding a conflict of interest in this situation. Researching standards set by state boards of occupational therapy practice and AOTA might guide Lloyd's responses to this situation.

How should Lloyd resolve his discomfort with carrying out Ed's suggestions to keep clients on his caseload longer than Lloyd believed was appropriate and warranted? First, Lloyd needed to decide whether a client had reached maximum benefit in collaboration with the occupational therapist. Lloyd's professional and ethical responsibility in collaboration with the occupational therapist is discussed in RSCs 1H (terminate services when goals have been met), 4D (advocate for just, fair, ethical treatment), 5B (refrain from false, fraudulent, or deceptive communication), and 4O (ensure that documentation is in accordance with regulations) of the Code. Keeping clients on one's caseload who have reached their goals and are no longer benefitting from occupational therapy intervention is a violation of these standards.

Government Agency Relations

In addition to compliance with federal, state, and local laws, employees are required to be compliant with rules and requirements of government agencies, even when the relationship is not contractual. This obligation is relevant to federal grants and cooperative agreements (U.S. Code of Federal Regulations, 1999). State laws vary, and all practicing occupational therapy practitioners should be aware of the laws and regulations that govern practice in their state. The state licensure board and membership in the state occupational therapy association are recommended as sources of information on state laws, regulations, and information concerning requirements of state funding sources. Occupational therapy practitioners may engage with government agencies in many ways.

Local, state, and federal agencies, including hospitals and universities, have rules regarding the use of human research participants. For example, in 1991, the *Federal Policy for the Protection of Human Subjects,* or "Common Rule," was adopted as regulations that are applicable across many federal agencies (Office for Human Research Protections, DHHS, 2005). Ethical principles are identified in the Belmont Report, which formed the basis for the federal policy (see U.S. Department of Education, 2011).

The U.S. Department of Education's Rehabilitation Services Administration, in conjunction with states, provides grant funding to support the work of centers for independent living (CILs). Occupational therapy students and practitioners are sometimes involved with CILs as volunteers, staff, or board members. People with disabilities must form 51% of the members of the board of directors of a CIL. This percentage requirement also is applied to community boards, advisory councils, and commissions. The government also may pose requirements for racial and geographic diversity on boards.

The federal government, through the Individuals with Disabilities Education Act of 1990, helps families and individualized education program team members (which include occupational therapy practitioners) resolve ethical and legal disputes with the help of a mediator. The impartial mediator is considered external to the occupational therapist and his or her role. For example, if parents request an increase in the frequency and intensity of occupational therapy services for their child that is not supported by the school, a mediator may help the parties resolve the dispute (Scott, 2007).

In Case Study 20.5, an occupational therapy researcher must decide how to handle communication with the funders of his research regarding the difficulties he encounters in his study.

Case Study 20.5. Dealing Ethically With Funding Agencies and Organizations

Paul was an occupational therapist with a doctoral degree in disability studies. He was a faculty member and researcher in the occupational therapy department of a large university, where he was seeking tenure. Following a pilot study, Paul received a federal research grant to examine occupational therapy's role in health promotion in a program integrating primary care and behavioral health (e.g., mental health and substance abuse) to serve the needs of people diagnosed with serious and persistent behavioral health disorders. The research study protocol required patient consent and had defined selection criteria for diagnosis and level of functioning of each research participant. In his proposal, Paul indicated that in his 3-year study, he would enroll 75 participants in a subgroup of the program that had an occupational therapist working as the health promotion specialist and 75 control participants in another subgroup in which social workers provided the health promotion services. Previously, social workers had run other health promotion activities in a nonintegrated behavioral health system, but the program saw limited change in participants' overall health status.

Because of hiring and licensing difficulties, Paul's research program had a slow start. In addition, the program experienced difficulties integrating services because of differences in organizational culture between the primary care and behavioral health care practices.

In the program's 8th month, the occupational therapist was hired and began providing services to clients who entered the integrated practice and elected to join the health promotion group program on a rolling basis. By the end of the 2nd year, trends indicating an improvement in health status were noted in the research group; the lack of a statistically significant difference was attributed to the small size of the group run by the occupational therapist because of low enrollment in the overall integrated program. Paul's government project officer (GPO) and his department director were concerned about the low enrollment of participants in the research study. Paul tried numerous tactics to increase enrollment in the health promotion group program, but to no avail. He was counting on success in this study to further his aspirations for tenure and demonstrate that he could responsibly administer and use federal funds.

A colleague suggested that "there are ways" for Paul to seem to improve his results, in spite of low enrollment. This colleague had tenure and several significant grants completed in his portfolio and might potentially be on the committee that reviewed Paul's dossier for tenure. Paul wondered whether he could improve his results through alternate means but stay within the confines of his study parameters. He realized that most of the questions he faced could be answered through a review of the Code and a discussion with the GPO or grants manager.

Paul considered the options of falsifying his outcomes, lowering the study's entry criteria, or changing the methods used in his groups. RSC 2F of the Code reminded Paul to remain objective because altering the admission criteria might have a negative impact on the type and benefit of participation; RSC 2F states, "Avoid dual relationships, conflicts of interest, and situations in which a practitioner, educator, researcher, or employer is unable to maintain clear professional boundaries or objectivity" (AOTA, 2015c, p. 3). If Paul altered the selection criteria or the group interventions, the study outcomes also would be altered. If he decided to "fudge" the outcomes, future study participants might not be helped.

(Continued)

Case Study 20.5. Dealing Ethically With Funding Agencies and Organizations *(Cont.)*

If the admission criteria or group interventions were weakened to produce better outcomes, current or future participants might be harmed. If future researchers attempted to replicate Paul's work and wasted time and money, this might ultimately harm the public's perception of occupational therapy. RSC 1J states, "Conduct and disseminate research in accordance with currently accepted ethical guidelines and standards for the protection of research participants" (p. 3).

He also reflected on RSCs 5A and 5B, which address misrepresentation of the facts. The expectation articulated in these RSCs is to "represent the credentials, qualifications, education, experience, training, roles, duties, competence, contributions, and findings accurately in all forms of communication" and "refrain from using or participating in the use of any form of communication that contains false, fraudulent, deceptive, misleading, or unfair statements or claims" (AOTA, 2015c, p. 6).

Even though Paul was motivated to establish a positive working relationship with participants, faculty, his project officer, and potential funding agencies, it was imperative that Paul familiarize himself with all relevant policies, institutional and ethical, that might affect his work. His understanding was clarified after reading RSC 4L: "Collaborate with employers to formulate policies and procedures in compliance with legal, regulatory, and ethical standards and work to resolve any conflicts or inconsistencies" (AOTA, 2015c, p. 5).

If any of Paul's colleagues also were occupational therapy practitioners, Paul should share the Code with them (RSC 4E). If Paul believed that his colleagues were engaged in wrongdoing, his first step would be to follow RSC 6J (attempt to resolve violations using internal conflict resolution resources first). He also had to consider the implications of RSCs 1J (ensure that research is conducted in line with ethical guidelines) and 4K (report acts that appear unethical or illegal) before revealing his personal and ethical conflicts with this situation. This information might highlight to Paul's colleagues vulnerabilities in their thinking and behavior while keeping Paul compliant with the Code. If Paul's colleagues were to threaten him with a negative tenure review recommendation, Paul would need to follow up with his supervisor and attempt to handle the situation locally without escalating to the SRB, AOTA's Ethics Commission, or NBCOT, unless necessary.

There are still more questions in this complex case. What should Paul have told his GPO? What were his ethical responsibilities to the federal government for accepting the grant funds? Are there any differences in responsibilities to government funders versus private foundations? Principle 5, Veracity, of the Code states, "Occupational therapy personnel shall provide comprehensive, accurate, and objective information when representing the profession" (AOTA, 2015c, p. 6). Occupational therapy practitioners represent themselves and the profession in a wide variety of situations in which they are communicating information. They have an obligation to deliver reports, testimony, research outcomes, recommendations, and verbal and written materials in an honest and factual manner. Falsifying one's credentials or experiences is unethical and likely a breach of one's licensure law.

On further discussion, Paul believed that what his colleague was suggesting was unethical, and he considered how he might proceed. For both his government and private funders, Paul decided to contact the GPO and grants manager and accurately communicate the problems and difficulties he was experiencing as early as possible so they were aware of the situation and could suggest ways for Paul to proceed within the confines of his funding. Waiting for an extended period for things to improve might result in negative results and a lack of further support. Communication might be through a phone call, report, or other type of communication. This communication could result in positive assistance. For example, Paul's GPO might suggest he meet with the staff working on implementing the overall integrated project to determine why their enrollment was so low and explore ways to improve engagement of clients in the health promotion program that

(Continued)

Case Study 20.5. Dealing Ethically With Funding Agencies and Organizations *(Cont.)*

were ethical and allowed by the funding agency or organization.

Note. This vignette originally appeared in "External relationships: Ethical issues in interactions among institutions," by M. K. Scheinholtz and Janie B. Scott. In J. B. Scott and S. M. Reitz (Eds.), *Practical Applications for the Occupational Therapy Code of Ethics and Ethics Standards*, pp. 241–253. Copyright © 2010 by the American Occupational Therapy Association. Reprinted with permission.

Summary

Occupational therapy practitioners have a role to play in fostering healthy, meaningful relationships in the workplace (Glennon & Van Oss, 2010) and in professional organizations. This proactive preventive behavior is supported by the Code, specifically Principle 1, Beneficence; Principle 2, Nonmaleficence; and Principle 6, Fidelity.

As a profession, we communicate strategies to the public to prevent bullying of school-age students (AOTA, 2008, 2011, 2012, 2015d); we also need to consider what we can do as a profession to stop bullying, sabotaging, and mobbing at the workplace and among ourselves. We must always be vigilant and reflective to avoid engaging in behaviors that take time and attention from our responsibilities to students and clients. If we become aware of any such behaviors, we must be prepared to confront the perpetrators and take appropriate action consistent with the Code and the *Enforcement Procedures for the Occupational Therapy Code of Ethics* (AOTA, 2015b). Our profession and those we serve deserve nothing less.

Occupational therapy practitioners engage in numerous external relationships throughout their academic and professional lives. These relationships are established through organizations, agencies, governments, and institutions that have policies, procedures, and regulations that occupational therapy students and practitioners must follow. In addition to compliance with each set of standards, practitioners must adhere to ethical principles governing occupational therapy during service delivery. Occupational therapy practitioners are encouraged to continually update their knowledge of guidelines that have an impact on their relationships with external entities.

Reflective Questions

1. Lolita was angry about the outcome of a supervision meeting and disclosed to Darlene later that she had discretely taped their meeting on this and other occasions. Darlene knew it was against state law to audiotape anyone without his or her permission. She reinforced this to Lolita and then received verbal threats from her.
   - What steps should Darlene take?
   - Which Principles in the Code are relevant in this situation?
2. You have just been appointed to the transition team for your school system. Identify the types of interprofessional collaboration that may be required to help your students' transition post high school.
3. Your state occupational therapy association has invited you to represent the association on a statewide planning committee composed of organizations and state agencies whose mission is to analyze existing productive aging services and collaborate in planning for this population's future needs.
   - What barriers and opportunities do you see in this process?
   - How do you distinguish occupational therapy but ensure your participation is as an interprofessional team member?
4. Refer to the definition of interprofessionality. Describe which areas of the Code speak to the kind of interactions that are required across disciplines and how occupational therapy practitioners can ensure their roles are consistent with the Code and our scope of practice.

References

American Medical Association. (2011, August). One in five medical school grads report mistreatment; AMA taking action. *AMA MedEd Update.* Retrieved from www.ama-assn.org/ama/pub/meded/2011-august/2011-august.shtml

American Occupational Therapy Association. (2008). AOTA's societal statement on youth violence. *American Journal of Occupational Therapy, 62,* 709–710. https://doi.org/10.5014/ajot.62.6.709

American Occupational Therapy Association. (2011). *Mental health in children and youth: The benefit and role of occupational therapy* [Fact sheet]. Retrieved from http://www.aota.org/-/media/Corporate/Files/AboutOT/Professionals/WhatIsOT/MH/Facts/MH%20in%20Children%20and%20Youth%20fact%20sheet.pdf

American Occupational Therapy Association. (2012). *Children and youth: Bullying.* Retrieved from http://www.aota.org/practice/children-youth/emerging-niche/bullying.aspx

American Occupational Therapy Association. (2013). *AOTA forum on interprofessional team-based care.* Retrieved from http://www.aota.org/~/media/corporate/files/secure/advocacy/health-care-reform/forum-report.pdf

American Occupational Therapy Association. (2014). Occupational therapy's commitment to nondiscrimination and inclusion. *American Journal of Occupational Therapy, 68,* S23–S24. https://doi.org/10.5014/ajot.2014.686S05

American Occupational Therapy Association. (2015a). *2015 AOTA salary and workforce study.* Bethesda, MD: AOTA Press.

American Occupational Therapy Association. (2015b). Enforcement procedures for the *Occupational Therapy Code of Ethics. American Journal of Occupational Therapy, 69*(Suppl. 3), 6913410012. https://doi.org/10.5014/ajot.59.6.643

American Occupational Therapy Association. (2015c). Occupational therapy code of ethics (2015). *American Journal of Occupational Therapy, 69*(Suppl. 3), 6913410030. https://doi.org/10.5014/ajot.2015.696S03

American Occupational Therapy Association. (2015d) *Pediatric virtual chats: Prevention of and intervention for bullying* [Audio presentation]. Retrieved from https://otconnections.aota.org/galleries/aota_podcasts/m/pediatric_virtual_chats/120996.aspx

American Occupational Therapy Association Ethics Commission. (2011). *Everyday ethics: Core knowledge for occupational therapy practitioners and educators* (CEonCD; 2nd ed.). Bethesda, MD: American Occupational Therapy Association.

Austin, D. L. (2016). Ethical considerations when occupational therapists engage in business transactions with clients. In D. Y. Slater (Ed.), *Reference guide to the occupational therapy code of ethics* (2015 ed., pp. 161–165). Bethesda, MD: AOTA Press

Briles, J. (1994). *The Briles Report on Women in Healthcare: Changing conflict to collaboration in a toxic workplace.* San Francisco: Jossey-Bass.

Canadian Interprofessional Health Collaborative. (February, 2010). *A national interprofessional competency framework.* Retrieved from http://www.cihc.ca/files/CIHC_IPCompetencies_Feb1210.pdf

Clark, F. (2009). *The Centennial Vision: Power, branding, and OT state associations* (PowerPoint presentation at the Spring Program Directors Meeting). Bethesda, MD: American Occupational Therapy Association.

Engleberg, A. N., & Wynn, D. R. (2007). *Working in groups* (4th ed.). Boston: Houghton Mifflin.

Fuimano-Donley, J. (2011). What is "lateral violence"? *Advance for Occupational Therapy Practitioners, 27*(16), 5–6.

Glennon, T. J., & Van Oss, T. V. (2010). Identifying and promoting professional behavior. *OT Practice, 15*(17), 13–16.

The Joint Commission. (2009). *The Joint Commission code of conduct.* Oakdale, IL: Joint Commission Resources. Retrieved from http://www.jointcommission.org/assets/1/18/TJC_Code_of_Conduct_09

Kinsella, E. A., Park, A. J., Appiagyei, J., Chang, E., & Chow, D. (2008). Through the eyes of students: Ethical tensions in occupational therapy practice. *Canadian Journal of Occupational Therapy, 75*(3), 176–183. https://doi.org/10.1177/000841740807500309

Lovell, B. L., & Lee, R. T. (2011). Impact of workplace bullying on emotional and physical well-being: A longitudinal collective case study. *Journal of Aggression, Maltreatment and Trauma, 20,* 344–357. https://doi.org/10.1080/10926771.2011.554338

Merriam-Webster. (n.d.). *Conflict of interest.* Retrieved from https://www.merriam-webster.com/dictionary/conflict+of+interest

Mobbing-USA. (2010). *Definition: Mobbing is . . . emotional abuse in the workplace.* Retrieved from www.mobbing-usa.com

Niedhammer, I., David, S., Degioanni, S., Drummond, A., Philip, P., Acquarone, D., . . . Vital, N. (2011). Workplace bullying and psychotropic drug use: The mediating role of physical and mental health status. *American Occupational Hygiene, 55,* 152–163. https://doi.org/10.1093/annhyg/meq086

Office for Human Research Protections, U.S. Department of Health and Human Services. (2005). *Protection of human subjects.* 45 C.F.R. §46.111. Retrieved from http://www.hhs.gov/ohrp/humansubjects/guidance/45cfr46.html/

Scheinholtz, M. K., & Scott, J. B. (2010). External relationships: Ethical issues in interactions among institiutions. In. J. B. Scott & S. M. Reitz (Eds.), *Practical applications for the occupational therapy Code of ethics and ethics standards* (pp. 241–254). Bethesda, MD: AOTA Press.

Scott, J. B. (2007). Ethical issues in school based and early intervention practice. In L. L. Jackson (Ed.), *Occupational therapy services for children and youth under IDEA* (3rd ed., pp. 213–227). Bethesda, MD: AOTA Press.

Seeley, K., Tombari, M. L., Bennett, L. J., & Dunkle, J. B. (2011). Bullying in schools: An overview. *Juvenile Justice Bulletin.* Retrieved from https://www.ojjdp.gov/pubs/234205.pdf

Slater, D. Y. (Ed.). (2016). *Reference guide to the Occupational Therapy Code of Ethics* (2015 ed.). Bethesda, MD: AOTA Press.

Small, C. R., Porterfield, S., & Gordon, G. (2015). Disruptive behavior within the workplace. *Applied Nursing Research, 28*(2), 67–71. http://dx.doi.org/10.1016/j.apnr.2014.12.002

Southern Poverty Law Center. (2005). *Responding to everyday bigotry: Speak up!* Montgomery, AL: Author.

U.S. Code of Federal Regulations, 45, Part 72 and Part 94. Revised as of October 1, 1999. Retrieved from https://www.archives.gov/federal-register/cfr/subject-title-45.html

U.S. Department of Education. (2011). *Information about the protection of human subjects in research supported by the Department of Education—Overview.* Retrieved from http://www2.ed.gov/policy/fund/guid/humansub/overview.html

Workplace Bullying Institute. (2010). *The WBI U.S. workplace bullying survey.* Retrieved from http://workplacebullying.org/multi/pdf/WBI_2010_Natl_Survey.pdf

Workplace Bullying Institute. (2014). *The WBI definition of workplace bullying.* Retrieved from http://www.workplacebullying.org/individuals/problem/definition/

Chapter 21.

CULTURE AND ETHICAL PRACTICE

Shirley A. Wells, DrPH, OTR, FAOTA

Learning Objectives

By the end of the chapter, readers will be able to

- Describe the influence and effect of culture on ethical clinical decisions,
- Determine the unique ethical considerations when providing services to different cultural groups, and
- Apply cultural and ethical dimensions to decision making in occupational therapy practice.

Key Terms and Concepts

- ✧ Advance directive
- ✧ Autonomy
- ✧ Beneficence
- ✧ Compensatory justice
- ✧ Cultural bioethics
- ✧ Cultural effectiveness
- ✧ Distributive justice
- ✧ Ethic of diversity framework
- ✧ Ethical decision making
- ✧ Ethical dilemma
- ✧ Ethics
- ✧ Health care ethics
- ✧ Informed consent
- ✧ Justice
- ✧ Nonmaleficence
- ✧ Social justice
- ✧ Veracity

Ethics are by nature an extension of culture. The term *ethics* comes from the Greek word *ethos,* meaning "cultural custom or habit." ***Ethics*** is "a systemic study of rules of conduct that is rounded in philosophical principles and theory; character and customs of societal values and norms that are assumed in a given cultural, professional, or institutional setting as ways of determining right and wrong" (Slater, 2016, p. 291).

In the presence of cultural differences, health care practitioners frequently confront choices that depend more on moral and ethical values than on medical knowledge. The moral consequences of not respecting differences within a multicultural society are raising difficult questions for ethicists, policymakers, researchers, and practitioners. This chapter

Note. This chapter is adapted from "Culture and Clinical Practice," by S. A. Wells. In S. A. Wells, R. M. Black, & J. Gupta (Eds.), *Culture and Occupation: Effectiveness for Occupational Therapy Practice, Education, and Research* (3rd ed.), pp. 189–204. Bethesda, MD: AOTA Press.

examines how culture influences the ethics of health care decision making and policy. The ethical responsibilities of occupational therapy practitioners and the rights of the client and family also are explored.

Ethical Decision Making

Good intentions alone are insufficient to guide moral decision making: Consequences matter when applying moral principles and making a judgment. ***Ethical decision making*** is the mode of reasoning used to recognize, analyze, and clarify ethical problems and decide the right thing to do in a particular case (Pozgar, 2016; Purtilo & Doherty, 2011). It requires reflection and logical judgment and involves gathering relevant information, correctly applying ethical knowledge and skills (Purtilo & Doherty, 2011), and reflecting on one's actions from the perspective of moral theories.

According to Callahan (1995), good individual moral decision making encompasses three elements: (1) self-knowledge, (2) knowledge of moral theories and principles, and (3) cultural perception. Self-knowledge is fundamental to ethical decision making because one's feelings, motives, inclinations, and interests both enlighten and obscure moral understanding. Understanding moral theories and principles supports one's ability to make good decisions when dealing with people who hold different values. Understanding general ethical principles can help one foster dialogue and facilitate a resolution (Morris, 2003).

Cultural perception can challenge and influence ethical decision making. Stereotyping, bias, and ethnocentricity all involve cultural perceptions that can lead one to prejudge people, apply negative generalities about a group unfairly to members of an entire population, or prevent one from making an impartial judgment (Fremgen, 2012).

People are cultural and social beings, reflecting a particular culture at a particular time that shapes how they understand themselves, how they perceive moral problems, and what they view as plausible and feasible responses to moral problems. Recognizing that one's own behaviors are shaped and defined by one's specific culture can lead to collaboration and cooperation in making sound ethical decisions (Wells, 2016). Ethical decision making involves choice and balance. It is not easy when there are multiple routes to take (Chmielewski, 2004; Pozgar, 2016).

Health Care Context

What are occupational therapy practitioners' duties and obligations to the people whose lives and well-being may be affected by their actions? What do practitioners owe to the common good or the public interest? An ethical decision in health care is different from general ethical decisions because the domains of health care are different from other areas of human life and because medicine has its own moral approaches and traditions (Pellegrino & Thomasma, 1981). All health care practitioners have written standards of care that detail what is minimally required of them, and standards of care typically address ethical decision making.

Proponents of differences between general and health care ethical decision making argue that making a decision in a health care context requires a detailed and sensitive appreciation of the characteristics of health care practice and of the unique features of sick, injured, and dying people. The medical ethical literature emphasizes the imperative that health care practitioners keep a focus on the well-being of the whole person. Bishop and Scudder (2001) described the core of the health care practitioner as a "caring presence"—that is, a personal presence that assures the other of the practitioner's concern for his or her well-being. Therefore, practitioners must bring trustworthiness to the relationship. It is not that the ethical principles and virtues of medicine are different from the more general principles of ethics; it is the combination of general ethical principles and the context of health care that give health care ethics special consideration.

Health care ethics is the set of moral principles, beliefs, and values that guide practitioners in making choices about medical care. The ethical aspects of health care decisions help practitioners to make choices that are right, good, fair, and just (Kirsch, 2009).

Ethical Dilemmas in Health Care

An ***ethical dilemma*** arises when ethical principles and values are in conflict (Pozgar, 2016). Conflict occurs when competing interests create a problem; the dilemma occurs after the problem has been created. A dilemma arises when a person's concepts of what is right and wrong conflict with what he or she is supposed to do (Allen, 2013). It involves both ethical conflict and conduct. As Purtilo and Doherty (2011) described it, "an ethical dilemma occurs when a moral agent is faced with two or more conflicting courses of action but only one can be chosen as the agent attempts to bring about an outcome consistent with the professional goal of a caring response" (p. 60).

On the basis of cultural context and beliefs, when two values present themselves and one chooses one value rather than the other, one says that that value is more important than the other. For example, a respect for client autonomy that stresses the right of competent clients to make their own choices on the basis of their cultural context can conflict with the Principle of Beneficence if a client's choice may be harmful.

Professional ethics documents cannot make a practitioner ethical; they can only inform and guide. Occupational therapy practitioners need to develop and continually refine their cultural effectiveness in order to practice in an ethical manner. ***Cultural effectiveness*** is the ability to interact effectively with people and systems of different cultures and socioeconomic backgrounds by integrating and transforming knowledge about people and groups of people to increase the quality of services and better outcomes. The ethical Principles of the *Occupational Therapy Code of Ethics (2015)* (referred to as the "Code"; American Occupational Therapy Association [AOTA], 2015) most relevant to cultural effectiveness (Wells, Black, & Gupta, 2016) are

- *Principle 1, Beneficence.* "Occupational therapy personnel shall demonstrate a concern for the well-being and safety of the recipients of their services" (p. 2).
- *Principle 4, Justice.* "Occupational therapy personnel shall promote fairness and objectivity in the provision of occupational therapy services" (p. 5).
- *Principle 6, Fidelity.* "Occupational therapy personnel shall treat client, colleagues, and other professionals with respect, fairness, discretion, and integrity" (p. 7).

Wells (2016) recognized that culture may influence how people cope with problems and interact with each other. The perspectives of both practitioners and clients are influenced by the social and cultural factors that define each person. Each individual's background and experiences influence their personal beliefs and moral codes. If not handled correctly they will adversely affect the interaction. Therefore, the ways in which occupational therapy services are planned and implemented need to be culturally sensitive to be culturally effective.

Occupational therapy practitioners have an ethical responsibility to be culturally effective practitioners. Specifically, a Related Standard of Conduct (RSC) for Principle 3, RSC 3J, autonomy, which reads "Facilitate comprehension and address barriers to communication (e.g., aphasia; differences in language, literacy, culture) with the recipient of service (or responsible party), student, or research participant" (AOTA, 2015, p. 5), clearly articulates the responsibility to address the cultural needs of a client. The Code challenges occupational therapy practitioners to acknowledge and respect cultural diversity and find common grounds of morality.

Culture and Ethics

Ethical dilemmas and conflicts arise frequently in culturally pluralistic settings. Health care dilemmas often occur when there are alternative choices, limited resources, and differing values among clients, family members, and caregivers (Pozgar, 2016). Most questions center on whether health care practitioners are obligated to act in accordance with contemporary medical ethics in the United States or with respect for the cultural differences of their clients and their families' wishes (Ho, 2006; Jotkowitz, Glick, & Gezundheit, 2006; Paasche-Orlow, 2004). Problems arise when participants in the health care setting have different interpretations of illness and intervention, hold disparate values in relation to death and dying, and use language or decision-making frameworks differently (Kleinman & Benson, 2006).

Cultural bioethics refers to ethical questions in relation to the historical, ideological, cultural, and social context in which bioethical principles are expressed. Culture has become important in bioethics because of divergent viewpoints and judgments from various cultures regarding the many bioethical problems (Beck, 2014). Which practice among the many different practices in many cultures is the right one? Occupational therapy practitioners are obligated to fulfill their duties by respecting clients' attitudes and behaviors, but they should also observe common ethical standards with a special interpretation for different backgrounds and various cultures (Zahedi & Larijani, 2009).

Four commonly accepted principles of health care ethics, from Beauchamp and Childress (2013), form the core of a cross-cultural common morality:

1. ***Autonomy:*** Respect for the decision-making capacity of the individual;
2. ***Nonmaleficence:*** Avoidance of causing harm;
3. ***Beneficence:*** Provision of benefits and balancing of benefits, burdens, and risks; and
4. ***Justice:*** Fairness in the distribution of benefits and risks.

Although these principles can take different forms in different cultural contexts, they can be useful to consider in judging rightness and wrongness of beliefs and behaviors (Ebbesen, 2011; Zahedi & Larijani, 2009).

Autonomy

The law recognizes and upholds a person's right to make his or her own decisions about health care. People also have the right to know the risks and benefits of and alternatives to recommended procedures (Pozgar, 2016). The Principle of Autonomy and individual rights can be at odds with the values of some cultures and religions, and a focus on individuality can overshadow the interconnectedness of social relationships. Autonomy is relational and situated rather than a matter of individual choice (Zahedi, 2011).

Much of the world embraces a value system that places the family, the community, or society as a whole above the individual. In some cases, the good or primacy of the community may take precedence over the individual's autonomy (Crow, Matheson, & Steed, 2000; Zahedi, 2011). In Vignette 21.1, the patient and family are from a culture in which health care practitioners typically inform the family, rather than the patient, about a diagnosis.

Clients from all cultures want and need the support of their families. Recognizing the culturally prescribed role that families play when a loved one is ill demonstrates respect for individual values and wishes and supports the Principle of Autonomy (Jotkowitz et al., 2006; Kleinman & Benson, 2006; Zahedi, 2011).

To respect cultural differences when encountered, health care practitioners need to develop a level of comfort with client autonomy. Practitioners can accept a range of views and refrain from assuming that their clients share their own perspectives (Paasche-Orlow, 2004). Individual beliefs and reactions to illness cannot be ascertained or presumed on the basis of the client's language, education, class, or ethnicity. Issues of autonomy and individual rights, ethical and cultural value systems, and family processes are important in influencing the position and assumptions that clients and health care practitioners carry into and throughout the delivery of health care.

Autonomy is at the center of medical decision making regarding truth telling, informed consent, and advance directives (Glannon, 2005; Pozgar, 2016; Zahedi, 2011).

Truth telling (veracity)

The Principle of ***Veracity*** (i.e., the duty to tell the truth) is central to the practitioner–client relationship. It binds the practitioner to honesty (Purtilo & Doherty, 2011). Veracity is not about disclosing a unilateral truth to the client; it is about an ongoing process of communication

Vignette 21.1. Autonomy

A 52-year-old Nigerian immigrant, **Akoni,** had an abiding fear of cancer. He visited his doctor because of a small growth on his lip. The pair had a long-standing patient–physician relationship, and the doctor was aware of the patient's fear of cancer.

When the biopsy was completed, the physician informed Akoni's son and daughter of the Akoni's diagnosis and terminal prognosis. They asked that all information be withheld from the patient and one other daughter. They reported a strong cultural prohibition against the telling of bad news, explaining that disclosure would discourage hope and might hasten their father's death. They also expressed the fear that if their sister learned of the prognosis, it would place her unborn child at risk.

Did this physician have an obligation to inform the patient of the diagnosis, placing autonomy above all other values? Or was the physician obligated to follow the family's wish, thereby respecting their cultural custom?

with the client (Jotkowitz et al., 2006; Surbone & Zwitter, 2000). The ethical justification for truth telling exists in the legal requirement for complete disclosure and the necessity of avoiding malpractice (Pozgar, 2016).

Cross-cultural differences in truth-telling attitudes and practices have become a major source of debate. The application of truth telling can become a quagmire when multiple cultural views, values, beliefs, and practices are operative. The predominant practice in the United States of disclosing a diagnosis of serious illness to the patient is not considered appropriate by individuals of some ethnic and religious cultures (Fallowfield & Jenkins, 2004). Many Mexican Americans, for example, endorse the view that doctors should not discuss death and dying with their patients because doing so could be harmful to the patient, and this population also tends to place emphasis on family-centered decision-making styles (Candib, 2002). Similarly, Eastern cultures place more emphasis on the collective role of the family in decision making and disclosure.

Lai (2006) argued that truth telling is influenced by four major social–cultural and ethical factors:

1. Family as a key player in medical-related decision making
2. Harmony as an essential value for both the individual and family
3. Taboos about discussing death and related issues
4. Ethical concerns in truth telling (e.g., the predominant value of nonmaleficence [i.e., to do no harm] may lead to not telling the truth).

Surbone (2006) has suggested that imposing the truth on unprepared patients whose cultural expectation is to be shielded from painful medical information is culturally disrespectful or ineffective.

Advocates of truth telling believe that sharing information strengthens a trusting client–practitioner relationship (Zahedi, 2011). It is the duty of health care practitioners to ask clients if they wish to receive information and make decisions or if they prefer that their families handle such matters. In recent years, U.S. health care practitioners have learned to use listening skills and to let clients communicate what and how much they want to learn about their disease or condition. It is obligatory for health care practitioners to know how to provide information in a kind and considerate manner (Jotkowitz et al., 2006; Kleinman & Benson, 2006; Paasche-Orlow, 2004).

Informed consent

Informed consent is a legal and ethical concept that consists of two components: (1) the disclosure of all medical information to the patient, and (2) the right of competent patients to decide whether to accept or forgo treatment on the basis of the information given (Glannon, 2005). Although informed consent provides clients with the right to know the potential risks, benefits, and alternatives of a proposed treatment (Pozgar, 2016), it may be inapplicable to members of ethnic groups that traditionally make collective decisions among the family or tribal group (Ho, 2006).

Disclosing risks during an informed consent discussion and offering clients the opportunity to make advance directives can pose problems for adherents to traditional cultural beliefs. For example, the structure of the language in advance directives can be culturally insensitive. The traditional Navajo belief is that health is maintained and restored through positive ritual language. When health care practitioners disclose the risks of any intervention in an informed consent discussion, they speak in a negative way, thereby violating the Navajo value of thinking and speaking in a positive way. The Navajo traditionally have believed that thought and language have the power to shape and control events (Jotkowitz et al., 2006; Sico, 2013). Health care providers, including occupational therapy practitioners, have a responsibility to make sure that the client understands the possible and probable outcomes of refusing the proposed intervention.

Case Study 21.1 explores an occupational therapist's ethical decision making regarding the provision of informed consent. Occupational therapy practitioners should attempt to understand the basis for the person's refusal and address those concerns and any misperceptions the person or their family may have. Enlisting the aid of a leader in the person's cultural or religious community may be helpful.

Given the increasing diversity of clients, waiving informed consent or refusing family requests to withhold information from a patient cannot be taken lightly. It is important to open the channels of communication rather than impose an individualist

Case Study 21.1. Informed Consent

Bonita, a 55-year-old Spanish-speaking woman, status post-rotator cuff repair, arrives at the occupational therapy clinic with orders for passive range of motion (PROM) of the shoulder. She has limited understanding of English. Before the intervention begins, **Jessica,** the occupational therapist, describes and demonstrates to Bonita the procedures for passive manipulation of the shoulder. Jessica informs Bonita of the risks associated with this procedure, such as tearing of the repair, subluxation, pain, and impingement. The use of shoulder pulleys is also explained as an alternative treatment. Jessica explains that passive manipulation is the preferred intervention because the risk factors would be diminished as she would be able to prevent overly stressing the repair through her on-going assessment.

Can Bonita truly give an informed consent for occupational therapy? What if Bonita refuses the intervention? The next week, Jessica deviates from the original intervention plan requiring the use of a different modality, a form of manipulation added to the other procedures. Will this require a new consent from Bonita?

Bonita informs Jessica that she is seeing a "curandero" to heal her shoulder from the surgery. Jessica is uncomfortable with this and believes that this traditional practitioner can impede Bonita's progress. What should Jessica do? See Table 21.1.

TABLE 21.1. Decision Table for Case Study 21.1

Possible Action	Positive Outcomes	Negative Consequences
Take no action.	Bonita progresses with no problems.	Bonita heals at a slow pace or experiences complications from curandero's care.
Learn about the traditional belief and healer.	Acknowledgment of client's cultural belief and improved therapeutic relationships.	Bonita's compliance with therapy is poor due to stronger belief in traditional healer.
Take Bonita's request to work collaboratively with the curandero seriously.	Formulate a plan that is acceptable to Bonita, and Jessica. Bonita progresses in healing and regaining PROM.	Curandero may be offended and not want to collaborate. Bonita may cease therapy.

Note. PROM = passive range of motion.

approach to informed consent that could exacerbate the patient's and family's vulnerability and disharmony (Ho, 2006). Before sharing health information, health care practitioners need to assess the wishes of the patient, including whether the patient wants others present when information is provided (Crow et al., 2000).

Health care practitioners are not morally obligated to provide modalities or procedures that they do not believe offer a benefit to the patient or which may harm the patient nor should they offer interventions they do not believe competent to provide. (This is supported by Principles 1, Beneficence and 2, Nonmaleficence.) It is important to take the patient's request seriously, consider accommodating requests that will not harm the patient or others, and attempt to formulate a plan that would be acceptable to both the patient and provider (Diekema, 2013).

Advance directives

An ***advance directive*** allows people to make their wishes known regarding health decisions that must be made when they are legally incompetent, especially in the case of illness that will end in death (Purtilo & Doherty, 2011). Advance directives are processes accompanied by forms to help reassure clients that their wishes will be honored as much as possible. A key concept underlying advance directives is respect for a patient's right to give informed consent to health-related examination and intervention (Scott, 2013). These directives guide choices for practitioners and caregivers if the patient is terminally

Vignette 21.2. End of Life

John is a home health patient with a diagnosis of testicular cancer that has metastasized to his brain and lungs. On your recent home health visit, he said, "This will be your last time coming. No tribe members or family have visited in 3 days. And I do not want anyone present when the spirit leaves my body."

How would you respond to John's statement? Is it ethical for everyone to withdraw from the client? What would you tell the home health agency?

ill, seriously injured, in a coma, in the late stages of dementia, or near the end of life (see Vignette 21.2).

The realities of death and attempts to make plans for end-of-life scenarios may cause some ethnic groups, such as Mexican Americans and Korean Americans, to shy away from planning because they do not believe that preparing advance directives will bring them or their family any benefit in a situation they believe is out of their hands (Sico, 2013).

Nonmaleficence

The Principle of Nonmaleficence requires that health care practitioners not intentionally harm or injure the client, either through commission or omission in the performance of their job responsibilities (McCormick, 2013). The obligation to avoid or minimize the risk of harm is supported not only by commonly held moral convictions but also by the laws of society. Western societies place greater importance on harmful acts done with deliberate intent than out of neglect or ignorance (Purtilo & Doherty, 2011). Harm can extend beyond physical or psychological harm and may include harm to one's reputation, liberty, or property.

What constitutes harm may differ among clients as well as among health care practitioners (Garrett, Braillie, & Garrett, 2010). This Principle affirms the need for competence. Mistakes in health care occur; however, this Principle articulates a fundamental commitment to protect clients from harm.

Beneficence

Beneficence involves actions used to help other people. Occupational therapy practitioners have a duty to "prevent harm, remove harm when it is being inflicted and bring about positive good" (Purtilo & Doherty, 2011, p. 83). Occupational therapy practitioners must make an active decision to act with compassion, communicate with clients about what is going to happen, and consider the client's needs and feelings. Clients assume that practitioners are there for their benefit and will act with charity and kindness toward them (Purtilo & Doherty, 2011). Yet, what a practitioner may think is good for the client may not be what the client wants or thinks is good for him or her (Kornblau & Burkhardt, 2012).

The goal of providing benefit is at the very heart of population health care: to promote the welfare of people. Should all members of society receive all the health care they need? Should immunization be mandatory for children regardless of personal or religious belief? Beneficence entails an awareness of the inequality in some social structures (Allen, 2013). Doctors Without Borders, which provides medical care to the less fortunate around the world, is an example of an organization with beneficence as its foundation.

All occupational therapy practitioners must strive to improve their clients' health, to do the most good for all clients in every situation. But what is good for one client may not be good for another, so occupational therapy practitioners must consider each situation individually, taking into account cultural values that might conflict with the Code's Principles. See Case Study 21.2 concerning respect for cultural norms.

Justice

The Principle of Justice demands that occupational therapy practitioners be as fair as possible when offering interventions and allocating scarce health care resources. It is a form of fairness, giving to each person his or her due. If a patient arrives at the emergency room with a broken arm before another patient with a broken arm, the one who arrives first would expect to be seen first. However, if the patient who arrives second is bleeding profusely, the first patient would expect that person to be seen first. Practitioners should be able to justify their actions in every situation. The caring response is achieved when individuals or groups are treated fairly and equitably (McCormick, 2013; Purtilo & Doherty, 2011; Slater, 2016; Zahedi & Larijani, 2009).

Justice requires special concern for the poor and individuals from diverse backgrounds. These groups

Case Study 21.2. Respect for Cultural Norms

Brandi was at the end of her work day and had been treating clients since the 7:30 a.m. dressing program. She had lunch at her desk while completing paperwork. She couldn't wait to go home, take her new puppy for a walk, and just relax and rest to refuel for tomorrow's hectic schedule.

But as she was walking out the door, a local physician called and asked Brandi to conduct an evaluation. The client was a 45-year-old man with multiple sclerosis who is Muslim. (*Note.* During clinical examinations or procedures, Muslim men and women may be reluctant to expose their bodies. Health professionals should request permission before uncovering any part of the body and this should be limited to the minimum that is necessary.) Brandi is aware that to conduct the evaluation in a respectful manner will increase the time needed to between 1 and 2 hours.

Following the Principles of Nonmaleficence and Beneficence, what actions are available to Brandi? Complete a decision table to weigh alternative options.

are the least likely to have access to health resources and most likely to receive unequal care. Eliminating disparities in quality of care and addressing cultural preferences should form the basis of making health care decisions, which produces the best outcomes (Kluge, 2007; Scheunemann & White, 2011). The primary social obligation of health care providers is to ensure everyone has access to a tier of services that effectively promotes normal functioning and thus protects equal opportunity (see Vignette 21.3).

Distributive justice is concerned with the distribution of health care goods and services. It hinges on the fact that some goods and services are in short supply; when there is not enough to go around, some fair means of allocating resources must be determined. Is everyone entitled to receive health care benefits, and if so, is everyone entitled to the same amount? Distributive justice is the strong motivation behind health care reform to address the needs of the entire population. Distributive justice is based on the use of medical conditions to justify the allocation of resources such as in Medicare (McCormick, 2013; Purtilo & Doherty, 2011).

Compensatory justice assumes that the allocation of resources should be based on more than need alone. The individual's position in society also is a relevant factor (e.g., union, workers' compensation, nonprofit organizations). ***Social justice*** focuses on disparities in health and health care allocations such as differences between racial and ethnic groups in health insurance coverage, access to and use of care, and quality of care (Purtilo & Doherty, 2011).

Approaches to the Principle of Justice foster the societal goals of providing care in the face of limited resources. For occupational therapy practitioners, the Principle of Justice is applied when consulting at the bedside of individual patient; participating in business arrangements; selling products; choosing technology for clients; supervising students; and complying with laws, rules and policies, and is also addressed in systemically following laws and policies that govern the access of populations to health care (Slater, 2016).

The reasoning behind justice in occupational therapy is that practitioners should show due respect for people and avoid making absolute, prejudicial, or unsound distinctions (Purtilo & Doherty, 2011). Nor should they discriminate against people because of culture, religious, and lifestyle differences in the provision of occupational therapy services.

Occupational Therapy Practice

The challenge in providing ethical and culturally competent care is in the diversity of meanings that

Vignette 21.3. Nondiscrimination: Justice

Michelle, the director of occupational therapy, was notified that a new patient had been admitted to the rehabilitation floor for therapy. The patient was transgender, an anatomical male living as a female, who appears, speaks, and dresses as a woman. The patient requested a female occupational therapist for her activities of daily living training. There is only one female occupational therapist available to take on a new patient. What if this occupational therapist refuses to work with this patient on religious grounds? Consider the Principle of Justice. What should Michelle do to ensure equality in care?

can be applied to similar constructs and principles (Iwama, 2003). The meanings people assign to ideas and concepts are culturally based and culturally driven. Culture shapes people's views of illness and well-being in both the physical and spiritual realms and affects their perceptions of health care and the outcome of intervention. Occupational therapy practitioners may be comfortable with the idea of respecting cultural difference when the client is a competent adult, but when children are involved they may be unwilling to tolerate decisions that result in what they perceive to be compromised care or harm, even when these decisions make sense in the context of a particular culture (Jotkowitz et al., 2006). Cultural effectiveness is key to making sound, ethical, culturally appropriate decisions in clinical practice.

Practitioners and clients may not agree on a common set of cultural values. What may be regarded as morally wrong in one culture may be morally praiseworthy in another (Ho, 2006). For example, the sick role in occupational therapy is viewed as an active role, one in which clients achieve their optimal level of functioning through active participation. In other societies, however, the sick role is a passive role. In Chinese society, for example, it is sometimes believed that a person is chronically ill because of sins committed by family members. Thus, family members may try to do everything for the sick person, encouraging maximum dependence (Zahedi, 2011).

Beliefs and values serve as a basis for moral decision making and vary by culture. Ethics are greatly influenced by the cultural framework in which an interpersonal encounter takes place. Practitioners must be aware of the value assumptions embodied in biomedical approaches and in the culture, power, and ethics of medicine to identify how these assumptions play out in practice (Coward & Hartrick, 2000; Paasche-Orlow, 2004). Clients and their families, as well as occupational therapy practitioners, bring many different cultural models of morality and moral reasoning to the clinical setting. Constantly overlapping and interacting cultures can create daily conflicts and dilemmas when providing health care services.

Because present bioethical concepts of moral deliberation offer little insight into how to develop meaningful responses to cultural pluralism, religious diversity, and normal conflicts, Wells (2005) proposed an ***ethic of diversity framework*** with moral principles and rules of human conduct for finding resolutions in a pluralistic environment (see Exhibit 21.1). This framework, which includes the principles of understanding, tolerance, standing up to evil, fallibility, respect, cultural competence, justice, and care, can be used to guide decisions when conflicts arise in a multicultural setting. It can help health care practitioners and students engage in moral reasoning and test their moral opinions against those of others. It supports the expectation

Exhibit 21.1. Ethic of Diversity Framework

The following principles can be used to protect clients against harm and to help identify the good of people. These principles collectively assist occupational therapy practitioners in acknowledging differences as "norms."

- *Principle of understanding:* We seek to understand other cultures before we pass judgment on them.
- *Principle of tolerance:* We recognize that there are important areas in which intelligent people of good will, in fact, differ.
- *Principle of standing up to evil:* We recognize that at some point we must stand up against evil, even when it is outside of our own bodies.
- *Principle of fallibility:* We recognize that, even with the best of intentions, our judgment may be flawed and mistaken.
- *Principle of respect:* We recognize that all human beings are worthy of respect simply because they are human.
- *Principle of cultural competence:* We seek self-exploration, knowledge, and skills to interact effectively and humanely with people different from ourselves.
- *Principle of justice:* We seek to deal with everyone fairly and equitably in the distribution of goods and services.
- *Principle of care:* We recognize that the needs of others play a part in all ethical decision making.

These principles can be used to protect individuals against harm and to help identify the good of people. These principles collectively assist in acknowledging differences as the "norms."

Source. From "An Ethic of Diversity," by S. A. Wells, in *Educating for Moral Action: A Sourcebook in Health and Rehabilitation Ethics* (pp. 31–41), by R. B. Purtilo, G. M. Jensen, & C. B. Royeen (Eds.), 2005, Philadelphia: F. A. Davis.

of differences in all interactions within the health care system.

The values of ethical relativism and pluralism hold that practitioners respect the moral choices clients make in light of their culture or religious beliefs (Haddad, 2001; Paasche-Orlow, 2004; Zahedi & Larijani, 2009). Embracing these values increases learning opportunities and facilitates cultural effectiveness. Using the ethic of diversity framework as a guideline offers practitioners an opportunity to extend human knowledge by finding wisdom in dissimilar cultural practices. It allows them to teach clients what, from a medical point of view, may damage health and to learn more about the rationale for and techniques of many traditional practices. It assists practitioners in discovering ways to give care to people who have different values and lifestyles in their practice setting.

A cross-cultural ethical conflict may not have a single, ethically correct resolution but rather many possible resolutions, each with ethical costs and advantages (Pozgar, 2016; Purtilo & Doherty, 2011). Which resolution is ultimately chosen depends on which voices are included in the dialogue. Paasch-Orlow (2004) stated that culturally effective ethical decisions involve learning about culture, embracing pluralism, and minimizing the negative consequences of difference. A sound moral decision requires occupational therapy practitioners to reflect on their own values and biases, interpret the cultures involved, and acknowledge the contributions and principles of moral reasoning.

Summary

Clients and their families bring cultural, religious, and ideological beliefs to every client–practitioner relationship. If health care practitioners' views on the ethical principles that govern decision making conflict with the values held by clients, their families, or their communities, disagreement over cultural values may lead to confrontation. Respecting the beliefs and values of the client is important in establishing an effective therapeutic relationship. Conflicts based on cultural difference can be mediated using strategies that allow both the client and the practitioner the opportunity to clarify their values.

Each health care practitioner must embody an ethic of caring and respect for all groups, a responsibility to condemn unjust medical practices, and a humility and an empathy regarding human suffering. We must discover how to see each person as a cultural being, take the time to learn how the client and family define ethical values, and give weight to alternative values, social systems, and decision-making styles. As we face the ethical challenges of today—health care reform, widening health disparities, chronic disease management, and electronic medical records (Lachman, 2012)—let's not forget to be ethical and culturally effective occupational therapy practitioners.

Reflective Questions

1. How are occupational therapy practitioners in your practice setting made aware of existing client advance directives?
2. Identify and discuss ethical challenges that may affect occupational therapy practitioners in providing culturally effective care.
3. Which RSCs would support occupational therapy practitioners' commitment to being an ethical practitioner in multicultural settings?

References

Allen, J. F. (2013). *Health law and medical ethics for healthcare professionals.* Boston: Pearson.

American Occupational Therapy Association. (2015). Occupational therapy code of ethics (2015). *American Journal of Occupational Therapy, 69*(Suppl. 3), 6913410030. https://doi.org/10.5014/ajot.2015.696S03

Beauchamp, T. L., & Childress, J. F. (2013). *Principles of biomedical ethics* (7th ed.). New York: Oxford University Press.

Beck, D. (2014). Between relativism and imperialism: Navigating moral diversity in cross-cultural bioethics. *Developing World Bioethics, 15,* 162–171. https://doi.org/10.1111/dewb.12059

Bishop, A., & Scudder, J. (2001). Caring presence. In *Nursing ethics: Holistic caring practice* (2nd ed., pp. 41–65). Sudbury, MA: Jones & Bartlett.

Callahan, D. (1995). History of bioethics. In W. T. Reich (Ed.), *Encyclopedia of bioethics* (2nd ed., pp. 248–256). New York: Macmillan Reference.

Candib, L. M. (2002). Truth telling and advance planning at the end of life: Problems with autonomy in a multicultural world. *Families, Systems, and Health, 20,* 213–228. https://doi.org/10.1037/h0089471

Chmielewski, C. (2004). *Values and cultures in ethical decision-making.* Retrieved from http://www.nacada.ksu.edu/Resources/Clearinghouse/View-Articles/Values-and-culture-in-ethical-decision-making.aspx

Coward, H., & Hartrick, G. (2000). Perspectives on health and cultural pluralism: Ethics in medical education. *Clinical and Investigative Medicine, 23,* 261–266.

Crow, K., Matheson, L., & Steed, A. (2000). Informed consent and truth-telling: Cultural directions for healthcare providers. *Journal of Nursing Administration, 30,* 148–152. http://dx.doi.org/10.1097/00005110-200003000-00007

Diekema, D. S. (2013). Cross-cultural issues and diverse belief. *Ethics in Medicine*. Seattle: University of Washington School of Medicine.

Ebbesen, M. (2011). Cross cultural principles for bioethics. In G. D. Gargiulo (Ed.), *Advanced biomedical engineering* (pp. 207–214). Rijeka, Croatia: InTech. Retrieved from http://www.intechopen.com/books/advanced-biomedical-engineering/cross-cultural-principles-for-bioethics

Fallowfield, L., & Jenkins, V. (2004). Communicating sad, bad, and difficult news in medicine. *Lancet, 363,* 312–319.

Fremgen, B. F. (2012). *Medical law and ethics* (4th ed.). Boston: Pearson.

Garrett, T. M., Braillie, H. W., & Garrett, R. M. (2010). *Health care ethics: Principles and problems* (5th ed.). Upper Saddle River, NJ: Pearson Prentice Hall.

Glannon, W. (2005). *Biomedical ethics.* New York: Oxford University Press.

Haddad, A. (2001). Ethics in action. *RN, 64*(3), 21–24.

Ho, A. (2006). Family and informed consent in multicultural setting. *American Journal of Bioethics, 6,* 6–28. https://doi.org/10.1080/15265160500394531

Iwama, M. (2003). Toward culturally relevant epistemologies in occupational therapy. *American Journal of Occupational Therapy, 57,* 582–588. https://doi.org/10.5014/ajot.57.5.582

Jotkowitz, A., Glick, S., & Gezundheit, B. (2006). Truth-telling in a culturally diverse world. *Cancer Investigation, 24,* 786–789. https://doi.org/10.1080/07357900601063972

Kirsch, N. R. (2009). The nature of healthcare ethics. *Topics in Geriatric Rehabilitation, 25*(4), 277–281. https://doi.org/10.1097/TGR.0b013e3181bdd6af

Kleinman, A., & Benson, P. (2006). Anthropology in the clinic: The problem of cultural competency and how to fix it. *PLoS Medicine, 3,* 1673–1676. https://doi.org/10.1371/journal.pmed.0030294

Kluge, E. W. (2007). Resource allocation in healthcare: Implications of models of medicine as a profession. *MedGenMed, 9*(1), 57.

Kornblau, B. L., & Burkhardt, A. (2012). *Ethics in rehabilitation: A clinical perspective* (2nd ed.). Thorofare, NJ: Slack.

Lachman, V. D. (2012). Ethical challenges in the era of health care reform. *MEDSURG Nursing, 21,* 248–250, 245.

Lai, Y. (2006, July). *Views from Asia: Truth telling in cancer diagnosis and progress in Taiwan.* Paper presented at the World Cancer Congress of the Union for International Cancer Control, Washington, DC.

McCormick, T. R. (2013). *Principles of bioethics.* Retrieved from https://depts.washington.edu/bioethx/tools/princpl.html#prin2

Morris, J. F. (2003, February 24). Is it possible to be ethical? *OT Practice,* pp. 18–23.

Paasche-Orlow, M. (2004). The ethics of cultural competence. *Academic Medicine, 79,* 347–350. https://doi.org/10.1097/00001888-200404000-00012

Pellegrino, E. D., & Thomasma, D. C. (1981). *A philosophical basis of medical practice: Toward a philosophy and ethic of the healing professions.* New York: Oxford University Press.

Pozgar, G. D. (2016). *Legal and ethical issues for health professionals* (4th ed.). Boston: Jones & Bartlett.

Purtilo, R. B., & Doherty, R. F. (2011). *Ethical dimensions in the health professions* (5th ed.). St. Louis: Elsevier/Saunders.

Purtilo, R. B., Jensen, G. M., & Royeen, C. B. (Eds.) (2005). *Educating for moral action: A sourcebook in health and rehabilitation ethics.* Philadelphia: F. A. Davis.

Scheunemann, L. P., & White, D. B. (2011). The ethics and reality of rationing in medicine. *CHEST, 140*(6), 1625–1632. https://doi.org/10.1378/chest.11-0622

Scott, R. W. (2013). *Legal, ethical, and practical aspects of patient care documentation: A guide for rehabilitation professionals* (4th ed.). Burlington, MA: Jones & Bartlett.

Sico, R. (2013). End-of-life care: The legal, cultural, and interdisciplinary barriers hindering the effective use of advance directives. *Annals of Health Law, 22,* 44–63.

Slater, D. Y. (2016). Appendix A: Glossary of ethics terms. In D. Y. Slater (Ed.), *Reference guide to the Occupational Therapy Code of Ethics and Ethics Standards* (pp. 291–292). Bethesda, MD: AOTA Press.

Surbone, A. (2006). Telling the truth to patients with cancer: What is the truth? *Lancet Oncology, 7,* 944–950. https://doi.org/10.1016/S1470-2045(06)70941-X

Surbone, A., & Zwitter, M. (2000). Communication with the cancer patient: Information and truth. In *Annals of the New York Academy of Sciences* (2nd ed., pp. 109–118). New York: Johns Hopkins University.

Wells, S. A. (2005). An ethic of diversity. In R. B. Purtilo, G. M. Jensen, & C. B. Royeen (Eds.), *Educating for moral action: A sourcebook in health and rehabilitation ethics* (pp. 31–41). Philadelphia: F. A. Davis.

Wells, S. A. (2016). Cultural competency and ethical practice. In D. Y. Slater (Ed.), *Reference guide to the Occupational Therapy Code of Ethics.* (2015 ed., pp. 155–160). Bethesda, MD: AOTA Press.

Wells, S. A., Black, R. M., & Gupta, J. (Eds.). (2016). *Culture and occupation: Effectiveness for occupational therapy practice, education, and research* (3rd ed.). Bethesda, MD: AOTA Press.

Zahedi, F. (2011). The challenge of truth telling across cultures: A case study. *Journal of Medical Ethics and History of Medicine, 4,* 11.

Zahedi, F., & Larijani, B. (2009). Common principles and multiculturalism. *Journal of Medical Ethics and History of Medicine, 2,* 6.

Part IV.

TRENDS

INTRODUCTION TO PART IV

Janie B. Scott, MA, OT/L, FAOTA

The profession of occupational therapy evolves in response to the infusion of evidence into practice, regulatory changes, demographics (e.g., increased aging population), and incorporation of new technologies into communities and daily living. Chapters in Part IV are new to this edition and devoted to current trends and those that are anticipated for occupational therapy practice.

As the profession becomes more globally relevant and connected, Chapter 22, "Ethics in International Practice," provides readers with perspectives on international practice and introduces the utility of the Ethics in Cross-Cultural Human Occupational Emergent Situation (ECHOES) model that integrates with the principles articulated in the *Occupational Therapy Code of Ethics (2015)* (referred to as the "Code"; American Occupational Therapy Association [AOTA], 2015).

Chapter 23, "Environmental Modification: Ethics of Assessment and Intervention," explores different settings in which occupational therapy practitioners can evaluate environments, the skills they need, and ethical challenges that may be inherent in this practice area.

In Chapter 24, "Autism Across the Lifespan: Ethical Considerations," the authors consider the complexities of delivering ethical occupational therapy services to individuals with autism and their families as they transition through different life stages. Chapter 25, "Technology: Ethics in Service Delivery," informs readers about the past, current, and future uses of technologies by occupational therapy practitioners. In this chapter, external influences, interprofessional collaborations, competency, and certification are explored through an ethical lens.

Issues related to reimbursement and how it affects occupational therapy practice are discussed in Chapter 26, "Reimbursement: Ethical Considerations for Getting Paid—and Fairly." Payment mechanisms, regulations governing reimbursement, and application of ethical reasoning to complex systems are explored in this chapter.

Finally, in Chapter 27, "Current and Future Ethical Trends," the authors take a macro-level approach to the ethical dilemmas that current and future occupational therapy practitioners may face. It is important to appreciate where occupational therapy occurs from a demographic perspective (i.e., where services are and will be delivered by occupational therapy practitioners), as well as where current leaders and stakeholders envision the profession through *Vision 2025* (AOTA, 2016). Knowledge of the Code will assist occupational therapy practitioners to face the opportunities and challenges of the future.

References

American Occupational Therapy Association. (2015). Occupational therapy code of ethics (2015). *American Journal of Occupational Therapy, 69*(Suppl. 3), 6912310030. https://doi.org/10.5014/ajot.2015.696S03

American Occupational Therapy Association. (2016). *Vision 2025*. Retrieved from https://www.aota.org/AboutAOTA/Get-Involved/ASD/npp.aspx

Chapter 22.

INTERNATIONAL PRACTICE: ETHICS OF INTERNATIONALIZATION

Liliana Alvarez Jaramillo, PhD, MSc, OT, and Susan Coppola, MS, OTR/L, BCG, FAOTA

One cannot expect positive results from an educational or political action program [that] fails to respect the particular view of the world held by the people. Such a program constitutes cultural invasion, good intentions notwithstanding."
—Paulo Freire (1970, p. 76)

Learning Objectives

By the end of the chapter, readers will be able to

- Explain how self-awareness serves as a central component of ethical conduct when practicing internationally,
- Discuss ways in which understanding temporality serves to inform cross-cultural work that is both sustainable and ethical,
- Describe the importance of embracing uncertainty to act ethically in international contexts,
- Provide examples of how international practice calls for shifts in how occupational therapy practitioners enact key Principles of the AOTA *Occupational Therapy Code of Ethics (2015),* and
- Describe how the Ethics in Cross-Cultural Human Occupational Emergent Situations (ECHOES) model integrates transactional principles with the AOTA Code.

Key Terms and Concepts

- ✧ Cultural imperialism
- ✧ Cultural safety
- ✧ Ethical pragmatism
- ✧ Moral relativism
- ✧ Outcome bias
- ✧ Self-awareness
- ✧ Temporality
- ✧ Transactions
- ✧ Uncertainty

What comes to mind when you think about the ethics of international and cross-cultural practice? What images do those words evoke?

Perhaps a common image when it comes to an international situation is that of a bridge. Indeed, the notion of building a cultural bridge that rests upon the pillars of ethical principles illustrates some crucial components of navigating a cross-cultural exchange. Two cultures stand on opposite sides of a gap (i.e., ethical conflict). The Principles of Beneficence, Nonmaleficence, Autonomy, Justice, Veracity, and Fidelity can help bridge cultural distance and the resulting ethical tensions in the field.

These principles are understood, weighted, valued, and represented in fundamentally different ways among cultures. Perhaps the image of building a bridge to bypass the messy gap between two cultural shores overlooks the notion that avoiding ethical tensions in cross-cultural exchanges may not be possible or even desirable. After all, this difference draws occupational therapy practitioners to seek international collaborations and experiences and to reach beyond their professional comfort zones.

To address the ways in which occupational therapy practitioners can prepare themselves to navigate the ethical tensions that can arise in an international experience, this chapter proposes a model that can help practitioners approach cross-cultural ethical tensions. This model incorporates the Principles outlined in the *Occupational Therapy Code of Ethics (2015)* (hereinafter referred to as the "Code"; American Occupational Therapy Association [AOTA], 2015) but also integrates elements that are unique to intercultural experiences. The chapter discusses a series of case studies that expose readers to some of the potential ethical conflicts that can arise and the ways in which the Code can inform the necessary reasoning and decision.

Intentionally navigating the ethical landscape of an international professional experience requires an appraisal of its inherent complexity. Further, AOTA members are expected to abide by the Principles and Related Standards of Conduct (RSCs) within the Code, regardless of their geographical location. Thus, occupational therapy students and practitioners can benefit from a guiding model that can assist them in framing the critical elements of ethical conduct in international settings and can guide the necessary consideration on the practical application of the Principles outlined in the Code.

ECHOES Model

The ECHOES (*E*thics in *C*ross-Cultural *H*uman *O*ccupational *E*mergent *S*ituations) model is a guiding framework to approach cross-cultural ethics in occupational therapy. The model is based on a transactional philosophy that views humans as relational beings engaged in dynamic processes in the stream of time. In this view, each moment is co-constituted of people within a present situation as well as their history and intentions. Having a transactional approach refers to thinking about the ever-changing and interdependent nature of humans, the complexity of factors that are in each situation, and the uncertainty of the future.

The ECHOES model offers a transactional perspective for occupational therapy practice as a way to approach the uncertain and complex issues surrounding the ethics of internationalization as well as the practical application of the Code (AOTA, 2015). The model invites practitioners to consider the following elements as critical to navigating cross-cultural ethical tension: self-awareness, temporality, uncertainty, and transactions. Each is further explained below. In addition, the model guides practitioners through how each Principle outlined in the Code can be better applied in an international context if the above-mentioned elements are considered first.

It is worth noting that, like the Code, this model is not meant to be exhaustive. Occupational therapy practitioners who embark on an international experience are likely to face varying political, social, economic, and cultural complexities that this model cannot fully capture. However, we hope that this model will serve as a starting point, a safe harbor from which to begin a journey toward ethical conduct in international settings, and a guiding compass when embracing and navigating ethical tensions in the field. Figure 22.1 portrays the ECHOES model as a pinwheel, anchored in the process of self-awareness.

In the ECHOES model, ***self-awareness*** is a process of continuous and conscious reflection about one's own values, belief systems, identities, and lived experiences, and constitutes a central starting point for occupational therapy practitioners to act and interact ethically in a cross-cultural setting. From a place of self-awareness, practitioners must embrace

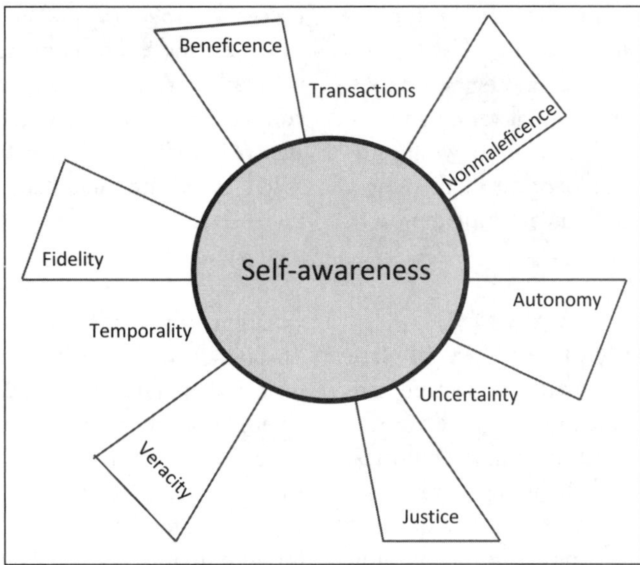

FIGURE 22.1

ECHOES model.

- Transactions,
- Temporality, and
- Uncertainty.

These essential elements can help practitioners understand the culturally informed shifts in the enactment of ethical conduct. Anchored in self-awareness and mobilized by the three elements, the Principles outlined in the Code project outward as moving blades. Ethical principles remain constant, but like moving blades, their meaning or practical application may shift as we characterize these same principles in the context of different cultures, societies, and communities. An echo reverberating in time and space is a metaphor for the infinite possibilities and effects of action.

Later in this chapter, the ECHOES model will be applied to examples of practices in underresourced areas because of the inherent power imbalances. Specific countries are not mentioned so that focus is maintained on the situation, rather than on specifics that may elicit biases from personal experiences.

Readers also are encouraged to consider applying ECHOES when practicing with immigrants and refugees as well as cross-cultural situations in high-resource countries. We refer readers to the *World Federation of Occupational Therapists Code of Ethics* (World Federation of Occupational Therapists [WFOT], 2005), which addresses ethical conduct, and related position statements on such topics as human rights (WFOT, 2006), international professionalism (WFOT, 2014b), diversity and culture (WFOT, 2014a), and telehealth (WFOT, 2014c).

Self-Awareness

Impartiality is rarely more unattainable than when it comes to cross-cultural exchanges. Regardless of our levels of awareness, occupational therapy practitioners enter cross-cultural interactions shaped by our values; political, social, and spiritual identities; and the experiences that make up the fabric of our lives. Learned habits of thinking form a bias embedded in the very things we value and the weight we give to certain factors over others. Thus, eliminating bias when exposed to a different culture is unrealistic at best.

Instead, self-awareness provides an opportunity for practitioners to recognize their belief system and identify the ways in which their own personal and cultural history has shaped what they believe to be right, true, good, and just. In turn, self-awareness allows us to grasp the ways in which other people's views are equally shaped by their personal and cultural histories. By engaging in continual reflection to distinguish and assess one's judgments and the consequences of the actions that emanate from them, occupational therapy practitioners become equipped to negotiate the unavoidable ethical tensions that arise in an international or cross-cultural context.

The process of developing self-awareness enables practitioners to notice when personal values and beliefs are projected onto others. In doing so, we are empowered to uphold the Principles of the Code using a culturally sensitive and contextually relevant approach.

Transactions

The construct of ***transactions*** holds a central place in the ECHOES model. Human transactions are complex, interdependent interactions that are under constant negotiation within familiar cultures. Transactions can be quite challenging in unfamiliar contexts. In international exchanges, occupational therapy practitioners may face a common tension that exists between two opposing views of cross-cultural bioethics. On one hand is an inclination toward enforcing the culture and values of a dominant group, historically that of Western societies, as universally applicable; this is known as ***cultural imperialism.*** The opposite view is that all moral claims can be considered relative, and ethical principles are applicable only in the cultures and context for which they are derived, referred to as ***moral relativism*** (Beck, 2015).

In a cross-cultural exchange, practitioners may find themselves inexorably pressed to decide whether their own views of morality and ethical conduct should dominate their view of the situation or whether the situation calls for an acceptance of cultural norms. The pitfall of this dichotomy is the well-established historical predominance of Western, middle-class, and anglophone perspectives on what guides and characterizes occupational therapy (Jull & Giles, 2012; Rudman & Dennhardt, 2008; Talero, Kern, & Tupé, 2015). The tendency is to opt, perhaps unknowingly, for an outcome bias in ethical conduct. An ***outcome bias*** (Baron & Hershey, 1988) is a tendency to judge the wisdom and appropriateness of a conduct based on the ultimate outcome it produces, perceived as good or bad. Case Study 22.1 illustrates the impact of a transactional approach to cross-cultural ethics.

Case Study 22.1. Ethics Embedded in Transactions

Anna, an occupational therapist, was serving for 6 months in a remote area of a foreign country. The local culture had patriarchal views of community and family leadership. Women's traditional roles included caring for children and older adults as well as preparing meals and housekeeping. Men were viewed as providers and protectors of the community; they worked long hours and did not get significantly involved with family affairs. Anna's responsibilities led her to a home visit with **Stella,** who had experienced a stroke after which she was dependent on her husband for most activities of daily living.

After their home visit, Anna was convinced that she could help Stella transition to greater independence, starting with bathing and dressing. However, Stella expressed a desire to remain dependent on her husband for these specific activities. Stella felt that her dependence greatly increased their intimacy and her husband's demonstration of love in his daily selfless caring for her. Stella was afraid that if she regained independence with bathing and dressing, her husband would be expected to return to the field instead of being supported by the other men while caring for her. Anna convinced Stella that independence should be her goal because it would increase her sense of autonomy and well-being. The husband was not included in the discussion or decision making because Anna felt this was something Stella should decide as a capable woman.

There were two possible outcomes of Anna's plan. Stella may believe Anna was right and be happy she agreed to this plan. Stella would then become more independent and return to her roles, and her husband would be encouraged by the outcome of his devoted care, after which he is more respected in the community. Based on that outcome, most people would agree that Anna's conduct was ethical as reflected in the Code's RSCs 4B, 4C, 4D, 4E, and 6J, among others.

Or, after regaining her independence, Stella could find herself facing feelings of loneliness and abandonment after her husband feels he must return to his traditional roles. The husband might start to work even longer hours than before. Stella

(Continued)

Case Study 22.1. Ethics Embedded in Transactions *(Cont.)*

and her husband might grow further apart, and Stella spiral into feelings of depression and isolation. What is your judgment on Anna's ethical decision making and conduct in this scenario? Although Anna's process was the same, we may feel justified in judging Anna's conduct as breaching RSCs 2A, 3A, 3C, 3J, and 4F.

What would it look like for Anna to engage in a comprehensive appraisal of the transactions that take place in this cultural exchange in which she finds herself practicing? First, it may help to recognize that in this context, the process of ethical deliberation means, by its very nature, that this is not Anna's situation; rather it is, at the very least, both Stella and Anna's situation. Any approach should provide space and opportunity for them to navigate their mutual options and beliefs. After engaging in a process of self-awareness and reflective inquiry, Anna will need to identify her own set of beliefs. She may ask herself questions such as, Do I believe personal independence has greater value than interpersonal intimacy? Why do I believe that Stella should make this decision by herself?

Figure 22.2 illustrates how Anna might apply ethical deliberation in a professional transaction to include her perspective and Stella's.

This ethical process begins with imagining possible scenarios that are uncomfortable relative to local cultural perspectives. Anna identifies her own personal and cultural beliefs and moral views of the scenario from a personal and professional standpoint. She enters into a deliberation with Stella (and possibly her husband) to understand her beliefs and goals, after which collaborative goal setting is based on Stella's desired outcomes.

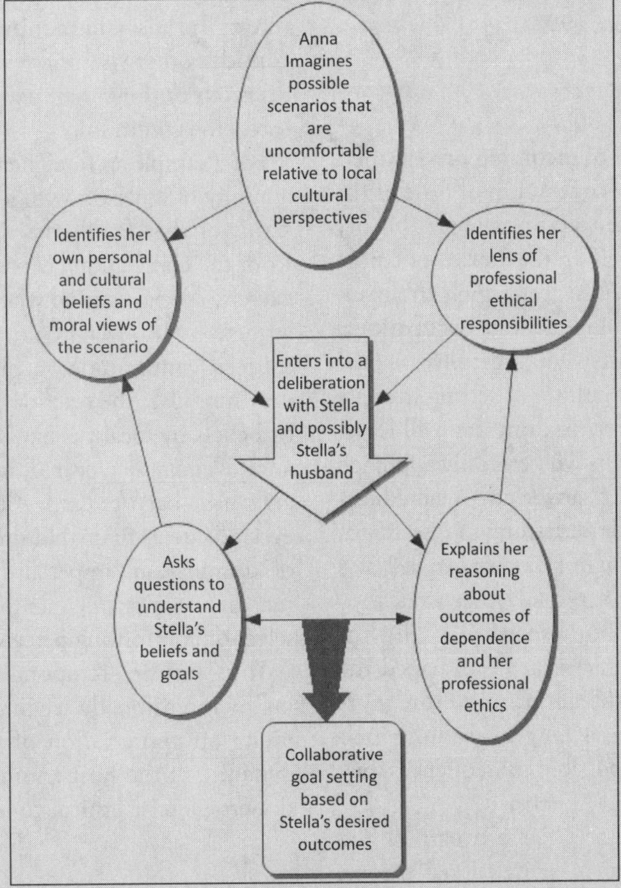

FIGURE 22.2

Anna's ethics embedded in professional transaction.

If understood as a transactional and reflective interaction, the ethics of internationalization do not need to favor imperialism or moral relativism. A transactional approach to cross-cultural ethics in occupational therapy involves a creative, imaginative, deliberative process of inquiry in which personal interpretation of ethical principles is not considered as a moral absolute but rather "hypothesis for action" (Dewey, 1922/2008; Fesmire, 2003; Vaughn, 2013). The practical application of ethical principles in such an approach involves Dewey's ***ethical pragmatism,*** which is

> a set of virtues which the agent or practical reasoner should possess: a willingness to work within the concrete circumstances in which he finds himself; a preparedness to examine the sources and consequences of his own dispositions; an openness to criticism and to the modification of desires and intentions in the light of new knowledge, and of the exercise of intelligence and imagination. (Festenstein, 1997, p. 45)

Temporality

Temporality is the ability of incoming practitioners to place themselves in the continuum of time of the international setting, understanding the past history of the local people as well as the future potential effects of their conduct. When engaging in an international cross-cultural interaction, occupational therapy practitioners must place themselves in the continuum of time of the culture or setting they are currently in, about to enter, and one day will leave. In other words, practitioners who ethically approach an international exchange of any kind—be it educational, service provision, or pertaining to research or volunteering—must, through awareness of self and transactions, be mindful of the fact that what they witness and experience is but a snapshot of the historical and cultural dynamics that have shaped the people, their physical world, and their culture. Further, practitioners must be willing to examine their actions in the light of the possible consequences they will have in the short and long term.

Understanding how past events are part of the current situation is central to transactional theory; however, temporality is highlighted in the ECHOES model to emphasize its importance in international contexts. For example, a history of charity model services in many regions has created harmful dependency patterns that require intensive and thoughtful work to develop true collaboration and trust. If occupational therapy services in the past have not been comprehensive, such as providing only sensory integration or neuro-motor interventions, then it may take a long time to change expectations of what the profession has to offer. If foreign occupational therapists have made local practitioners seem inadequate to local people, much damage must be undone. Future impact may be characterized along a continuum that begins with short-term direct service that is intermittent or taken away; to exchanges and education that eventually fade; to the sustained benefit of empowering and building local capacity such as an occupational therapy education program for locals. Needless to say, the most ethical approach is for sustained benefit, which requires far more time and investment than short-term approaches.

To uphold the Code in an international context, practitioners must consider temporality in actions and decision making. Knowledge of the history and culture of the host community can guide practitioners to consider otherwise unforeseen consequences of their decisions or those that may arise after the practitioner leaves the community.

For example, a foreigner having a homestay with a family of a person with a disability may elevate the status of that family or cause them to be excluded from the community. Moreover, practitioners should exercise special caution when it comes to unseen consequences. In several cultures, especially in underresourced communities, a practitioner's very presence may modulate the reactions or expressions of opinion or beliefs by local people. They may choose compliancy over conflict, even if they believe cultural boundaries have been crossed. Although this is not true in every context, many cultures are shaped by histories of domination, imperialism, and power dynamics that may prevent people from advocating for themselves or confronting perceived unethical actions.

Thus, infusing temporality in their ethical reasoning by intentionally seeking information and developing an appreciation of the history and cultural dynamic of the host communities will help practitioners exercise ethical conduct.

Uncertainty

Embrace ***uncertainty.*** A culture's set of values and beliefs is displayed in everything from time management to what stakeholders expect will result from a meeting and the time and pace at which things will progress and decisions will be made. Even when taking a proactive approach to preparing for an international, cross-cultural practice experience, practitioners must realize that critical elements of the culture and professional expectations of the host culture may remain uncertain and may even remain unspoken by the very nature of the local belief system.

Culture may vary within groups and families (Mattingly, 2010). Thus, uncertainty is perhaps the most common experience for which all occupational therapy practitioners engaging in an international, cross-cultural practice situation, regardless of geographical location and local history and culture, can prepare. Occupational therapy best practices in Africa are different from those in North America (Crouch, 2010; Sherry, 2010). Letting go of a position of control that overvalues knowledge obtained in a U.S. context enables practitioners to ethically engage in international transactions. Doing so provides an opportunity to embrace a new worldview, benefit from the local knowledge and experience, and grow in upholding professional conduct expectations and expanded human experience.

Ethical Principles in the Context of ECHOES

Throughout this chapter are descriptions and applications of the Code in international contexts. Additional resources that have informed ECHOES are the Capabilities approach (Bailliard, 2014; Hocking, 2013; Sen, 1979) and Young's work (1990) on diverse inclusive networks. Readers also are referred to Noddings (2003) and Van Amburg (1997) to learn about a relational approach to ethics. Given the diverse political, cultural, geographic, and economic situations internationally, sample scenarios and constructs that allow readers to consider how ethical principles can illuminate moral challenges in indeterminate situations are provided. Through the scenarios, the four-part anchor of the ECHOES model—self-awareness, transactions, temporality, and uncertainty—are reinforced.

Principle 1: Beneficence

Beneficence is practitioners' demonstrated "concern for the well-being and safety of recipients of their services" (AOTA, 2015, p. 2). International contexts require the understanding of beneficence not only in terms of physical well-being and safety but also cultural safety.

Cultural safety is a construct developed in New Zealand by nurses working with people of the Maori culture to address spiritual, emotional, and social safety (Williams, 1999). This construct informs our understanding of power imbalances for service recipients of a different cultural group than the provider (Gerlach, 2012). In occupational therapy, recognizing that all behavior has an ethical dimension, ethical practitioners must be mindful of power imbalances and avoid demeaning or dismissing another person's culture. Cultural safety requires a finely tuned sensitivity to subtle micro-aggressions that could detract from respectful exchanges. That sensitivity extends to culturally appropriate dress, body language, eye contact, and touching.

Principle 2: Nonmaleficence

Nonmaleficence requires occupational therapy practitioners to "refrain from actions that cause harm" (AOTA, 2015, p. 3). Considerable judgment and knowledge of the local context are needed to foresee subtle potential harm in cross-cultural situations. A perception that people from the United States have more advanced skills and techniques creates possible exploitation for financial or status gains for visitors, even when the information provider believes they are helping. Ethical problems are obvious when a person or organization knowingly participates in exploitation. Regardless of intent, the practitioner is responsible for avoiding nonmaleficence by educating themselves on the local context and reasoning through potential adverse consequences of actions.

Principle 3: Autonomy

A challenge that occupational therapy practitioners often face outside of the United States is a clash of communal rather than individualistic perspectives. The United States is known for having the freedom of opportunities and choices in work and leisure occupations. The occupational therapy profession is founded on these Westernized beliefs in occupational rights and choices for individuals (Kantartzis & Molineux, 2011).

Encounters with a culture that prioritizes group interests over individual preferences or needs can be a dissonant but transformative learning experience for people from the United States. Scholars in occupational therapy note that we are only beginning to understand the complexity of collectivist and individualistic occupations within cultures (Ramugondo & Kronenberg, 2013). Thus, each visitor must seek to understand family traditions, community interests, power relationships, and religious beliefs that may take precedence over an individual's interests.

For example, Buddhist temples have a threshold board on the floor to prevent ghosts and asuras from entering temples and sacred structures because it is believed that ghosts travel on a subground level. When considering physical accessibility, it is appropriate to recommend alternatives to access other than suggesting the board be removed for wheelchair users.

Self-awareness requires a realization of the ways individualistic views are but one perspective. Further, advocacy can take varied forms. A baby with little chance of survival may not be given the food or attention required by another child who, if well fed, can thrive and eventually provide for the family's survival. This situation, referred to as *lifeboat ethics,* can create dissonance for foreigners from the United States or other Western countries. If the baby has no hope of survival, the mother's strong bond to that child may heighten her grief at a time when she is overwhelmed with care for her other children. There is clearly no simple or correct answer to this dilemma. Providing the most for the weakest is too simplistic for such a context. In contrast, visitors to the United States are often appalled to learn that so many older people live in institutions rather than with their families.

The risk of breaching confidentiality increases when working with translators across language and cultural barriers. Great efforts are needed, for example, to gain truly informed consent for photographs, intervention, and research participation. Further, consent may reside beyond the individual and require permission by community and family leaders.

Principle 4: Justice

Human rights are a central tenet of U.S. laws, but constructs of justice can be enacted more strongly in other countries. For example, in countries where all people have access to health care, occupational therapy personnel may have more freedom to provide needed services.

However, a country's abundant resources do not ensure ethical distribution of services. Where there is competition for scarce resources and a history of oppression and corruption, human rights are often violated. When the practitioner is a visitor to such a region, enacting justice in the face of injustices and human rights violations can be overwhelming. If adequately prepared, foreign occupational therapy practitioners can be in a key position to provide care to underserved or marginalized groups and partner with local service providers or communities to promote culturally sensitive, contextually relevant, occupation-centered alternatives. Vignettes 22.1 and 22.2 provide positive examples of ethical international occupational therapy practice.

Knowledge of procedural contexts of international practice requires considerable research, as illustrated in Vignette 22.2. This research is consistent with RSCs 2A, 2D, 2H, 3D, 4B, 6B, 6F, 6G, 6H, 6I, 6J, and 6L.

Practice in another country is often in partnership with a university, a nongovernmental organization, or a business. A practitioner must know the mission, vision, and ethics of that organization, and those systems should align with the Code. Problematic examples are outlined in Exhibit 22.1.

Vignette 22.1. Using Occupational Therapy Skills to Address Problem of Justice

While visiting a homeless shelter for older adults, **Cyndi,** a visiting occupational therapist, noted a blind older adult with dementia tied by a sheet to his chair and a column in the building. Cyndi controlled her inclination to untie him or criticize the staff and asked if the restraint helped him stay safe and comfortable. She then asked if she could try some activities that would help him feel safer. Working with a staff member, Cyndi identified ways the man could be occupied and get sensory experiences that helped him remain calm and could occur during the limited time the staff could spend with him.

Vignette 22.2. Ethics of Respect and Collaboration With Local Occupational Therapists

Michael planned a visit to a country for a service project with people with HIV/AIDS. He inquired with the WFOT website resource guide for practicing in that country and learned the country required a $100 fee to the Ministry of Health to practice there, but had no licensure requirement. Next he found the website for a national occupational therapy organization and sent an e-mail to share his plans and ask for advice and collaboration. He asked if there was a shortage of occupational therapy practitioners or if there were occupational therapy practitioners currently out of work from whom he would be taking a job.

Well in advance, Michael gathered information on daily occupations, culture, religion, disability, and other sociopolitical information. He took an intensive course in the language and culture so he could communicate effectively. When he got to the country, he found a local occupational therapy practitioner with whom he had worked and focused his efforts on building collaboration and shared learning to support the practice of the local occupational therapist. This process was consistent with RSCs 3D, 4E, 4N, 6I, and 6L.

Exhibit 22.1. Examples of Problematic Misalignment Between the Code and an Organization's Mission and Vision

- An organization that operates on a charity model with services that promote dependency instead of building capacity for the local people to become self-sustaining, provide for themselves, or work as employees of the organization. (Beneficence)
- An organization that has a religious or evangelical mission in which occupational therapy service recipients must adopt beliefs, rituals, or other duties to receive services. (Justice)
- An organization that obscures the sources and use of funds and resources. (Veracity)
- An organization that exploits service recipients, such as use of photos without true informed consent. (Autonomy)
- An organization that brings foreigners in to do work rather than trains and employs locals. (Beneficence)

Principle 5: Veracity

The Principle of Veracity refers to the responsibility of occupational therapy practitioners to provide comprehensive, accurate, and objective information when representing the profession. Although this has clear applications in a relationship with an individual client, in international contexts, this Principle must be carefully enacted, especially in areas where occupational therapy services have not yet been established. International practitioners must be mindful of the breadth and scope of practice of occupational therapy and the importance of culturally relevant occupations.

When representing the profession in an international context, occupational therapy practitioners must carefully provide an accurate representation of the profession's scope of practice. Particular caution should be exercised to avoid approaches that overvalue foreign knowledge without regard of local needs, traditions, knowledge, and resources. In a favorable scenario, the presenting occupational therapist in Vignette 22.3 could work collaboratively with the national occupational therapy organization on a conference for occupational therapists and present sensory integration as one of many tools in occupation-centered practice.

Principle 6: Fidelity

The Principle of Fidelity requires practitioners to treat others with respect, discretion, and integrity. This is especially difficult when navigating an international

Vignette 22.3. Representing the Profession's Occupational Core

An **expert in sensory integration** was invited to present in a country that had few occupational therapists. That person provided a workshop to occupational therapists, practitioners from other disciplines, and laypersons. Some attendees then established sensory clinics in various locations and received pay from parents to provide services. Those clinics advertised that they were providing occupational therapy in regions that did not regulate the profession. Occupational therapists in the country then had difficulty establishing a full range of occupation-based services because parents and others believed that sensory integration was occupational therapy rather than just a small part of the profession. As a result, some occupational therapists could not find work or were just pressured to provide sensory integration for all clients despite their unique needs.

setting where limited awareness of the local customs and values can result in unintended offenses. Thus, practitioners should reflect on their own values and beliefs (i.e., self-awareness) but also be sensitive to the values and belief systems of local practitioners, clients, and communities.

To uphold the Principle of Fidelity in an international context, practitioners must ensure that they fulfill acquired commitments and that realistic expectations are adequately discussed and agreed on. Making unrealistic commitments is a common ethical tension that international practitioners face, exemplified in Vignette 22.4. Setting common goals while carefully considering the opportunities and barriers can provide a starting point to negotiate ethical tensions arising from Fidelity. Readers are referred to the AOTA International Interests portion of the AOTA website (AOTA, 2016) for up-to-date documents about international fieldwork.

Vignette 22.5 illustrates how a practitioner can proactively prepare for an international experience from an ethical standpoint, including being ready to enact the Code, which can be used to promote ethical engagement in international contexts.

Summary

The ECHOES model for thinking about ethics in a cross-cultural context in which relational ethics may be more relevant has been shared in this chapter. The model illustrates how a Principle-based approach of the Code can be enacted by allowing application of those Principles in dynamic and unfamiliar situations. From a core of self-awareness and mobilized by understanding complex transactions, recognizing temporality, and embracing uncertainty, the visiting occupational therapy practitioner is more likely to act ethically.

Reflective Questions

1. Reflect on and give examples of the cultural values that you uphold related to ethical Principles such as Autonomy, Veracity, and Fidelity. How might you adapt to function in a culture that has significantly different values from yours?
2. How might you apply the ECHOES model to preparing and delivering a workshop on your

Vignette 22.4. Setting Expectations

A **group of occupational therapy students** planned a learning experience to an underresourced area that included a homeless shelter for children with disabilities. They, like other groups who visit this hospital, were excited about opportunities to learn handling and physical intervention for children with disabilities. After a successful experience, one of the clients asked the student who had been working with her if he could promise to come back. The student, passionate about the experience and committed to the sustainability of the experience, hesitated to answer. After carefully reflecting on ethical conduct and the Principles of Veracity and Fidelity, he explained that he could not commit to returning because he was uncertain about the feasibility of such a commitment. The student discussed the client's request with the staff, and together they developed a strategy to promote and strengthen the experience among other students committed to international practice.

Vignette 22.5. Embedding Ethics Into Preparation and Readiness

An international opportunity in an underresourced international practice arose. **Students** were asked to apply for the experience by writing an essay about what they hoped to do. The **faculty** gained a sense of the students' ethical readiness using a rubric for scoring the survey based on the students' ability to

- Understand how the experience would benefit and transform them, rather than focus on changing or helping people who were less resourced;
- Demonstrate an interest in collaborative partnerships, instead of educating others on the ways of practice in the United States;
- Display flexibility for an unfolding process defined by the hosts, instead of expecting particular opportunities, such as hands-on experience;
- Recognize the power imbalance that is perpetuated when bringing objects like toys or gifts to underresourced areas;
- Focus on sustainability and potential unexpected consequences rather than short-term benefits of direct intervention; and
- Honor the host culture above personal need for self-expression.

area of occupational therapy expertise in another country?

3. Given that best practices are occupation and client centered, how and to what extent should a visiting occupational therapy practitioner learn culturally relevant occupations in preparation for work in that country?
4. Imagine or role play a scenario in which you explain your occupations through a translator to a person from a remote village in a far-off country with no technology. What can be learned from this exercise that will help you understand occupations in cross-cultural situations?

References

American Occupational Therapy Association. (2015). Occupational therapy code of ethics (2015). *American Journal of Occupational Therapy, 69*(Suppl. 3), 69134100301. https://doi.org/10.5014/ajot.2015.696S03

American Occupational Therapy Association. (2016). *International interests.* Retrieved from http://www.aota.org/practice/manage/intl.aspx

Bailliard, A. (2014). Justice, difference, and the capability to function. *Journal of Occupational Science, 20*(4), 3–16. https://doi.org/10.1080/14427591.2014.957886

Baron, J., & Hershey, J. C. (1988). Outcome bias in decision evaluation. *Journal of Personality and Social Psychology, 54,* 569–579. https://doi.org/10.1037/0022-3514.54.4.569

Beck, D. (2015). Between relativism and imperialism: Navigating moral diversity in cross-cultural bioethics. *Developing World Bioethics, 15,* 162–171. https://doi.org/10.1111/dewb.12059

Crouch, R. (2010). The relationship between culture and occupation in Africa. In V. Alers & R. Crouch (Eds.), *Occupational therapy: An African perspective* (pp. 50–59). Johannesburg, South Africa: Shorten.

Dewey, J. (2008). *Human nature and conduct.* New York: Barnes and Noble. (Original work published 1922)

Fesmire, S. (2003). *John Dewey and moral imagination: Pragmatism in ethics.* Bloomington: Indiana University Press.

Festenstein, M. (1997). *Pragmatism and political theory: From Dewey to Roty.* Chicago: University of Chicago Press.

Freire, P. (1970). *Pedagogy of the oppressed.* New York: Herder & Herder.

Gerlach, A. J. (2012). A critical reflection on the concept of cultural safety. *Canadian Journal of Occupational Therapy, 79*(3), 151–8. https//doi.org/10.2182/cjot.2012.79.3.4

Hocking, C. (2013). Book review [Review of the book *Health Justice: An Argument from the Capabilities Approach*]. *Journal of Occupational Science, 22*(4), 508. https://doi.org/10.1080/14427591.2013.864222

Jull, J. E., & Giles, A. R. (2012). Health equity, aboriginal peoples and occupational therapy. *Canadian Journal of Occupational Therapy, 79*(2), 70–6. Retrieved from http://search.proquest.com/openview/5520e2fe687af581394ee387082edbe9/1?pq-origsite=gscholar

Kantartzis, S., & Molineux, M. (2011). The influence of Western society's construction of a healthy daily life on the conceptualisation of occupation. *Journal of Occupational Science, 18*(1), 62–80. https://doi.org/10.1080/14427591.2011.566917

Mattingly, C. (2010). *The paradox of hope.* Berkeley: University of California Press.

Noddings, N. (2003). *Caring: A feminine approach to ethics and moral education.* Berkeley: University of California Press.

Ramugondo, E., & Kronenberg, F. (2013). Explaining collective occupations from a human relations perspective: Bridging the individual–collective dichotomy. *Journal of Occupational Science, 22*(1), 3–16. https://doi.org/10.1080/14427591.2013.781920

Rudman, D. L., & Dennhardt, S. (2008). Shaping knowledge regarding occupation: Examining the cultural underpinnings of the evolving concept of occupational identity. *Australian Occupational Therapy Journal, 55*(3), 153–62. https://doi.org/10.1111/j.1440-1630.2007.00715.x

Sen, A. (1979, May). *Equality of what?* Paper presented at the Tanner lectures on human values, Stanford University. Retrieved from http://tannerlectures.utah.edu/_documents/a-to-z/s/sen80.pdf

Sherry, K. (2010). Voices of occupational therapists in Africa. In V. Alers & R. Crouch (Eds.), *Occupational therapy: An African perspective* (pp. 26–47). Johannesburg, South Africa: Shorten.

Talero, P., Kern, S., & Tupé, D. (2015). Culturally responsive care in occupational therapy: An entry-level educational model embedded in service-learning. *Scandinavian Journal of Occupational Therapy, 22*(2), 95–102. https://doi.org/10.3109/11038128.2014.997287

Van Amburg, R. (1997). A Copernican revolution in clinical ethics: Engagement versus disengagement. *American Journal of Occupational Therapy, 51,* 186–190. https://doi.org/10.5014/ajot.51.3.186

Vaughn, L. (2013). *Doing ethics: Moral reasoning and contemporary issues* (3rd ed.). New York: W.W. Norton.

Williams, R. (1999). Cultural safety—What does it mean for our work practice? *Australian and New Zealand Journal of Public Health, 23*(2), 213–214. https://doi.org/10.1111/j.1467-842X.1999.tb01240.x

World Federation of Occupational Therapists. (2005). *World Federation of Occupational Therapists (WFOT) code of ethics.* Retrieved from http://www.wfot.org/ResourceCentre.aspx

World Federation of Occupational Therapists. (2006). *Position statement on human rights*. Retrieved from http://www.wfot.org/ResourceCentre.aspx

World Federation of Occupational Therapists. (2014a). *Position statement on diversity and culture*. Retrieved from http://www.wfot.org/ResourceCentre.aspx

World Federation of Occupational Therapists. (2014b). *Position statement on international professionalism*. Retrieved from http://www.wfot.org/ResourceCentre.aspx

World Federation of Occupational Therapists. (2014c). *Position statement on telehealth*. Retrieved from http://www.wfot.org/ResourceCentre.aspx

Young, J. M. (1990). *Justice and the politics of difference*. Princeton, NJ: Princeton University Press.

Chapter 23.

ENVIRONMENTAL MODIFICATION: ETHICS OF ASSESSMENT AND INTERVENTION

Rochelle J. Mendonca, PhD, OTR/L; Noralyn D. Pickens, PhD, OT; and Roger O. Smith, PhD, OT, FAOTA, RESNA Fellow

Learning Objectives

By the end of the chapter, readers will able to

- Describe the skills and training needed to perform a comprehensive ethical evaluation and interpretation leading to intervention recommendations;
- Articulate the decision-making relationships and required team functioning among the homeowner, family or caregiver, occupational therapy practitioner, occupational therapy student, and other providers in environmental and home assessments and interventions;
- Explain the importance and requirements for ethical practice related to measuring intervention needs and documenting outcomes of environmental interventions;
- Describe unique ethical challenges to environmental evaluation and intervention specific to the home environment; and
- Identify potential acts of comission and acts of omission that could lead to ethical issues in occupational therapy practice related to environmental assessments and interventions.

Key Terms and Concepts

- ✧ Acts of comission
- ✧ Contexts
- ✧ Environmental assessment
- ✧ Environments
- ✧ Gerotechnologies
- ✧ Interdisciplinary team
- ✧ Omitted activities
- ✧ Social context

This chapter describes the scope of practice and the interdisciplinary nature of environmental assessments and interventions. Adherence to the *Occupational Therapy Code of Ethics (2015)* (hereinafter referred to as the "Code"; American Occupational Therapy Association [AOTA], 2015b), promotes ethical occupational therapy practice in this and other practice arenas.

The diversity of contexts and environments that need to be considered during environmental interventions and the importance of a comprehensive approach to assessment, intervention, and outcome measurement are discussed. The importance of considering the client's social network, the fiscal possibilities and constraints, and the therapist's responsibility to see the project to completion during the process of home modifications also are covered. This chapter also discusses the importance of educating entry-level occupational therapy practitioners about home and environmental evaluation and intervention both in the classroom and through field experience.

Scope of Practice in Environmental Assessments and Interventions

Environmental assessments and interventions encompass the physical, sensory, cognitive, and social needs of individuals, groups, and populations in the built and natural environments (AOTA, 2010, 2014b). ***Environmental assessment*** is defined as the process of using specific tools, instruments, or systems to collect data on the environment inclusive of both physical and social environments.

Occupational therapy practitioners are well suited to conduct environmental assessments and interventions in both private and public spaces because of the profession's holistic educational model and client-centered approaches. The holistic approach is facilitated by prerequisite knowledge in physical motor rehabilitation, psychology, measurement, and lifespan development gained through completion of an accredited occupational therapy educational program. The profession's emphasis on activity analysis through the lens of motor, cognitive, sensory, and psychosocial skills provides a basis for understanding how people engage in occupation in different environments.

Interdisciplinary Teams for Environmental Assessment and Intervention

Environmental assessments and interventions are complex and interdisciplinary. Principle 6, Fidelity (Related Standards of Conduct [RSCs] H, I), requires occupational therapists to work with interprofessional teams when needed to provide the best quality outcomes for clients. A unidisciplinary approach is almost guaranteed to fail. Although occupational therapy practitioners have a broad background and a rich foundation on which to perform environmental assessments, the addition of a team facilitates a more comprehensive outcome.

Interdisciplinary team members, including builders or contractors, designers, social services experts, occupational therapy practitioners, and of course, the owner or resident, are essential for most environmental needs assessments and implementations. An important additional member of the team could be an occupational therapy student. Home environments serve as rich learning sites for occupational therapy students, who also can contribute substantially to the services with appropriate support and guidance.

When a complete team is not available, the core service provider members must be aware of their limitations so appropriate referrals can be solicited. Moreover, when outside team members, such as contractors, are included, the occupational therapy practitioner often becomes the team coordinator, organizing the team's activities to produce a successful outcome.

To be an effective team, all team members must understand the perspectives and assets of each possible contributor. Occupational therapy practitioners often must concertedly research the backgrounds of available home remodelers, social services experts, family members, homeowners, funders, designers, and architects and then include each in a given home evaluation and intervention as appropriate. It also is critical to understand the differences in perspectives and authority between the building owner, who views the longer term use of a home, versus a resident. Sometimes the resident may own the home, while other times the resident may be renting the space.

Case Study 23.1 depicts an occupational therapist using client-centered ethical decision making to secure community partners for simple environmental modifications, keeping expenses low for the homeowner.

Diversity of Contexts and Areas for Environmental Assessments and Interventions

Occupational therapy practitioners have a responsibility to evaluate and intervene with clients across contexts, environments, and practice areas. According to the AOTA's *Occupational Therapy Practice*

Case Study 23.1. Limitations of Going It Alone

Aimee received a referral from her home health agency to evaluate a new client, with a specific request to evaluate the home. Upon driving up to the home, Aimee saw that the concrete around the home was broken up, the front gate latch was held together with a rope, and a front porch light was without a bulb.

Mrs. McGee answered the door, using her walker for mobility. Mrs. McGee was clear and direct in her communication, had plans to "get used to this darn walker," and wanted to make her home easier to get around. Since returning home from a short stay at a skilled nursing facility, she had attempted to move furniture, but with continued pain from her rheumatoid arthritis, she was limited in what she could do. Mrs. McGee told Aimee she had "looked up everything she needs" and had a good sense of basic adaptive equipment options for her home.

Aimee assessed Mrs. McGee moving about the home, performing basic transfers, and doing homemaking activities. Widowed for 16 years and living alone, Mrs. McGee was accustomed to taking care of herself and her home. Aimee and Mrs. McGee discussed options and equipment that could make her home safer, including installing grab bars and handrails, improving lighting, exchanging round doorknobs for lever handles, and swapping current small drawer and cabinet knobs for longer pulls.

Mrs. McGee started crying as Aimee wrapped up her recommendations. "I am so tired of doing this all alone," Mrs. McGee said. Aimee used her therapeutic skills to support Mrs. McGee in expressing her stresses and promised to return to facilitate the modifications.

Although Mrs. McGee had some savings to put toward the needed changes, she was on a tight fixed budget. Aimee belonged to a worship community that had a group of volunteers who did basic home maintenance and cleanup for shut-in seniors.

Aimee's use of the Decision Table helped her determine her options for helping Mrs. McGee while maintaining client-centered ethical conduct (Table 23.1). Her task was to identify the possible actions and outcomes and which ethical principles would be relevant. She used the Code to identify the Principles and RSCs associated with the options that she considered.

Table 23.1. Decision Table for Case Study 23.1

Possible Action	Positive Outcomes	Negative Consequences
Call on friends from her worship community to complete basic home modifications (Justice RSC 4C; Core Value Altruism).	Recommendations completed with minimal cost (Beneficence; Justice RSC 4C).	Questionable skill set to accomplish recommendations and requires more team coordination. Potential conflict of interest because of perceived/ misperceived attempt to proselytize (Nonmaleficence RSC 2J; Fidelity RSC 6D).
Call on home modification contractor to complete basic home modifications (Beneficence RSC 1).	Recommendations are completed accurately (Beneficence RSC 1).	Higher costs, added financial stress, and requires more team coordination (Autonomy RSCs 3B, 3C, 3D; Justice RSC 4C).
Find social services agencies that have sliding scale for donated equipment (Justice RSC 4C).	Equipment provided at a lower cost (Justice RSC 4B).	Donated equipment may not be an appropriate fit for Mrs. McGee because of the limited options available. Requires vigilant follow-up (Nonmaleficence RSCs 2A, 2C).
Contact colleague at DME vendor to ask for discount (Justice RSC 4C).	Equipment provided at higher quality and most appropriate fit for Mrs. McGee (Beneficence RSC 1A).	Discount may still result in high costs (Autonomy RSC 3B).

(Continued)

Case Study 23.1. Limitations of Going It Alone *(Cont.)*

Table 23.1. Decision Table for Case Study 23.1 (*Cont.*)

Possible Action	Positive Outcomes	Negative Consequences
Post request for equipment donations on social media (Justice RSCs 4B, 4C; Core Values Altruism and Prudence).	Widens the opportunity to find equipment (Justice RSCs 4B, 4C).	Potential breach of confidentiality. Requires vigilant follow-up (Autonomy RSCs 3H, 3I).
Document in home health care record that Mrs. McGee appears overwhelmed and possibly depressed. Make referral to psychologist (Beneficence RSC 1I).	Mrs. McGee will get the intervention needed and in return will have reduced stress (Beneficence RSC 1A).	Additional costs for intervention and transportation (Nonmaleficence RSC 2A).
Refer Mrs. McGee to local support group for widows (Justice RSC 4C).	A supportive outlet to relieve stress and no longer experiencing life alone (Justice RSC 4C).	Additional transportation to and from support group meetings (Nonmaleficence RSC 2A).
Visit with Mrs. McGee 1 to 2 times per month when in the neighborhood with other clients (Nonmaleficence RSC 2B).	Informal check-ins for the therapist to provide Mrs. McGee with reassurance that the equipment and recommendations provided are helping (Nonmaleficence RSC 2B; Fidelity RSC 6K).	Lack of professional boundaries. Could cause Mrs. McGee to develop a dependence on the therapist's presence (Nonmaleficence RSC 2F).

Note. DME = durable medical equipment; RSCs = Related Standards of Conduct.

Framework, environments and contexts are distinct aspects that influence an individual's participation and engagement (AOTA, 2014a). ***Environments*** are the physical and social aspects of one's surroundings, while ***contexts*** are elements around a client that are less tangible, yet exert a significant influence on performance such as the cultural context, virtual context, personal context, and temporal context (AOTA, 2014a).

Occupational therapy practitioners must understand and holistically include all aspects of environments and contexts when performing environmental assessments and interventions. Occupational therapy practitioners also need to consider and evaluate contexts in all practice areas, including acute care, rehabilitation, skilled nursing, long-term care, assistive living, and home care. When evaluating the home, it must be considered in the larger context of the community, including neighborhood supports and resources.

In addition to recognizing how contexts affect the person–environment transaction, including cultural, personal, temporal, and virtual contexts, ongoing continuing education in assistive technologies and building design and construction deepens occupational therapy practitioners' skill set for environmental assessment. Environmental modifications are inherently about doing what is right and good for the client's safety and occupational performance. The ethical Principle of Beneficence is evident when occupational therapists are competent to complete environmental assessments and interventions as supported by RSCs 1D, 1E, and 1G. The client may have complex needs or the simple desire to age in place. Different levels of knowledge and skill are required to serve different client groups within a range of contexts.

Comprehensive Approach to Environmental Modifications

A comprehensive approach to environmental modifications includes evaluation, intervention, and outcome measurement. The evaluation should include assessment of the person, environment, and occupation. This should be done using data collection tools or instruments that can be used for evaluating needs; determining modifications to the environment, occupation, or need for technology; and establishing baseline measures. Interventions for environmental modifications should always consider the client's priorities and recommend services and products that are needed for optimal occupational performance. On completion of implementing interventions, it is important to measure outcomes that can document the effectiveness of the interventions and modifications.

Evaluation

Environmental modification begins with an assessment of the person, environment, and occupation. An environmental assessment collects data on both the physical and social the environment. Ecological models of practice serve as theoretical foundations for assessment and intervention approaches. The Ecology of Human Performance model emphasizes context to best understand a person's performance (Dunn, Brown, & McGuigan, 1994). Occupational performance of a task is influenced by the person's characteristics; the person's physical, social, and cultural environment; and the nature of the task itself (Weeks, Lamb, & Pickens, 2010).

The Person–Environment–Occupation (PEO) model emphasizes the interaction of person (e.g., mind, body, spirit), environment (e.g., social, physical), and occupation (e.g., fulfilling roles, demands) to produce occupational performance. The more harmonious the transaction, the better the PEO fit (Law et al., 1996). Most assessment tools for the home environment are client centered, although arguably some more than others (Weeks et al., 2010). Maintaining a client-centered approach addresses potential ethical concerns around Principle 3, Autonomy, and how much control the client has over the assessment and interventions.

Beginning with an occupational profile, the occupational therapist seeks to understand the person for whom the evaluation is being conducted. The client's responses to the occupational therapist's questions capture how the person lives in the home environment and what occupations the individual is able and unable to do or has difficulty doing because of the home environment's constraints. The evaluation includes viewing the physical aspects of the home and observing the client performing activities or skills in the environment.

A comprehensive evaluation can take considerable time and can create an undue burden on a client and other team members. Practitioners have access to new technologies for assessment that can reduce the homeowner's time and effort; for example, web-based assessments facilitate capturing data beyond paper and pencil. However, as with any electronic data collection and transfer, the occupational therapy practitioner must take care to protect the homeowner's privacy. Principle 3, Autonomy, RSC 3H states that "occupational therapy personnel shall maintain the confidentiality of all . . . communications, in compliance with all applicable laws" (AOTA, 2015b, p. 4). Web access also offers the practitioner and homeowner more product choices (Sanford, 2010).

Assessment tools serve different purposes in practice. Diagnostic and descriptive assessments provide information about problems, including severity of the problem. Comparative and conclusive assessments monitor progress and determine the effectiveness of interventions (Hinojosa & Kramer, 2014). The former help determine intervention approaches and specific modifications to the environment, occupation, or need for technology, whereas the latter determine the effects of interventions as outcome measures. These assessments provide scores that can be compared after the intervention is complete and serve as outcome measures.

The reliability and validity of environmental assessments can be tenuous. Many therapists use their own homemade checklists and assessments. Although this can be effective for informal data collection and intervention planning, it is always more ethical to use an instrument that has been tested for its effectiveness (RSC 1C) when one is available. Examining reliability and validity documentation or using tools with evidence of acceptable reliability and validity are two methods to comply with ethical assessment protocols. Law and colleagues have compiled and published numerous comparative charts (Law et al., 1996; Letts et al., 1994). However, new assessments continue to be developed, many as mobile apps. Although these have not yet been formally tested, they are likely to lead to more efficient and effective environmental assessments and interventions.

A unique challenge to measuring the impact of occupational therapy in environmental intervention is the lack of control the occupational therapy practitioner generally has over the intervention. Although the recommendations may be clearly detailed by an experienced evaluator, contractors or equipment vendors implement the environmental modifications. When possible, the occupational therapy practitioner needs to follow up with the homeowner to confirm recommendations were implemented accurately and to train the homeowner in the products or explain how to safely move about in remodeled spaces (RSC 1B).

Intervention

Occupational therapy practitioners must be sensitive to clients' priorities regarding the recommendations for environmental modification. Clients should be the ultimate decision makers (RSCs 3A, 3B, 3D, 3E). Homeowners can experience a loss of control and a disruption to routines because of the modification design (Tanner, Tilse, & Jonge, 2008). If occupational therapy practitioners implement technology without understanding clients' daily routines, they neglect important aspects of homeowners' lives (Riikonen, Paavilainen, & Salo, 2013).

Principle 4, Justice, requires recommending products and services that are deemed necessary for occupational performance in and around the home. According to RSC 4M, occupational therapy practitioners are expected to "bill and collect fees legally and justly in a manner that is fair, reasonable, and commensurate with services delivered" (AOTA, 2015b, p. 5).

Principle 5, Veracity, requires being clear about the actual costs for the intervention options as well as costs for the evaluation services. Disclosing costs, laws, and city ordinances allows the homeowner to make informed decisions. A societal dimension to environmental modifications includes "the political and economic conditions which affect the resources and control that people have over their home" (Aplin, de Jonge, & Gustafsson, 2013, p. 107). Limiting homeowners' experience of control may affect their occupational well-being and negatively change the experience of home. Vignette 23.1 demonstrates challenges of doing what is best for the homeowner when constrained by funding.

In addition to developing an intervention to improve occupational performance, the occupational therapy practitioner must consider how the house is a home. Homes are closely related to identity: how a person or family decorates, freely moves about the home, or creates areas for inviting others in from the community. Many clients' attitudes toward home modifications are influenced by personal and social meaning and perceived independent status. Kruse and colleagues (2010) found that older adults who had fallen in their homes were unaware of the safety issues. Although their homes were potentially unsafe and home modifications would have aided in preventing future falls, the older adults preferred not to make changes. Homes reflect self-image and promote emotional well-being despite the potential health risks.

Recent advances in technologies and a growing older adult population have created a market for "gerotechnologies." ***Gerotechnologies*** are assistive technology devices that promote independence in old age and allow older adults to age in place (Künemund & Tanschus, 2013; Rodeschini, 2011). Examples of these assistive technologies applied to older populations range from medication timers to environmental sensors that monitor falls or health. These technologies, recommended to reduce caregiver burden and homeowner dependency, need to be used with caution because they have both positive and negative outcomes.

Rural areas may benefit from technological means to provide health care services; however, a network of family and caregiver support is often in place (Bowman, Hooker, Steggell, & Brandt, 2013). Technology within the homes of elderly people may impair their quality of life by impeding on privacy and

Vignette 23.1. Costly Best Options

Ms. Mims contacted a local nonprofit home rehabilitation organization for help after her kitchen ceiling collapsed following a heavy rain. The **home rehabilitation team** found that not only was the kitchen in need of help, but Ms. Mims had been living without a functional bath or shower for more than 3 years. She claimed that even if the tub were functional, she couldn't use it because of her arthritis. The home rehab team called in an **occupational therapist** who evaluated the home and Ms. Mims's occupational performance.

The occupational therapist provided two options: repair the tub and provide a tub transfer bench and long-handled shower head, or remove the tub and gut that area of the bathroom to create a curbless shower. The latter was the preferred option because of Ms. Mims's small stature and severe arthritis. However, she lived on Social Security disability and did not have funds for such a project. The plan was beyond the scope of the home rehabilitation organization's mission.

decreasing face-to-face interactions with both professional and family caregivers (Demiris & Hensel, 2009; Mahmood, Yamamoto, Lee, & Steggell, 2008). Technology has the potential to violate Principle 3, Autonomy, and Principle 5, Veracity (RSC 5J), specifically regarding privacy and self-determination.

Outcomes

Whether the homeowner or client is an older adult aging in place or a youth with a complex developmental disability needing flexible and dynamic technologies, occupational therapy practitioners have the knowledge and skills to evaluate and recommend improvements for the homeowner's occupational performance in and around the home. Principle 1, Beneficence, requires the therapist to use valid and reliable measures to guide decision making. However, one of the weakest areas of environmental assessment and intervention concerns outcomes documentation and outcomes measurement. The field of environmental modifications has revolved around intervention implementation and intervention decision making. Part of the reason for this is that documenting outcomes requires ongoing contact with the owners or residents and returning to the environment for data collection. This is an added cost, and most practices do not support this comprehensive service.

Moreover, outcomes documentation is usually only indirectly funded, making outcomes measurement and documentation particularly challenging. This does not condone the behavior of neglecting outcomes because it is critical to understand that interventions work in general, and specifically for each client.

Social Context and Environmental Modification

Occupational therapy practitioners need to consider several factors during environmental assessments and interventions, including the client's social network, the fiscal possibilities and constraints, and the therapist's responsibility to see the project to completion.

Social Context

The client's social environment and network play a critical role in the success of assessing and intervening in a client's environment. The ***social context*** consists of both the immediate social context, such as family, caregivers, and friends, and the extended social context, including groups and populations with whom the client interacts.

From an occupational therapist's perspective, the social context often includes activities that have a social element as well as social support from family or caregivers. This social context significantly influences health outcomes (James, Wilson, Barnes, & Bennett, 2011; Krueger et al., 2009; Maillot, Perrot, & Hartley, 2012; Small, Dixon, McArdle, & Grimm, 2012). Being holistic, occupational therapy practitioners also would be attuned to the homeowner's psychological needs. Does the homeowner feel safe retrieving mail or taking garbage to the curb? Are they at risk because of neighborhood instability? Meeting only the homeowner's physical needs without addressing the psychological needs would violate Principle 2, Nonmaleficience.

Home modifications may be a team effort, which could result in added stress for the homeowner when the home environment feels less than the individual's own. Involving the homeowner in each decision and every process mitigates this concern. Principle 6, Fidelity (RSC 6H) requires occupational therapists to work collaboratively with other professionals to promote quality and safety for clients. The process of environmental assessment and intervention might include builders, contractors, designers, social services experts, and physical therapists, all of whom form part of the client's social context.

Vignette 23.2 demonstrates the sometimes competing needs within the home and those of home-dwellers. Understanding the occupational needs of all who live in the home is critical to a successful modification.

The value of the team approach in Vignette 23.2 is demonstrated through positive outcomes for both the husband, for whom the modification was intended, and for the wife, whose occupational performance would be affected by the same modifications. The team members respected each other's roles and responsibilities in collaborating in best practice (RSCs 6C, 6G, 6H, 6I).

Fiscal Considerations

Occupational therapy practitioners should also consider fiscal constraints. Fiscal factors often guide the type of evaluation, intervention, and outcome measurement that is completed for a client. Although using fiscal constraints as a guideline for

Vignette 23.2. Whose Bathroom Is It Anyway?

Ted, a veteran with a T-8 spinal cord injury, was receiving services to make his bathroom more accessible for him. Although he had a private bathroom off the master bedroom, he was unable to easily maneuver in the space to transfer safely to the toilet or tub bench. Additionally, he found it easier to do bowel care in the bedroom than the bathroom because of lack of counter and storage space.

The **home modifications team** included an occupational therapist, contractor, and the homeowners—Ted, the client, and his wife, **Taylor.** The contractor and occupational therapist worked easily with Ted; together they determined they would gut the bathroom and take out a wall to open a closet that originally was accessed from the hallway. Closing off this door and opening the space allowed for an additional 4 feet of length, creating space for a roll-under sink, roll-in shower (with saddle curb to hold water), and adequate space to turn around and safely transfer to the toilet, even with the shower chair stationed next to the toilet.

As the team excitedly discussed surfaces and design measurements, Taylor looked cautiously around the room. It would have a "spa feel" with the amenities being described; however, something seemed lacking. The occupational therapist caught and followed her gaze: There was no storage for her. The spa features of open space and minimalistic details created an accessible space for her husband but resulted in a complete loss of function for her. The occupational therapist spoke this aloud, and Taylor frowned, stating she wanted it to work for Ted; she could "figure something out."

This scenario demonstrates a conflict between ethical principles of Beneficence and Nonmaleficence: making the bathroom accessible for Ted, but reducing the usability of the space for Taylor. The team responded by recommending a simple floor-to-ceiling custom-built shelf-and-cabinet unit tucked next to the toilet, which although shallow in depth, created 6 square feet of storage for her. Being alert to the needs of all who live in the home is imperative for the occupational performance of the whole family.

determining interventions or modifications that might be made for a specific client is not a best practice, it is the reality of the current practice environment. Therefore, it becomes the occupational therapy practitioner's responsibility, to a large extent, to innovatively determine how to implement as many environmental interventions as possible given the client's fiscal constraints (RSCs 2A, 2B, 4B, 4C, 4D). Additionally, fiscal constraints often result in the lack of outcome measurements and follow-up with clients to ensure that the implemented interventions are effective.

See It Through

Occupational therapists have an ethical responsibility to see the project through until the interventions have been implemented and tested by the clients; the practitioners can then make additional recommendations or provide training as needed according to Principle 2, Nonmaleficence. However fiscal reimbursement, time requirements, and occasionally social pressures, might prevent occupational therapists from seeing projects to successful completion.

Training

Academic programs have a responsibility to educate entry-level practitioners about home modifications. The Accreditation Council for Occupational Therapy Education (ACOTE, 2012) and others (AOTA, 2015a, 2015c) highlight the importance of the role of occupational therapy practitioners in evaluating, modifying, and adapting the client's contexts and environments to support and maximize function and participation.

ACOTE standards (ACOTE, 2012) require that entry-level occupational therapy programs provide education and training for students to evaluate a client in context and in different environments (B.4.4); understand factors that could bias assessment results, including variables related to the context (B.4.7); be able to design interventions that address the context and environment (B.5.1); modify and adapt process and environments (B.5.9); and teach use of compensatory strategies to support performance (B.5.24).

The role of occupational therapy practitioners in evaluating, modifying, choosing, and using environments to support maximal participation of clients, families, groups, and communities has been clarified in AOTA policy documents (AOTA, 2015a, 2015c). However, educational strategies used to teach environmental assessments and interventions lack consistency. Experiential learning alongside an expert in home modifications is recommended as a major component of the learning experience (DuBroc & Pickens, 2015). Nonprofit organizations, such as Rebuilding Together, welcome occupational therapy practitioners to train students while providing in-home evaluations and recommendations.

Beyond basic practice, therapists are encouraged to develop skills in design, construction, and assistive technology so they can be recognized and credentialed through the AOTA Specialty Certificate in Environmental Modification (2014b) or the National Association of Home Builders Certified Aging in Place Specialist credential. With additional training and expertise, an occupational therapy practitioner credentialed in assistive technology, for example, can provide high-tech product recommendations along with environmental modifications for the home and occupational performance (Beneficence, RSCs 1D, 1E; Justice, 4G). As with all practice, maintaining competency and staying abreast of new technologies is critical to advanced practice in environmental modifications (Beneficence, RSC 1G).

Recognizing limits of knowledge and skills is an ethical responsibility of therapists as shown in the Vignette 23.3 below.

Ethics of Comission and Omission

Acts of commission are deliberate acts performed with the intention of being proactive (Reamer, 2015). Acts of comission, discussed throughout the chapter, are recognizable; however, it is essential to remember that ***omitted activities*** are also unethical, such as not providing additional community resource information, or not providing a full assessment when needed. This is particularly important in the area of environmental assessment and intervention because most occupational therapy practice occurs in clinics or schools. However, environmental assessments and interventions occur in

Vignette 23.3. Can She Do It?

Vanessa learned about home modifications in school and did some work with a nonprofit organization while a student and new graduate. Her mother, proud of Vanessa's endeavors, asked her to evaluate a townhome on the block for a new neighbor. Vanessa was thinking about specializing in home environmental modifications, so she took on the request.

Vanessa met the **homeowner** at the new house a couple of weeks before the move. The homeowner was moving from a state with 3 children, including an 11-year-old daughter with cerebral palsy, which severely impaired the girl's ability to be independently mobile. The daughter required a self-directed power chair and was unable to shower independently, but she could do basic morning care. Additionally, the daughter's eyesight was less than 20/200 (threshold for legally blind), although she had already received mobility and orientation services.

Case Study 23.2. Distant Home

Mrs. Rosa was in a skilled nursing facility for rehabilitation after suffering multiple fractures to her ribs, pelvis, and left femur in a motor vehicle accident. Although she had made good improvement, she experienced moderate pain and would continue to require a wheeled walker after discharge home. Additionally, her home would need modification for her to live independently.

Mrs. Rosa had two children, a son who lived in her same town 1 hour away, and a daughter who lived 1,000 miles away. The **rehab team** was unable to go to her home for a home assessment but, with Mrs. Rosa's permission, established communication with her son (RSC 3B) and instructed him to take photos and a video of specific areas of the home to share with the team. The areas were selected based on the occupational therapist using a psychometrically sound assessment tool to establish areas of the home that had potential problems (RSC 1C).

Reviewing the photos provided some answers to equipment questions but prompted more questions about Mrs. Rosa's functional ability in the home. The physician agreed to allow Mrs. Rosa to return home on a day pass with her son. During that day, she moved through her home while the son Skyped her movement to the **occupational therapist** (RSC 3H). This new information was enough to write up recommendations (RSC 1A) for a local community group that provided basic home repair and modifications (RSC 4B) on a sliding payment scale.

the community or in the home where occupational therapy practitioners must take initiative to perform the needed assessments and interventions. This often requires administrative creativity to generate economic mechanisms to drive these services. A significant piece of a practitioner's responsibility also includes identifying issues that might be beyond the scope of one's expertise and making referrals to therapists with more experience in home modifications (RSCs 1E, 1I).

Using technology has potential to facilitate environmental assessment as shown in Case Study 23.2.

Summary

Environmental modification is a burgeoning practice area for occupational therapy. Therapists are frequently called on to complete environmental assessments in a range of practice contexts from simple home assessment for rehabilitation discharge planning to home health care intervention.

Occupational therapists can pursue additional training and credentials to enhance their practice and develop expertise to address complex client needs. Ethical practice requires therapists to practice within their expertise, call on experts as needed, be knowledgeable in community resources, and work collaboratively with the client and family.

Reliable and valid assessment tools provide comprehensive and accurate information needed to implement timely and cost-effective interventions, while forecasting future needs. Occupational therapy practitioners need to be sensitive to the complex and sometimes subtle ethical challenges in environmental assessment to ensure best practices.

Reflective Questions

1. What potential ethical issues are currently or could become relevant in your own practice setting related to environmental assessment and intervention? For example, in higher education, what content is incorporated into the curriculum? In subacute rehabilitation, what outcomes data are documented in your program, or what team members do you involve in your environmental assessments and interventions?
2. If you identify ethical issues around environmental assessment and intervention in your program, what steps might you attempt to resolve them?
3. What skills or training does an occupational therapy practitioner need to obtain before engaging in private environmental modifications practice to assure consumers of their competence?
4. Review Vignette 23.1. What is the occupational therapist's role in carrying the plan through to completion? What Principles and RSCs would apply in this situation?
5. Review Vignette 23.3. What are Vanessa's options? What Principles and RSCs from the Code would apply in this situation?
6. Review Case Study 23.2. What did the occupational therapist do successfully for Mrs. Rosa? What Principles and RSCs would apply in this situation?

References

Accreditation Council for Occupational Therapy Education. (2012). 2011 Accreditation Council for Occupational Therapy Education (ACOTE) standards. *American Journal of Occupational Therapy, 66*(6 Suppl.), S6–S74. https://doi.org/10.5014/ajot.2012.66S6

American Occupational Therapy Association. (2010). Specialized knowledge and skills in technology and environmental interventions for occupational therapy practice. *American Journal of Occupational Therapy, 64*(Suppl.), S44–S56. https://doi.org/10.5014/ajot.2010.64S44-64S56

American Occupational Therapy Association. (2014a). Occupational therapy practice framework: Domain and process (3rd ed.). *American Journal of Occupational Therapy, 68*(Suppl. 1), S1–S48. https://doi.org/10.5014/ajot.2014.682006

American Occupational Therapy Association. (2014b). *Specialty certification in environmental modification.* Retrieved from http://www.aota.org/Education-Careers/Advance-Career/Board-Specialty-Certifications/EnvironmentalModification.aspx

American Occupational Therapy Association. (2015a). Complex environmental modifications. *American Journal of Occupational Therapy, 69*(Suppl. 3), 6913410010p1–p7. https://doi.org/10.5014/ajot.2015.696S01

American Occupational Therapy Association. (2015b). Occupational therapy code of ethics (2015). *American Journal of Occupational Therapy, 69*(Suppl. 3), 6912310030. https://doi.org/10.5014/ajot.2015.696S03

American Occupational Therapy Association. (2015c). Occupational therapy's perspective on the use of environments and contexts to facilitate health, well-being, and participation in occupations. *American Journal of Occupational Therapy, 69*, 6913410050p1–13. https://doi.org/10.5014/ajot.2015.696S05

Aplin, T., de Jonge, D., & Gustafsson, L. (2013). Understanding the dimensions of home that impact on home modification decision making. *Australian Occupational Therapy Journal, 60*, 101–109. https://doi.org/10.1111/1440-1630.12022

Bowman, S., Hooker, K., Steggell, C. D., & Brandt, J. (2013). Perceptions of communication and monitoring technologies among older rural women: Problem or panacea? *Journal of Housing for the Elderly, 27*, 48–60. https://doi.org/10.1080/02763893.2012.754814

Demiris, G., & Hensel, B. (2009). "Smart homes" for patients at the end of life. *Journal of Housing for the Elderly, 23*(1/2), 106–115. https://doi.org/10.1080/02763890802665049

DuBroc, W., & Pickens, N. D. (2015). Becoming "at home" in home modifications: Professional reasoning across the expertise continuum. *Occupational Therapy in Health Care, 29*(3), 316–329. https://doi.org/10.3109/07380577.2015.1010129

Dunn, W., Brown, C., &, McGuigan, A. (1994). The ecology of human performance: A framework for considering the effect of context. *American Journal of Occupational Therapy, 48*, 595–607. https://doi.org/10.5014/ajot.48.7.595

Hinojosa, J., & Kramer, P. (Eds.).(2014). *Evaluation: Obtaining and interpreting data* (4th ed.). Bethesda: AOTA Press.

James, B. D., Wilson, R. S., Barnes, L. L., & Bennett, D. A. (2011). Late-life social activity and cognitive decline in old age. *Journal of the International Neuropsychological Society, 17*, 998–1005. https://doi.org/10.1017/S1355617711000531

Krueger, K. R., Wilson, R. S., Kamenetsky, J. M., Barnes, L. L., Bienias, J. L., & Bennett, D. A. (2009). Social engagement and cognitive function in old age. *Experimental Aging Research, 35*(1), 45–60. https://doi.org/10.1080/03610730802545028

Kruse, R. L., Moore, C. M., Tofle, R. B., LeMaster, J. W., Aud, M., Hicks, L. L., . . . Mehr, D. R. (2010). Older adults' attitudes toward home modifications for fall prevention. *Journal of Housing for the Elderly, 24*(2), 110–129. https://doi.org/10.1080/02763891003757031

Künemund, H., & Tanschus, N. (2013). Gerotechnology: Old age in the electronic jungle. In K. Komp & M. Aartsen (Eds.), *Old age in Europe: A textbook of gerontology* (pp. 97–112). Heidelberg, Germany: Springer.

Law, M., Cooper, B., Strong, S., Stewart, D., Rigby, P., & Letts, L. (1996). The Person–Environment–Occupation model: A transactional approach to occupational performance. *Canadian Journal of Occupational Therapy, 63*, 9–23. https://doi.org/10.1177/000841749606300103

Letts, L., Law, M., Rigby, P., Cooper, B., Stewart, D., & Strong, S. (1994). Person–environment assessments in occupational therapy. *American Journal of Occupational Therapy, 48*(7), 608–618. https://doi.org/10.5014/ajot.48.7.608

Mahmood, A., Yamamoto, T., Lee, M., & Steggell, C. (2008). Perceptions and use of gerotechnology: Implications for aging in place. *Journal of Housing for the Elderly, 22*(1/2), 104–126. https://doi.org/10.1080/02763890802097144

Maillot, P., Perrot, A., & Hartley, A. (2012). Effects of interactive physical-activity video-game training on physical and cognitive function in older adults. *Psychology and Aging, 27*(3), 589–600. https://doi.org/10.1037/a0026268

Reamer, F. G. (2015). Eye on ethics: *Omission and Comission in social work.* Retrieved from http://bit.ly/2jwZush

Riikonen, M., Paavilainen, E., & Salo, H. (2013). Factors supporting the use of technology in daily life of home-living people with dementia. *Technology and Disability, 25*, 233–243. https://doi.org/10.3233/TAD-130393

Rodeschini, G. (2011). Gerotechnology: A new kind of care for aging? An analysis of the relationship between older people and technology. *Nursing and Health Sciences, 13*, 521–528. https://doi.org/10.1111/j.1442-2018.2011.00634.x

Sanford, J. (2010). The physical environment and home health care. In S. A. Rapporteur (Ed.), *The role of human factors in home health care: Workshop summary* (pp. 201–246). Washington, DC: National Academies Press.

Small, B. J., Dixon, R. A., McArdle, J. J., & Grimm, K. J. (2012). Do changes in lifestyle engagement moderate cognitive decline in normal aging? Evidence from the Victoria longitudinal study. *Neuropsychology, 26*(2), 144–155. https://doi.org/10.1037/a0026579

Tanner, B., Tilse, C., & Jonge, D. (2008). Restoring and sustaining home: The impact of home modifications on the meaning of home for older people. *Journal of Housing for the Elderly, 22*(3), 195–215. https://doi.org/10.1080/02763890802232048

Weeks, A. L., Lamb, E. A., & Pickens, N. D. (2010). Home modification assessments: Clinical utility and treatment context. *Physical and Occupational Therapy in Geriatrics: Current Trends in Geriatric Rehabilitation, 28*(4), 396–409. https://doi.org/10.3109/02703180903528405

Chapter 24.

AUTISM ACROSS THE LIFESPAN: ETHICAL CONSIDERATIONS

Lisa Crabtree, PhD, OTR/L, FAOTA, and Janet DeLany, DEd, OTR/L, FAOTA

Learning Objectives

By the end of the chapter, readers will be able to

- Apply the *Occupational Therapy Practice Framework: Domain and Process* and the *Occupational Therapy Code of Ethics (2015)* to guide ethical occupational therapy services for people on the autism spectrum and their families;
- Describe characteristics of autism and contextual and environmental factors that contribute to ethical dilemmas when providing services to people on the autism spectrum and their families;
- Apply ethical decision-making models to identify and determine potential solutions to ethical dilemmas when providing services to people on the autism spectrum and their families; and
- Access resources that inform occupational therapy practitioners about best practices, current resources, and emerging research related to autism.

Key Terms and Concepts

✧ Autism
✧ Autism spectrum disorder
✧ Neurodevelopmental disorders
✧ Neurodiversity

Autism, officially identified as ***autism spectrum disorder*** (ASD) by the American Psychiatric Association (APA; 2013), is a neurodevelopmental disorder that involves difficulties with social communication and social interactions, restricted or repetitive behaviors, and interests. The purpose of this chapter is to apply the *Occupational Therapy Code of Ethics (2015)* (referred to as the "Code"; American Occupational Therapy Association [AOTA], 2015h) to guide ethical practice for occupational therapy practitioners as they collaborate with people on the autism spectrum and their families to promote engagement in meaningful and purposeful occupations.

Autism Overview

Leo Kanner, a psychiatrist, first described *autism* in 1943 through his case descriptions of 11 children who demonstrated unusual patterns of withdrawal and insistence on consistent patterns (Blacher & Christensen, 2011). Initially considered a low-incidence condition, its reported prevalence began to escalate in the late 1990s internationally (World Health Organization [WHO], 2013). APA (2013) uses the term *ASD* in the *Diagnostic and Statistical Manual for Mental Disorders, 5th Edition (DSM–5)* and includes the disorder under the category of neurodevelopmental disorders.

Neurodevelopmental disorders have an onset during early childhood and are characterized by developmental discrepancies in "personal, social, academic, or occupational functioning" (APA, 2013, p. 31). The characterization of autism as a neurodevelopmental disorder is based on brain, physiological, and genetic research that has identified complexities that contribute to the diagnosis, instead of solely relying on observation of behavioral characteristics (Interagency Autism Coordinating Committee [IACC], 2014).

The *DSM–5* lists two general diagnostic criteria for ASD. The first describes persistent deficits in social communication and social interaction across multiple contexts, and the second identifies restricted, repetitive patterns of behaviors, interests, or activities, including sensory differences. Additionally, the *DSM–5* has included descriptions of specifiers that define characteristics such as intellectual disability, co-occurrence with another behavioral or genetic disorder, and severity of symptoms. The severity levels describe an individual as requiring support, substantial support, or very substantial support.

Groups such as Autism Speaks (2015) have strongly advocated for finding a cure. Autism Speaks uses a puzzle piece in its logo to reflect its mission to identify and solve the puzzle of ASD. In contrast, people who consider themselves autistic self-advocates view autism as a form of ***neurodiversity*** of the human genome—that is, normal variations in neurological structures (Kapp, Gillespie-Lynch, Sherman, & Hutman, 2013). They believe that the focus should be on accepting rather than curing autism and autistic behaviors and on recognizing people with autism as a minority group (Autistic Self Advocacy Network, 2015).

Common to both groups is the goal to support the ability of individuals with autism to lead fulfilling lives. Occupational therapy, whose disciplinary focus is to promote people's successful and meaningful engagement in occupations of daily life, is strategically situated to provide the expertise necessary to achieve this goal.

Autism Demographics

As reported by the Centers for Disease Control and Prevention (CDC) in 2014, the autism prevalence rate in the United States for 2013 was estimated to be 1.25%, or 1 in 68. However, revisions in ordering the questions in the National Health Interview Survey (Zablotsky, Black, Maenner, Schieve, & Blumberg, 2015) resulted in a higher autism prevalence rate of 2.24%, or 1 in 45. WHO (2013) estimates 1 in 160 people worldwide are on the autism spectrum. Although the causes of autism are not firmly identified, evidence suggests that hereditary and environmental factors contribute to its prevalence.

Occupational Therapy for People on the Autism Spectrum and Their Families

The *Occupational Therapy Practice Framework: Domain and Process* (*Framework;* AOTA, 2014), coupled with occupational therapy practice models, provides a structure for outlining the purview, processes, and belief systems that guide the delivery of ethical occupational therapy services for people on the autism spectrum. Occupational therapy practitioners need to concurrently respect the individuality of the person on the autism spectrum and the centrality of the family within the person's daily life by posing the following questions when providing occupational therapy services:

- What are the person's values, beliefs, interests, needs, and experiences? How do they influence the person's engagement in occupations? How are they influenced by the person's autism characteristics?
- What occupations are meaningful and important to the person, and what occupations does the person need and want to learn or master to participate in daily life?
- How do the characteristics of autism and coexisting health conditions and learning differences manifest themselves in this person?
- What are the person's level and complexity of performance skills and performance patterns for engaging in these occupations, and how does autism enhance, alter, or limit these performance skills and patterns?

- What contexts, environments, and resources surround and influence the person to support or hinder engagement in these occupations?
- What accommodations and adaptions to the performance skills, performance patterns, contexts, environments, and occupations are feasible to facilitate the engagement in the occupations? (AOTA, 2014)

Consistent with the Code's Related Standard of Conduct (RSC) 1A to "provide appropriate evaluation and plan of intervention for recipients of occupational therapy services specific for their needs" (AOTA, 2015h, p. 3), the answers to these broad questions are based on data integrated as part of the assessment process from relevant observations, interviews, and evaluation tools. Given the characteristics of autism and the likelihood of coexisting health conditions and learning differences, the answers will be distinct for each person and reflect varying patterns of talents and needs across and within the person's occupations. The person's performance skills and capacities in one area of occupational performance may not necessarily align with those in other areas.

For example, some people on the autism spectrum who have limited verbal communication skills may be cognitively gifted, while others may have cognitive limitations. Some individuals may be talented artists or mathematicians but struggle to manage routine self-care and household tasks. Thus, as part of the assessment process, observations should occur across occupations and in the contexts in which they occur. Interviews should include the person and, when applicable, significant family members, caregivers, and other relevant professionals and community members.

The analysis of the responses to the broad questions asked during the occupational therapy assessment process is to be grounded within current research and evidence. Doing so adheres to RSC 1C, which directs occupational therapy practitioners to "use to the extent possible, evaluation, planning, intervention techniques, assessments, and therapeutic equipment that are evidence based, current, and within the recognized scope of occupational therapy practice" (AOTA, 2015h, p. 3). Such analysis provides the foundation for the development, implementation, and evaluation of an intervention plan with targeted outcomes that are determined in collaboration with the person and other significant people in the person's life. To promote collaboration and build consensus may require artful negotiation, particularly when conflicting perspectives arise between the person and the other significant people regarding the priorities for and viability of the targeted outcomes.

During such deliberations, occupational therapy practitioners are to "establish a collaborative relationship with the recipient of service and relevant stakeholders, to promote shared decision making" (RSC 3D; AOTA, 2015h, p. 5), "respect and honor the expressed wishes of recipients of service" (RSC 3A; AOTA, 2015h, p. 5), and "maintain awareness of current laws and AOTA policies and Official Documents that apply to the profession of occupational therapy" (RSC 4E; AOTA, 2015h, p. 6). Case Studies 24.1 and 24.2 highlight some potential conflicts that arise from the varying perspectives of the stakeholders and suggest ethical principles that can be used to guide conflict resolution.

Evidence-Based Practice

Historically, occupational therapy interventions focused on the needs of children on the autism spectrum. However, as knowledge about autism has evolved, the scope of services has expanded to include adolescents, young adults, and older adults on the autism spectrum and their families. AOTA (2015i) published a statement titled *Scope of Occupational Therapy Services for Individuals With an Autism Spectrum Disorder Across the Life Course.* Included in the statement are examples of how autism affects occupational engagement differently throughout a person's life in response to changing occupational complexities and aspirations, performance skills, and environmental influences. Examples of occupational therapy interventions that support occupational engagement of people on the autism spectrum throughout their lives in response to these changes are provided.

Yet, in spite of increased recognition within health care systems about the prevalence of adults on the autism spectrum and their needs, programs and services remain underdeveloped, underresearched, and underfunded. However, AOTA, through the Code, encourages occupational therapy practitioners to "advocate for changes to systems and policies that are discriminatory or unfairly limit or prevent access to occupational therapy services" (RSC 4D; AOTA, 2015h, p. 6) and other community and health services. Using available resources to support the role of advocate is ethical and essential.

Case Study 24.1. Occupational Therapy Services in Early Intervention

Nuna worked as an occupational therapist in an early intervention program that included home- and center-based services. The center-based program used an inclusionary model that brought together young children on the autism spectrum and typically developing children. Using play as the primary modality for learning, activities were tailored to foster the children's individualized cognitive, social, physical, and emotional development.

Jacque was a 4-year-old on the autism spectrum, and he was making limited progress compared to the other children in the program. Mondays were particularly challenging for him. He needed significant prompting to dress or feed himself. He communicated primarily through single words and body actions and punched and bit the other children and staff when he was frustrated. Other families asked that Jacque not be permitted to continue in the center-based program.

Jacque's father, **Jeremiah,** worked long hours to earn money for food and shelter for the family. He wanted his son to attend kindergarten at the local school next year. Jacque's grandmother, **Annalisa,** was the primary caregiver for Jacque and his two sisters. Because of his special needs, Annalisa believed Jacque was a gift from the Almighty and that it was her responsibility to do everything for him. Jacque and his sisters visited their mother, **Sarafine,** on Sundays. She was coping with depression, and caring for the children overwhelmed her. Thus, she placed few behavioral expectations on them.

Step 1. Gather facts.
To understand the ethical dilemma, Nuna first asked the following questions:

- Who is the primary recipient of my occupational therapy services? Jacque? The family? Does this include Sarafine? Should I initiate a referral for separate services for her?
- What is my responsibility to the safety of the other children and staff in the program?
- How do the family members' expectations for Jacque coincide or conflict with those of the program, the local school, and the occupational therapy profession?
- Are Jacque's disruptive behaviors a form of communication, bullying, or family-accepted behavior?

Nuna reviewed Part C of the Individuals with Disabilities Education Improvement Act of 2004 (IDEA; P. L. 108–44.) that addresses family-focused services for young children; center guidelines and polices related to the classroom, scope of services, and referral for additional services; the Code (AOTA, 2015h); and literature about culturally based child-rearing practices, children's disruptive behaviors, and maternal depression.

Step 2. Analyze possible courses of action.
Nuna concluded that Jacque and his family were her primary recipients of services as related to the scope of early intervention programs for him (Principle 1, Beneficence). As an employee of the program, she was responsible for the safety of the children and staff (Principle 2, Nonmaleficence, and Principle 6, Fidelity). She needed to collect additional data from observations and discussions with staff and family members to accurately assess Jacque's performance skills, determine intervention plans (Principle 1, Beneficence), and promote shared decision making among Jacque's family members and program staff (Principle 3, Autonomy). She also needed to address Sarafine's occupational performance needs as a parent and recommend that she seek mental health services (Principle 1, Beneficence, and Principle 4, Justice).

Step 3. Select and implement a course of action.
Nuna implemented a temporary plan to manage Jacque's behaviors that allowed him to remain in the center program and to keep the other children and staff safe until a more comprehensive plan was developed (Principle 2, Nonmaleficence, and Principle 6, Fidelity). She conducted further observations and evaluations at the center and at Jacque's home and met with family members to assess Jacque's performance skills and environmental and contextual

(Continued)

Case Study 24.1. Occupational Therapy Services in Early Intervention *(Cont.)*

factors influencing that performance (Principle 1, Beneficence, and Principle 3, Autonomy).

She arranged meetings among the family members and select staff to prioritize their immediate and long-term aspirations for Jacque and negotiated strategies they could collectively implement to help him achieve those goals (Principle 3, Autonomy). Nuna identified community support systems that could help Annalisa understand how to fulfill her cultural role as a caring grandmother while also promoting Jacque's growth and development (Principle 3, Autonomy, and Principle 4, Justice).

She arranged for Annalisa and Sarafine to participate in the center-based activities so they and the staff could learn effective approaches from each another to promote Jacque's development. Nuna composed a list of mental health providers for Sarafine and financial and transportation resources for accessing them (Principle 1, Beneficence, and Principle 4, Justice). In response to Sarafine's request, Nuna arranged the initial contact (Principle 2, Nonmaleficence).

Step 4. Evaluate the results of the action.
Nuna reviewed her actions and concluded that they adhered to federal regulations, program guidelines, and Principles 1, 2, 3, 4, and 6 of the Code (AOTA, 2015h). She determined that because of the complexity of Jacque's needs, he and his family would benefit from continued services. She arranged for continuation of home-based programming, routine monitoring of progress, and periodic family–staff meetings.

Case Study 24.2. Information Sharing

Ogechi was an occupational therapist working with students on the autism spectrum who were ages 14 to 18 years. He formed a fathers group to help them with parenting and promoting the successful occupational engagement of their children.

During the sessions, the fathers talked about their frustrations with particular school personnel who were not helping their children prepare for life after graduation. They also shared that they felt disenfranchised from their role as fathers because they had little input into their child's life at school or home.

Ogechi faced an ethical dilemma regarding what information he could share with the fathers that he learned from the students and the school personnel, and what information he could share with the students and the school personnel that he learned from the fathers. His goal was to address the men's concerns and promote shared decision making about services for the students.

Step 1. Gather facts.
To resolve this ethical dilemma, Ogechi posed the following questions:

- Who are the primary recipients of my services? What are my therapeutic responsibilities to the students and the fathers, and what are my professional responsibilities to the school personnel?
- What information is confidential, and what information can be shared with the school personnel, the fathers, and the students about the students' family life and school experiences?
- What are the conflicting perspectives of the different constituents, and how can I promote shared decision making?
- What is the scope of my expertise in working with family concerns, and what other resources are available in the school system and the community that I should consider?

Ogechi reviewed the Code (AOTA, 2015h), the *Framework* (AOTA, 2014), IDEA, the Family Education Rights and Privacy Act (FERPA; P. L. 93–380), and the Health Insurance Portability and Accountability Act of 1996 (HIPAA; P. L. 104–191) to determine ethical guidelines, the purview of occupational therapy practice, and confidentiality requirements for the adolescents and the fathers. He also reviewed literature about best practices for adolescents on the autism spectrum and consulted with his supervisor to ensure that his concerns and courses of action were consistent with the school's

(Continued)

Case Study 24.2. Information Sharing *(Cont.)*

mission and policies. Concluding that the family dynamics related to home life were beyond his area of expertise, he investigated resources within the school and community that provided family counseling.

Step 2. Analyze possible courses of action. Ogechi concluded that this situation involved all the principles of the Code (AOTA, 2015h). He used a Decision Table (Table 24.1) to frame possible courses of action.

Step 3. Select and implement a course of action. Ogechi dismissed the second option as violating Principles 1, 2, 3, 5, and 6. He discussed the remaining options with the fathers, who requested that he provide them with the information in option 4. They gave written permission to share their collective concerns and to arrange a joint meeting with the school personnel to identify potential solutions. After the joint meeting, Ogechi arranged individual meetings so each father could meet with designated school personnel, the son or daughter, and other family members to prioritize the school-based services and targeted outcomes. Ogechi met with the students to educate them about their rights and roles in these meetings and to help them prepare questions they wanted to ask and statements they wanted to make. The fathers agreed to invite a family counselor to one of their meetings to better understand the family counseling process and determine whether they wanted to individually seek such services.

Step 4. Evaluate the results of the action. Ogechi concluded that his actions adhered to the Principles of Beneficence, Nonmaleficence, Autonomy, and Justice with respect to the fathers and the students and the Principle of Fidelity with respect to school personnel. The actions also abided by federal regulations related to FERPA, HIPAA, and IDEA and created a path for shared decision making related to school-based services for the adolescents and the fathers' autonomy in decision making.

Table 24.1. Decision Table for Case Study 24.2

Possible Action	Positive Outcomes	Negative Outcomes
Take no action.	Protects the confidentiality of the fathers (Principle 3, Autonomy) and abides by HIPAA. Protects the confidentiality of the students and abides by FERPA regulations for those 18 years or older.	Fathers' concerns remain unresolved, potentially violating Principle 1, Beneficence, and Principle 2, Nonmaleficence.
Report the fathers' individual concerns about particular school personnel and about their lack of school–home involvement to school authority.	Brings the fathers' concerns to the attention of the school (Principle 1, Beneficence).	Without receiving fathers' written permission, this action violates HIPAA regulations and Principle 3, Autonomy. Because the fathers' claims have not been verified (Principle 5, Veracity), colleagues' reputations could be harmed, violating Principle 6, Fidelity, and family issues could be exacerbated, violating Principle 2, Nonmaleficence.
Discuss the concerns with the school personnel in general terms without identifying particular fathers or students.	Protects the confidentiality of the fathers (Principle 3, Autonomy) while bringing the general concerns to school personnel (Principle 4, Justice).	Without providing specific details, school personnel may not understand the complexities or engage in collaborative relations with the fathers and family members to find solutions, thus violating Principle 3, Autonomy.

(Continued)

Case Study 24.2. Information Sharing *(Cont.)*

Table 24.1. Decision Table for Case Study 24.2 ***(Cont.)***

Possible Action	Positive Outcomes	Negative Outcomes
Provide information to the fathers about current school practice, other evidence-based practice models, IDEA, FERPA, HIPAA, and family counseling options, and assist them in framing the actions they wish to pursue.	Addresses rather than ignores the fathers' concerns (Principle 1, Beneficence, and Principle 2, Nonmaleficence). Provides fathers with information (Principle 5, Veracity) to understand their choices, the laws protecting their rights and those of their children (Principle 4, Justice), and consequences of actions (Principle 3, Autonomy). Allows for referral to other professionals (Principle 1, Beneficence).	Requires additional time, resources, and personnel to implement the plan (Principle 6, Fidelity) and potential exacerbation of family issues (Principle 2, Nonmaleficence).

Note. FERPA = Family Educational Rights and Privacy Act of 1974; HIPAA = Health Insurance Portability and Accountability Act of 1996; IDEA = Individuals with Disabilities Education Improvement Act of 2004.

AOTA provides access to databases, research groups, and online forums to inform occupational therapy practitioners about best practices, current resources, and emerging research related to autism. A document to guide practitioners in advocating for occupational therapy services specifically for individuals on the autism spectrum has been developed (AOTA, 2015e). Membership in AOTA allows for ready access to the *AOTA Evidence-Based Practice and Research* website (AOTA, 2015f) where occupational therapy practitioners can search the *Evidence-Based Resource Directory* for databases and Internet sites related to autism (AOTA, 2015g).

Occupational therapy practitioners also can access *AOTA's Evidence Exchanges* on the website (AOTA, 2015a) and review Critically Appraised Papers (CAPs) related to autism under the headings of "Children and Youth" and "Mental Health." CAPs are peered-reviewed critiques of individual research studies. Occupational therapy practitioners also can access evidence briefs, called "Critically Appraised Topics" (CATs; AOTA, 2015d), that address interventions for people with autism such as sensory and motor processing, social interactions and social skills, behavioral management, and home-based programs. Additional CATs related to autism can be found under the headings of "Early Intervention–Early Childhood," "Sensory Processing and Sensory Integration," and "School-Based Practice." From the Autism Resource webpage, practitioners can access information related to school participation and high school and college success (AOTA, 2015c).

The AOTA has created a series of robust educational opportunities for occupational therapy practitioners who work with individuals on the autism spectrum and their families. According to RSC 1E, occupational therapy practitioners are to "provide occupational therapy services, including education and training that are within each practitioner's level and scope of practice" (AOTA, 2015h, p. 3). According to RSC 1G, occupational therapy practitioners are to "maintain competency by ongoing participation in education relevant to one's practice area" (AOTA, 2015h, p. 3).

As robust as these resources are, additional research and evidence-based data are needed for occupational therapy practitioners to advance their level of competency. For example, more research needs to be conducted to understand how to support the health, well-being, and productive aging of people on the autism spectrum throughout their lives; how to promote their success within work and industry; and how to address other rehabilitation and disability needs that may arise as part of the aging process, such as cerebral vascular accidents, cardiovascular disease, diabetes, and dementia. Vignettes 24.1 and 24.2 depict dilemmas related to competent ethical practice.

Vignette 24.1. Providing Necessary Resources

Lanfen was an occupational therapy practitioner who specialized in working with school-age children with behavioral health challenges. Her cousin, **Ming,** emigrated from China to the United States 2 years ago and was developing an understanding of the English language. Ming had a 1-year-old son, **Jiang,** who inconsistently responded to his name, tolerated eating only a few foods, stared at light patterns for extended periods of time, and was not yet babbling. Ming was proud of Jiang and his ability to entertain himself for extended periods of time. Ming reported that at Jiang's 9-month checkup, the physician said he was healthy. Lanfen had concerns that Jiang may be exhibiting early signs of autism.

Step 1. Gather the facts and specify the dilemma.
Before sharing her concerns with Ming, Lanfen asked herself the following questions:

- As a family member, what is my responsibility to share my concerns with Ming?
- As an occupational therapy practitioner, what expertise do I have for identifying early signs of autism?
- What information can I provide to Ming about childhood development?
- How should I respond to Ming's statement that the physician said Jiang was healthy?

Lanfen then reviewed state licensure guidelines, the Code (AOTA, 2015h), literature about autism on the AOTA website, and resources available for parents on the CDC's *Learn the Signs. Act Early.* website (CDC, 2015) that describe childhood development and expectations for the 12-month well-baby checkup.

Step 2. Analyze possible courses of action.
Lanfen concluded that her relationship with her cousin was familial rather than professional and that she had general rather than expert knowledge about autism in infants and young children (Principle 2, Nonmaleficence). She was knowledgeable about childhood development and the differences in culturally based child-rearing practices in China versus the United States (Principle 1, Beneficence, and Principle 4, Justice). She knew of reputable, free resources available for family members to monitor the development of their young children and checklists parents could use to communicate with the physician during well-baby checkups (Principle 1, Beneficence).

Step 3. Select and implement a course of action.
Lanfen shared the resources with Ming about childhood development and well-baby checkups and agreed to translate the printed material for Ming (Principle 1, Beneficence; Principle 3, Autonomy; and Principle 4, Justice). At Ming's request, Lanfen accompanied Ming and Jiang to the next well-baby checkup to facilitate communication between Ming and the physician and to provide a detailed description of Jiang's observed behaviors (Principle 3, Autonomy, and Principle 5, Veracity).

Step 4. Evaluate the results of the action.
Lanfen's actions maintained the separation between her family and her professional roles while providing Ming with the resources and support to seek appropriate health care for her son.

Advocacy on Behalf of and in Partnership With Individuals on the Autism Spectrum and Their Families

Autism is unique among disability categories because it can be considered as both a disability and an asset. Disability can be viewed as a psychiatric disability category (APA, 2013) or as a social construct limitation (Krcek, 2013). In contrast, many autism advocates view the unique characteristics and abilities of those on the autism spectrum to be assets from the standpoint of neurodiversity (Kapp et al., 2013). Autism advocates suggest that health professionals should provide support for inclusion and participation of individuals on the autism spectrum rather than solely focus on remediating behaviors considered to be unacceptable to society.

The delicate balance between these perspectives creates distinctive ethical challenges for practitioners who want to provide meaningful and ethical services to individuals on the autism spectrum and their families. This is particularly challenging when considering the needs of adults and older adults as individuals age out of pediatric health care systems and take on the challenges of adulthood in society, including higher education, employment, and community-based activities.

Case Study 24.3 highlights some of the challenges in balancing ethical issues with meeting the needs of transition-aged young adults on the autism spectrum, their family members, and school personnel.

Vignette 24.2. Fidelity in Programming

Raouf assumed the role of director of occupational therapy and speech therapy services for children on the autism spectrum in a public school system. Previously, he worked as a director of occupational therapy services in a hospital-affiliated school program that was at the forefront of using research to implement evidence-based and transdisciplinary educational and therapeutic services for children and youth on the autism spectrum.

Raouf was excited to share his expertise and to advance services for children with autism in the public school system (Principle 1, Beneficence, and Principle 4, Justice). After conducting a review of the therapeutic services and meeting with therapy and educational staff, he concluded that within the public school system,

- Education programs and therapeutic services are individualized for each student and are provided primarily on a one-to-one basis or in parallel group structures;
- Educational approaches primarily are based on behavioral management systems;
- Occupational therapy focuses on sensory integration, educational readiness (e.g., fine and gross motor skills, prereading and prewriting skills, basic organizational skills), and self-care skills; and
- Speech therapy uses a pullout model and focuses on language acquisition and communication systems.

Raouf was concerned that missing were

- Integrated educational and therapeutic service plans for each child across disciplines (Principle 1, Beneficence, and Principle 6, Fidelity); and
- Integrated occupational therapy and speech therapy service models that also focus on the students' occupational engagement, social participation, and communication competencies within the context of students' school and daily life occupations (Principle 1, Beneficence, and Principle 6, Fidelity).

Raouf debated whether he should abandon or move forward with his plan to implement evidence-based, integrated therapeutic services that address students' occupational engagement, social participation, and communication competencies within the context of their school and daily life occupations. As part of his deliberations, he examined whether changing well-established education and therapy delivery methods at the school would benefit or disrupt the children's educational progress (Principle 2, Nonmaleficence). He assessed the evidence about the efficacy of the proposed changes; the staff's knowledge base and competency to provide integrated services; the education and time they would require to learn and transition to the new integrated system; and the cost of, and resources available to provide, the services (Principle 1, Beneficence; Principle 5, Veracity; Principle 6, Fidelity).

He also met with the children's parents to ascertain the potential impact of the school changes on the child at home and in the community (Principle 3, Autonomy). Understanding the importance of program assessment, he drafted a plan to evaluate the immediate and sustained effects of the program changes on the students' learning, occupational engagement, social participation, and communication competencies (Principle 1, Beneficence; Principle 2, Nonmaleficence), and the plan's compliance with state and federal education policies (Principle 4, Justice).

Health Disparities in the Transition From Pediatric to Adult Services

Often young adults ages of 18 and 21 years transition from the care of a pediatrician to the care of an adult primary care physician. Similarly, occupational therapy practitioners differentiate their practice into areas, including children and youth and adult services. The transition in services and practitioners can be particularly challenging for youth on the autism spectrum and their families. The continuity of care for adults on the autism spectrum is limited, and preliminary research identifies that adults on the autism spectrum are not receiving the same level of preventive health services as adults without disabilities (AOTA, 2015b; Bruder, Kerins, Mazzarella, Sims, & Stein, 2012).

Often, occupational therapy practitioners who work with adults do not have extensive knowledge regarding specific supports and needs of adults on the autism spectrum, although they have received significantly more education and training in this area than physicians (Ousseny, Massolo, Qian, & Croen, 2015). At a meeting of IACC (2015), public comments included statements of concern and frustration regarding the dearth of services and supports for adults on the autism spectrum. One parent wrote, "We have no caregivers, we can't find anyone. We even pay a lot, but no one knows how or what to do" (IACC, 2015, p. 32).

Case Study 24.3. Support for Transition-Aged Young Adults

Tabitha was a newly hired occupational therapist for a local high school program for young adults aged 18 to 21 years on the autism spectrum. Her primary role on the educational team was to support and prepare individuals in their transition to college, the workforce, community living, or a combination of those upon completion of high school. The team chair informed Tabitha that the students were rarely included in the IEP meetings because of behavioral and communication challenges. Most of the young adults in the program were under legal guardianship of their parents, who typically made the decisions.

The first team meeting to develop a new IEP for **Leo,** a 19-year-old man on Tabitha's assigned caseload, was scheduled for a month later. Tabitha met with Leo to identify goals for his occupational therapy intervention, using the Canadian Occupational Performance Measure (COPM; Law et al., 1998) and the TEACCH Transition Assessment Profile (TTAP; Mesibov, Thomas, Chapman, & Schopler, 2007) to guide her understanding of his priorities and needs. Tabitha's analysis of the evaluation results suggested that Leo was interested in music as a career; wanted to develop friendships and have a girlfriend; and might consider living on his own in the future, although at the time he was dependent on his parents. He did not drive, had never held a paid job, and did not get together with other students outside of the school setting.

Tabitha wanted to work with Leo to present his priorities and goals at the team meeting but was hesitant to introduce new procedures. She used an ethical decision-making model to guide her as she considered the following questions:

- How should she introduce her concerns to the education team regarding the lack of a specific transition plan for Leo and other students on her caseload?
- What are the best strategies to involve Leo in participating in development of IEP- and transition-related goals?
- What are the best strategies to involve the family in the IEP and transition planning?

Step 1. Gather facts.
To understand how to best address these questions, Tabitha first identified specific facts and information that would assist her.

- Tabitha consulted the IDEA website, the AOTA document related to *Guidance and Trends* (AOTA, 2015e), and the guidelines for occupational therapy practice in the school district. She confirmed that the IDEA 2004 mandates a transition plan be in place before the age of 16. Leo's current transition plan was not specific to his identified priorities, and Tabitha wondered if the team was aware of his stated preferences.
- Tabitha also found evidence in the documents to support Leo's participation in the team meeting and weighed this information against the high school's established protocols of including only parents and guardians at the meetings. Results of the TTAP included information from Leo's parents and teachers, which highlighted his communication and behavior challenges, but did not identify his interest in music.

Step 2. Analyze possible courses of action.
Based on her review, Tabitha believed it was her role as an occupational therapist to advocate for Leo's right to be included in planning his future, advocating for himself, and participating in goal determination (Principle 3, Autonomy, and Principle 4, Justice). She used a Decision Table (Table 24.2) to frame her options for various actions she could implement.

Step 3. Select and implement a course of action.
Tabitha reviewed all of her options and considered her responsibility to provide appropriate intervention services for Leo and his family (RSC 1A and RSC 4D) and to promote shared decision making at the IEP meeting with Leo and his family (RSC 3D). Tabitha concluded that by including Leo in a supported way in the IEP meeting and the transition planning, the team could better identify his interests, strengths, preferences, and aptitudes (Principle 2, Nonmaleficence). She discussed her plans individually with Leo, who was excited about taking a greater role

(Continued)

Case Study 24.3. Support for Transition-Aged Young Adults *(Cont.)*

in the process, and also discussed the opportunity with his mother, who supported the plan. During occupational therapy sessions, Tabitha outlined intervention goals with Leo, and together they developed a transition plan to present as a PowerPoint to the team at his IEP meeting.

Step 4. Evaluate the results of the action.
When presented with Tabitha's proposed plan for the team meeting, team members were interested in the intervention strategies that she planned to implement to support Leo's autonomy. They were impressed with her advocacy actions based on evidence and supported the process by revising the timeframe to better accommodate Leo's participation in the meeting. Tabitha felt that the guidance she gained from her review of the Code (AOTA, 2015g) and her review of the literature related to autism and the transition process strengthened her position. She upheld the Principles of Beneficence, Nonmaleficence, Autonomy, and Justice and laid the groundwork for similar practices with other students on her caseload.

Table 24.2. Decision Table for Case Study 24.3

Possible Action	Positive Outcomes	Negative Outcomes
Take no action. Report the results of the evaluation at the team meeting on Leo's behalf.	Tabitha would meet RSCs 6H and 6K, Fidelity, by communicating collaboratively as a member of the team and by abiding by the school's policies, procedures, and protocols.	Possible violation of RSC 3D, Autonomy, by neglecting to promote shared decision making with Leo.
Discuss alternative strategies to Leo's participation in the team meeting with the chair of the IEP team and other team members, including Leo's family members.	Provides appropriate services (Principle 1, Beneficence) and advocates for changes in policy that are in line with IDEA and best practices (Principle 4, Justice). Addresses practice that violates the spirit of IDEA transition planning (Principle 2, Nonmaleficence).	Discussing Leo's potential participation in the meeting without his or his parents' permission may violate Principle 3, Autonomy.
Notify the team of the best practice recommendations for transitioning youth and present evidence related to IDEA 2004 compliance regarding participation in team meetings. Coach Leo in presenting his issues at the IEP meeting in a way that he feels comfortable and empowered.	Promoting fairness and advocating for Leo upholds Principle 4, Justice. Establishes a collaborative relationship with Leo and team members and encourages his autonomy (Principle 3, Autonomy).	Tension among team members who are not in agreement with a change in policy related to team meetings may violate Principle 2, Nonmaleficence.

Note. IDEA = Individuals with Disabilities Education Improvement Act; IEP = individualized education program; RSC = Related Standard of Conduct.

Examples of resources to help expand occupational therapy practitioners' knowledge of adults on the autism spectrum include *Adults With Intellectual and Developmental Disabilities: Strategies for Occupational Therapy* (Haertl, 2014), *Transitions Across the Lifespan: An Occupational Therapy Approach* (Orentlicher, Schefkind, & Gibson, 2015), and *Scope of Occupational Therapy Services for Individuals Across the Life Course* (AOTA, 2015i).

As more youth on the autism spectrum age into adulthood, occupational therapy practitioners who work with adults need to pay specific attention to the Principles of Beneficence, Nonmaleficence, Autonomy, and Justice, and how they relate to

Vignette 24.3. Ethical Decision Making in Acute Care

Bayani had worked with an adult neurological population in acute care at a large metropolitan hospital for 5 years after spending several years working with children and youth in a school system. His supervisor asked him to consult with the orthopedic staff because they had just admitted a 38-year-old man named **Armando** who had a diagnosis of autism and had sustained fractures to his right femur, ankle, wrist, and humerus in a hit-and-run car accident. Medical staff also wanted to rule out a possible head injury and were trying to determine if the behaviors Armando was exhibiting were related to autism or might have been the result of a head injury from the accident.

Armando had minimal communication strategies and used an iPad to communicate simple responses to questions. He was sedated after surgery to reset the bones in his arm and leg. The hospital staff was concerned about how to provide the most effective care for Armando because no one had experience treating adults on the autism spectrum. Because of Bayani's previous experiences with autism in a school system, his supervisor asked him to provide advice and support to the staff on strategies for communication and intervention.

Bayani's experiences were specific to children and youth on the autism spectrum, and he was unsure if he could ethically provide appropriate support for the staff as well as for Armando (RSC 2A). However, he realized that he had more experience than others and wanted to ensure that Armando received an appropriate evaluation and intervention consistent with Principle 1, Beneficence. Also, he was concerned that if he did not comply with his supervisor's request, he might be violating RSC 2B by abandoning the service recipient. He wanted to ensure that he was able to exercise appropriate professional judgment by applying principles from interventions for youth on the autism spectrum to an adult. Bayani analyzed principles in the Code (AOTA, 2015h), conducted a preliminary appraisal of CATs related to autism on AOTA's website (www.aota.org), and reviewed information on the Autism Speaks website (www.autismspeaks.org) about adults on the autism spectrum.

Bayani decided to meet Armando, review his history, and provide the staff with basic information regarding the characteristics of autism. He also provided the staff with a summary of resources that he deemed useful. Bayani consulted with Armando's mother, who was his legal guardian, about his particular needs, routines, and effective strategies. He gained her approval of and support for a plan of action, in line with Principle 6, Fidelity. Addressing RSC 6H, promoting collaborative actions to facilitate quality care for clients, Bayani believed he could outline a preliminary plan of care for the orthopedic staff and act as a consultant regarding strategies and approaches specific to autism.

Note. CATs = critically appraised topics; RSCs = Related Standards of Conduct.

their practice. In Vignette 24.3, an occupational therapy practitioner considers these ethical principles in his role as a team member in a hospital setting.

Summary

Because of the neurodevelopmental, ideological, political, and social complexities associated with autism, ethical dilemmas exist on the best way to provide services for people on the autism spectrum and their families. The Code (AOTA, 2015h), in addition to the multitude of resources available on the AOTA website that are supported by evidence identified in the literature, can guide an ethical decision-making process. Currently available resources focus primarily on children and youth, although the increase in the prevalence of autism worldwide has given rise to a greater need to develop resources, programs, and effective interventions for adults on the autism spectrum. Occupational therapy practitioners are poised to address this need and be a great resource for those on the autism spectrum.

Reflective Questions

1. How do your current knowledge, experiences, and value systems create ethical dilemmas for you when working with people on the autism spectrum and their families?
2. Using the structure of the Decision Table in Case Studies 24.1 and 24.3, what actions might you take to address the dilemmas identified in Question 1, and what could be the potential outcomes of those actions?
3. How do current occupational therapy practices contribute to ethical dilemmas when working with professionals from other disciplines to provide services for people on the autism spectrum and their families?
4. What ethical dilemmas might arise as aging adults who are on the autism spectrum seek occupational therapy services?

References

American Occupational Therapy Association. (2014). Occupational therapy practice framework; Domain and process (3rd ed.). *American Journal of Occupational Therapy, 68*(Suppl. 1), S1–S48. https://doi.org/10.5014/ajot.2014.682006

American Occupational Therapy Association. (2015a). *AOTA's Evidence Exchange*. Retrieved from http://www.aota.org/Practice/Researchers/Evidence-Exchange.aspx

American Occupational Therapy Association. (2015b). *Autism in adults*. Retrieved from http://www.aota.org/Practice/Rehabilitation-Disability/Emerging-Niche/Autism.aspx

American Occupational Therapy Association. (2015c). *Autism resources*. Retrieved from http://www.aota.org/Practice/Children-Youth/Autism.aspx

American Occupational Therapy Association. (2015d). *Autism spectrum disorder critically appraised topics*. Retrieved from http://www.aota.org/practice/children-youth/evidence-based.aspx#autism

American Occupational Therapy Association. (2015e). *Autism spectrum disorders: Guidance and trends*. Retrieved from http://www.aota.org/Practice/Children-Youth/Autism/Guidance-Trends.aspx

American Occupational Therapy Association. (2015f). *Evidence-based practice and research*. Retrieved from http://www.aota.org/Practice/Researchers.aspx

American Occupational Therapy Association. (2015g). *Evidence-based practice resource directory*. Retrieved from http://www.aota.org/Practice/Researchers/EBP-Resource-Directory.aspx

American Occupational Therapy Association. (2015h). Occupational therapy code of ethics (2015). *American Journal of Occupational Therapy, 69*(Suppl. 3), 6913410030. https://doi.org/10.5014/ajot.2015.696S03

American Occupational Therapy Association. (2015i). Scope of occupational therapy services for individuals with autism spectrum disorder across the life course. *American Journal of Occupational Therapy, 69*(Suppl. 3), 6913410054. https://doi.org/10.5014/ajot.2015.696S18

American Psychiatric Association. (2013). *Diagnostic and statistical manual of mental disorders* (5th ed.). Washington, DC: Author.

Autism Speaks. (2015). *Ten years of progress: A life of hope*. Retrieved from https://www.autismspeaks.org/

Autistic Self Advocacy Network. (2015). *Position statements*. Retrieved from http://autisticadvocacy.org/policy-advocacy/position-statements/

Blacher, J., & Christensen, L. (2011). Sowing the seeds of the autism field: Leo Kanner (1943). *Intellectual and Developmental Disabilities, 49*(3), 172–191. https://doi.org/10.1352/1934-9556-49.3.172

Bruder, M., Kerins, G. Mazzarella, C., Sims, J., & Stein, N. (2012). Brief Report: The medical care of adults with autism spectrum disorders: Identifying the needs. *Journal of Autism and Developmental Disorders, 42,* 2498–2504. https://doi.org/10.1007/s10803-012-1496-x

Centers for Disease Control and Prevention. (2014, March 28). Prevalence of autism spectrum disorders among children aged 8 years–Autism and Developmental Disabilities Monitoring Network, 11 sites, United States, 2010. *Morbidity and Mortality Weekly Report, 63,* SS–2. Retrieved from http://www.cdc.gov/mmwr/preview/mmwrhtml/ss6302a1.htm

Centers for Disease Control and Prevention. (2015). *Learn the signs: Act early.* Retrieved from http://www.cdc.gov/ncbddd/actearly/

Family Educational Rights and Privacy Act of 1974, Pub. L. 93–380, 20 U.S.C. § 1232g; 34 CFR Part 99.

Haertl, K. (Ed.). (2014). *Adults with intellectual and developmental disabilities: Strategies for occupational therapy.* Bethesda, MD: AOTA Press.

Health Insurance Portability and Accountability Act of 1996, Pub. L. 104–191, 110 Stat. 136.

Individuals with Disabilities Education Improvement Act of 2004, Pub. L. 108–446, 20 U.S.C. 1400–1482

Interagency Autism Coordinating Committee. (2014). *2013 IACC summary of advances in autism spectrum disorder research.* Retrieved from http://iacc.hhs.gov/summary-advances/2013/index.shtml

Interagency Autism Coordinating Committee. (2015). *Written public comments.* Retrieved from https://iacc.hhs.gov/events/2015/comments/written_public_comments_111715.pdf

Kanner, L. (1943). Autistic disturbances of affective contact. *Nervous Child, 2,* 217–250. Retrieved from http://www.neurodiversity.com/library_kanner_1943.html

Kapp, S. K., Gillespie-Lynch, K., Sherman, L. E., & Hutman, T. (2013). Deficit, difference, or both? Autism and neurodiversity. *Developmental Psychology, 49,* 59–71. https://doi.org/10.1037/a0028353

Krcek, T. E. (2013). Deconstructing disability and neurodiversity: Controversial issues for autism and implications for social work. *Journal of Progressive Human Services, 24*(1), 4–22. https://doi.org/10.1080/10428232.2013.740406

Law, M., Baptiste, S., Carswell, A., McColl, M. A., Polatajko, H., & Pollock, N. (1998). *Canadian occupational performance measure* (3rd ed.). Ottawa, ON: CAOT Publications ACE.

Mesibov, G., Thomas, J. B., Chapman, S. M., & Schopler, E. (2007). *TEACCH Transition Assessment Profile [TTAP]* (2nd ed.). Austin, TX: Pro-Ed.

Orentlicher, M., Schefkind, S., & Gibson, R. (Eds.). (2015). *Transitions across the lifespan: An occupational therapy approach.* Bethesda, MD: AOTA Press.

Ousseny, Z., Massolo, M. L., Qian, Y., & Croen, L. A. (2015). A study of physician knowledge and experience with autism in adults in a large integrated healthcare system. *Journal of Autism and Developmental Disorders, 45,* 4002–4014. https://doi.org/10.1007/s10803-015-2579-2

World Health Organization. (2013). *Autism spectrum disorders and other developmental disorders: From raising awareness to building capacity.* Retrieved from http://apps.who.int/iris/bitstream/10665/103312/1/9789241506618_eng.pdf

Zablotsky, B., Black, L. I., Maenner, M. J., Schieve, L. A., & Blumberg, S. J. (2015). Estimated prevalence of autism and other developmental disabilities following questionnaire changes in the 2014 National Health Interview Survey. *National Health Statistics Reports No 87.* Hyattsville, MD: National Center for Health Statistics.

Chapter 25.

TECHNOLOGY: ETHICS OF SERVICE DELIVERY

Mary Ellen Buning, PhD, OTR/L, ATP/SMS, RESNA Fellow

Learning Objectives

By the end of the chapter, readers will be able to

- Understand the unique contributions that occupational therapy practice can make in the evaluation and support of clients who can benefit from assistive technology (AT),
- Describe how the Principles and Related Standards of Conduct within in the *Occupational Therapy Code of Ethics (2015)* protect and enable consumers when practice includes or should include AT,
- Apply occupational therapy ethical principles when functioning within an interdisciplinary AT model, and
- Associate continuing education and AT certifications with practice specialization and capacity for advanced-level practice.

Key Terms and Concepts

- ✧ Assistive technology
- ✧ Assistive technology device
- ✧ Assistive Technology Professional certification
- ✧ Assistive technology service
- ✧ Empowerment model
- ✧ Information and communication technologies
- ✧ Rehabilitation Engineering and Assistive Technology Society of North America
- ✧ Specialty Certification in Environmental Modification
- ✧ Technology
- ✧ Technology-Related Assistance for Individuals With Disabilities Act of 1988

Occupational therapy has always incorporated technology into its practice. This is evident in the definition of the word ***technology,*** which "is the application of scientific knowledge for practical purposes" (Oxford University Press, n.d., para. 1). ***Assistive technology (AT)*** includes "devices and services that make it possible for people with disabilities to participate in everyday tasks" (DeCoste, 2013, p. 499).

Occupational therapy practitioners have always modified common technologies, tools, and materials of the day to adapt valued activities like weaving, wood working, and cooking. Inspired by creativity and their knowledge of physics, kinesiology, and activity analysis, they used these technologies to achieve therapeutic goals such as increasing strength, relearning skills, adapting daily environments, and enabling self-care tasks.

Our present understanding of technology is influenced by today's world. To most people, the word *technology* describes devices that are based on microprocessors, digital signals, and wireless communication with all types of user interfaces that produce amazing outputs. As the technology revolution continues, today's occupational therapy practitioners will discover even more ways to use it to enable functional task performance, support learning and other cognitive processes, and compensate for missing body structures and functions. This chapter provides an overview of technology in occupational therapy, legal definitions, and ethical challenges.

Legal Definitions

Although occupational therapy practitioners used technologies as intervention tools for years, lawmakers, via the ***Technology-Related Assistance for Individuals With Disabilities Act of 1988*** (Tech Act; P. L. 100–407), created the definition that is most relevant for this chapter. An ***AT device*** is defined as "any item, piece of equipment, or product system, whether acquired commercially, modified, or customized, that is used to increase, maintain, or improve functional capabilities of individuals with disabilities" (§2202[2]). AT can be

- Low-tech (e.g., communication boards made of cardboard or fuzzy felt);
- High-tech (e.g., special-purpose computers);
- Hardware (e.g., prosthetics, attachment devices such as mounting systems, positioning devices);
- Computer hardware (e.g., special switches, keyboards, pointing devices);
- Computer software (e.g., screen-readers, communication software);
- Inclusive or specialized learning materials, curriculum aids, and software; and
- Much more, including digital devices, standard manual and ultralight manual wheelchairs or powered wheelchairs with custom complex seating and user interfaces, or computers and communication devices controlled with speech recognition, eye-gaze, and head trackers. (Adapted from Assistive Technology Industry Asociation, 2016, para. 2)

An ***AT service*** is "any service that directly assists an individual with a disability in the selection, acquisition, or use of an assistive technology device" (§1308[2]). Examples of AT services taken from the Tech Act include

- Evaluating a person's AT needs, including a functional evaluation of how AT would help him or her;
- Purchasing, leasing, or otherwise providing an AT device;
- Selecting, designing, fitting, customizing, adapting, applying, maintaining, repairing, replacing, or donating an AT device;
- Coordinating and using therapies (e.g., occupational therapy) with AT devices under an educational, rehabilitative, or vocational plan;
- Training or technical assistance for people with a disability and their family members, guardians, advocates, or authorized representatives;
- Training or technical assistance for educational or rehabilitation professionals, AT device manufacturers, employers, training and employment services providers, and others who help people with disabilities; and
- Providing a service that expands access to technology, including email and the Internet, to people with disabilities.

The Tech Act is aligned with occupational therapy's Core Values of Altruism, Equality, Freedom, Justice, Dignity, Truth, and Prudence (American Occupational Therapy Association [AOTA], 2015). The Tech Act's purpose was to support inclusion and participation by individuals with disabilities by eliminating barriers, enabling choice, and placing the dignity and empowerment of the individual's desire for meaningfulness and life satisfaction at the center of the AT intervention.

Information and Communication Technologies

Today, decades after the Tech Act was passed and reauthorized, technology is even more integral to daily life because it supports and drives all types of human enterprise. ***Information and communication technologies*** (ICTs) is an umbrella term that includes any communication device or application, encompassing "radio, television, cellular phones, computer and network hardware and software, satellite systems and so on, as well as the various services and applications associated with them, such as videoconferencing and distance learning" (Rouse, 2005, para. 1). ICTs are usually discussed within a particular context such as education, health care, or business.

Given this fact, AT could be viewed as the digital equivalent of ramping an entrance, making toilets accessible, or ensuring that websites comply with World Wide Web Consortium (WC3) standards (Berners-Lee, 2016). Berners-Lee, recognizing the importance of including everyone in the revolution brought about by the web, initiated the development of the WC3 to guide the development of webpages and websites to offer accessibility features and ensure the Internet's long-term growth and usability.

AOTA considers technology to be an element of the practice context and categorizes it as "a virtual context," because technology interactions occur absent of physical contact (AOTA, 2014, p. S9). The profession acknowledges that this "virtual context is becoming increasingly important for clients as well as occupational therapy practice" (AOTA, 2014, p. S9).

AT also can be seen as interventions that provide clients with opportunities to develop specific performance skills needed to participate in key human occupations such as social participation, education, play, and work, (AOTA, 2014). AT is more than context when it enables print literacy through digital tools and software that compensate for dyslexia or enable text entry, choice selection, and self-determination in the presence of total paralysis. AT is more than preparation for a new digital reality; it has the potential to allow development of motor, process, and social interaction skills as well.

As technology continues to develop, the profession may need to consider new constructs and language. Not fully preparing for technology's influence and potential will lead to harm to those we serve as exemplified in Principle 1, Beneficence (Related Standards of Conduct [RSCs] 1A–1G, 1I); Principle 2, Nonmaleficence (RSCs 2A, 2B); and Principle 3, Autonomy (RSC 3J; *Occupational Therapy Code of Ethics (2015)*, hereinafter referred to as the "Code"; AOTA, 2015).

Empowerment Model

The Tech Act is compatible with occupational therapy practice. It is grounded in the concept of client-centered decision making within an interdisciplinary team and is related to reducing the impact of impairment on skills development. The Act states that the process of acquiring AT should use a person-centered or ***empowerment model.*** Psychologist Carl Rogers (1989) pioneered the concept of the *empowerment model* with his focus on the client as an individual who possess goals, abilities, and strengths. AT intervention is envisioned as having the potential to create "congruence" as a result of a skilled match for the individual that augments abilities and minimizes impairment. Congruence is possible through the unique ability of technologies to enable compensation in powerful new ways so people's potential is allowed to surface. This technological compensation gives individuals the power to achieve goals and self-actualize (Rogers, 1989).

In the empowerment model, occupational therapy practitioners are facilitators who collaborate with clients and others to evaluate, plan, and use new tools to help clients achieve goals. Most commonly, members of the AT team blend their knowledge and skills to benefit the client. Early AT adopters often cross-trained, so professional delineation was not always exact. For example, occupational therapy practitioners learned about communication devices, and speech–language therapists learned about adaptations for user interface. Interdisciplinary, client-centered teams are central to AT service delivery because diverse skill sets are needed to implement complex solutions.

Applying Occupational Therapy Ethical Principles in an Interdisciplinary AT Model

Ethical issues can arise in every area of occupational therapy practice, but as occupational therapists move to further develop competence within AT service delivery, they may find themselves facing issues that require application of ethical behavior and decision making in an unfamiliar realm. Guidelines need to be developed to promote self-assessment of skills and knowledge. In addition, opportunities to acquire specialty knowledge, to stay updated about new devices, and to obtain guidance in applying them to specific functional limitations are needed.

ACOTE Standards

AT content is required as part of the profession's educational standards as seen in Accreditation Council for Occupational Therapy Education (ACOTE; 2012) Standards B.5.10, B.5.11–13, and B5.23–24. ACOTE standards include statements such as "articulate principles of and be able to design, fabricate, apply, fit, and train in assistive technologies and devices (e.g., electronic aids to daily living, seating and positioning systems) used to enhance occupational performance and foster participation and well-being" (p. S45). Students attracted to practice specializing in these areas need to be encouraged to further develop skills and knowledge by pursuing advanced-level practice and connecting with occupational therapy practitioners who have this specialization.

ACOTE standards also include, within the Foundational Content section, ACOTE Standard B.1.8, "Demonstrate an understanding of the use of technology to support performance, participation, health and well-being. This technology may include, but is not limited to, electronic documentation systems, distance communication, virtual environments, and telehealth technology" (ACOTE, 2012, pp. S34–S35). Hopefully, student learning within these broader forms of ICT will expose them to usability, technology problem solving, using tech support and learning how software features can affect performance. Attention to these areas is supported in the Code (AOTA, 2015) by Principle 1, Beneficence (RSCs 1A–1G, 1I), Principle 2, Nonmaleficence (RSC 2B); Principle 3, Autonomy (RSC 3B); Principle 4, Justice (RSC 4C, 4D); and Principle 6, Fidelity (RSCs 6D, 6H, 6I, 6K).

Beneficence

Occupational therapy practitioners, unaware of the range or sophistication of AT options, may not recognize the potential benefits for a client and so fail to refer them for AT services. These challenges may arise because of inadequate educational preparation, personal discomfort with technology, time and productivity pressures in practice settings, or limited access to AT expertise. Practitioners may find it easier to use interventions they relied on in the past.

Occupational therapists always need to be aware of the boundaries of their competence. Many AT resources can be located with plain-language queries on search engines or YouTube. Often consumer-oriented organizations such as the Christopher and Dana Reeve Foundation (Wilderotter, 2016) or Autism Speaks (Geiger, 2016) offer advice and reviews. A client assessment that points to difficulty in meeting occupational goals should motivate the occupational therapist to consider the possibility of AT or a consultation with an AT specialist to discuss alternate options for reaching a goal.

Vignette 25.1 illustrates how learning more about the evidence related to keyboarding or speech recognition as compensation for impaired visual–motor perception skills may support achievement of academic goals.

Nonmaleficence

The rapid evolution of ICT can create ethical challenges when practitioners have incomplete or out-of-date knowledge of terminology, options in user interface technologies, products, resources, and the interoperability of microprocessor-driven devices. An information deficit leaves occupational therapy practitioners vulnerable to making poor decisions based on biased or outdated information sources, thus wasting resources. It is common for novice practitioners to be overly influenced by enthusiastic

Vignette 25.1. Lack of AT Device Knowledge

Consider the **school-based therapist** who repeatedly submits annual individualized education program (IEP) handwriting goals for a fourth-grader who is still failing to meet written language standards. The practitioner should explore the evidence about using keyboarding or speech recognition as a better tool for developing written language proficiency. Or, think about the **pediatric therapist** who recommends manual wheeled mobility for a toddler with spastic tetraplegia. This therapist may be uneducated or overwhelmed by the complexity of trying to learn about the process of developing driving skills with a power chair and its associated benefits for perception, socialization, self-concept, and learning that comes from independent access to the environment (Deitz, Swinth, & White, 2002; Nilsson, Eklund, Nyberg, & Thulesius, 2011). These situations relate to the Principle of Beneficence and RSCs 1B, C, and F.

product representatives. Suppliers and marketers may be equipment experts, but a practitioner should be the expert on the client and on his or her function. Data from evaluation and goal setting should enable the practitioner to represent the client's strengths and limitations and then help select product features and technology outputs. The practitioner's knowledge of the client's occupations, environments, supports, and access to transportation also are issues to consider.

Vignette 25.2 illustrates how the rapid progression of the availability of more consumer-oriented devices can save money and enable tech-savvy family members to provide ongoing support to a family member with a common visual impairment.

Autonomy

Principle 3, Autonomy, respects clients' desires and supports their self-determination. AT does not succeed by itself but relies on a range of community supports to make the outcome possible, as explained in Vignette 25.3. The following success story about Tom relies not only on his therapist's AT knowledge but also on his therapist's advanced occupational therapy practice skills, knowledge of systems, leadership, and advocacy and collaboration with Tom's family and others on his school AT team. With these tools and services, Tom developed the skills to arrive at an amazing outcome.

Justice

In contrast to Tom's experience, individuals with significant impairments commonly have limited options for independent living. Many live lives of passive dependence on the edge of poverty. State Medicaid programs have Home and Community Support Waivers and are developing more user-driven options as alternatives to nursing homes (Centers for Medicare and Medicaid Services, 2016). According to the National Council on Disability (NCD), state agencies often leave federal funds on the table because the required state-level matches were not allocated. This can be true for vocational rehabilitation, too—a key source of funding for AT devices and services for training and employment (NCD, 2010).

Occupational therapy practitioners are often on the front lines and see the consequences of limitations in the use of AT services; however, they also understand how AT devices could assist in the remedy of such injustice. Advocacy can become a critical professional role when the alternative is injustice. In this situation, Principle 4, Justice (RSCs 4B, 4D, 4I), would guide the practitioner (AOTA, 2015).

Veracity

Occupational therapy practitioners demonstrate ethical behavior when they show respect for the developers of software, hardware, and other forms of intellectual property. Although sometimes protected by educational use, school districts and other practice settings should not excuse unlicensed distribution of illegal copies or educational resources. The population of those who require adaptive hardware and software is relatively small, and the inventors' rights need to be respected so inventors can remain in business and financially support themselves and future clients with this important work.

Veracity is based on honesty and candor as well as the objective transfer of information. School-based occupational therapy practitioners on AT teams may recognize a related situation. Some school districts do not allow school AT team members to specify a particular AT, augmentative and alternative communication device (AAC), or mobility device in the results section of an AT evaluation. Practitioners are warned that naming AT equipment will obligate the school system to pay for the specified device as part of a student's IEP and so exhaust a school system budget. Practitioners with knowledge of the potential benefit of AT devices often fear repercussions from special education managers and avoid putting this information into a child's

Vignette 25.2. Using AT Knowledge to Guide Decisions

An **occupational therapist** working in a geriatric setting is persuaded by a product sales to recommend that a family make a private-pay purchase of a specialized low vision device for a parent with sudden-onset macular degeneration. A more knowledgeable therapist might have suggested a much less expensive option (e.g., tablet). Mass market products often offer built-in accessibility options like audible books, voice output for text messages, large print, and even the ability to photograph a page of text and translate it into speech, and more. This alternative could provide more value for the client and avoid violating RSCs 2A, 2C, and 2 D (AOTA, 2015).

Vignette 25.3. Opening the Door to Self-Determination

Today **Tom** lives in his own apartment in the same town as his parents. He had this option because the AT devices and services introduced during his school years allowed him to compensate for his unintelligible speech and inability to walk. Without AT, Tom would never have had the opportunity for the independence, self-directedness, and quality of life he has today. At age 25 years, he lives in a wheelchair-accessible apartment with staff support. His apartment has modifications that make it easy for staff to help with showers and transfers. He can direct his personal care assistants because he started using an AAC in elementary school. His family supported his device mastery by waiting for him to use his device rather than anticipating his needs.

Learning to use a power chair in wheelchair-friendly environments allowed Tom to develop visual–perceptual and cognitive skills like wayfinding and remembering directions. Powered mobility helped him learn to manage time and develop a sense of personal efficacy. After integrated control was set up, Tom could use his wheelchair joystick to control the cursor on his AAC device. This meant the AAC device was always handy and he could more quickly find its stored language.

If we eavesdropped on Tom's life today, we would consider him a master at using his AAC device. He is ready for any interaction. It has allowed his educational inclusion and enabled him to develop friendships and learn community living skills. These two forms of AT have supported the development of important performance skills and are continuing to support him with new activities like using accessible public transportation, having a part-time job at the YMCA, and going to movies with friends.

If left to their own knowledge and resources, Tom's parents could never have envisioned this kind of life for their son. They always wanted the best for Tom and relied on his occupational therapist, **Cyndi,** for guidance. Cyndi linked the family with others in educational and community support networks to help Tom incrementally build the skills that led to his self-determined life. This vignette demonstrates the potential of AT when used well and exemplifies the Code's (AOTA, 2015) Principle 1, Beneficence (RSCs 1A–1D); Principle 2, Nonmaleficence (RSC 2B); Principle 3, Autonomy (RSCs 3A, 3D, 3J); and Principle 4, Justice (RSC 4A).

IEP. Thus students and their concerned parents languish without important equipment because school-based occupational therapy practitioners withhold information. This situation points toward violation of Principle 4, Justice (RSC 4B), and Principle 5, Veracity (RSC 5G), of the Code (AOTA, 2015).

Fidelity

Many AT practitioners have been in the situation in which steps taken to reach a final goal with a client suddenly seem out of reach. A practitioner's fear that the proposed AT solution will fail can create panic. Can technical problems with a new AT device be resolved? Is the elementary school student who has been so successful with math software doomed because nobody can find software that handles algebra equations? What should happen when a client with multiple needs arrives on a caseload and the needed AT resources are not available?

Fidelity to client needs will lead an ethical occupational therapy practitioner to search for greater expertise, a continuing education class, a help line, or an equipment loan bank. Knowledgeable mentors and resources exist; they can take the form of a consultation with a colleague with advanced practice skills or via an e-mail group, a product help desk, a search on a remote database, or a face-to-face demonstration via video conferencing. These are the powerful tools and advantages of serving clients within the arena of digital assistive technologies. These actions demonstrating a practitioner's determination to acquire information arise from Principle 6, Fidelity (RSCs 6H, 6I), of the Code (AOTA, 2015).

AT in Occupational Therapy Practice

Across practice settings, there are individuals who could and perhaps should benefit from an introduction to AT. Occupational therapy practitioners with AT skills can support interaction through learning; they can also help these individuals regain mobility-related independence and move ahead with participation in education vocation and community living (AOTA, 2016). As wireless technology becomes increasingly commonplace, the average person will use it and rely on it more. Occupational therapy is poised to be to be the health care profession most capable of adapting and modifying wireless technology to enable the occupations of everyday life.

Occupational therapy practitioners use the Core Values of Altruism and Prudence to guide their use of specific AT with different populations across practice settings. In using technology as a practice tool, practitioners need to be aware of the multiple individual and contextual issues at play.

Practitioners must determine whether their AT intervention skills are at the beginner, intermediate, or advanced levels.

Early efforts to define levels of competence within AT service delivery for occupational therapy practitioners were initiated but never formally adopted (Hammel & Angelo, 1996). Guidelines were proposed to help academic programs teach entry-level practice skills and to serve as the baseline for future work (Hammel & Angelo, 1996; Hammel & Smith, 1993). AOTA (2010) took this work further, creating a matrix of skills defining beginner and advanced levels for occupational therapy practitioners.

Behavioral objectives still need to be developed to promote the use of these competencies to help practitioners self-assess their skill level and support their compliance with Principle 1, Beneficence (RSC 1E), and Principle 2, Nonmaleficence (RSC 2A).

ATP Certification as Evidence of AT Practice Skills

The ***Rehabilitation Engineering and Assistive Technology Society of North America*** (RESNA), an interdisciplinary member organization dedicated to the use of technology to "promote the health and well-being of people with disabilities," has developed service delivery knowledge and skills (RESNA, 2015, para. 1). Founded in the late 1970s by a group of Canadian and U.S. rehabilitation engineers interested in designing and refining products to be used by individuals with impairment, RESNA's focus on technology and disability enables a variety of health care professionals to acquire AT knowledge and skills through continuing education.

AOTA does not offer certification in AT, so occupational therapy practitioners who want to distinguish themselves as having advanced knowledge and specialized practice skills in AT earn an ***Assistive Technology Professional*** (ATP) ***certification*** through RESNA. The organization also offers a more advanced certification, the Seating and Mobility Specialist certification. These certifications indicate that practitioners have met established criteria, which include passing certification exams, pursuing continuing education, and complying with RESNA's Code of Ethics and Standards of Practice, which apply to interactions with clients, colleagues, employers, and payers (RESNA, 2000, 2008). They allow occupational therapists to self-identify as having focused on developing skills in AT. Certifications indicate knowledge of devices, services, and funding streams as well as competence in evaluating consumer needs, assisting in selection of appropriate AT devices, and training and integrating devices into roles and activities.

Many occupational therapy practitioners with RESNA credentials teach other occupational therapy practitioners about AT by lecturing in ACOTE-certified educational programs, providing workplace in-services, hosting webinars, presenting at conferences, and serving as education specialists for a wide range of AT manufacturers. These more experienced colleagues support others in acquiring greater knowledge and in developing their critical-thinking, problem-solving, and decision-making skills in the area of AT.

SCEM Certification as a Support to Delivery AT Devices and Services

AOTA (2013) developed a ***Specialty Certification in Environmental Modification*** (SCEM). As discussed previously, environmental modification is essential for the successful implementation and integration of AT device use into everyday life. In many ways, the ability to determine environmental needs and provide intervention strategies, suggest devices, and recommend space adaptations is also a part of AT service delivery. The SCEM reflects the person–environment fit, which enhances occupational performance and maximizes participation, safety, accessibility, and independence (Caplan, 1987). An occupational therapy practitioner's commitment to a specialty area of practice allows great satisfaction, continual challenges, and the development of a unique set of professional occupational therapy skills.

Digital assistive technologies are constantly changing, and clients may need to rely heavily on human and nonhuman (i.e., environmental) supports. For example, the best power wheelchair has little value without an accessible environment. Those who successfully learn to use AAC devices need communication partners who expect them to use their device and are willing to teach social language pragmatics (American Speech–Language–Hearing Association, 2016; Fried-Oken, Beukelman, & Hux, 2011).

Human behavior, the socioeconomic realities of home life, cultural attitudes about disability, access to health insurance, transportation options, and access to wi-fi are examples of human and nonhuman supports that are potential barriers to or facilitators of service delivery and the full integration of AT devices into human occupations. This kind of awareness of the effect of environment on successful intervention often comes with more advanced practice, which supports Principle 1, Beneficence (RSCs 1A, 1F), of the Code (AOTA, 2015).

Case Study 25.1, including Table 25.1, illustrate a situation that occurred when an occupational therapist with extensive experience with seating and mobility first interacted with a rehabilitation technology supplier who was accustomed to providing the most expedient device. This had been the vendor's style for many years, but it failed to take into consideration recommending a mobility device that best served a client with a progressive diagnosis or that enabled completion of valued daily life occupations.

Summary

AOTA offers wise guidance to its members and to those who interact with or are served by occupational therapy practitioners. The Code is broad enough to consider all aspects of service provision and the

Case Study 25.1. Unethical Wheelchair Sale

Kevin lived in the public housing tower near the rehabilitation hospital with its AT program that included a wheelchair seating and mobility clinic. Diagnosed with Ehlers-Danlos Syndrome, a progressive, hereditary connective tissue disorder, Kevin asked for a referral from his primary care physician for a wheelchair evaluation. In the last year he had become unsafe when driving in his heavy-duty three-wheeled scooter. The scooter, which he used extensively in the community, had tipped several times on poorly maintained sidewalks and left him struggling both to get up and to put the scooter back on its wheels. These falls led to two emergency room visits within 6 months.

Kevin lived with his mom in the public housing tower, and because of his outgoing, friendly personality, he knew many residents. Having a scooter and a helpful nature, he found an unexpected occupation. He often provided grocery-shopping services for his mom and soon, by word of mouth, he started doing this same errand for other elderly residents in their tower. With his scooter, he was able to get to a grocery store about 8 blocks from the tower. However, his scooter mishaps made him fearful about continuing to make these trips.

As **Trudy,** the occupational therapist, began her assessment, she started to question whether a scooter was still the best mobility device for Kevin. His Ehlers-Danlos symptoms had progressed so that he now had much greater joint pain, weakness, and increased risk of falls during transfers. At this point Kevin was even using his scooter inside the tiny two-bedroom apartment that he shared with his mom.

Trudy recognized how difficult it must be for Kevin to steer a large, full-sized scooter in the small spaces of a tower apartment. She opened the door to discussion about switching to a mid-wheel drive power chair that would be more powerful on community sidewalks, provide more needed postural support, and be easier to maneuver with his apartment. Trudy learned about what issues Kevin faced by forming a positive therapeutic relationship with him during his intake interview and their intervention planning session. Trudy complimented Kevin on his Gay Pride ball cap and asked whether he was in the recent community parade. Kevin said he had and eagerly shared his experience, reporting that he had carried his small dog between his feet on his scooter. Kevin was pleased to share this story and reported that he was ready to start looking for a new gay rights bumper sticker for the proposed new power chair. This exchange between Kevin and Trudy was emblematic of her efforts to establish support and a trusting relationship.

With this information recorded, Kevin returned to the clinic for a second visit and was introduced to **Ray,** a local rehabilitation technology supplier who worked for a large national wheelchair company. Trudy and Kevin told Ray about the need for a midwheel drive power chair to enable improved in-home mobility but that also had the power and durability to support Kevin's volunteer role in his public housing tower. The mobility device specifications were within the funding criteria for Kevin's Medicaid HMO plan. Extra time was spent discussing other options such as sturdy arm rests and an extra-wide foot plate.

(Continued)

Case Study 25.1. Unethical Wheelchair Sale *(Cont.)*

After this occupational therapy session, the evaluation and device feature justification report was finished, co-signed by Kevin's primary care physician, sent to Ray's company for attachment of a detailed product description for final physician signature, and then submitted to Medicaid for funding approval.

At no time did Ray disclose his difference of opinion about the product selection to Trudy. However, Trudy later learned that Ray had phoned Kevin, told him that Medicaid would likely deny the chair Trudy had recommended, and in getting a denial, he would likely lose approval for any replacement power chair. This scared Kevin and persuaded him to agree to Ray's option: a lesser-quality power chair with smaller motors and batteries and upholstered seating without the recommended postural supports for his regional lumbar pain.

In recommending his preferred chair, Ray avoided spending the unpaid time that might have been required for a Medicaid appeal. Ray also avoided the final fit session (required by Trudy) by failing to report that Medicaid had approved a power chair or that it was delivered directly to Kevin at his apartment "in response to Kevin's urgent need." Kevin ambivalently decided not to pursue Trudy's recommendation and agreed to Ray's plan out of gratitude for his willingness to consider his needs. Ray's phone communications had shaken Kevin's confidence in Trudy's competence and desire to meet his needs. Ray's unethical behavior was not discovered until 3 months later when Trudy happened to see Kevin on the street near the clinic and the story of Ray's subversion was unveiled. Three potential actions Trudy could take care analyzed in Table 25.1.

Table 25.1. Decision Table for Case Study 25.1

Action	Positive Outcomes	Negative Consequences
Trudy takes no action; dismisses the delivery of Kevin's new power chair as the result of "unfortunate" miscommunication. Violates Principles 1, 4, 5, and 6 (AOTA, 2015).	Kevin gets a new wheelchair but not the product best suited to his diagnosis, other health conditions, or his occupational needs.	Kevin gets an inferior wheelchair that does not provide effective postural support, increases his risk of skin breakdown, and will not hold up to contextual demands. Medicaid spends less money but makes a funding decision based on manipulated information.
Trudy calls Ray to confront him about his dishonesty. Ray dismisses her concern saying that he was focused on Kevin's welfare.	Trudy feels vindicated by confronting Ray with her discovery, but she also feels manipulated by Ray who says the client was happy. Trudy leaves the unethical behavior unresolved for fear of a future confrontation or argument resulting from categorizing his behavior as a violation of the RESNA Code of Ethics, which applies to him as an ATP. She decides she will never work with Ray again.	Ray feels free to proceed in his action because no penalty follows. He made more profit on the sale of Kevin's less expensive wheelchair. Ray views "time as money," and he reduced time spent with both the therapist and client and in a potential appeal for denial.
Trudy contacts the RESNA Professional Standards Board that regulates the RESNA Code of Ethics (RESNA, 2000) for those with ATP Certification. She files a formal complaint. Supports Principles 1, 3, 4, 5, and 6 (AOTA, 2015).	Ray's ATP credential is suspended by RESNA for 6 months and the Medicaid agency gets a notification. Ray changes his business plan so he works primarily with children and avoids adults likely to have Medicare. Medicare requires ATP certification, but state Medicaid does not.	Kevin was unwilling to upgrade his mobility device because he has high anxiety and fear of repercussions. Kevin has often been the target of bullying because of his gender identity. Due to his openness about his sexual orientation, he was concerned about potential retribution if he pressured Ray to upgrade his device.

Note. AOTA = American Occupational Therapy Association; ATP = Assistive Technology Professional; HMO = health maintenance organization; RESNA = Rehabilitation Engineering and Assistive Technology Society of North America.

settings in which it occurs, yet it is specific enough to guide practitioners in the most specific area of the intervention dyad. This wisdom allows the Code to easily apply to a newer area of practice such as AT.

The challenge in this relatively new area of practice is to recognize the need for ethics in situations that can and do arise because of a client's need for specific AT solutions or AT accommodations that are beyond the norm for a particular setting. Situations like these will demand new learning or consultation and potential referral to others who have the skills and knowledge needed to ensure client success.

Reflective Questions

1. What opportunities do today's telecommunication technologies provide to assist a novice occupational therapy practitioner in making informed decisions and avoiding doing harm?
2. What are some important decision-making safeguards to remember and use when trying to decide among competing claims from AT product or device manufacturers?
3. How do occupational therapy practitioners know or judge when they need to refer a client to a practitioner with greater knowledge or experience (e.g., how do you know when you do not have enough knowledge or experience)?
4. What are some options for finding someone with more expertise who can assist? What are some options when travel distance is great or resources are low?

References

Accreditation Council for Occupational Therapy Education. (2012). 2011 Accreditation Council for Occupational Therapy Education (ACOTE) standards. *American Journal of Occupational Therapy, 66*(6 Suppl.), S6–S74. https://doi.org/10.5014/ajot.2012.66S6

American Occupational Therapy Association. (2010). Specialized knowledge and skills in technology and environmental interventions for occupational therapy practice. *American Journal of Occupational Therapy, 64*, 544–556. https://doi.org/10.5014/ajot.2010.64S44

American Occupational Therapy Association. (2013). *Specialty certification in environmental modification.* Retrieved from http://www.aota.org/education-careers/advance-career/board-specialty-certifications/environmentalmodification.aspx

American Occupational Therapy Association. (2014). Occupational therapy practice framework: Domain and process (3rd ed.). *American Journal of Occupational Therapy, 68*(Suppl. 1), S1–S48. https://doi.org/10.5014/ajot.2014.682006

American Occupational Therapy Association. (2015). Occupational therapy code of ethics (2015). *American Journal of Occupational Therapy, 69*(Suppl. 3), 6913410030. https://doi.org/10.5014/ajot.2015.696S03

American Occupational Therapy Association. (2016). Assistive technology and occupational performance. *American Journal of Occupational Therapy, 70,* 7012410030. https://doi.org/10.5014/ajot.2016.706S02

American Speech–Language–Hearing Association. (2016). Social language use (Pragmatics). *Topic Index.* Retrieved from http://www.asha.org/topicindex/

Assistive Technology Industry Association. (2016). *What is AT?* Retrieved from http://www.atia.org/at-resources/what-is-at/

Berners-Lee, T. (2016). *World Wide Web Consortium (W3C).* Retrieved from http://www.w3.org/

Caplan, R. D. (1987). Person–environment fit theory and organizations: Commensurate dimensions, time perspectives and mechanisms. *Journal of Vocational Behavior, 31,* 247–267. https://doi.org/10.1016/0001-8791(87)90042-X

Centers for Medicare and Medicaid Services. (2016). *1915(c) Request for information—Provision of timely and quality home and community based services.* Retrieved from https://www.medicaid.gov/medicaid/hcbs/guidance/index.html

DeCoste, D. C. (2013). Best practices in the use of assistive technology to enhance participation. In G. Frolek Clark & B. Chandler (Eds.), *Best practices for occupational therapy in school* (pp. 499–512). Bethesda, MD: AOTA Press.

Deitz, J., Swinth, Y., & White, O. (2002). Powered mobility and preschoolers with complex developmental delays. *American Journal of Occupational Therapy, 56,* 86–96. https://doi.org/10.5014/ajot.56.1.86

Fried-Oken, M., Beukelman, D. R., & Hux, K. (2011). Current and future AAC research considerations for adults with acquired cognitive and communication impairments. *Assistive Technology, 24*(1), 56–66. https://doi.org/10.1080/10400435.2011.648713

Geiger, A. (2016). *Autism Speaks: Resource guide.* Retrieved from https://www.autismspeaks.org/family-services/resource-library

Hammel, J., & Angelo, J. A. (1996). Technology competencies for occupational therapy practitioners. *Assistive Technology, 8,* 34–42. https://doi.org/10.1080/10400435.1996.10132271

Hammel, J. M., & Smith, R. O. (1993). The development of technology competencies and training guidelines for occupational therapists. *American Journal of Occupational Therapy, 47,* 970–979. https://doi.org/10.5014/ajot.47.11.970

National Council on Disability. (2010). *Vocational rehabilitation (VR) funding*. Retrieved from https://www.ncd.gov/publications/2010

Nilsson, L., Eklund, M., Nyberg, P., & Thulesius, H. (2011). Driving to learn in a power wheelchair: The process of learning joystick used in people with profound cognitive disabilities. *American Journal of Occupational Therapy, 65*, 652–660. https://doi.org/10.5014/ajot.2011.001750

Oxford University Press. (n.d.). *Technology*. Retrieved from https://en.oxforddictionaries.com/definition/technology

Rehabilitation Engineering and Assistive Technology Society of North America. (2000). *RESNA code of ethics*. Retrieved from http://www.resna.org/sites/default/files/legacy/certification/RESNA_Code_of_Ethics.pdf

Rehabilitation Engineering and Assistive Technology Society of North America. (2008). *RESNA Standards of practice for assistive technology professionals*. Retrieved from http://www.resna.org/sites/default/files/legacy/certification/Standards_of_Practice_final_10_10_08.pdf

Rehabilitation Engineering and Assistive Technology Society of North America. (2015). *RESNA policy position statement*. Retrieved from http://www.resna.org/knowledge-center/government-relations/resna-policy-position-statement

Rogers, C. R. (1989). *The Carl Rogers reader*. Boston: Houghton Mifflin.

Rouse, M. (2005). *Definition: ICT (information and communications technology—or technologies)*. Retrieved from http://searchcio.techtarget.com/definition/ICT-information-and-communications-technology-or-technologies

Technology-Related Assistance for Individuals With Disabilities Act of 1988, Pub. L. 100–407, U.S.C. 2201–2217

Wilderotter, P. J. (2016). *Christopher and Dana Reeve Foundation*. Retrieved from https://www.christopherreeve.org/living-with-paralysis

Chapter 26.

REIMBURSEMENT: ETHICAL CONSIDERATIONS FOR GETTING PAID—AND FAIRLY

Wayne L. Winistorfer, MPA, OTR

Learning Objectives

By the end of the chapter, readers will be able to

- Describe how a variety of health care service reimbursement mechanisms apply to occupational therapy practice environments,
- Apply Principles of the *Occupational Therapy Code of Ethics (2015)* to analyze conflicts generated while striving to adhere to reimbursement rules and organizational directives,
- Differentiate among alternative decisions and actions that best resolve ethical dilemmas encountered in occupational therapy reimbursement, and
- Use the Code and Related Standards of Conduct to guide future decision making applicable to reimbursement of occupational therapy services.

Key Terms and Concepts

- ✧ Beneficence
- ✧ Episode-of-care reimbursement
- ✧ Fee-for-service reimbursement
- ✧ Prospective payment
- ✧ Reimbursement
- ✧ Reimbursement systems

In general, consumers make conscious choices about the goods and services we purchase based on a variety of factors, including preferences, convenience, and price. However, when it comes to health care, consumers have few choices, and we face economic transactions unlike any others. In the world of fine dining, some exclusive restaurants don't list prices on the menu. Unless we are very wealthy, most of us do not frequent restaurants of this ilk. The phrase "If you have to ask, you can't afford it!" speaks to the rational, economic reasoning that cost considerations often take priority ahead of quality, or our cravings for an exceptionally fine experience.

When told we need a health service or procedure, patients almost never get to review a full list of services and the corresponding prices. We have limited voice in selecting the medical services we want or need. Health care workers are woefully unprepared to supply an accurate bill, and we often wait months before we receive the bill for our appointments, tests, or treatments.

When we assume the role of patient, our skills as savvy shoppers often fail or are simply not applicable to health care transactions. We typically have limited choices of where we may access health services. Our bodies may be subjected to tests and procedures performed by health care providers we will never meet or won't remember because we are in pain or are sedated. It is also rare to know, in advance of receiving the service, exactly what we will eventually be required to pay. In other routine purchases and other service transactions, we would not tolerate businesses that fail to disclose their prices and bill customers as health care services do.

Health care funding and reimbursement are complex and unique. Health care services constitute a large service industry. Health care products and services have a massive scope, and who is responsible for payment is far different than other services.

In this chapter, occupational therapy reimbursement will be viewed from two perspectives:

1. The occupational therapy practitioner's perspective on the systems of payment encountered, requirements of these systems, and ethical challenges encountered.
2. The client's perspective on the challenges of accessing occupational therapy services and collaborating in ways that respect autonomy and unique desires and contexts.

Both viewpoints bring forth the potential for conflicts of values and ethical challenges. Limited choices and financial constraints require decision making in which the "right" choice is often not evident.

The *Occupational Therapy Code of Ethics (2015)* (hereinafter referred to as the "Code"; American Occupational Therapy Association [AOTA], 2015) describes the core values of the profession. The Related Standards of Conduct (RSCs) delineate specific strategies and behaviors to address situations and common dilemmas encountered by occupational therapy practitioners. The Code is an important tool to inform, illuminate, and guide choices that are ethically sound.

What Is "Reimbursement," and Why Should We Care?

The term ***reimbursement*** implies compensation or repayment after an expense has been incurred or after services have been rendered. In the United States, most payments for health services are, in fact, paid after some proof of services (e.g., medical records, claim forms) is submitted and accepted. A very small percentage of health services are paid for before or at the time of service. Reimbursement for occupational therapy services is a topic of concern because getting paid represents a paycheck for the therapist.

Reimbursement results in profitability, or at least a positive financial return, for the organizations employing occupational therapy practitioners and certainly for those who operate their own private practice. Reimbursement represents sustainability for both the therapist and the organization to continue to provide services. The complexity of ***reimbursement systems***—the processes that must be followed and regulations that dictate the type, intensity, and duration of services—presents challenges for occupational therapy practitioners.

Noncompliance with requirements because of processing errors or ignorance may result in rejection of submitted claims and denial of payment. Overt violation of rules and regulations can result in civil and criminal penalties.

The challenges of reimbursement present ethical dilemmas for occupational therapy practitioners. A variety of reimbursement mechanisms, including fee for service, episode of care, and self-pay, are explored in this chapter, and an assortment of ethical dilemmas that may be encountered are identified.

Double Win: Benefits and Rewards

Occupational therapy practitioners can typically share their story of why they were drawn to their profession. These stories invariably include an explicit or implied values statement of a desire to help others. Beneficence is an important ethical principle of the occupational therapy profession (AOTA, 2015). ***Beneficence*** "includes all forms of action intended to benefit other persons" and "connotes acts of mercy, kindness, and charity" (Beauchamp & Childress, 2013, as cited by AOTA, 2015, p. 2). Essential to the Principle of Beneficence is an action required to effectively help others by promoting good, preventing harm, and, in some instances, removing harm. Occupational therapy is a beneficent profession.

At the same time, individuals rarely enter this profession with abundant financial resources or an overriding altruistic intent to provide occupational therapy services on a charitable, uncompensated volunteer basis. Certainly, the time and expense devoted to successfully completing an occupational therapy education is deserving of rewards after the practitioner has entered the workforce. The rewards of a career in occupational therapy include professional engagement and personal satisfaction. Work in this field also provides compensation at a wage capable of supporting a satisfactory standard of living.

Occupational therapy practitioners are not unique from other workers who expect to be compensated for their efforts and paid fairly. Accepting compensation for services is coupled with our duty to conform to the realities of how occupational therapy services are reimbursed.

AOTA (2014) describes the profession's foundation of client-centered services and goals focused on enhancing the occupational engagement of those served. Occupational therapy practitioners also address the contexts and environments that restrict full engagement. The realities of the contexts in which some clients function may well include financial limitations, preventing full occupational engagement. Occupational therapy practitioners must deal with the array of regulations, requirements, mechanisms, and seeming idiosyncrasies of those who are paying the bills. In some instances, practitioners accept private payment from the client or simply opt out of the profession. Vignette 26.1 describes rules and challenges unique to reimbursement for rehabilitation professions.

Vignette 26.1. Reimbursement: Challenged Occupational Therapist

Occupational therapist **Mitch** recently accepted a job with high earning potential at a thriving outpatient private practice owned by **Sheila,** a respected physical therapist in their community. Mitch was hired to serve primarily a young adult population with commercial insurance or Workers' Compensation. Because of an influx of new clinic patients, Mitch was assigned several patients with Medicare as their main payment source. As usual, Mitch used standardized assessments to complete the initial evaluation and establish appropriate intervention plans for each patient.

Mitch entered the clinical documentation and submitted charges via the clinic's electronic record and management system. When Mitch exported the data, the electronic system generated red-flag reminders to prepare and send a Physician Plan of Care and to enter Medicare G-codes. Mitch vaguely recalled a discussion of Medicare Part B requirements, yet he bypassed the red flags. Mitch reasoned that because he didn't really understand the rules and the system allowed bypass of the red flags, they must not be important (AOTA, 2013).

At the beginning of the next month, Sheila reviewed the insurance denials as well as claims that had been rejected. She easily identified that nonpayable G-codes for functional limitations were missing from charges Mitch had submitted for his Medicare patients. Sheila confronted Mitch and directed him to fix the charges. Mitch asked Sheila to explain why the no-fee codes were important. He knew he had followed the standards of practice, used standardized evaluation tools, and had documented thoroughly. Sheila reminded Mitch about the impending Medicare Part B reimbursement changes based on value. "Though reimbursement is not yet based on this method, the functional reporting requirements will affect payment based on the level of change we accomplish during the course of therapy," Sheila said. "Claims that don't include the G-codes are simply rejected."

Sheila, who happened to be quite familiar with reimbursement regulations and, as the state Physical Therapy Association's ethics chairperson, was familiar with ethics principles, also informed Mitch that consistent with the Principle of Beneficence, the use of standardized assessments is a best practice and an approved method of quantifying functional limitations. Also the Principle of Justice requires compliance with regulations in documentation; red flags in the electronic documentation system, an error-proofing tool, are not to be ignored. The Principle of Fidelity requires stewardship of resources. Noncompliance with reimbursement requirements may result in nonpayment for services. Stewardship requires respect for the employer's financial interests.

Sheila also reminded Mitch that the compensation section of his employment contract was configured with a base wage plus a bonus formula factoring in volume and value, including outcomes and patient satisfaction. Sheila scolded Mitch, "When you ignore the rules, it's disrespectful of my business, violates my trust, and conflicts with the Principle of Veracity. If this business doesn't get paid, you don't get paid, at least not as well!" Sheila clarified that the "procedure count volume" for services that are not reimbursed because of avoidable error are ineligible for bonus. Mitch readily admitted his errors and thanked Sheila for setting him straight. Mitch decided he would improve his knowledge of and compliance with Medicare guidelines. Mitch recognized it was in his employer's and his best interest to be compliant.

Reimbursement: Duty to Inform

Occupational therapy's service model includes interventions ranging from one or more brief sessions to hours, weeks, months, or even years of services. As a result, occupational therapy practitioners may have more opportunity than many other health care providers, and therefore a higher duty, to provide clients with information and resources regarding reimbursement. Provisions in the Patient Protection and Affordable Care Act of 2010 (P. L. 111–148) and comparable changes in Medicare have resulted in an estimated 45% of older adults switching their insurance plan in the past two years (Fitteron, 2015). The amount of time spent with clients, coupled with the therapeutic and personal relationships developed, increase the likelihood that occupational therapy practitioners are asked, "Please help me! I don't understand my health insurance." The Principle of Veracity (AOTA, 2015) requires that occupational therapy practitioners implicitly promise to be truthful and not deceptive in communications. Furthermore, without also ensuring that the client understands the information provided, the transmission of the information is considered to be incomplete (AOTA, 2015). Vignette 26.2 depicts an occupational therapy client experiencing the challenges of knowing about and paying for health care services.

In most situations, we would consider Steve to be a smart shopper. Steve is probably asking reasonable questions. The Principle of Autonomy (AOTA, 2015), often referred to as the *self-determination principle,* conveys practitioners' duty to treat clients according to their desires, within the bounds of accepted standards of care. However, respecting a person's autonomy goes beyond acknowledging an individual as a mere agent; it acknowledges a person's right "to hold views, to make choices, and to take actions based on [his or her] values and beliefs" (Beauchamp & Childress, 2013, p. 106). Clients have a right to make decisions about their care on the basis of their personal circumstances, including financial constraints.

Consider your reactions and potential responses when clients express their autonomy:

- What should an intervention plan include when a client provides an absolute dollar limit they are willing or able to spend for occupational therapy services?
- What do you do if the client demands you accept their full and accurate payment for the day's visit at the end of each therapy session?
- Should you inform the client exactly how long each visit will last, and are you capable of declaring the exact number of visits that will be required to achieve full functional performance?

Vignette 26.2. Out-of-Pocket Expenses: Challenged Client

Steve suffered a non-work–related traumatic injury to his dominant right forearm and hand. After a surgical repair, Steve was referred to **Sally,** an occupational therapist with specialty certification as a hand therapist. The surgery and related services exhausted the maximum payable amount of Steve's high-deductible health insurance plan, and the plan's coverage for outpatient therapy services required significant out-of-pocket expense.

As soon as Sally introduced herself, Steve immediately requested a price list. Steve was adamant and explained, "When I take my car to the shop for an oil change or repairs, I see the price list posted above the service desk. I can even compare prices by checking the websites of other shops. My guys at the car repair shop always give me a price quote for the services they recommend. When they diagnose the cause of a noise my car is making, they always describe the problem and give me a detailed explanation of what it will take to fix it. They always tell me the estimated maximum cost of getting my car back to running safely and smoothly. Just last week they recommended several routine maintenance options that cost more than I can afford right now. I told them that I'm just too strapped for cash, and they helped me decide which repairs were most important. I was able to choose my car's 'treatment plan' based on what I could afford. So, Sally, before I start therapy, you need to understand that I'm paying for this out of my own pocket. You need to tell me what it is going to cost to get my arm and hand back in working order! And, by the way, what kind of a deal can you give me?!"

Sally's response was brief and accurate, yet inadequate to satisfy Steve's request. "It depends," she said. "I can tell what our rates are, but what we charge depends on your intervention plan, which modalities we use, the duration of each visit, and how long you continue to need therapy. It is possible that your insurance may actually pay a portion of your bill. And, by the way, we don't have sales, and you can't get discount coupons for my services. So all I can tell you is, 'It depends.' Paying for health care is different than paying for your car repairs."

Consider your response when clients asks for full information, such as a

- Charge list, including a; description of all services and the rate per service;
- Upfront price guarantee for each therapy visit;
- Detailed intervention plan with the list of the *Current Procedural Terminology*® codes (American Medical Association, 2014) that will be charged and the exact number of units that each procedure code will be charged at each visit; or
- Accurate quote of the portion of the total bill that will be their responsibility.

It is little wonder that in some outpatient settings, clients do not consistently comply with the established intervention plan, or they reduce visits and the duration of care without communication because of unknown costs. Sometimes the reality of the client's context and the choices the individual makes are driven by challenges of using occupational therapy services that are simply too expensive, and the client's financial constraints produce significant negative outcomes as they attempt to pay for other personal and family needs.

The Code includes several RSCs that address a client-centered respect for autonomy:

- *RSC 3C:* "Obtain consent after disclosing appropriate information and answering any questions posed by the recipient of service . . . to ensure voluntariness" (AOTA, 2015, p. 4); and
- *RSC 3E:* "Respect the client's right to refuse occupational therapy services temporarily or permanently, even when that refusal has potential to result in poor outcomes" (AOTA, 2015, p. 4).

Reimbursement: More Than Insurance

Today's occupational therapy practice environments involve a multitude of payment sources. Casto and Forrestal (2013) describe the two major categories of payment for health care reimbursement: (1) fee-for-service reimbursement and (2) episode-of-care reimbursement.

In ***fee-for-service reimbursement,*** specific fees are established and payments are made for each service rendered. Examples include self-pay options, traditional retrospective payment systems, and managed care methodologies used by commercial insurance and some government-sponsored insurance plans. Specific examples included in this chapter further describe these methods of reimbursement.

In ***episode-of-care reimbursement,*** providers receive one lump sum for all services they provide related to a condition, disease, or duration of treatment. Within episode-of-care methodology, capitated payments are fixed and are not tied to the actual volume or intensity of services provided.

Prospective payment methods of episode-of-care reimbursement mean payment rates are established in advance for a specific time period. Average levels of resources provided for certain types of patients, conditions, or health care settings are used to establish predetermined payment rates; these "relative weights" may result in higher rates of reimbursement for some services. Several U.S. federal payment programs use case-based prospective methods, including payments applicable to skilled nursing facilities, home health agencies, and inpatient rehabilitation facilities (Casto & Forrestal, 2013).

Some reimbursement sources have highly complex rules for patient eligibility and specific requirements for documentation. These frameworks, including Medicare and Medicaid, directly affect the types of services that may be provided, the organizational settings and environments in which the services are provided, and the quantity and duration of services delivered.

Some other sources of reimbursement may seem quite removed from daily practice, yet the funds allocated for programs and services have a direct impact on staffing resources and availability of supplies and equipment (e.g., occupational therapy services included in the daily rate for behavioral health programs). No single method or source of reimbursement is free of potential conflicts. In Case Study 26.1, an occupational therapist is challenged with balancing the demands of multiple roles and complying with rules of reimbursement.

In Case Study 26.1, Ted obviously violated several principles of the Code. By accepting the work at both nursing homes, Ted overcommitted to do more than he could possibly fit into his day. Instead of assertively notifying one or more of his employers that he was not able to accomplish the work within the available time, Ted violated the principle of Nonmaleficence and RSC 2C by failing to take appropriate action to remedy

Case Study 26.1. Reimbursement Challenges

Ted, an occupational therapist, considered himself to be a "free agent" as a PRN *(pro re nata)* therapist. He regularly scheduled for weekend shifts and accepted short-notice weekday requests from the rehabilitation services departments of three local skilled nursing facilities (SNFs). Ted liked the flexibility of his employment status, which allowed him to prioritize his family's demands and activities. Ted's spouse traveled for work, and together they were raising four active adolescents.

Early on a Friday morning, Ted received calls from two SNFs, both describing their staffing need as "desperate" because of sick calls from the permanent staff, new admissions, and the upcoming weekend. Ted recalled that he had a parent–teacher meeting scheduled for his troubled son at the end of the school day. Ted decided to accept the requests to work at both SNFs, performing occupational therapy evaluations before noon at Lakeside Villa and providing therapy interventions to a few residents in the afternoon at Golden Acres Care Center. Ted prided himself on being efficient, so he was confident he could fulfill these work assignments and still be on time for the meeting at his son's school. Besides, the extra income would help pay for driver's education classes for his nearly 16-year-old twins.

Upon arrival at Lakeside Villa, **Jill,** the rehab director, informed Ted of an additional resident admitted this morning, one more than was known at the time Ted was called in. Jill instructed Ted, "Because of the resident's managed care plan, you have to see him for an occupational therapy evaluation today. There's no wiggle room with this insurance." Ted completed the residents' evaluations and documented the findings. However, because of the time for the additional resident, the documentation was not at the standard of quality Ted expected of himself.

Checking the clock and realizing it was already after 1 p.m., Ted knew the residents scheduled at Golden Acres were waiting for him. Upon arriving and feeling the time crunch, Ted gathered the three residents on his schedule in the rehab gym. He briefly reviewed the individualized goals that had been established by the Golden Acres staff occupational therapist. Ted moved back and forth among the residents, doing his best to provide individualized attention. Ted thought that because no other therapists were in the department, no one would know whether he provided group or individual therapy, even though it was not consistent with the established intervention plans for the residents. Ted rationalized, "Better they get some therapy than none at all." Ted ended the therapy session in less than 1 hour and then documented each of the services provided in the resident's records. Ted felt okay about his actions because he was scheduled to work at Golden Acres on Saturday and was confident he could make up for the short session at that time.

Upon entering service charges, Ted realized that **Mrs. Merrick,** one of the residents he had just seen, was in the 7-day assessment period. Ted had missed the note requesting that Mrs. Merrick be seen for 53 minutes of occupational therapy to reach the 720-minute Ultra High (Resource Utilization Group) Level. Ted had had previous encounters with the SNF administrator and **Oscar,** the rehabilitation director. He had been called out the last time he had not provided the required minutes for a resident. Ted knew there would be trouble if the expected services were not delivered during the assessment period that established Mrs. Merrick's level of care.

Ted decided to enter four 15-minute charge units and record 53 minutes of occupational therapy service for Mrs. Merrick. During the therapy session, Mrs. Merrick kept falling asleep and repeatedly asked to go back to her room. Ted knew Mrs. Merrick could not have tolerated even 25 minutes of individual therapy and certainly not the 53 minutes that he recorded.

Ted left Golden Acres and arrived 25 minutes late for his appointment at his son's school. His spouse was angry that she had to deal with the school staff on her own. That evening, Ted apologized to his spouse and vowed to say "no" more often when he was called to work. He also shared that he hated being put in situations where he was asked to do too much because the quality of his work suffered and he ended up having to enter charges that were "not quite right."

personal problems and limitations that might cause harm to clients.

Ted also violated RSC 2H by compromising the rights or well-being of those served by falsifying documentation of the services provided. Ted violated the principle of Autonomy and RSC 3A, which requires honoring "the expressed wishes of recipients of services" (AOTA, 2015, p. 4), by ignoring Mrs. Merrick's requests to end the therapy session. Ted violated the Principle of Justice and RSC 4M, which stipulates billing and collecting fees must be done "legally and justly in a manner that is fair, reasonable, and commensurate with services delivered" (AOTA, 2015, p. 5), when he entered charges for services that were not provided and essentially committed fraud (Centers for Medicare and Medicaid Services, 2014).

The situations and environments that Ted encountered and in which he actively engaged are a major cause for concern in the occupational therapy profession, especially in SNFs. The Office of the Inspector General is taking notice (Levinson, 2015). Medicare rules are rife with opportunities for exploitation. Opportunities to violate the rules, because of personal and organizational challenges, also create opportunities for occupational therapy practitioners to violate ethical standards. Ted's behavior violated several ethical principles, violated the rights of those he served, and ultimately did not enhance the reputation of the occupational therapy profession.

Reimbursement and Patient Responsibility

Discussions of health care reimbursement typically center on the challenges faced by the occupational therapy practitioner or the organization. What about the challenges of reimbursement from the client's perspective? Clients (e.g., customers, patients, students, participants, members) have autonomous rights such as consent for intervention and consent to the components of a particular plan, including frequency and duration of the episode of care, choices about adherence to a home program, and decisions to use or abandon adaptive equipment. Clients also have some level of financial responsibility when they enter into a therapeutic transaction. This responsibility may include, but is not limited to, carrying an eligible insurance plan, paying their cost share as a co-pay at the time of service, making regular payments on their insurance deductible, subscribing to governmental health insurance programs for which they are eligible, and paying local, state, and federal taxes that support school-based services and community mental health programs. Case Study 26.2 highlights how clients may be

Case Study 26.2. Financially Challenged Parents

Feline, an 8-year-old with sensory processing disorders, was seen by the school-based occupational therapy team 3 times a week because she had an established "exceptional educational need." Feline's teachers, therapists, and parents all agreed that she was making great progress and the impact of occupational therapy interventions had been significant.

At the end-of-the-school-year interdisciplinary team meeting, Feline's parents asked that services be continued during the summer. The head of the Special Needs Program informed the parents that therapy services were not available during the summer break. Feline's parents expressed disappointment and demanded to know about other resources. **Nikki,** the occupational therapy assistant on the team, shared that the nearby hospital's outpatient therapy department, with **Dawn,** an occupational therapist with a specialty in pediatric rehabilitation, could be a good resource for Feline.

After the team meeting, the parents, who felt close to Nikki, asked if she would be willing to provide services privately to Feline over the summer. The parents shared their concerns about being able to afford Feline's summer day care expenses but still wanting to do the best for Feline. Knowing that Nikki loved the outdoors, they offered Nikki and her family a week at Feline's grandparent's lake cabin in return for her work with Feline. Table 26.1 provides

(Continued)

Case Study 26.2. Financially Challenged Parents *(Cont.)*

Table 26.1. Decision Table for Case Study 26.2

Possible Action	Positive Outcomes	Negative Consequences
Take No Action: Violates Principles of Beneficence and Nonmaleficence		
The Special Services Team ignores the parents' request for help. Nikki does not recommend options for services.	The staff expends no effort. "Thank goodness, summer break is here!"	The parents are frustrated and struggle with Feline's behavior as the summer progresses (RSCs 4B, 4C). Feline receives no occupational therapy services for 12 weeks, and her behavior deteriorates (see RSC 2B).
Ethically Suspect Actions: Violates principles of Beneficence, Nonmaleficence, and Fidelity		
Nikki decides to accept the parents' offer for 1 week at a lakeside cabin in exchange for providing services to Feline during the summer.	Feline receives services from a therapist she knows. The parents are relieved that Feline is benefitting from occupational therapy services. Feline is able to pursue existing goals and make some progress. Nikki's family enjoys their weeklong vacation.	Nikki struggles with professional concerns. There is no occupational therapist to consult. She wonders if Feline's intervention plan should be modified, based on the progress she observes (RSC 1E). Nikki experiences personal anxiety about ramifications at work if they discover she provided services to a student on her own time (RSCs 6C, 6K). Nikki experiences moral distress about bartering her time for a very expensive, weeklong lakeside cabin vacation (RSC 2J).
Dawn, an occupational therapist, performs the initial evaluation and initiates therapy. Dawn does not contact the parent's insurance company for prior authorization. (See details later in the discussion of this case study.)	Feline is seen 3 times a week for occupational therapy services, just as she is during the school year. Feline makes great progress. Dawn is satisfied that she made a difference for Feline and helped fill the gap created by the school system.	Insurance company denies payment as "non-covered service" because of "exclusion from Certificate of Coverage" (RSC 4B). Feline's parents are shocked to receive bills for occupational therapy services (RSC 4C). The parents can't pay the bills, and the bills are sent to collection (RSC 2A). The parents feel betrayed by Nikki's recommendation and for refusing to barter for the family cabin in return for providing therapy for Feline. The parents are angry with Dawn for not informing them of their responsibility (RSC 5D). Feline's parents tell other parents at the school about their bad experience (RSC 6L).
Ethically Sound Actions: Honors Principles of Beneficence, Nonmaleficence, Fidelity, and Justice		
Nikki offers an option for summer services.	Feline's parents pursue a viable option (RSCs 4B, 4C). Feline receives appropriate services and continues to make progress (Principle 1, Beneficence).	None.

(Continued)

Case Study 26.2. Financially Challenged Parents *(Cont.)*

Table 26.1. Decision Table for Case Study 26.2 (*Cont.*)

Possible Action	Positive Outcomes	Negative Consequences
Dawn takes steps to • Pursue prior authorization, investigate the family's eligibility for the hospital's self-pay program, and assist them in applying for the self-pay program. • Modify visit frequency and provide services at an acceptable frequency.	Feline receives appropriate services and makes progress (RSC 1A). The parents manage their finances and balance resources to meet their daughter's needs (RSC 4C). There are no surprises for the parents and no unplanned expenses (RSC 4B).	Feline does not receive occupational therapy services at the recommended intensity, so does not make as much progress as anticipated (RSC 2A).

an analysis of several options and potential outcomes of each action.

Nikki was tempted to accept the offer of the summer cabin, but declined knowing

- The complexity of Feline's challenges would be too much for her,
- There would be no occupational therapist in charge of the intervention plan,
- Accepting "payment" of a weeklong cabin stay would be a conflict of interest with her employment by a public school system, and
- Establishing a unique relationship with Feline and her family could cloud her objectivity with the family in the future.

Nikki decided the best way to advocate for Feline was to help make arrangements at the nearby outpatient clinic.

Feline's parents were relieved when they were able to schedule occupational therapy sessions for Feline at the outpatient clinic with Dawn, an occupational therapist specializing in sensory processing disorders. Dawn completed an initial evaluation with Feline and established an intervention plan that closely mirrored Feline's school-based service plan. Dawn was known for being diligent in making sure her services were covered, so she submitted a Prior Authorization request to the insurance company. The insurance company rejected the request on the basis of a determination of Feline's condition as developmental delay, a specific exclusion in the insurance plan's certificate of coverage.

Dawn discussed the situation with Feline's parents, who were persistent. They asked for Dawn's advice. Fortunately, Dawn's employer was a nonprofit, faith-based organization with the philosophy that "no one be denied needed services." The children served at the clinic often did not have commercial insurance because most were eligible for Medicaid, although reimbursement was typically below cost. Dawn was able to offer the parents the self-pay program, which her employer considered to be an important community service for children with disabilities.

This program charged at rates that just covered the expense of staff salary and benefits. The criteria for eligibility for this less-than-break-even program included the following:

- The client is "insurance eligible," but the insurance plan has denied coverage. (The insurance company is not billed for the service.)
- The client's physician orders occupational therapy.
- The parents desire ongoing therapy services for their child.
- The parents agree to pay out of pocket at the self-pay program rate.
- The family is charged for all occupational therapy services at a flat rate per visit.
- As an added incentive, charges are discounted 20% when payment is made on the date of service.

Although Feline's parents both worked full-time, they decided they could not afford the expense of 3 occupational therapy visits per week. The parents discussed their dilemma with Dawn, and together they modified the schedule to 3 visits every 2 weeks, a plan that was satisfactory to all involved.

challenged with the demands of paying for health care services.

The Code includes several RSCs that address the client-centered respect for autonomy displayed by both Nikki and Dawn in Case Study 26.2. For example, RSC 3D describes the duty to "establish a collaborative relationship with recipients of service and relevant stakeholders, to promote shared decision making" (AOTA, 2015, p. 4). Both Nikki and Dawn demonstrated behaviors consistent with the principle of Beneficence.

Nikki took actions consistent with the principle of Justice by addressing barriers to access by referring the parents to a local provider while services were not available at the school, declining the cabin barter deal, and offering choices within the parameters of organizational policies (RSC 4C). Other RSCs supporting these actions include

- *RSC 2I:* "Avoid exploiting any relationship established as an occupational therapy clinician . . . to further one's own . . . financial . . . interests at the expense of recipients of services" (AOTA, 2015, p. 4), and
- *RSC 2J:* "Avoid bartering for services when there is the potential for exploitation and conflict of interest" (AOTA, 2015, p. 4).

Dawn and the organization for which she worked are notable examples of justice in health care delivery. "The Principle of Justice relates to the fair, equitable, and appropriate treatment of persons" (Beauchamp & Childress, 2013, as cited by AOTA, 2015, p. 5). Dawn's efforts to serve Feline and collaborate with the parents display a concern for "equitable opportunity to achieve occupational engagement . . . and impartial consideration and consistent following of rules to promote unbiased decisions" (AOTA, 2015, p. 5).

The RSCs specific to the principle of Justice that Dawn honored include

- *RSC 4C:* "Address barriers in access to occupational therapy services by offering or referring clients to financial aid, charity care, or pro bono services within the parameters of organizational policies."
- *RSC 4M:* "Bill and collect fees legally and justly in a manner that is fair, reasonable, and commensurate with services delivered" (AOTA, 2015, p. 6).

Episode-of-Care Reimbursement

Reimbursement for health care services depends on the client's context (e.g., Does the client have health insurance?). Many large employers offer health insurance as part of an employee benefits package. Health insurance in the United States has been made available to help individuals and families offset expenses incurred from diagnosis and treatment of illnesses and injuries.

Health insurance was first established in 1929 when a group of Texas schoolteachers was covered for their health care expenses by Blue Cross. During World War II, the executive and judicial branches of the U.S. government issued a series of laws to address labor shortages. Limits on wage increases were supplanted by benefits programs that included employer-sponsored health insurance (Casto & Forrestal, 2013). This foundation of reimbursement remains today as one of the major methods of payment for health care services.

Health insurance plans typically pay for services per encounter or per procedure. As cost control measures are being implemented, single-payment "episode of care" reimbursement models, which require a new level of collaboration, are emerging, as described in Vignette 26.3.

Summary

Occupational therapy practitioners work in a wide variety of settings, and services are reimbursed through an array of methods. Being paid fairly requires knowing the regulations and requirements and following them. Yet, it is not quite that simple.

The black-and-white rules for documentation and service charges provide seemingly inflexible structure and guidance. Applying the rules consistently to daily practice requires judgment and flexibility. Some situations become ethical dilemmas when they do not exactly fit within the boundaries of strict rules. Following reimbursement guidelines while meeting the unique needs of the clients served may require a nuanced approach. Doing the right thing is not necessarily the easiest thing. Acting ethically may cause self-doubt, negative consequences in employment, organizational disruption, and, ultimately, moral distress for the occupational therapy practitioner (Slater & Brandt, 2016).

Vignette 26.3. Promoting a Collaborative, Interprofessional Work Environment

Alma, an occupational therapy assistant, worked at a local hospital that had managed care contracts for its Orthopedics Center of Excellence. About 2 weeks before elective joint replacement, patients attended Joint Camp, which helped patients and their family members understand what they could expect during recovery, helped them prepare their home environment, and provided a kit of adaptive equipment that they would need after surgery. Alma knew that the rehabilitation services department had worked with the orthopedic surgeons to establish protocols for this population. Each patient was to receive 3 post-surgical occupational therapy interventions, with 1 visit on the last day before discharge to a short-term rehabilitation setting or home.

A new **orthopedic surgeon** joined the hospital staff. Because the new surgeon had low seniority, she was assigned only afternoon blocks in the surgical suite. This resulted in her patients arriving back in their hospital room late in the day after surgery. The occupational therapist first saw these patients for occupational therapy evaluation early in the morning on Day 2 and typically placed the patients on Alma's schedule for the additional 2 intervention sessions, one in the afternoon of Day 2 and the last session before noon on Day 3.

The new surgeon approached Alma as she was finishing the 3rd and final occupational therapy session for one of the surgeon's patients. The surgeon stated, "Because of my surgery schedule, my patients aren't ready for discharge until the evening. They end up sitting around for hours on their last afternoon here. I don't think my patients get the full benefit of your services. I'm sure they could be more independent at home if you saw them one more time. I also know that your teaching about fall prevention is so very important. I want you to see all of my patients for an extra therapy session in the afternoon before they leave."

Alma appreciated that the orthopedic surgeon valued occupational therapy services. Alma interpreted the surgeon's request as consistent with the principle of Beneficence: The surgeon wanted the best for her patients. However, Alma knew the "one visit on Day 3" protocol was established as best and most efficient practice through collaboration with the orthopedic surgery group. Alma also recalled the **rehabilitation manager** referring to the visit limit as "cost containment" to manage the time and resources devoted to orthopedic patients and to generate the profit typical of this short-term orthopedics caseload. The rehabilitation manager had said, "Joint Camp isn't paid for, but it helps the patients get ready for the short hospital stay of our orthopedics program. The Inpatient Prospective Payment System pays our hospital the same whether we see the orthopedic patients for 1 visit or 6 visits." Alma also was aware that having to provide extra visits would be a challenge for the department, given the small number of occupational therapy staff members.

Alma conferred with the **supervising occupational therapist** and the rehabilitation manager. Consistent with the Principle of Justice, Alma advocated that instead of revising the protocol, an additional occupational therapy intervention session be provided to those patients not yet achieving the expected level of independence typically seen after 3 visits.

The rehabilitation manager liked Alma's reasoning. Together, the rehabilitation team met with the new orthopedic surgeon and collaborated in shared decision making, consistent with RSC 3D. All agreed that the decision to provide additional occupational therapy visits should be based on the best interest of each individual patient. An additional mandatory therapy visit, outside of the established protocol, could be redundant for some patients and a waste of resources. For others, the additional visit could be essential. The occupational therapy team commended the orthopedic surgeon for honoring the principle of Beneficence by facilitating quality care and honoring the Principle of Nonmaleficence through her concern for patient safety. The rehabilitation manager demonstrated the Principle of Fidelity by stewarding the available staff resources and promoting a collaborative, interprofessional work environment.

Reflective Questions

1. Would you consider developing an intervention plan that includes a pick list or menu of "options and outcomes" with a price quote for each potential intervention option and anticipated outcome, even if some of the outcomes are likely to be less than optimal? Which principles and RSCs support your response?
2. How do you address the challenge of knowing your client is in dir e need of your services, and perhaps even at great risk of harm, when the reimbursement source determines the client is no longer eligible for services?
3. How much time and effort should you expend to assist your client in understanding their insurance benefit? What ethical principles and RSCs might apply?
4. What are the challenges to the Principle of Veracity when providing information to a payer when a full description of the lack of progress is likely to result in denial of reimbursement for additional occupational therapy services? Does the insurance company need to know everything?

5. What are appropriate and ethical responses when a client asks about occupational therapy service fees and then asks how much you are being paid?

References

American Medical Association. (2014). *Current procedural terminology (CPT)*. Chicago: Author.

American Occupational Therapy Association. (2013). *Functional data collection requirements for outpatient therapy.* Retrieved from http://www.aota.org/Advocacy-Policy/Federal-Reg-Affairs/News/2013/Functional-Data-CY2013.aspx

American Occupational Therapy Association. (2014). Occupational therapy practice framework: Domain and process (3rd ed.). *American Journal of Occupational Therapy, 68*(Suppl. 1), S1–S48. https://doi.org/10.5014/ajot.2014.682006

American Occupational Therapy Association. (2015). Occupational therapy code of ethics (2015). *American Journal of Occupational Therapy, 69*(Suppl. 3), 6913410030p1. https://doi.org/10.5014/ajot.2015.696S03

Beauchamp, T. L., & Childress, J. F. (2013). *Principles of biomedical ethics* (7th ed.). New York: Oxford University Press.

Casto, A. B., & Forrestal, E. (2013). *Principles of health care reimbursement* (4th ed.). Chicago: American Health Information Management Association.

Centers for Medicare and Medicaid Services. (2014). *Medicare fraud and abuse: Prevention, detection, and reporting* [Fact Sheet]. Retrieved from http://www.cms.gov/Outreach-and-Education/Medicare-Learning-Network-MLN/MLNProducts/downloads/Fraud_and_Abuse.pdf

Fitteron, D. J. (2015). Who pays—and how? Advocates can help older adults navigate the complexities of American healthcare. *Generations, 39*(1), 69–71.

Levinson, D. R. (2015). *The Medicare payment system for skilled nursing facilities needs to be reevaluated.* Retrieved from https://oig.hhs.gov/oei/reports/oei-02-13-00610.pdf

Patient Protection and Affordable Care Act of 2010, Pub. L. 111–148, 42 U.S.C. § 18001.

Slater, D., & Brandt, L. (2016). Combating moral distress. In D. Y. Slater (Ed.), *Reference guide to the Occupational Therapy Code of Ethics (2015)* (pp. 117–123). Bethesda: AOTA Press.

Chapter 27.

CURRENT AND FUTURE ETHICAL TRENDS

Janie B. Scott, MA, OT/L, FAOTA, and S. Maggie Reitz, PhD, OTR/L, FAOTA

Learning Objectives

By the end of the chapter, readers will be able to

- Identify emerging practice areas and potential ethical dilemmas,
- Apply Principles and Related Standards of Conduct from the *Occupational Therapy Code of Ethics (2015)* to emerging practice trends, and
- Use a model for ethical decision making to analyze ethical dilemmas.

Key Terms and Concepts

✧ Emerging niches
✧ Habilitative services
✧ Occupational outlook
✧ Occupational therapy trends
✧ Vision 2025

Occupational therapy practice is constantly evolving. Occupational therapy students and practitioners exploring new and emerging practice areas must be prepared to address potential ethical dilemmas encountered in these developing environments. Several American Occupational Therapy Association (AOTA) official documents and other work of the Association and U.S. government agencies can help us identify emerging areas in health care and resultant shifts in practice. The *2015 AOTA Salary and Workforce Survey* (AOTA, 2015a), *Vision 2025* statement (AOTA, 2016), AOTA reports, and other documents related to this topic area will be reviewed. Projections from U.S. government agencies and works of professional and advocacy organizations and scholars external to occupational therapy will assist in painting a larger vista of issues that will affect the future of the occupational therapy profession.

This chapter explores trends in health care and emerging practice opportunities identified by the profession. Opportunities and challenges for ethical practice are discussed in various contexts across practice areas.

Emerging Niches and Trends

Emerging niches are potential areas for innovative responses to developing societal needs related to occupational performance. AOTA has produced several documents that explored emerging niches in occupational therapy practice within the following practice areas: children and youth; mental health; rehabilitation, disability, and participation; health and wellness; productive aging; education; and work and industry (Yamkovenko, 2015b).

As AOTA monitored the implementation and goal attainment of the *Centennial Vision* (AOTA, 2007), greater attention was placed on emerging trends for the profession. Many of the initial areas identified were actualized and integrated into practice. As this occurred, new opportunities grew, and emerging niches expanded. ***Occupational therapy trends*** are projections regarding the direction that occupational therapy practice may take in the future, including the demand for services and expanded service opportunities. Through the use of vignettes and case studies, this chapter explores some of these niche areas.

AOTA's ***Vision 2025*** states, "Occupational therapy maximizes health, well-being and quality of life for all people, populations, and communities through effective solutions that facilitate participation in everyday living" (AOTA, 2016, para. 1). As can be easily seen, *Vision 2025* embraces all of the trend areas identified above. For occupational therapy practitioners to identify effective solutions for those served, they must understand the evidence that informs each practice area and integrate this knowledge into practice interventions.

The U.S. Department of Labor's Bureau of Labor Statistics (BLS; 2016) is "responsible for measuring labor market activity, working conditions, and price changes in the economy" (para. 1). BLS (2016b) publishes the *Occupational Outlook Handbook* that includes information about a wide variety of occupational groups (e.g., health care). BLS presents information about the ***occupational outlook*** such as median pay, entry-level education, the number of new jobs, projected growth rate, and so forth. Under health care, the *Handbook* has separate categories for occupational therapists, occupational therapy assistants, and occupational therapy aides. "Employment of occupational therapists is projected to grow 27% from 2014 to 2024, much faster than the average for all occupations" (BLS, 2016b, para. 5). In the category of occupational therapy assistants and aides, the BLS (2015) projects a 40% growth during this same time period.

Emerging Trends in Productive Aging

One area in which explosive growth in the population and demand for occupational services will occur is aging. The aging population is expanding and will continue to do so (Administration on Aging, 2014; U.S. Census Bureau, 2014; White House Conference on Aging, 2015). The expectations for growth among this population create significant prospects for the occupational therapy profession.

Opportunities for occupational therapy practitioners will present themselves in the areas of work and industry, long-term care, home and community living, assistive and environmental technologies, and mental health—all areas of everyday living. Case Study 27.1 highlights one occupational therapist's hope of capitalizing on the growing opportunities within this practice area.

Emerging Trends in Rehabilitation, Disability, and Participation

Areas within rehabilitation, disability, and participation are considered as trending. This section presents information about habilitative services, adults living with autism, and veterans services.

Habilitative Services

A potential area of growth for occupational therapy practitioners in many practice areas is through the provision of habilitative services. ***Habilitative services*** are

> health care services that help you keep, learn, or improve skills and functioning for daily living. Examples include therapy for a child who isn't walking or talking at the expected age. These services may include physical and occupational therapy, speech–language pathology, and other services for people with disabilities in a variety of inpatient and/or outpatient settings. (Healthcare.gov, n.d., para. 1)

Case Study 27.1. Emerging Trends in Productive Aging: Alzheimer's Disease and Caregiving

Stephanie, an occupational therapist, had worked as an early interventionist for the past 10 years. She enjoyed being able to arrange her schedule around the needs of her family and working directly with families and caregivers.

Stephanie became intrigued about the growing numbers of individuals diagnosed with Alzheimer's disease (AD) and dementias after a report in a local newspaper. The article mentioned an elderly man with dementia who wandered away from his home. His wife, who was his primary caregiver, was interviewed for the story. The more Stephanie learned about this couple and the impact of AD on individuals and families, the more passionate she became.

Stephanie searched the web for the Centers for Disease Control and Prevention (CDC) at www.cdc.gov, the Alzheimer's Association (www.alz.org), AOTA (www.aota.org), the National Institute on Aging (www.nia.nih.gov), and other organizations for information about research, trends, and continuing education opportunities. Her research indicated that the projected number of individuals with dementias and the impact on families and society was an important trend. She was ready to give up her current practice and begin a business focused on the needs of people with dementia and their caregivers. Stephanie had not worked with adults, let alone individuals with dementia, since her Level II fieldwork experience.

What steps did Stephanie need to take to develop competence to work not only with people with dementia but their caregivers, too? She was overwhelmed thinking about what she needed to do to practice in a competent, ethical way. After completing preliminary research, she found a Decision Table to help her process the courses of action that were available to her and the positive and negative outcomes for each action in the context of her scope of practice and AOTA's (2015b) *Occupational Therapy Code of Ethics (2015)*. Table 27.1 reflects Stephanie's thought process that helped to guide her decision making.

Stephanie realized that moving forward without gaining knowledge and experience could endanger clients and violate the Code. She researched and developed a list of competencies that she would need, as well as strategies and timelines, to become an occupational therapist whose services would be valued by clients, the community, and the profession.

Table 27.1. Decision Table for Case Study 27.1

Possible Action	Positive Outcomes	Negative Consequences
Stephanie would quit her job and publicize her aging-in-place occupational therapy services. She would conduct research as needed and when time allowed.	Stephanie would receive more immediate, short-term gratification from her decision to change her career path.	Lacking adequate research and experience, Stephanie might provide inadequate care or potentially harm clients and violate the Code, specifically RSCs 1C, 1E, 1F, 2A, 5A, 5B, 5E, and 6L.
Stephanie would reduce her current work hours and work part-time for a home health company.	Stephanie would increase her knowledge base through on-the-job-training.	Stephanie may not obtain adequate supervision to provide needed services, potentially violating RSCs 1E and 2A.
Stephanie would delay her plans to quit until she gained knowledge and experience.	Stephanie upholds the Code, adhering to Principle 1, Beneficence; RSC 2A; Principle 3, Autonomy; and RSCs 5B, 5C, and 5F.	Stephanie might feel frustrated with her inability to make a faster transition. This frustration might negatively affect current clients.
Stephanie decides to abandon her plan because developing the skill set needed for this client population is too difficult and demanding.	Stephanie continues to practice occupational therapy and continues to benefit children, families, and the profession.	None.

Note. RSCs = Related Standards of Conduct.

Some states (e.g., Maryland) have passed legislation requiring insurers to provide coverage to individuals who are 19 years and younger through health insurance plans regulated by the state so their medically necessary services are covered. These services may benefit children and youth as well as adults and may one day be covered through large group insurance plans. When reporting on the Patient Protection and Affordable Care Act of 2010 (ACA; P. L. 111–148), Hooper (2015) explained that a habilitative service has been described as "helping a person to learn something for the first time" (p. 7). This expanded definition can be communicated through occupational therapy advocacy efforts and be beneficial for insurers, clients, and occupational therapy practitioners. This coverage will likely increase access to services and devices for covered individuals.

Advocacy and increasing access to needed services are addressed within Principle 4, Justice, and RSCs 4B, 4C, and 4D (AOTA, 2015b). It is important to be aware of these policy developments to help clients access occupational therapy services.

Adults Living With Autism

The benefit of occupational therapy services for individuals on the autism spectrum has been trending for some time. Much of the focus was placed on serving this population through early intervention and school-based practice. We now have developed greater appreciation for the lack of available services for people on the autism spectrum, such as housing, social opportunities, work, and transportation. As the profession looks to the future, expanded roles and opportunities become clear.

Furthermore, parents and caregivers for this population are aging, and some will become less able to care for individuals on the autism spectrum as the caregivers themselves develop disabling conditions and eventually die. Therefore, there will be a need for innovative alternative care structures to provide lifespan services for individuals living on the autism spectrum within a context that provides the greatest level of autonomy. Occupational therapy practitioners will have the opportunity to be leaders in the development of these structures as well as to provide ongoing consultative services.

These greater service opportunities and need for care underscore a growing demand for occupational therapy services. Vignette 27.1 describes a situation involving an occupational therapist and people on the autism spectrum.

As seen with Marcus, occupational therapy practitioners are sometimes faced with the challenge to maintain or improve their knowledge and skills in a particular practice area as supported by RSCs 1D, 1E, and 1F, or seek other employment opportunities. When presented with a major decision, each individual practitioner must weigh the pros and cons of opportunities for the good of the population served and adherence to the profession's values and beliefs.

Veterans Services

Health care services are provided to U.S. military veterans in various settings, including hospitals, community centers, among others (U.S. Department of Veterans Affairs, 2016). Occupational therapy practitioners work with veterans in these settings as well as in veteran's homes and private institutions.

Ethical challenges can exist with this population. Review Vignette 27.2, and consider which ethical principles and RSCs are at stake and how you might respond in this or similar situations.

Emerging Trends in Health and Wellness

Although occupational therapy has been providing preventive services related to health promotion since its inception (Reitz, 2010), new foci and opportunities have emerged over time. The American Occupational Therapy Foundation (2015) released its research priorities, the first of which focuses on "Health behaviors to prevent and manage chronic conditions" (para. 1). AOTA identified chronic disease management as one of its emerging trends (Yamkovenko, 2015a). Managing and preventing chronic conditions requires

- Knowledge of the etiology and progression of common chronic diseases as well as occupational therapy clinical and health promotion knowledge and skills;
- Proficiency in service coordination and advocacy;
- Commitment to client- and family-centered care;
- Ability to work with individuals to identify skills they want to gain to better manage care; and
- Skill as an interprofessional team member. (Moyers & Metzler, 2014)

Vignette 27.1. Emerging Trends in Rehabilitation, Disability, and Participation: Adults Living on the Autism Spectrum

Marcus worked for a center that provided comprehensive occupational therapy services to children and adults on the autism spectrum. Hired directly after graduating from his occupational therapy program, he didn't have experience working with people on the autism spectrum, particularly those who were significantly cognitively and behaviorally challenged with autism.

Marcus began his employment serving students ages 12–21 years. As he gained experience working with this population, he became more aware of the importance of transitioning and future employment opportunities for his students. Even though his caseload was expanding, he wanted to offer some prevocational experiences and ultimately guide the graduates and older adults to work experiences. Marcus saw this as an important future trend for occupational therapy and meeting the needs of individuals on the autism spectrum.

Marcus was creative and developed different work stations that students could try (e.g., administrative work, maintenance). The center and parents were grateful for any additional services that clients could receive. The center was reviewed by an accrediting agency that asked for program descriptions, standardized evaluations, and the evidence to support the occupational therapy and prevocational programming. Marcus attended the meeting but was unable to provide the documentation beyond general program descriptions. The agency offered the center 3 months to construct the documentation necessary for accreditation. Marcus wanted to comply with the requirements of the agency and center; however, he was uncertain about his ability to comply with them and whether he was ethically obligated to do so.

For example, chronic disease management has been an important component of managed care and the ACA. Chronic diseases include diabetes, heart disease, cancer, obesity, and arthritis (CDC, 2016). Occupational therapy students and practitioners have the opportunity to engage in research, practice, and care management in this important evolving area. Additional competencies may need to be acquired in order to provide these types of occupational therapy services; this is the topic of Case Study 27.2.

Trends in Technologies

Occupational therapy practice has a long history of promoting the use of technologies in driving, rehabilitation, work and industry, behavioral health, and

Vignette 27.2. Advocacy and Beneficence

Brian worked for an outpatient physical rehabilitation center providing a variety of occupational therapy services to children, youth, and adults. The center was part of a larger health care delivery system. He had worked at the center for 5 years and was proud of his work, especially with wounded warriors.

The new marketing vice president, **Ms. Flash,** had been spending increasing amounts of time at the center in patient care areas. When Brian expressed his concern to his supervisor, **Clarinda,** she responded that given the center's current dire fiscal circumstances, he should be happy to have the attention of the new vice president, who had previously turned around a cosmetic company's profits. Clarinda was looking forward to having the occupational therapy services showcased in order to increase referrals.

A week later, Brian arrived at work to see Ms. Flash and a photographer in the occupational therapy space. Brian was scheduled to provide services to **Thom,** a wounded warrior, in the next 30 minutes. Brian knew that Thom was always very quiet and a bit withdrawn, and he had previously stated that discussing his war experience and injuries made him anxious.

Brian sought out Clarinda but was told she went home sick. Brian set up a portable screen to provide a private space for him to work with Thom in alignment with RSCs 2A, 3A, and 3F. As he was ushering Thom to this space, Ms. Flash approached Thom. Brian stepped forward and asked her to leave the space. She did not listen and continued to approach Thom, flirting and making inappropriate comments in an attempt to get him to agree to be interviewed. Brian could see that Thom was becoming increasingly agitated and told Ms. Flash that she needed to leave or he would call the center's security personnel. Ms. Flash stalked out, saying, "You will regret this. You'd better dust off your résumé!"

Brian's first concern was Thom, so he asked Thom if he was up for the session; when Thom responded positively, they completed the planned intervention. Brian went home and turned to the Code for guidance.

Reflect on who Brian owed his primary responsibility to, Thom or Ms. Flash. Considering the situation, what would you do? How should Brian's manager intervene, if at all?

the environment. Occupational therapy students receive a fundamental orientation in the use of technology, and a small segment of occupational therapy practice uses technologies to "facilitate participation in everyday living" (AOTA, 2016, para. 10).

Vignette 27.3 promotes the importance of gathering evidence and resources when considering delivering new technology-based services in the community.

Summary

Occupational therapy is a holistic practice that works with individuals, families, communities, and populations through direct intervention, education, research, and consultation. This practice has grown over 100 years, and it continues to evolve.

We are at an exciting horizon in occupational therapy. However, responding to trends in health care in innovative ways may bring ethical challenges. To comply with laws, regulations, scope of practice, and the Code, occupational therapy practitioners must maintain vigilance in their practice. Many resources are available to aid in this journey; several are referenced in this chapter and text, and are available through AOTA.

Reflective Questions

1. Refer to Vignette 27.1. What guidance does the Code hold for Marcus? Are there obligations in the Code for occupational therapy practitioners to incorporate evidence into their daily practice? If Marcus refuses to comply with the directives from his employer, what would you anticipate the consequences to be? What Principles and RSCs address compliance with the laws, institutional policies, and so forth? Complete the Decision Table to help Marcus decide the appropriate and ethical courses of action. Include the Principles and RSCs found in the Code that will help guide his decision making.
2. Review Vignette 27.2. What ethical concerns do you believe were behind Brian's initial concern? When Ms. Flash appears at the beginning of Thom's next session, what course of action would

Case Study 27.2. Emerging Trends in Health and Wellness: Chronic Disease Management

Tenisha had years of experience as an administrator for a free-standing rehabilitation center. Through her recent readings, she learned about the Affordable Care Act's emphasis on developing new models of care using care management. Tenisha wanted to embrace these opportunities to expand services in this emerging practice area.

Tenisha visualized herself in the role of care coordinator, helping to manage care and services to people with chronic health conditions. She believed that she had the technology skills to help develop community networks to aid in service coordination. Although Tenisha hadn't provided direct occupational therapy services in 5 years, she hoped that her administrative skills could make up for her lack of clinical expertise.

Tenisha was enthusiastic and proposed this new position to her supervisor, **Hank.** Hank listened carefully to Tenisha's proposal and reviewed an *American Journal of Occupational Therapy* article and other literature that she provided explaining occupational therapy's role in the emerging practice area. Hank thought that incorporating care managers into the center's business model could improve care for clients and families and might lead to cost savings. He wondered if Tenisha had the necessary skills for a position like this. Hank asked her to make a list of the proficiencies and duties associated with the role of care coordinator and analyze whether she had the competencies to ethically represent the business and deliver the needed services to their client population.

Tenisha paused when Hank mentioned that he wanted her to outline her competencies related to this new position and whether they met the expectations articulated in the Code. She needed help summarizing her competencies and the expectations, so she turned to the Decision Table to help her process her questions and options. Put yourself in Tenisha's shoes and complete the Decision Table on her behalf. Include the principles and RSCs found in the Code that will help guide her decision making and subsequent actions.

Vignette 27.3. Exploring New Opportunities

The incorporation of technologies across all practice areas is expanding at a remarkable rate. Imagine that **you** and an **occupational therapy colleague** experienced in rehabilitation settings are interested in building a practice that would promote the use of technologies in the daily lives of the community, including individuals with disabilities. One strategy identified is to understand the feasibility of this venture by exploring the AOTA website (www.aota.org), participating in discussions on OTConnections, and gathering information through RESNA, especially its occupational therapy professional specialty group. You and your colleague also recognize the need to comply with the principles and RSCs in the Code, specifically 1F, among others.

Note. AOTA = American Occupational Therapy Association; RESNA = Rehabilitation Engineering and Assistive Technology Society of North America; RSCs = Related Standards of Conduct.

you recommend Brian take with Ms. Flash and later with Clarinda? What core values and principle(s) address this situation? Use the Decision Table to help Brian decide the appropriate and ethical courses of action. Include the principles and RSCs found in the Code that will help guide his decision making.

3. Refer to Vignette 27.3. Identify which principles or RSCs would be most relevant in your business exploration and implementation.

References

Administration on Aging. (2014). *Profile of older Americans: Future growth.* Retrieved from https://aoa.acl.gov/Aging_Statistics/Profile/index.aspx

American Occupational Therapy Association. (2007). AOTA's *Centennial Vision* and executive summary. *American Journal of Occupational Therapy, 61,* 613–614. https://doi.org/10.5014/ajot.61.6.613

American Occupational Therapy Association. (2015a). *2015 AOTA salary and workforce survey.* Bethesda: AOTA Press.

American Occupational Therapy Association. (2015b). Occupational therapy code of ethics (2015). *American Journal of Occupational Therapy, 64*(Suppl. 6), 6913410030. https://doi.org/10.5014/ajot.2015.696S03

American Occupational Therapy Association. (2016). *Vision 2025.* Retrieved from https://www.aota.org/AboutAOTA/vision-2025.aspx

American Occupational Therapy Foundation. (2015). *AOTF announces research priorities to support effective, evidence-based occupational therapy.* Retrieved from http://www.aotf.org/Portals/0/documents/news/pressreleases/research%20priorities-%2010%2021%202015.pdf

Centers for Disease Control and Prevention, U.S. Department of Health & Human Services. (2016). *Chronic disease prevention and health promotion: Chronic disease overview.* Retrieved from http://www.cdc.gov/chronicdisease/overview/index.htm

Healthcare.gov. (n.d.). *Habilitative/Habilitation services.* Retrieved from https://www.healthcare.gov/glossary/habilitative-habilitation-services/

Hooper, L. (2015). *A uniform definition for habilitative services.* Retrieved from http://www.aota.org/Advocacy-Policy/State-Policy/State%20Policy%20Resources%20and%20Factsheets/A-Uniform-Definition-for-Habilitative-Services.aspx

Moyers, P. A., & Metzler, C. A. (2014). Interprofessional collaborative practice in care coordination [Health Policy Perspectives]. *American Journal of Occupational Therapy, 68,* 500–505. https://doi.org10.5014/ajot.2014.6850020

Patient Protection and Affordable Care Act, Pub. L. No. 111-148, 42 U.S.C. § 18001 (2010).

Reitz, S. M. (2010). Historical and philosophical perspectives of occupational therapy's role in health promotion. In M. E. Scaffa, S. M. Reitz, & M. A. Pizzi (Eds.), *Occupational therapy in the promotion of health and wellness* (pp. 1–21). Philadelphia: F. A. Davis.

U.S. Census Bureau. (2014). *Fueled by aging Baby Boomers, nation's older population to nearly double in the next 20 years, Census Bureau reports.* Retrieved from http://census.gov/newsroom/press-releases/2014/cb14-84.html

U.S. Department of Labor, Bureau of Labor Statistics (2015). *Occupational outlook handbook: Occupational therapy assistants and aides.* Retrieved from http://www.bls.gov/ooh/healthcare/occupational-therapy-assistants-and-aides.htm

U.S. Department of Labor, Bureau of Labor Statistics (2016a). *About BLS.* Retrieved from http://www.bls.gov/bls/infohome.htm

U.S. Department of Labor, Bureau of Labor Statistics (2016b). *Occupational outlook handbook, 2016–2017 edition, occupational therapists.* Retrieved from http://www.bls.gov/ooh/healthcare/occupational-therapists.htm

U.S. Department of Veterans Affairs. (2016). *Health care.* Retrieved from https-3A__www.va.gov_&d=DQMFAg&c=euGZstcaTDllvimEN8b7jXrwqOf-v5A_CdpgnVfiiMM&r=5nWwFq9vrEBATqPV-jhaJA&m=li-E08MZhKhOhaxLjC-W4Ohv8rTQH1q2A8GJnL7XLN4&s=iJhb5ku2658lDDygNwaZz8NWiyJbgKGa2C9U3l8gjyE&e=" https://www.va.gov/

White House Conference on Aging. (2015). *White House Conference on Aging: Final report.* Retrieved from http://www.whitehouseconferenceonaging.gov/2015-WHCOA-Final-Report.pdf

Yamkovenko, S. (2015a). *Emerging niche in health and wellness.* Retrieved from http://www.aota.org/Practice/Health-Wellness/Emerging-Niche.aspx

Yamkovenko, S. (2015b). *The emerging niche: What's next in your practice area?* Retrieved from http://www.aota.org/Practice/Manage/Niche.aspx

Appendix A.

Occupational Therapy Code of Ethics (2015)

Preamble

The 2015 *Occupational Therapy Code of Ethics* (Code) of the American Occupational Therapy Association (AOTA) is designed to reflect the dynamic nature of the profession, the evolving health care environment, and emerging technologies that can present potential ethical concerns in research, education, and practice. AOTA members are committed to promoting inclusion, participation, safety, and well-being for all recipients in various stages of life, health, and illness and to empowering all beneficiaries of service to meet their occupational needs. Recipients of services may be individuals, groups, families, organizations, communities, or populations (AOTA, 2014b).

The Code is an AOTA Official Document and a public statement tailored to address the most prevalent ethical concerns of the occupational therapy profession. It outlines Standards of Conduct the public can expect from those in the profession. It should be applied to all areas of occupational therapy and shared with relevant stakeholders to promote ethical conduct.

The Code serves two purposes:

1. It provides aspirational Core Values that guide members toward ethical courses of action in professional and volunteer roles.
2. It delineates enforceable Principles and Standards of Conduct that apply to AOTA members.

Whereas the Code helps guide and define decision-making parameters, ethical action goes beyond rote compliance with these Principles and is a manifestation of moral character and mindful reflection. It is a commitment to benefit others, to virtuous practice of artistry and science, to genuinely good behaviors, and to noble acts of courage. Recognizing and resolving ethical issues is a systematic process that includes analyzing the complex dynamics of situations, weighing consequences, making reasoned decisions, taking action, and reflecting on outcomes. Occupational therapy personnel, including students in occupational therapy programs, are expected to abide by the Principles and Standards of Conduct within this Code. Personnel roles include clinicians (e.g., direct service, consultation, administration); educators; researchers; entrepreneurs; business owners; and those in elected, appointed, or other professional volunteer service.

The process for addressing ethics violations by AOTA members (and associate members, where applicable) is outlined in the Code's Enforcement Procedures (AOTA, 2014a).

Although the Code can be used in conjunction with licensure board regulations and laws that guide standards of practice, the Code is meant to be a free-standing document, guiding ethical dimensions of professional behavior, responsibility, practice, and decision making. This Code is not exhaustive; that is, the Principles and Standards of Conduct cannot address every possible situation. Therefore, before making complex ethical decisions that require further expertise, occupational therapy personnel should seek out resources to assist in resolving ethical issues not addressed in this document. Resources can include, but are not limited to, ethics committees, ethics officers, the AOTA Ethics Commission or Ethics Program Manager, or an ethics consultant.

Core Values

The profession is grounded in seven long-standing Core Values: (1) Altruism, (2) Equality, (3) Freedom, (4) Justice, (5) Dignity, (6) Truth, and (7) Prudence. *Altruism* involves demonstrating concern for the welfare of others. *Equality* refers to treating all people impartially and free of bias. *Freedom* and personal choice are paramount in a profession in which the values and desires of the client guide our interventions. *Justice* expresses a state in which diverse communities are inclusive; diverse communities are organized and structured such that all members can function, flourish, and live a satisfactory life. Occupational therapy personnel, by virtue of the specific nature of the practice of occupational therapy, have a vested interest in addressing unjust inequities that limit opportunities for participation in society (Braveman & Bass-Haugen, 2009).

Inherent in the practice of occupational therapy is the promotion and preservation of the individuality and *Dignity* of the client by treating him or her with respect in all interactions. In all situations, occupational therapy personnel must provide accurate information in oral, written, and electronic forms (*Truth*). Occupational therapy personnel use their clinical and ethical reasoning skills, sound judgment, and reflection to make decisions in professional and volunteer roles (*Prudence*).

The seven Core Values provide a foundation to guide occupational therapy personnel in their interactions with others. Although the Core Values are not themselves enforceable standards, they should be considered when determining the most ethical course of action.

Principles and Standards of Conduct

The Principles and Standards of Conduct that are enforceable for professional behavior include (1) Beneficence, (2) Nonmaleficence, (3) Autonomy, (4) Justice, (5) Veracity, and (6) Fidelity. Reflection on the historical foundations of occupational therapy and related professions resulted in the inclusion of Principles that are consistently referenced as a guideline for ethical decision making.

BENEFICENCE

Principle 1. Occupational therapy personnel shall demonstrate a concern for the well-being and safety of the recipients of their services.

Beneficence includes all forms of action intended to benefit other persons. The term *beneficence* connotes acts of mercy, kindness, and charity (Beauchamp & Childress, 2013). Beneficence requires taking action by helping others, in other words, by promoting good, by preventing harm, and by removing harm. Examples of beneficence include protecting and defending the rights of others, preventing harm from occurring to others, removing conditions that will cause harm to others, helping persons with disabilities, and rescuing persons in danger (Beauchamp & Childress, 2013).

RELATED STANDARDS OF CONDUCT

Occupational therapy personnel shall

A. Provide appropriate evaluation and a plan of intervention for recipients of occupational therapy services specific to their needs.

B. Reevaluate and reassess recipients of service in a timely manner to determine whether goals are being achieved and whether intervention plans should be revised.

C. Use, to the extent possible, evaluation, planning, intervention techniques, assessments, and therapeutic equipment that are evidence based, current, and within the recognized scope of occupational therapy practice.

D. Ensure that all duties delegated to other occupational therapy personnel are congruent with credentials, qualifications, experience, competency, and scope of practice with respect to service delivery, supervision, fieldwork education, and research.

E. Provide occupational therapy services, including education and training, that are within each practitioner's level of competence and scope of practice.

F. Take steps (e.g., continuing education, research, supervision, training) to ensure proficiency, use careful judgment, and weigh potential for harm when generally recognized standards do not exist in emerging technology or areas of practice.

G. Maintain competency by ongoing participation in education relevant to one's practice area.

H. Terminate occupational therapy services in collaboration with the service recipient or responsible party when the services are no longer beneficial.

I. Refer to other providers when indicated by the needs of the client.

J. Conduct and disseminate research in accordance with currently accepted ethical guidelines and standards for the protection of research participants, including determination of potential risks and benefits.

NONMALEFICENCE

Principle 2. Occupational therapy personnel shall refrain from actions that cause harm.

Nonmaleficence "obligates us to abstain from causing harm to others" (Beauchamp & Childress, 2013, p. 150). The Principle of *Nonmaleficence* also includes an obligation to not impose risks of harm even if the potential risk is without malicious or harmful intent. This Principle often is examined under the context of due care. The standard of *due care* "requires that the goals pursued justify the risks that must be imposed to achieve those goals" (Beauchamp & Childress, 2013, p. 154). For example, in occupational therapy practice, this standard applies to situations in which the client might feel pain from a treatment intervention; however, the acute pain is justified by potential longitudinal, evidence-based benefits of the treatment.

RELATED STANDARDS OF CONDUCT

Occupational therapy personnel shall

A. Avoid inflicting harm or injury to recipients of occupational therapy services, students, research participants, or employees.

B. Avoid abandoning the service recipient by facilitating appropriate transitions when unable to provide services for any reason.

C. Recognize and take appropriate action to remedy personal problems and limitations that might cause harm to recipients of service, colleagues, students, research participants, or others.

D. Avoid any undue influences that may impair practice and compromise the ability to safely and competently provide occupational therapy services, education, or research.

E. Address impaired practice and, when necessary, report it to the appropriate authorities.

F. Avoid dual relationships, conflicts of interest, and situations in which a practitioner, educator, student, researcher, or employer is unable to maintain clear professional boundaries or objectivity.

G. Avoid engaging in sexual activity with a recipient of service, including the client's family or significant other, student, research participant, or employee, while a professional relationship exists.

H. Avoid compromising the rights or well-being of others based on arbitrary directives (e.g., unrealistic productivity expectations, falsification of documentation, inaccurate coding) by exercising professional judgment and critical analysis.

I. Avoid exploiting any relationship established as an occupational therapy clinician, educator, or researcher to further one's own physical, emotional, financial, political, or business interests at the expense of recipients of services, students, research participants, employees, or colleagues.

J. Avoid bartering for services when there is the potential for exploitation and conflict of interest.

AUTONOMY

Principle 3. Occupational therapy personnel shall respect the right of the individual to self-determination, privacy, confidentiality, and consent.

The Principle of *Autonomy* expresses the concept that practitioners have a duty to treat the client according to the client's desires, within the bounds of accepted standards of care, and to protect the client's confidential information. Often, respect for Autonomy is referred to as the *self-determination principle.* However, respecting a person's autonomy goes beyond acknowledging an individual as a mere agent and also acknowledges a person's right "to hold views, to make choices, and to take actions based on [his or her] values and beliefs" (Beauchamp & Childress, 2013, p. 106). Individuals have the right to make a determination regarding care decisions that directly affect their lives. In the event that a person lacks decision-making capacity, his or her autonomy should be respected through involvement of an authorized agent or surrogate decision maker.

RELATED STANDARDS OF CONDUCT

Occupational therapy personnel shall

A. Respect and honor the expressed wishes of recipients of service.

B. Fully disclose the benefits, risks, and potential outcomes of any intervention; the personnel who will be providing the intervention; and any reasonable alternatives to the proposed intervention.

C. Obtain consent after disclosing appropriate information and answering any questions posed by the recipient of service or research participant to ensure voluntariness.

D. Establish a collaborative relationship with recipients of service and relevant stakeholders to promote shared decision making.

E. Respect the client's right to refuse occupational therapy services temporarily or permanently, even when that refusal has potential to result in poor outcomes.

F. Refrain from threatening, coercing, or deceiving clients to promote compliance with occupational therapy recommendations.

G. Respect a research participant's right to withdraw from a research study without penalty.

H. Maintain the confidentiality of all verbal, written, electronic, augmentative, and nonverbal communications, in compliance with applicable laws, including all aspects of privacy laws and exceptions thereto (e.g., Health Insurance Portability and Accountability Act [Pub. L. 104–191], Family Educational Rights and Privacy Act [Pub. L. 93–380]).

I. Display responsible conduct and discretion when engaging in social networking, including but not limited to refraining from posting protected health information.

J. Facilitate comprehension and address barriers to communication (e.g., aphasia; differences in language, literacy, culture) with the recipient of service (or responsible party), student, or research participant.

JUSTICE

Principle 4. Occupational therapy personnel shall promote fairness and objectivity in the provision of occupational therapy services.

The Principle of *Justice* relates to the fair, equitable, and appropriate treatment of persons (Beauchamp & Childress, 2013). Occupational therapy personnel should relate in a respectful, fair, and impartial manner to individuals and groups with whom they interact. They should also respect the applicable laws and standards related to their area of practice. Justice requires the impartial consideration and consistent following of rules to generate unbiased decisions and promote fairness. As occupational therapy personnel, we work to uphold a society in which all individuals have an equitable opportunity to achieve occupational engagement as an essential component of their life.

RELATED STANDARDS OF CONDUCT

Occupational therapy personnel shall

A. Respond to requests for occupational therapy services (e.g., a referral) in a timely manner as determined by law, regulation, or policy.

B. Assist those in need of occupational therapy services in securing access through available means.

C. Address barriers in access to occupational therapy services by offering or referring clients to financial aid, charity care, or pro bono services within the parameters of organizational policies.

D. Advocate for changes to systems and policies that are discriminatory or unfairly limit or prevent access to occupational therapy services.

E. Maintain awareness of current laws and AOTA policies and Official Documents that apply to the profession of occupational therapy.

F. Inform employers, employees, colleagues, students, and researchers of applicable policies, laws, and Official Documents.

G. Hold requisite credentials for the occupational therapy services they provide in academic, research, physical, or virtual work settings.

H. Provide appropriate supervision in accordance with AOTA Official Documents and relevant laws, regulations, policies, procedures, standards, and guidelines.

I. Obtain all necessary approvals prior to initiating research activities.

J. Refrain from accepting gifts that would unduly influence the therapeutic relationship or have the potential to blur professional boundaries, and adhere to employer policies when offered gifts.

K. Report to appropriate authorities any acts in practice, education, and research that are unethical or illegal.

L. Collaborate with employers to formulate policies and procedures in compliance with legal, regulatory, and ethical standards and work to resolve any conflicts or inconsistencies.

M. Bill and collect fees legally and justly in a manner that is fair, reasonable, and commensurate with services delivered.

N. Ensure compliance with relevant laws, and promote transparency when participating in a business arrangement as owner, stockholder, partner, or employee.

O. Ensure that documentation for reimbursement purposes is done in accordance with applicable laws, guidelines, and regulations.

P. Refrain from participating in any action resulting in unauthorized access to educational content or exams (including but not limited to sharing test questions, unauthorized use of or access to content or codes, or selling access or authorization codes).

VERACITY

Principle 5. Occupational therapy personnel shall provide comprehensive, accurate, and objective information when representing the profession.

Veracity is based on the virtues of truthfulness, candor, and honesty. The Principle of *Veracity* refers to comprehensive, accurate, and objective transmission of information and includes fostering understanding of such information (Beauchamp & Childress, 2013). Veracity is based on respect owed to others, including but not limited to recipients of service, colleagues, students, researchers, and research participants.

In communicating with others, occupational therapy personnel implicitly promise to be truthful and not deceptive. When entering into a therapeutic or research relationship, the recipient of service or research participant has a right to accurate information. In addition, transmission of information is incomplete without also ensuring that the recipient or participant understands the information provided.

Concepts of veracity must be carefully balanced with other potentially competing ethical principles, cultural beliefs, and organizational policies. Veracity ultimately is valued as a means to establish trust and strengthen professional relationships. Therefore, adherence to the Principle of Veracity also requires thoughtful analysis of how full disclosure of information may affect outcomes.

RELATED STANDARDS OF CONDUCT

Occupational therapy personnel shall

A. Represent credentials, qualifications, education, experience, training, roles, duties, competence, contributions, and findings accurately in all forms of communication.

B. Refrain from using or participating in the use of any form of communication that contains false, fraudulent, deceptive, misleading, or unfair statements or claims.

C. Record and report in an accurate and timely manner and in accordance with applicable regulations all information related to professional or academic documentation and activities.

D. Identify and fully disclose to all appropriate persons errors or adverse events that compromise the safety of service recipients.

E. Ensure that all marketing and advertising are truthful, accurate, and carefully presented to avoid misleading recipients of service, research participants, or the public.

F. Describe the type and duration of occupational therapy services accurately in professional contracts, including the duties and responsibilities of all involved parties.

G. Be honest, fair, accurate, respectful, and timely in gathering and reporting fact-based information regarding employee job performance and student performance.

H. Give credit and recognition when using the ideas and work of others in written, oral, or electronic media (i.e., do not plagiarize).

I. Provide students with access to accurate information regarding educational requirements and academic policies and procedures relative to the occupational therapy program or educational institution.

J. Maintain privacy and truthfulness when using telecommunication in the delivery of occupational therapy services.

FIDELITY

Principle 6. Occupational therapy personnel shall treat clients, colleagues, and other professionals with respect, fairness, discretion, and integrity.

The Principle of Fidelity comes from the Latin root *fidelis,* meaning loyal. *Fidelity* refers to the duty one has to keep a commitment once it is made (Veatch, Haddad, & English, 2010). In the health professions, this commitment refers to promises made between a provider and a client or patient based on an expectation of loyalty, staying with the client or patient in a time of need, and compliance with a code of ethics. These promises can be implied or explicit. The duty to disclose information that is potentially meaningful in making decisions is one obligation of the moral contract between provider and client or patient (Veatch et al., 2010).

Whereas respecting Fidelity requires occupational therapy personnel to meet the client's reasonable expectations, the Principle also addresses maintaining respectful collegial and organizational relationships (Purtilo & Doherty, 2011). Professional relationships are greatly influenced by the complexity of the environment in which occupational therapy personnel work. Practitioners, educators, and researchers alike must consistently balance their duties to service recipients, students, research participants, and other professionals as well as to organizations that may influence decision making and professional practice.

RELATED STANDARDS OF CONDUCT

Occupational therapy personnel shall

A. Preserve, respect, and safeguard private information about employees, colleagues, and students unless otherwise mandated or permitted by relevant laws.

B. Address incompetent, disruptive, unethical, illegal, or impaired practice that jeopardizes the safety or well-being of others and team effectiveness.

C. Avoid conflicts of interest or conflicts of commitment in employment, volunteer roles, or research.

D. Avoid using one's position (employee or volunteer) or knowledge gained from that position in such a manner as to give rise to real or perceived conflict of interest among the person, the employer, other AOTA members, or other organizations.

E. Be diligent stewards of human, financial, and material resources of their employers, and refrain from exploiting these resources for personal gain.

F. Refrain from verbal, physical, emotional, or sexual harassment of peers or colleagues.

G. Refrain from communication that is derogatory, intimidating, or disrespectful and that unduly discourages others from participating in professional dialogue.

H. Promote collaborative actions and communication as a member of interprofessional teams to facilitate quality care and safety for clients.

I. Respect the practices, competencies, roles, and responsibilities of their own and other professions to promote a collaborative environment reflective of interprofessional teams.

J. Use conflict resolution and internal and alternative dispute resolution resources as needed to resolve organizational and interpersonal conflicts, as well as perceived institutional ethics violations.

K. Abide by policies, procedures, and protocols when serving or acting on behalf of a professional organization or employer to fully and accurately represent the organization's official and authorized positions.

L. Refrain from actions that reduce the public's trust in occupational therapy.

M. Self-identify when personal, cultural, or religious values preclude, or are anticipated to negatively affect, the professional relationship or provision of services, while adhering to organizational policies when requesting an exemption from service to an individual or group on the basis of conflict of conscience.

References

American Occupational Therapy Association. (2014a). Enforcement procedures for the *Occupational therapy code of ethics and ethics standards*. *American Journal of Occupational Therapy, 68*(Suppl. 3), S3–S15. http://dx.doi.org/10.5014/ajot.2014.686S02

American Occupational Therapy Association. (2014b). Occupational therapy practice framework: Domain and process (3rd ed.). *American Journal of Occupational Therapy, 68*(Suppl. 1), S1–S48. http://dx.doi.org/10.5014/ajot.2014.682006

Beauchamp, T. L., & Childress, J. F. (2013). *Principles of biomedical ethics* (7th ed.). New York: Oxford University Press.

Braveman, B., & Bass-Haugen, J. D. (2009). Social justice and health disparities: An evolving discourse in occupational therapy research and intervention. *American Journal of Occupational Therapy, 63*, 7–12. http://dx.doi.org/10.5014/ajot.63.1.7

Purtilo, R., & Doherty, R. (2011). *Ethical dimensions in the health professions* (5th ed.). Philadelphia: Saunders/Elsevier.

Veatch, R. M., Haddad, A. M., & English, D. C. (2010). *Case studies in biomedical ethics*. New York: Oxford University Press.

Ethics Commission

Yvette Hachtel, JD, OTR/L, *Chair (2013–2014)*
Lea Cheyney Brandt, OTD, MA, OTR/L, *Chair (2014–2015)*
Ann Moodey Ashe, MHS, OTR/L *(2011–2014)*
Joanne Estes, PhD, OTR/L *(2012–2015)*
Loretta Jean Foster, MS, COTA/L *(2011–2014)*
Wayne L. Winistorfer, MPA, OTR *(2014–2017)*
Linda Scheirton, PhD, RDH *(2012–2015)*
Kate Payne, JD, RN *(2013–2014)*
Margaret R. Moon, MD, MPH, FAAP *(2014–2016)*
Kimberly S. Erler, MS, OTR/L *(2014–2017)*
Kathleen McCracken, MHA, COTA/L *(2014–2017)*
Deborah Yarett Slater, MS, OT/L, FAOTA, *AOTA Ethics Program Manager*

Adopted by the Representative Assembly 2015AprilC3.

Note. This document replaces the 2010 document *Occupational Therapy Code of Ethics and Ethics Standards (2010)*, previously published and copyrighted in 2010 by the American Occupational Therapy Association in the *American Journal of Occupational Therapy, 64*, S17–S26. http://dx.doi.org/10.5014/ajot.2010.64S17

Citation. American Occupational Therapy Association. (2015). Occupational therapy code of ethics (2015). *American Journal of Occupational Therapy, 69*(Suppl. 3), 6913410030. http://dx.doi.org/10.5014/ajot.2015.696S03

Appendix B.

Enforcement Procedures for the *Occupational Therapy Code of Ethics*

1. Introduction

The principal purposes of the *Occupational Therapy Code of Ethics* (hereinafter referred to as the Code) are to help protect the public and to reinforce its confidence in the occupational therapy profession rather than to resolve private business, legal, or other disputes for which there are other more appropriate forums for resolution. The Code also is an aspirational document to guide occupational therapists, occupational therapy assistants, and occupational therapy students toward appropriate professional conduct in all aspects of their diverse professional and volunteer roles. It applies to any conduct that may affect the performance of occupational therapy as well as to behavior that an individual may do in another capacity that reflects negatively on the reputation of occupational therapy.

The *Enforcement Procedures for the Occupational Therapy Code of Ethics* have undergone a series of revisions by the Association's Ethics Commission (hereinafter referred to as the EC) since their initial adoption. This public document articulates the procedures that are followed by the EC as it carries out its duties to enforce the Code. A major goal of these *Enforcement Procedures* is to ensure objectivity and fundamental fairness to all individuals who may be parties in an ethics complaint. The *Enforcement Procedures* are used to help ensure compliance with the Code which delineates enforceable Principles and Standards of Conduct that apply to Association members.

Acceptance of Association membership commits individuals to adherence to the Code and cooperation with its *Enforcement Procedures.* These are established and maintained by the EC. The EC and Association's Ethics Office make the *Enforcement Procedures* public and available to members of the profession, state regulatory boards, consumers, and others for their use.

The EC urges particular attention to the following issues:

1.1. **Professional Responsibility**—All occupational therapy personnel have an obligation to maintain the Code of their profession and to promote and support these ethical standards among their colleagues. Each Association member must be alert to practices that undermine these standards and is obligated to take action that is appropriate in the circumstances. At the same time, members must carefully weigh their judgments as to potentially unethical practice to ensure that they are based on objective evaluation and not on personal bias or prejudice, inadequate information, or simply differences of professional viewpoint. It is recognized that individual occupational therapy personnel may not have the authority or ability to address or correct all situations of concern. Whenever feasible and appropriate, members should first pursue other corrective steps within the relevant institution or setting and discuss ethical concerns directly with the potential Respondent before resorting to the Association's ethics complaint process.

1.2. **Jurisdiction**—The Code applies to persons who are or were Association members at the time of the conduct in question. Later nonrenewal or relinquishment of membership does not affect Association jurisdiction. The *Enforcement Procedures* that shall be utilized in any complaint shall be those in effect at the time the complaint is initiated.

1.3. **Disciplinary Actions/Sanctions (Pursuing a Complaint)**—If the EC determines that unethical conduct has occurred, it may impose sanctions, including reprimand, censure, probation (with terms) suspension, or permanent revocation of Association membership. In all cases, except those involving only reprimand (and educative letters), the Association will report the conclusions and sanctions in its official publications and also will communicate to any appropriate persons or entities. If an individual is on either the Roster of Fellows (ROF) or the Roster of Honor (ROH), the EC Chairperson (via the EC Staff Liaison) shall notify the VLDC Chairperson and Association Executive Director (ED) of their membership suspension or revocation. That individual shall have their name removed from either the ROF or the ROH and no longer has the right to use the designated credential of FAOTA or ROH during the period of suspension or permanently, in the case of revocation.

The EC Chairperson shall also notify the Chairperson of the Board for Advanced and Specialty Certification (BASC) (via Association staff liaison, in writing) of final disciplinary actions from the EC in which an individual's membership has been suspended or revoked. These individuals are not eligible to apply for or renew certification.

The potential sanctions are defined as follows:

1.3.1. **Reprimand**—A formal expression of disapproval of conduct communicated privately by letter from the EC Chairperson that is nondisclosable and noncommunicative to other bodies (e.g., state regulatory boards [SRBs], National Board for Certification in Occupational Therapy® [NBCOT®]). Reprimand is not publicly reported.

1.3.2. **Censure**—A formal expression of disapproval that is publicly reported.

1.3.3. **Probation of Membership Subject to Terms**—Continued membership is conditional, depending on fulfillment of specified terms. Failure to meet terms will subject an Association member to any of the disciplinary actions or sanctions. Terms may include but are not limited to

a. Remedial activity, applicable to the violation, with proof of satisfactory completion, by a specific date; and

b. The corrected behavior which is expected to be maintained.

Probation is publicly reported.

1.3.4. **Suspension**—Removal of Association membership for a specified period of time. Suspension is publicly reported.

1.3.5. **Revocation**—Permanent denial of Association membership. Revocation is publicly reported.

1.4. **Educative Letters**—If the EC determines that the alleged conduct may or may not be a true breach of the Code but in any event does not warrant any of the sanctions set forth in Section 1.3. or is not completely in keeping with the aspirational nature of the Code or within the prevailing standards of practice or professionalism, the EC may send a private letter to educate the Respondent about relevant standards of practice and/or appropriate professional behavior. In addition, a different private educative letter, if appropriate, may be sent to the Complainant.

1.5. **Advisory Opinions**—The EC may issue general advisory opinions on ethical issues to inform and educate the Association membership. These opinions shall be publicized to the membership and are available in the *Reference Guide to the Occupational Therapy Code of Ethics* as well as on the Association website.

1.6. **Rules of Evidence**—The EC proceedings shall be conducted in accordance with fundamental fairness. However, formal rules of evidence that are used in legal proceedings do not apply to these

Enforcement Procedures. The Disciplinary Council (see Section 5) and the Appeal Panel (see Section 6) can consider any evidence that they deem appropriate and pertinent.

1.7. Confidentiality and Disclosure—The EC develops and adheres to strict rules of confidentiality in every aspect of its work. This requires that participants in the process refrain from any communication relating to the existence and subject matter of the complaint other than with those directly involved in the enforcement process. Maintaining confidentiality throughout the investigation and enforcement process of a formal ethics complaint is essential in order to ensure fairness to all parties involved. These rules of confidentiality pertain not only to the EC but also apply to others involved in the complaint process. Beginning with the EC Staff Liaison and support staff, strict rules of confidentiality are followed. These same rules of confidentiality apply to Complainants, Respondents and their attorneys, and witnesses involved with the EC's investigatory process. Due diligence must be exercised by everyone involved in the investigation to avoid compromising the confidential nature of the process. Any Association member who breaches these rules of confidentiality may become subject to an ethics complaint/investigatory process himself or herself. Non–Association members may lodge an ethics complaint against an Association member, and these individuals are still expected to adhere to the Association's confidentiality rules. The Association reserves the right to take appropriate action against non–Association members who violate confidentiality rules, including notification of their appropriate licensure boards.

1.7.1. Disclosure—When the EC investigates a complaint, it may request information from a variety of sources. The process of obtaining additional information is carefully executed in order to maintain confidentiality. The EC may request information from a variety of sources, including state licensing agencies, academic councils, courts, employers, and other persons and entities. It is within the EC's purview to determine what disclosures are appropriate for particular parties in order to effectively implement its investigatory obligations. Public sanctions by the EC, Disciplinary Council, or Appeal Panel will be publicized as provided in these *Enforcement Procedures.* Normally, the EC does not disclose information or documentation reviewed in the course of an investigation unless the EC determines that disclosure is necessary to obtain additional, relevant evidence or to administer the ethics process or is legally required.

Individuals who file a complaint (i.e., *Complainant*) and those who are the subject of one (i.e., *Respondent*) must not disclose to anyone outside of those involved in the complaint process their role in an ethics complaint. Disclosing this information in and of itself may jeopardize the ethics process and violate the rules of fundamental fairness by which all parties are protected. Disclosure of information related to any case under investigation by the EC is prohibited and, if done, will lead to repercussions as outlined in these *Enforcement Procedures* (see Section 2.2.3.).

2. Complaints

2.1. Interested Party Complaints

2.1.1. Complaints stating an alleged violation of the Code may originate from any individual, group, or entity within or outside the Association. All complaints must be in writing, signed by the Complainant(s), and submitted to the Ethics Office at the Association headquarters. Complainants must complete the Formal Statement of Complaint Form at the end of this document. All complaints shall identify the person against whom the complaint is directed (the Respondent), the ethical principles that the Complainant believes have been violated, and the key facts and date(s) of the alleged ethical violations. If lawfully available, supporting documentation should be attached. Hard-copy complaints must be sent to the address indicated on the complaint form.

Complaints that are emailed must be sent as a pdf attachment, marked "Confidential" with "Complaint" in the subject line to ethics@aota.org and must include the complaint form and supporting documentation.

2.1.2. Within 90 days of receipt of a complaint, the EC shall make a preliminary assessment of the complaint and decide whether it presents sufficient questions as to a potential ethics violation that an investigation is warranted in accordance with Section 3. Commencing an investigation does not imply a conclusion that an ethical violation has in fact occurred or any judgment as to the ultimate sanction, if any, that may be appropriate. In the event the EC determines at the completion of an investigation that the complaint does rise to the level of an ethical violation, the EC may issue a decision as set forth in Section 4 below. In the event the EC determines that the complaint does not rise to the level of an ethical violation, the EC may direct the parties to utilize other conflict resolution resources or authorities via an educative letter. This applies to all complaints, including those involving Association elected/volunteer leadership related to their official roles.

2.2. Complaints Initiated by the EC

2.2.1. The EC itself may initiate a complaint (a *sua sponte* complaint) when it receives information from a governmental body, certification or similar body, public media, or other source indicating that a person subject to its jurisdiction may have committed acts that violate the Code. The Association will ordinarily act promptly after learning of the basis of a *sua sponte* complaint, but there is no specified time limit.

If the EC passes a motion to initiate a *sua sponte* complaint, the Association staff liaison to the EC will complete the Formal Statement of Complaint Form (at the end of this document) and will describe the nature of the factual allegations that led to the complaint and the manner in which the EC learned of the matter. The Complaint Form will be signed by the EC Chairperson on behalf of the EC. The form will be filed with the case material in the Association's Ethics Office.

2.2.2. ***De Jure* Complaints**—Where the source of a *sua sponte* complaint is the findings and conclusions of another official body, the EC classifies such *sua sponte* complaints as *de jure*. The procedure in such cases is addressed in Section 4.2.

2.2.3. The EC shall have the jurisdiction to investigate or sanction any matter or person for violations based on information learned in the course of investigating a complaint under Section 2.2.2.

2.3. Continuation of Complaint Process—If an Association member relinquishes membership, fails to renew membership, or fails to cooperate with the ethics investigation, the EC shall nevertheless continue to process the complaint, noting in its report the circumstances of the Respondent's action. Such actions shall not deprive the EC of jurisdiction. All correspondence related to the EC complaint process is in writing and sent by mail with signature and proof of date received. In the event that any written correspondence does not have delivery confirmation, the Association Ethics Office will make an attempt to search for an alternate physical or electronic address or make a second attempt to send to the original address. If the Respondent does not claim correspondence after two attempts to deliver, delivery cannot be confirmed or correspondence is returned to the Association as undeliverable, the EC shall consider that it has made good-faith effort and shall proceed with the ethics enforcement process.

3. EC Review and Investigations

3.1. Initial Action—The purpose of the preliminary review is to decide whether or not the information submitted with the complaint warrants opening the case. If in its preliminary review of the complaint the EC determines that an investigation is not warranted, the Complainant will be so notified.

3.2. Dismissal of Complaints—The EC may at any time dismiss a complaint for any of the following reasons:

3.2.1. Lack of Jurisdiction—The EC determines that it has no jurisdiction over the Respondent (e.g., a complaint against a person who is or was not an Association member at the time of the alleged incident or who has never been a member).

3.2.2. Absolute Time Limit/Not Timely Filed—The EC determines that the violation of the Code is alleged to have occurred more than 7 years prior to the filing of the complaint.

3.2.3. Subject to Jurisdiction of Another Authority—The EC determines that the complaint is based on matters that are within the authority of and are more properly dealt with by another governmental or nongovernmental body, such as an SRB, NBCOT®, an Association component other than the EC, an employer, educational institution, or a court.

3.2.4. No Ethics Violation—The EC finds that the complaint, even if proven, does not state a basis for action under the Code (e.g., simply accusing someone of being unpleasant or rude on an occasion).

3.2.5. Insufficient Evidence—The EC determines that there clearly would not be sufficient factual evidence to support a finding of an ethics violation.

3.2.6. Corrected Violation—The EC determines that any violation it might find already has been or is being corrected and that this is an adequate result in the given case.

3.2.7. Other Good Cause.

3.3. Investigator and EC (Avoidance of Conflict of Interest)—The investigator chosen shall not have a conflict of interest (i.e., shall never have had a substantial professional, personal, financial, business, or volunteer relationship with either the Complainant or the Respondent). In the event that the EC Staff Liaison has such a conflict, the EC Chairperson shall appoint an alternate investigator who has no conflict of interest. Any member of the EC with a possible conflict of interest must disclose and may be recused.

3.4. Investigation—If an investigation is deemed warranted, the EC Chairperson shall do the following within thirty (30) days: Appoint the EC Staff Liaison at the Association headquarters to investigate the complaint and notify the Respondent by mail (requiring signature and proof of date of receipt) that a complaint has been received and an investigation is being conducted. A copy of the complaint and supporting documentation shall be enclosed with this notification. The Complainant also will receive notification by mail (requiring signature and proof of date of receipt) that the complaint is being investigated.

3.4.1. Ordinarily, the Investigator will send questions formulated by the EC to be answered by the Complainant and / or the Respondent.

3.4.2. The Complainant shall be given thirty (30) days from receipt of the questions (if any) to respond in writing to the investigator.

3.4.3. The Respondent shall be given thirty (30) days from receipt of the questions to respond in writing to the Investigator.

3.4.4. The EC ordinarily will notify the Complainant of any substantive new evidence adverse to the Complainant's initial complaint that is discovered in the course of the ethics investigation and allow the Complainant to respond to such adverse evidence. In such cases, the Complainant will be given a copy of such evidence and will have fourteen (14) days in which to submit a written response. If the new evidence clearly shows that there has been no ethics violation, the

EC may terminate the proceeding. In addition, if the investigation includes questions for both the Respondent and the Complainant, the evidence submitted by each party in response to the investigatory questions shall be provided to the Respondent and available to the Complainant on request. The EC may request reasonable payment for copying expenses depending on the volume of material to be sent.

3.4.5. The Investigator, in consultation with the EC, may obtain evidence directly from third parties without permission from the Complainant or Respondent.

3.5. Investigation Timeline—The investigation will be completed within ninety (90) days after receipt of notification by the Respondent or his or her designee that an investigation is being conducted, unless the EC determines that special circumstances warrant additional time for the investigation. All timelines noted here can be extended for good cause at the discretion of the EC, including the EC's schedule and additional requests of the Respondent. The Respondent and the Complainant shall be notified in writing if a delay occurs or if the investigational process requires more time.

3.6. Case Files—The investigative files shall include the complaint and any documentation on which the EC relied in initiating the investigation.

3.7. Cooperation by Respondent—Every Association Respondent has a duty to cooperate reasonably with enforcement processes for the Code. Failure of the Respondent to participate and/or cooperate with the investigative process of the EC shall not prevent continuation of the ethics process, and this behavior itself may constitute a violation of the Code.

3.8. Referral of Complaint—The EC may at any time refer a matter to NBCOT®, the SRB, ACOTE®, or other recognized authorities for appropriate action. Despite such referral to an appropriate authority, the EC shall retain jurisdiction. EC action may be stayed for a reasonable period pending notification of a decision by that authority, at the discretion of the EC (and such delays will extend the time periods under these *Procedures*). A stay in conducting an investigation shall not constitute a waiver by the EC of jurisdiction over the matters. The EC shall provide written notice by mail (requiring signature and proof of date of receipt) to the Respondent and the Complainant of any such stay of action.

4. EC Review and Decision

4.1. Regular Complaint Process

4.1.1. Decision—If at the conclusion of the investigation the EC determines that the Respondent has engaged in conduct that constitutes a breach of the Code, the EC shall notify the Respondent and Complainant by mail with signature and proof of date received. The notice shall describe in sufficient detail the conduct that constitutes a violation of the Code and indicate the sanction that is being imposed in accordance with these *Enforcement Procedures.*

4.1.2. Respondent's Response—Within 30 days of notification of the EC's decision and sanction, if any, the Respondent shall

4.1.2.1. Accept the decision of the EC (as to both the ethics violation and the sanction) and waive any right to a Disciplinary Council hearing, or

4.1.2.2. Accept the decision that he/she committed unethical conduct but within thirty (30) days, submit to the EC a statement (with any supporting documentation) setting forth the reasons why any sanction should not be imposed or reasons why the sanction should be mitigated or reduced.

4.1.2.3. Advise the EC Chairperson in writing that he or she contests the EC's decision and sanction and requests a hearing before the Disciplinary Council.

Failure of the Respondent to take one of these actions within the time specified will be deemed to constitute acceptance of the decision and sanction. If the Respondent requests a Disciplinary Council hearing, it will be scheduled. If the Respondent does not request a Disciplinary Council hearing but accepts the decision, the EC will notify all relevant parties and implement the sanction. Correspondence with the Respondent will also indicate that public sanctions may have an impact on their ability to serve in Association positions, whether elected or appointed, for a designated period of time.

4.2. *De Jure* Complaint Process

4.2.1. The EC Staff Liaison will present to the EC any findings from external sources (as described above) that come to his or her attention and that may warrant *sua sponte* complaints pertaining to individuals who are or were Association members at the time of the alleged incident.

4.2.2. Because *de jure* complaints are based on the findings of fact or conclusions of another official body, the EC will decide whether or not to act based on such findings or conclusions and will not ordinarily initiate another investigation, absent clear and convincing evidence that such findings and conclusions were erroneous or not supported by substantial evidence. Based on the information presented by the EC Staff Liaison, the EC will determine whether the findings of the public body also are sufficient to demonstrate an egregious violation of the Code and therefore warrant taking disciplinary action.

4.2.3. If the EC decides that a breach of the Code has occurred, the EC Chairperson will notify the Respondent in writing of the violation and the disciplinary action that is being taken. Correspondence with the Respondent will also indicate that public sanctions may have an impact on their ability to serve in Association positions, whether elected or appointed, for a designated period of time. In response to the *de jure sua sponte* decision and sanction by the EC, the Respondent may

4.2.3.1. Accept the decision of the EC (as to both the ethics violation and the sanction) based solely on the findings of fact and conclusions of the EC or the public body, and waive any right to a Disciplinary Council hearing;

4.2.3.2. Accept the decision that the Respondent committed unethical conduct but within thirty (30) days submit to the EC a statement (with any supporting documentation) setting forth the reasons why any sanction should not be imposed or reasons why the sanction should be mitigated or reduced; or

4.2.3.3. Within thirty (30) days, present information showing the findings of fact of the official body relied on by the EC to impose the sanction are clearly erroneous and request reconsideration by the EC. The EC may have the option of opening an investigation or modifying the sanction in the event they find clear and convincing evidence that the findings and the conclusions of the other body are erroneous.

4.2.4. In cases of *de jure* complaints, a Disciplinary Council hearing can later be requested (pursuant to Section 5 below) only if the Respondent has first exercised Options 4.2.3.2 or 4.2.3.3.

4.2.5. Respondents in an ethics case may utilize Options 4.2.3.2 or 4.2.3.3 (reconsideration) once in responding to the EC. Following one review of the additional information submitted by the Respondent, if the EC reaffirms its original sanction, the Respondent has the option of accepting the violation and proposed sanction or requesting a Disciplinary Council hearing. Repeated requests for reconsideration will not be accepted by the EC.

5. Disciplinary Council

5.1. Purpose—The purpose of the Disciplinary Council (hereinafter to be known as the Council) hearing is to provide the Respondent an opportunity to present evidence and witnesses to answer and refute the decision and/or sanction and to permit the EC Chairperson or designee to present evidence and witnesses in support of his or her decision. The Council shall consider the matters alleged in the complaint; the matters raised in defense as well as other relevant facts, ethical principles, and federal or state law, if applicable. The Council may question the parties concerned and determine ethical issues arising from the factual matters in the case even if those specific ethical issues were not raised by the Complainant. The Council also may choose to apply Principles or other language from the Code not originally identified by the EC. The Council may affirm the decision of the EC or reverse or modify it if it finds that the decision was clearly erroneous or a material departure from its written procedure.

5.2. Parties—The parties to a Council Hearing are the Respondent and the EC Chairperson.

5.3. Criteria and Process for Selection of Council Members

5.3.1. Criteria

5.3.1.1. Association Administrative Standard Operating Procedures (SOP) and Association Policy 2.6 shall be considered in the selection of qualified potential candidates for the Council, which shall be composed of qualified individuals and Association members drawn from a pool of candidates who meet the criteria outlined below. Members ideally will have some knowledge or experience in the areas of activity that are at issue in the case. They also will have experience in disciplinary hearings and/or general knowledge about ethics as demonstrated by education, presentations, and/or publications.

5.3.1.2. No conflict of interest may exist with either the Complainant or the Respondent (refer to Association Policy A.13—Conflict of Interest for guidance).

5.3.1.3. No individual may serve on the Council who is currently a member of the EC or the Board of Directors

5.3.1.4. No individual may serve on the Council who has previously been the subject of an ethics complaint that resulted in a public EC disciplinary action within the past three (3) years.

5.3.1.5. The public member on the Council shall have knowledge of the profession and ethical issues.

5.3.1.6. The public member shall not be an occupational therapist or occupational therapy assistant (practitioner, educator, or researcher.)

5.4. Criteria and Process for Selection of Council Chairperson

5.4.1. Criteria

5.4.1.1. Must have experience in analyzing/reviewing cases.

5.4.1.2. May be selected from the pool of candidates for the Council or a former EC member who has been off the EC for at least three (3) years.

5.4.1.3. The EC Chairperson shall not serve as the Council Chairperson.

5.4.2. Process

5.4.2.1. The Representative Assembly (RA) Speaker (in consultation with EC Staff Liaison) will select the Council Chairperson.

5.4.2.2. If the RA Speaker needs to be recused from this duty, the RA Vice Speaker will select the Council Chairperson.

5.5. Process

5.5.1. Potential candidates for the Council pool will be recruited through public postings in official publications and via the electronic forums. Association leadership will be encouraged to recruit qualified candidates. Potential members of the Council shall be interviewed to ascertain the following:

a. Willingness to serve on the Council and availability for a period of three (3) years and

b. Qualifications per criteria outlined in Section 5.3.1.

5.5.2. The President and EC Staff Liaison will maintain a pool of no fewer than six (6) and no more than twelve (12) qualified individuals.

5.5.3. The President, with input from the EC Staff Liaison, will select from the pool the members of each Council within thirty (30) days of notification by a Respondent that a Council is being requested.

5.5.4. Each Council shall be composed of three (3) Association members in good standing and a public member.

5.5.5. The EC Staff Liaison will remove anyone with a potential conflict of interest in a particular case from the potential Council pool.

5.6. Notification of Parties (EC Chairperson, Complainant, Respondent, Council Members)

5.6.1. The EC Staff Liaison shall schedule a hearing date in coordination with the Council Chairperson.

5.6.2. The Council (via the EC Staff Liaison) shall notify all parties at least forty-five (45) days prior to the hearing of the date, time, and place.

5.6.3. Case material will be sent to all parties and the Council members by national delivery service or mail with signature required and/or proof of date received.

5.7. Hearing Witnesses, Materials, and Evidence

5.7.1. Within thirty (30) days of notification of the hearing, the Respondent shall submit to the Council a written response to the decision and sanction, including a detailed statement as to the reasons that he or she is appealing the decision and a list of potential witnesses (if any) with a statement indicating the subject matter they will be addressing.

5.7.2. The Complainant before the Council also will submit a list of potential witnesses (if any) to the Council with a statement indicating the subject matter they will be addressing. Only under limited circumstances may the Council consider additional material evidence from the Respondent or the Complainant not presented or available prior to the issuance of their proposed sanction. Such new or additional evidence may be considered by the Council if the Council is satisfied that the Respondent or the Complainant has demonstrated the new evidence was previously unavailable and provided it is submitted to all parties in writing no later than fifteen (15) days prior to the hearing.

5.7.3. The Council Chairperson may permit testimony by conference call (at no expense to the participant), limit participation of witnesses in order to curtail repetitive testimony, or prescribe other reasonable arrangements or limitations. The Respondent may elect to appear (at Respondent's own expense) and present testimony. If alternative technology options are available for the hearing, the Respondent, Council members, and EC Chairperson shall be so informed when the hearing arrangements are sent.

5.8. Counsel—The Respondent may be represented by legal counsel at his or her own expense. Association Legal Counsel shall advise and represent the Association at the hearing. Association Legal Counsel also may advise the Council regarding procedural matters to ensure fairness to all parties. All parties and the Association Legal Counsel (at the request of the EC or the Council) shall have the opportunity to question witnesses.

5.9. Hearing

5.9.1. The Council hearing shall be recorded by a professional transcription service or telephone recording transcribed for Council members and shall be limited to two (2) hours.

5.9.2. The Council Chairperson will conduct the hearing and does not vote.

5.9.3. Each person present shall be identified for the record, and the Council Chairperson will describe the procedures for the Council hearing. An oral affirmation of truthfulness will be requested from each participant who gives factual testimony in the Council hearing.

5.9.4. The Council Chairperson shall allow for questions.

5.9.5. The EC Chairperson shall present the ethics complaint, a summary of the evidence resulting from the investigation, and the EC decision and disciplinary action imposed against the Respondent.

5.9.6. The Respondent may present a defense to the decision and sanction after the EC presents its case.

5.9.7. Each party and/or his or her legal representative shall have the opportunity to call witnesses to present testimony and to question any witnesses including the EC Chairperson or his or her designee. The Council Chairperson shall be entitled to provide reasonable limits on the extent of any witnesses' testimony or any questioning.

5.9.8. The Council Chairperson may recess the hearing at any time.

5.9.9. The Council Chairperson shall call for final statements from each party before concluding the hearing.

5.9.10. Decisions of the Council will be by majority vote.

5.10. Disciplinary Council Decision

5.10.1. An official copy of the transcript shall be sent to each Council member, the EC Chairperson, the Association Legal Counsel, the EC Staff Liaison, and the Respondent and his or her counsel as soon as it is available from the transcription company.

5.10.2. The Council Chairperson shall work with the EC Staff Liaison and the Association Legal Counsel in preparing the text of the final decision.

5.10.3. The Council shall issue a decision in writing to the Association ED within thirty (30) days of receiving the written transcription of the hearing (unless special circumstances warrant additional time). The Council decision shall be based on the record and evidence presented and may affirm, modify, or reverse the decision of the EC, including increasing or decreasing the level of sanction or determining that no disciplinary action is warranted.

5.11. Action, Notification, and Timeline Adjustments

5.11.1. A copy of the Council's official decision and appeal process (Section 6) is sent to the Respondent, the EC Chairperson, and other appropriate parties within fifteen (15) business days via mail (with signature and proof of date received) after notification of the Association ED.

5.11.2. The time limits specified in the *Enforcement Procedures for the Occupational Therapy Code of Ethics* may be extended by mutual consent of the Respondent, Complainant, and Council Chairperson for good cause by the Chairperson.

5.11.3. Other features of the preceding *Enforcement Procedures* may be adjusted in particular cases in light of extraordinary circumstances, consistent with fundamental fairness.

5.12. Appeal—Within thirty (30) days after notification of the Council's decision, a Respondent upon whom a sanction was imposed may appeal the decision as provided in Section 6. Within thirty (30) days after notification of the Council's decision, the EC also may appeal the decision as provided in Section 6. If no appeal is filed within that time, the Association ED or EC Staff Liaison shall publish the decision in accordance with these procedures and make any other notifications deemed necessary.

6. Appeal Process

6.1. Appeals—Either the EC or the Respondent may appeal. Appeals shall be written, signed by the appealing party, and sent by mail requiring signature and proof of date of receipt to the Association ED in care of the Association Ethics Office. The grounds for the appeal shall be fully explained in this document. When an appeal is requested, the other party will be notified.

6.2. Grounds for Appeal—Appeals shall generally address only the issues, procedures, or sanctions that are part of the record before the Council. However, in the interest of fairness, the Appeal Panel may consider newly available evidence relating to the original complaint only under extraordinary circumstances.

6.3. Composition and Leadership of Appeal Panel—The Vice-President, Secretary, and Treasurer shall constitute the Appeal Panel. In the event of vacancies in these positions or the existence of a conflict of interest, the Vice President shall appoint replacements drawn from among the other Board of Directors members. If the entire Board has a conflict of interest, the Board Appeal process (Attachment C of EC SOP) shall be followed. The President shall not serve on the Appeal Panel. No individual may serve on the Council who has previously been the subject of an ethics complaint that resulted in a specific EC disciplinary action.

The Appeal Panel Chairperson will be selected by its members from among themselves.

6.4. Appeal Process—The Association ED shall forward any letter of appeal to the Appeal Panel within fifteen (15) business days of receipt. Within thirty (30) days after the Appeal Panel receives the appeal, the Panel shall determine whether a hearing is warranted. If the Panel decides that a hearing is warranted, timely notice for such hearing shall be given to the parties. Participants at the hearing shall be limited to the Respondent and legal counsel (if so desired), the EC Chairperson, the Council Chairperson, the Association Legal Counsel, or others approved in advance by the Appeal Panel as necessary to the proceedings.

6.5. Decision

6.5.1. The Appeal Panel shall have the power to (a) affirm the decision; (b) modify the decision; or (c) reverse or remand to the EC, but only if there were procedural errors materially prejudicial to the outcome of the proceeding or if the Council decision was against the clear weight of the evidence.

6.5.2. Within thirty (30) days after receipt of the appeal if no hearing was granted, or within thirty (30) days after receipt of the transcript of an Appeal hearing if held, the Appeal Panel shall notify the Association ED of its decision. The Association ED shall promptly notify the Respondent, the original Complainant, appropriate Association bodies, and any other parties deemed appropriate (e.g., SRB, NBCOT®). For Association purposes, the decision of the Appeal Panel shall be final.

7. Notifications

All notifications referred to in these *Enforcement Procedures* shall be in writing and shall be delivered by national delivery service or mail with signature and proof of date received.

8. Records and Reports

At the completion of the enforcement process, the written records and reports that state the initial basis for the complaint, material evidence, and the disposition of the complaint shall be retained in the Association Ethics Office for a period of five (5) years.

9. Publication

Final decisions will be publicized only after any appeal process has been completed.

10. Modification

The Association reserves the right to (a) modify the time periods, procedures, or application of these *Enforcement Procedures* for good cause consistent with fundamental fairness in a given case and (b) modify its *Code* and/or these *Enforcement Procedures*, with such modifications to be applied only prospectively.

Adopted by the Representative Assembly 2015NovCO13 as Attachment A of the Standard Operating Procedures (SOP) of the Ethics Commission.

Reviewed by BPPC 1/04, 1/05, 9/06, 1/07, 9/09, 9/11, 9/13, 9/15

Adopted by RA 4/96, 5/04, 5/05, 11/06, 4/07, 11/09, 12/13

Revised by SEC 4/98, 4/00, 1/02, 1/04, 12/04, 9/06

Revised by EC 12/06, 2/07, 8/09, 9/13, 9/15

This document replaces the 2014 document *Enforcement Procedures for the Occupational Therapy Code of Ethics and Ethics Standards,* previously published and copyrighted in 2014 by the American Occupational Therapy Association in the *American Journal of Occupational Therapy, 68*(Suppl. 3), S3–S15. http://dx.doi.org/10.5014/ajot.2014.686S02

Citation: American Occupational Therapy Association. (2015). Enforcement procedures for the *Occupational Therapy Code of Ethics. American Journal of Occupational Therapy, 69*(Suppl. 3), 6913410012. http://dx.doi.org/10.5014/ajot.2014.696S19

AMERICAN OCCUPATIONAL THERAPY ASSOCIATION
ETHICS COMMISSION

Formal Complaint of Alleged Violation of the *Occupational Therapy Code of Ethics*

If an investigation is deemed necessary, a copy of this form will be provided to the individual against whom the complaint is filed.

Date ______________________

Complainant: (Information regarding individual filing the complaint)

NAME	SIGNATURE
ADDRESS	TELEPHONE
	E-MAIL ADDRESS

Respondent: (Information regarding individual against whom the complaint is directed)

NAME	SIGNATURE
ADDRESS	TELEPHONE
	E-MAIL ADDRESS

1. **Summarize** in a written attachment the **facts and circumstances, including dates and events,** that support a violation of the *Occupational Therapy Code of Ethics* and this complaint. Include steps, if any, that have been taken to resolve this complaint before filing.

2. **Please sign and date all documents you have written and are submitting.** *Do not include confidential documents such as patient or employment records.*

3. **If you have filed a complaint about this same matter with any other agency (e.g., NBCOT®; SRB; academic institution; any federal, state, or local official), indicate to whom it was submitted, the approximate date(s), and resolution if known.**

I certify that the statements/information within this complaint are correct and truthful to the best of my knowledge and are submitted in good faith, not for resolution of private business, legal, or other disputes for which other appropriate forums exist.

Signature ______________________

Send completed form, with accompanying documentation, **IN AN ENVELOPE MARKED *CONFIDENTIAL* to**

Ethics Commission
American Occupational Therapy Association, Inc.
Attn: Ethics Program Manager/Ethics Office
4720 Montgomery Lane, Suite 200
Bethesda, MD 20814-3449

OR email all material in pdf format to ethics@aota.org with "Complaint" in subject line

Office Use Only:

Membership Verified? ❑ **Yes** ❑ **No**

By: ______________________

Appendix C.

NBCOT® CANDIDATE/CERTIFICANT CODE OF CONDUCT

NBCOT expects both certificants and applicants to uphold the organization's Code of Conduct Principles:

Principle 1

Certificants shall provide accurate and truthful representations to NBCOT concerning all information related to aspects of the Certification Program, including, but not limited to, the submission of information:

- On the examination and certification renewal applications, and renewal audit form;
- Requested by NBCOT for a disciplinary action situation; or
- Requested by NBCOT concerning allegations related to
  - Test security violations and/or disclosure of confidential examination material content to unauthorized parties;
  - Misrepresentations by a certificant regarding his/her credential(s) and/or education;
  - The unauthorized use of NBCOT's intellectual property, certification marks, and other copyrighted materials, including all NBCOT exam preparation tools e.g., practice exams.

Principle 2

Certificants who are the subject of a complaint shall cooperate with NBCOT concerning investigations of violations of the NBCOT Practice Standards, including the collection of relevant information.

Principle 3

Certificants shall be accurate, truthful, and complete in any and all communications, direct or indirect, with any client, employer, regulatory agency, or other parties as relates to their professional work, education, professional credentials, research, and contributions to the field of OT.

Principle 4

Certificants shall comply with state and/or federal laws, regulations, and statutes governing the practice of occupational therapy.

Principle 5

Certificants shall not have been convicted of a crime, the circumstances of which substantially relate to the practice of occupational therapy or indicate an inability to engage in the practice of occupational therapy safely and/or competently.

Principle 6

Certificants shall not engage in behavior or conduct, lawful or otherwise that causes them to be, or reasonably perceived to be, a threat or potential threat to the health, well-being, or safety of recipients or potential recipients of occupational therapy services.

Principle 7

Certificants shall not engage in the practice of occupational therapy while one's ability to practice is impaired due to chemical (i.e., legal and/or illegal) drug or alcohol abuse.

Principle 8

Certificants shall not electronically post personal health information or anything, including photos, that may reveal a patient's/client's identity or personal or therapeutic relationship. All statements, regardless of intent, about a patient/client can potentially contain sufficient information for a member of a community to recognize the patient/client, thus violating the state and/or federal law (i.e., Health Insurance Portability and Accountability Act).

Appendix D.

PROCEDURES FOR THE ENFORCEMENT OF THE *NBCOT® CANDIDATE/ CERTIFICANT CODE OF CONDUCT*

SECTION A. Preamble

In exercising its responsibility for promoting and maintaining standards of professional conduct in the practice of occupational therapy and in order to protect the public from those practitioners whose behavior falls short of these standards, the National Board for Certification in Occupational Therapy, Inc. ("NBCOT®," formerly known as "AOTCB") has adopted a Candidate/Certificant Code of Conduct. The NBCOT has adopted these enforcement procedures for resolving issues arising under the Candidate/Certificant Code of Conduct with respect to persons who have been certified by the NBCOT or who have applied for such certification. These procedures are intended to enable the NBCOT, through its Qualifications and Compliance Review Committee ("QCRC"), comprised of both professional and public members, QCRC Chair, (or Co-Chair when Chair is unavailable) and Staff to act fairly in the performance of its responsibilities to the public as a certifying agency, and to ensure that the rights of candidates and certificants are protected.

SECTION B. Basis for Sanction

A violation of the Candidate/Certificant Code of Conduct provides basis for action and sanction under these Procedures.

SECTION C. Sanctions

1. Violations of the Candidate/Certificant Code of Conduct may result in one or more of the following sanctions:
   a. Ineligibility for certification, which means that an individual is barred from becoming certified by the NBCOT, either indefinitely or for a certain duration.
   b. Reprimand, which means a formal expression of disapproval, which shall be retained in the certificant's file, but shall not be publicly announced.
   c. Censure, which means a formal expression of disapproval which is publicly announced.
   d. Probation, which means continued certification is subject to fulfillment of specified conditions, e.g., monitoring, education, supervision, and/or counseling.

e. Suspension, which means the loss of certification for a certain duration, after which the individual may be required to apply for reinstatement.
f. Revocation, which means permanent loss of certification.

2. All sanctions other than reprimand shall be announced publicly, in accordance with Section D.9. All sanctions other than reprimand shall be disclosed in response to inquiries in accordance with Section D.9.

SECTION D. Procedures for the Enforcement of the Candidate/Certificant Code of Conduct

1. Jurisdiction

The NBCOT has jurisdiction over all individuals who have been certified as an OCCUPATIONAL THERAPIST REGISTERED OTR (OTR®) henceforth OTR, or CERTIFIED OCCUPATIONAL THERAPY ASSISTANT COTA (COTA®) henceforth COTA, or who have applied for certification, or have applied for Occupational Therapist Eligibility Determination (OTED) to take the NBCOT Certification Examination for OTR. In addition, NBCOT has jurisdiction over all individuals who have applied for an Early Determination Review to determine eligibility to take the Certification Examination for OTR or COTA; Jurisdiction, in this case, is for the limited purpose of acting upon a request for an Early Determination.

2. Initiation of the Review Process

The NBCOT Staff ("Staff") shall initiate the process upon receipt by the NBCOT of information indicating that an individual subject to NBCOT's jurisdiction may have violated the Candidate/Certificant Code of Conduct. Receipt of such information shall be considered a complaint for the purposes of these procedures, regardless of the source.

3. Staff Investigation and Action

a. Staff shall evaluate all complaints and determine whether to dismiss the case or propose a sanction, as deemed appropriate.
b. Staff may review any evidence, which it deems appropriate and relevant.
c. If Staff determines that the evidence does not support the allegation(s), no file shall be opened and the complainant shall be notified of the Staff's decision.
d. If the complaint has also been made to the regulatory authority but no decision has been rendered, Staff may stay action pending a decision by the regulatory authority.
e. When a regulatory authority has imposed disciplinary action and Staff determines that the evidence does support the allegation(s) and the matter should be reviewed by NBCOT, the subject of the complaint shall be notified. This notification shall be in writing and shall include a brief description of the complaint. The subject of the complaint shall have thirty (30) days from the date notification is sent to respond in writing to the complaint. The Staff may extend this period up to an additional thirty (30) days upon request, provided sufficient justification for the extension is given.
f. When a regulatory authority has not imposed disciplinary action, (such as in the case of an OTED applicant, Early Determination Review, exam candidate who has responded affirmatively on the examination application to a character question or a third party complaint) Staff has the discretion to gather information in order to either dismiss the case, impose one or more sanctions, or refer to the QCRC for further review.
g. Upon completion of its investigation, Staff may take action based on the evidence and violation of NBCOT guidelines. Staff shall either:
   i. Dismiss the case due to insufficient evidence, the matter being insufficiently serious, or other reasons as may be warranted; or

ii. Notify the subject of the complaint that NBCOT will not pursue further action against the subject's certification due to appropriate action taken by the state; or

iii. Notify the subject of the complaint of the proposed sanction in writing. When disciplinary action is proposed, the subject of the complaint shall have thirty (30) days from the date notification is sent to accept the sanction or request a hearing in writing. Staff may extend this period up to an additional thirty (30) days upon request, provided sufficient justification for the extension is given.

h. Staff will review with QCRC chair all proposals for Revocation or Ineligibility for Certification prior to sending notification to the subject.

i. Staff will advise the QCRC Chair, on a periodic basis, of all imposed sanctions.

j. If any sanction other than reprimand is imposed, public notice may be given in accordance with Section D.9 of these procedures.

4. Voluntary Forfeiture

The subject of a complaint may voluntarily forfeit his or her certification. This forfeiture must be submitted in writing and can be made, at any time, while the complaint is either being reviewed or when disciplinary action has been taken by the NBCOT but the terms of the sanction remain incomplete.

Staff will advise the Qualifications and Compliance Review Committee (QCRC) Chair of any voluntary forfeiture.

If the subject requests reinstatement of certification, after voluntary forfeiture, the subject must meet all of the following requirements:

a. submit reinstatement of certification request in writing,
b. satisfy current certification examination eligibility requirements (including academic and fieldwork requirements),
c. re-take and pass the national certification examination and
d. comply with proposed sanction agreement and/or other informational requests, which will be resumed upon request to regain certification.

If the subject's certification is voluntarily forfeited, public notice may be given in accordance with Section D.9 of these procedures.

5. Failure to Respond to Investigative Inquiry

Individuals who are non-responsive on a timely basis to NBCOT investigative inquiries will have their certification automatically suspended for a period of up to three (3) years and during such period, CANNOT a) identify themselves to the public as an OCCUPATIONAL THERAPIST REGISTERED (OTR) or CERTIFIED OCCUPATIONAL THERAPY ASSISTANT (COTA) or b) use the OTR or COTA credential after their name. If no response is received within the suspension period, NBCOT certification shall automatically be revoked.

If the subject requests to be reinstated during the suspension, the subject shall:

a. submit reinstatement of certification request in writing,
b. satisfy current certification renewal requirements,
c. cooperate with and provide written response and supporting documentation to the NBCOT proposed sanction and/or other informational requests and
d. provide documentation by the state board confirming the current status of subject's license upon request.

Upon receipt of a request to satisfy these requirements, the complaint will be handled in accordance with these Enforcement procedures, except that NBCOT certification status will remain in suspended status until the matter is resolved.

6. Procedures for the Sanction Agreement Letter

Upon receipt of the proposed sanction letter, the subject may either:

a. Accept the sanction as proposed and thereby waive his/her right to a hearing. To accept the sanction, the subject must sign, date and return the sanction letter to NBCOT. Upon the subject's acceptance of the sanction agreement, the qualifications and compliance process shall be considered closed. The public notification standards of Section D.9 are applicable if the settlement contains a sanction that warrants such announcement be made; or
b. Not accept the sanction as proposed and request a hearing before the QCRC. Request for a hearing must be submitted by the subject in writing. Hearing requests must include subject's reasons for requesting a hearing and may also include any additional information or documentation which the subject wishes to provide in support of his/her position.
c. If the subject fails to respond to the sanction agreement letter, within thirty (30) days after the agreement has been sent to the subject, conditions and terms of the proposed agreement take effect immediately.

Prior to the hearing:

i. Staff shall prepare a case report of its review to the Hearing Panel.
ii. The report shall include any written responses, or other materials submitted by the subject or any other individual in relation to the complaint. A copy of the report shall be provided to the subject at least thirty (30) days prior to the hearing.
iii. Additional information may be requested by the Hearing Panel prior to the hearing.

At the hearing:

i. The subject of the complaint may be represented at the hearing by his/her legal counsel, or any other individual of his or her choosing.
ii. The subject of the complaint shall be solely responsible for all of his/her own expenses related to the hearing. Hearings can be conducted via teleconference call or in person at the sole discretion of the QCRC. Should the subject cancel the hearing, he/she must notify the QCRC of the cancellation no less than fifteen (15) days prior to the hearing date. Should the subject cancel the hearing within fifteen (15) days of the hearing date or not appear at the scheduled hearing, all costs associated with the preparation of the hearing shall be paid by the subject (e.g., court reporting fees, teleconference fees, hearing manual preparation fees).
iii. The subject of the complaint shall provide the QCRC with any and all materials he/she may wish to include for the hearing no less than fifteen (15) days prior to the hearing date.

Following the hearing, Staff shall notify (in writing) the complainant and the subject of the complaint of the QCRC's decision within thirty (30) days of the decision. The decision shall take effect immediately unless otherwise provided by the QCRC.

7. Appeals Process

Within thirty (30) days after the notification of the QCRC's decision, any individual(s) sanctioned by the QCRC at the hearing may appeal the hearing decision to the NBCOT Directors. A notice of appeal, which must be in writing and signed by the subject, shall be sent by the subject to the NBCOT Chairperson in care of the President/Chief Executive Officer. The basis for the appeal shall be fully explained in this notice.

The Chairperson of the Board of Directors shall form a three (3) person Appeals Panel within 30 days after receipt of the notice of appeal. At least one (1) member of the Appeals Panel shall be a member of the QCRC who did not serve on the Hearing Panel. No member of the QCRC who participated in the hearing shall serve on the Appeals Panel nor shall the QCRC Chair serve on the Appeals Panel if the Chair participated in the decision to offer a proposed sanction. Two-three members of the Board of Directors will be selected by the Chairperson of the Board of Directors to fill out the Panel.

An appeal must relate to evidence, issues and procedures that are part of the record of the QCRC hearing and decision. The appeal may also address the substance of the disciplinary action. However, the Panel may in its discretion consider additional evidence.

Within fifteen (15) days after the notice of appeal is received by the Appeals Panel, the Panel shall provide the subject with an opportunity to schedule an appeals hearing. The subject may be represented at the hearing by legal counsel or any other individual of his/her choosing. The subject shall be solely responsible for all of his/her own expenses related to the hearing.

Within fifteen (15) days after the appeals hearing or if the subject elects not to request a formal hearing, the Panel shall decide the appeal and notify the Chairperson of its decision.

The Appeals Panel may either:

a. Affirm the QCRC's sanction agreement;
b. Deny the QCRC's sanction agreement;
c. Refer the case back to the Staff for further investigation and resolution with full right of appeal; or
d. Modify the QCRC's sanction agreement, but not in a manner that would be more adverse to the subject.

The Chairperson shall promptly notify the subject of the Appeals Panel's decision. The decision of the Appeals Panel shall be final.

8. Cooperation with NBCOT Enforcement Procedures

Failure to respond to any aspect of the Enforcement Procedures, will be considered a violation of the Candidate/Certificant Code of Conduct, Principle 2, and is sufficient grounds for the imposition of sanction by the NBCOT.

9. Announcement of Sanction

If an individual's certification status is voluntarily forfeited, suspended or revoked, or he/she is censured or placed on probation, occupational therapy state regulatory bodies shall be notified and an announcement included in NBCOT's online resources and in one or more publications of general circulation to persons engaged or otherwise interested in the profession of occupational therapy. The NBCOT may also disclose its final decision, including ineligibility for certification, to others as it deems appropriate, including, but not limited to, persons inquiring about the status of an individual's certification, employers, third party payers and the general public.

10. Notification

All notifications referred to in these procedures shall be in writing and if the subject does not respond, shall be by confirmation of signature, return receipt mail, unless otherwise indicated. Subjects of complaints who live outside of the U.S. may be given additional time to respond to any notifications they are sent, as determined by the Staff in its discretion.

11. Records and Reports

At the completion of this procedure, all records and reports shall be returned to the Staff. The complete files in the qualifications and compliance review proceedings shall be maintained.

12. Expedited Action

The NBCOT may expedite a matter by shortening any notice or response period provided for under these procedures if the responsible party determines in its sole discretion that shortening the period is appropriate in order to protect against the possibility of harm to recipients of occupational therapy services.

In matters where the severity of the allegations and evidence provided warrant such action in order to protect the public, the NBCOT may authorize immediate suspension/revocation of certification. The subject will be duly notified of the action and given fifteen (15) days to contest the suspension or revocation.

13. Standard of Proof

The NBCOT shall take disciplinary action against an individual only where there is clear and convincing evidence of a violation of the Candidate/Certificant Code of Conduct.

14. Accommodations

The NBCOT recognizes the definition of disability as defined by the Americans with Disabilities Act (ADA) and acknowledges the provisions and protections of the Act. The NBCOT shall offer hearings related to qualifications and compliance review or the appeals process in a site and manner, which is architecturally accessible to persons with disabilities or offer alternative arrangements for such individuals.

An individual with a documented disability may request accommodations for a hearing by providing reasonable advance notice to the NBCOT of his or her disability and of the modifications or aids needed at the hearing at his or her own expense.

15. Amendment to Procedures

These procedures may be amended at any time by the NBCOT Directors.

Revision: February 21, 2015.

Appendix E.

ETHICS RESOURCES

Document Resources

American Occupational Therapy Association. (2015). Enforcement procedures for the *Occupational Therapy Code of Ethics. American Journal of Occupational Therapy, 69*(Suppl. 3), 6913410012. https://doi.org/10.5014/ajot.2014.696S19

American Occupational Therapy Association. (2015). Occupational therapy code of ethics (2015). *American Journal of Occupational Therapy, 69*(Suppl. 3), 6912310030. https://doi.org/10.5014/ajot.2015.696S03

American Occupational Therapy Association. (2015). Standards for continuing competence. *American Journal of Occupational Therapy, 69*(Suppl. 3), 6913410055. https://doi.org/10.5014/ajot.2015.696S16

Barker, P. (Ed.). (2011). *Mental health ethics: The human context.* New York: Routledge.

Beauchamp, T. L., & Childress, J. F. (2013). *Principles of biomedical ethics* (7th ed.). New York: Oxford University Press.

College of Occupational Therapists. (2015). *College of Occupational Therapists: Code of ethics and professional conduct.* Retrieved from https://www.cot.co.uk/sites/default/files/publications/public/CODE-OF-ETHICS-2015.pdf

Corey, G., Schneider-Corey, M., & Callanan, P. (2011). *Issues and ethics in the helping professions* (8th ed.). Pacific Grove, CA: Brooks/Cole.

Kornblau, B. L., & Burkhardt, A. (2012). *Ethics in rehabilitation: A clinical perspective* (2nd ed.). Thorofare, NJ: Slack.

Kyler, P. (2010). Ethical issues in evaluation. In J. Hinojosa, P. Kramer, & P. Crist (Eds.), *Occupational therapy evaluation: Obtaining and interpreting data* (3rd ed., pp. 295–319). Bethesda, MD: AOTA Press.

Penny, N. E., Bires, S. J., Bonn, E. A., Dockery, A. N., & Pettit, N. L. (2016). Moral Distress Scale for Occupational Therapists: Part 1. Instrument development and content validity. *American Journal of Occupational Therapy, 70*, 7004300020. https://doi.org/10.5014/ajot.2015.018358

Purtilo, R., & Doherty, R. F. (2011). *Ethical dimensions in the health professions* (5th ed.). St. Louis: Elsevier.

Purtilo, R., & Jensen, G., & Royeen, C. (Eds.). (2005). *Educating for moral action: A sourcebook in health and rehabilitation ethics.* Philadelphia: F. A. Davis.

Romano, J. L. (2011). *Legal rights of the seriously ill and injured: A family guide.* Pittsburgh: Author.

Slater, D. Y. (Ed.). (2016). *Reference guide to the Occupational Therapy Code of Ethics (2015).* Bethesda, MD: AOTA Press.

World Federation of Occupational Therapists. (2016). *Code of ethics.* Retrieved from http://www.wfot.org/ResourceCentre.aspx

World Federation of Occupational Therapists. (2016). *Position statement: Ethics, sustainability and global experiences.* Retrieved from http://www.wfot.org/ResourceCentre.aspx

Online Resources

- **American Medical Association Ethics Resource Center:** http://bit.ly/2hJWqeC
- **American Occupational Therapy Association (AOTA):** www.aota.org
  - AOTA ethics resources: http://bit.ly/2h4qsGa
  - AOTA evidence-based practice and research resources: http://www.aota.org/ebp
  - AOTA professional development tool: http://bit.ly/2hJX6Rt
- **Applied ethics resources:** http://bit.ly/2hzX8YW
- **Clinical ethics resources:** http://clinicalethics.info/
- **Consumers Union:** Doctor accountability, Safe Patient Project: http://safepatientproject.org
- **Global ethics:** http://www.globethics.net/
- **Hastings Center:** http://www.thehastingscenter.org/
- **Institutional Review Boards:** http://www.hhs.gov/ohrp/assurances/irb/index.html
- **International Center for Academic Integrity:** http://bit.ly/2dtBsKm
- Kennedy Institute of Ethics: http://kennedyinstitute.georgetown.edu
- **National Board for Certification in Occupational Therapy (NBCOT):** http://www.nbcot.org
  - NBCOT certificant attestation: http://bit.ly/2hzV836
  - NBCOT *Certification Examination Handbook:* http://bit.ly/2gP4j0G
  - NBCOT certification renewal: http://bit.ly/2hzXyP0
  - NBCOT Certification Renewal Log: http://bit.ly/2hK67K4
  - NBCOT Disciplinary Action Information Exchange Network: http://bit.ly/2hRUNHU
  - NBCOT Practice Standards/ Code of Conduct: http://bit.ly/2hRZvFp
- **National Center for Ethics in Health Care:** http://www.ethics.va.gov/
- **World Federation of Occupational Therapists ethics:** http://bit.ly/2hxN59k

Appendix F.

Guidelines for Supervision, Roles, and Responsibilities During the Delivery of Occupational Therapy Services

This document is a set of guidelines describing the supervision, roles, and responsibilities of occupational therapy practitioners. Intended for both internal and external audiences, it also provides an outline of the roles and responsibilities of occupational therapists, occupational therapy assistants, and occupational therapy aides during the delivery of occupational therapy services.

General Supervision

These guidelines provide a definition of supervision and outline parameters regarding effective supervision as it relates to the delivery of occupational therapy services. The guidelines themselves cannot be interpreted to constitute a standard of supervision in any particular locality. Occupational therapists, occupational therapy assistants, and occupational therapy aides are expected to meet applicable state and federal regulations, adhere to relevant workplace and payer policies and to the *Occupational Therapy Code of Ethics and Ethics Standards* (American Occupational Therapy Association [AOTA], 2010), and participate in ongoing professional development activities to maintain continuing competency.

Within the scope of occupational therapy practice, *supervision* is a process aimed at ensuring the safe and effective delivery of occupational therapy services and fostering professional competence and development. In addition, in these guidelines, supervision is viewed as a cooperative process in which two or more people participate in a joint effort to establish, maintain, and/or elevate a level of competence and performance. Supervision is based on mutual understanding between the supervisor and the supervisee about each other's competence, experience, education, and credentials. It fosters growth and development, promotes effective utilization of resources, encourages creativity and innovation, and provides education and support to achieve a goal.

Supervision of Occupational Therapists and Occupational Therapy Assistants

Occupational Therapists

Based on education and training, occupational therapists, after initial certification and relevant state licensure or other governmental requirements, are autonomous practitioners who are able to deliver occupational therapy services independently. Occupational therapists are responsible for all aspects of occupational therapy service delivery and are accountable for the safety and effectiveness of the occupational therapy services and service delivery process. Occupational therapists are encouraged to seek peer supervision and mentoring for ongoing development of best practice approaches and to promote professional growth.

Occupational Therapy Assistants

Based on education and training, occupational therapy assistants, after initial certification and meeting of state regulatory requirements, must receive supervision from an occupational therapist to deliver occupational therapy services. Occupational therapy assistants deliver occupational therapy services under the supervision of and in partnership with occupational therapists. Occupational therapists and occupational therapy assistants are equally responsible for developing a collaborative plan for supervision. The occupational therapist is ultimately responsible for the implementation of appropriate supervision, but the occupational therapy assistant also has a responsibility to seek and obtain appropriate supervision to ensure proper occupational therapy is being provided.

General Principles

1. Supervision involves guidance and oversight related to the delivery of occupational therapy services and the facilitation of professional growth and competence. It is the responsibility of the occupational therapy assistant to seek the appropriate quality and frequency of supervision to ensure safe and effective occupational therapy service delivery. It is the responsibility of the occupational therapist to provide adequate and appropriate supervision.
2. To ensure safe and effective occupational therapy services, it is the responsibility of occupational therapists to recognize when they require peer supervision or mentoring that supports current and advancing levels of competence and professional growth.
3. The specific frequency, methods, and content of supervision may vary and are dependent on the
    a. Complexity of client needs,
    b. Number and diversity of clients,
    c. Knowledge and skill level of the occupational therapist and the occupational therapy assistant,
    d. Type of practice setting,
    e. Requirements of the practice setting, and
    f. Other regulatory requirements.
4. Supervision of the occupational therapy assistant that is more frequent than the minimum level required by the practice setting or regulatory requirements may be necessary when
    a. The needs of the client and the occupational therapy process are complex and changing,
    b. The practice setting provides occupational therapy services to a large number of clients with diverse needs, or
    c. The occupational therapist and occupational therapy assistant determine that additional supervision is necessary to ensure safe and effective delivery of occupational therapy services.
5. There are a variety of types and methods of supervision. Methods can include but are not limited to direct, face-to-face contact and indirect contact. Examples of methods or types of supervision that involve direct face-to-face contact include observation, modeling, client demonstration, discussions, teaching, and instruction. Examples of methods or types of supervision that involve indirect contact include phone conversations, written correspondence, and electronic exchanges.
6. Occupational therapists and occupational therapy assistants must abide by facility and state requirements regarding the documentation of a supervision plan and supervision contacts. Documentation may include the
    a. Frequency of supervisory contact,
    b. Methods or types of supervision,
    c. Content areas addressed,

   d. Evidence to support areas and levels of competency, and
   e. Names and credentials of the persons participating in the supervisory process.

7. Peer supervision and mentoring related to professional growth, such as leadership and advocacy skills development, may differ from the peer supervision mentoring needed to provide occupational therapy services. The person providing this supervision, as well as the frequency, method, and content of supervision, should be responsive to the supervisee's advancing levels of professional growth.

Supervision Outside the Delivery of Occupational Therapy Services

The education and expertise of occupational therapists and occupational therapy assistants prepare them for employment in arenas other than those related to the delivery of occupational therapy. In these other arenas, supervision may be provided by non-occupational therapy professionals.

1. The guidelines of the setting, regulatory agencies, and funding agencies direct the supervision requirements.
2. The occupational therapist and occupational therapy assistant should obtain and use credentials or job titles commensurate with their roles in these other employment arenas.
3. The following can be used to determine whether the services provided are related to the delivery of occupational therapy:
   a. State practice acts;
   b. Regulatory agency standards and rules;
   c. *Occupational Therapy Practice Framework: Domain and Process* (AOTA, 2014) and other AOTA official documents; and
   d. Written and verbal agreement among the occupational therapist, the occupational therapy assistant, the client, and the agency or payer about the services provided.

Roles and Responsibilities of Occupational Therapists and Occupational Therapy Assistants During the Delivery of Occupational Therapy Services

Overview

The focus of occupational therapy is to assist the client in "achieving health, well-being, and participation in life through engagement in occupation" (AOTA, 2014, p. S2). Occupational therapy addresses the needs and goals of the client related to engaging in areas of occupation and considers the performance skills, performance patterns, context and environment, and client factors that may influence performance in various areas of occupation.

1. The occupational therapist is responsible for all aspects of occupational therapy service delivery and is accountable for the safety and effectiveness of the occupational therapy service delivery process. The occupational therapy service delivery process involves evaluation, intervention planning, intervention implementation, intervention review, and targeting of outcomes and outcomes evaluation.
2. The occupational therapist must be directly involved in the delivery of services during the initial evaluation and regularly throughout the course of intervention, intervention review, and outcomes evaluation.
3. The occupational therapy assistant delivers safe and effective occupational therapy services under the supervision of and in partnership with the occupational therapist.

4. It is the responsibility of the occupational therapist to determine when to delegate responsibilities to an occupational therapy assistant. It is the responsibility of the occupational therapy assistant who performs the delegated responsibilities to demonstrate service competency and also to not accept delegated responsibilities that go beyond the scope of an occupational therapy assistant.
5. The occupational therapist and the occupational therapy assistant demonstrate and document service competency for clinical reasoning and judgment during the service delivery process as well as for the performance of specific techniques, assessments, and intervention methods used.
6. When delegating aspects of occupational therapy services, the occupational therapist considers the following factors:
   a. Complexity of the client's condition and needs,
   b. Knowledge, skill, and competence of the occupational therapy assistant,
   c. Nature and complexity of the intervention,
   d. Needs and requirements of the practice setting, and
   e. Appropriate scope of practice of an occupational therapy assistant under state law and other requirements.

Roles and Responsibilities

Regardless of the setting in which occupational therapy services are delivered, occupational therapists and occupational therapy assistants assume the following general responsibilities during evaluation; intervention planning, implementation, and review; and targeting and evaluating outcomes.

Evaluation

1. The occupational therapist directs the evaluation process.
2. The occupational therapist is responsible for directing all aspects of the initial contact during the occupational therapy evaluation, including
   a. Determining the need for service,
   b. Defining the problems within the domain of occupational therapy to be addressed,
   c. Determining the client's goals and priorities,
   d. Establishing intervention priorities,
   e. Determining specific further assessment needs, and
   f. Determining specific assessment tasks that can be delegated to the occupational therapy assistant.
3. The occupational therapist initiates and directs the evaluation, interprets the data, and develops the intervention plan.
4. The occupational therapy assistant contributes to the evaluation process by implementing delegated assessments and by providing verbal and written reports of observations, assessments, and client capacities to the occupational therapist.
5. The occupational therapist interprets the information provided by the occupational therapy assistant and integrates that information into the evaluation and decision-making process.

Intervention Planning

1. The occupational therapist has overall responsibility for the development of the occupational therapy intervention plan.
2. The occupational therapist and the occupational therapy assistant collaborate with the client to develop the plan.
3. The occupational therapy assistant is responsible for being knowledgeable about evaluation results and for providing input into the intervention plan, based on client needs and priorities.

Intervention Implementation

1. The occupational therapist has overall responsibility for intervention implementation.
2. When delegating aspects of the occupational therapy intervention to the occupational therapy assistant, the occupational therapist is responsible for providing appropriate supervision.
3. The occupational therapy assistant is responsible for being knowledgeable about the client's occupational therapy goals.
4. The occupational therapy assistant in collaboration with the occupational therapist selects, implements, and makes modifications to occupational therapy interventions, including, but not limited to, occupations and activities, preparatory methods and tasks, client education and training, and group interventions consistent with demonstrated competency levels, client goals, and the requirements of the practice setting.

Intervention Review

1. The occupational therapist is responsible for determining the need for continuing, modifying, or discontinuing occupational therapy services.
2. The occupational therapy assistant contributes to this process by exchanging information with and providing documentation to the occupational therapist about the client's responses to and communications during intervention.

Targeting and Evaluating Outcomes

1. The occupational therapist is responsible for selecting, measuring, and interpreting outcomes that are related to the client's ability to engage in occupations.
2. The occupational therapy assistant is responsible for being knowledgeable about the client's targeted occupational therapy outcomes and for providing information and documentation related to outcome achievement.
3. The occupational therapy assistant may implement outcome measurements and provide needed client discharge resources.

Supervision of Occupational Therapy Aides[1]

An *aide,* as used in occupational therapy practice, is an individual who provides supportive services to the occupational therapist and the occupational therapy assistant. Aides do not provide skilled occupational therapy services. An aide is trained by an occupational therapist or an occupational therapy assistant

[1]Depending on the setting in which service is provided, aides may be referred to by various names. Examples include, but are not limited to, *rehabilitation aides, restorative aides, extenders, paraprofessionals,* and *rehab techs* (AOTA, 2009).

to perform specifically delegated tasks. The occupational therapist is responsible for the overall use and actions of the aide. An aide first must demonstrate competency to be able to perform the assigned, delegated client and non-client tasks.

1. The occupational therapist must oversee the development, documentation, and implementation of a plan to supervise and routinely assess the ability of the occupational therapy aide to carry out non–client- and client-related tasks. The occupational therapy assistant may contribute to the development and documentation of this plan.
2. The occupational therapy assistant can supervise the aide.
3. *Non–client-related tasks* include clerical and maintenance activities and preparation of the work area or equipment.
4. *Client-related tasks* are routine tasks during which the aide may interact with the client. The following factors must be present when an occupational therapist or occupational therapy assistant delegates a selected client-related task to the aide:
    a. The outcome anticipated for the delegated task is predictable.
    b. The situation of the client and the environment is stable and will not require that judgment, interpretations, or adaptations be made by the aide.
    c. The client has demonstrated some previous performance ability in executing the task.
    d. The task routine and process have been clearly established.
5. When performing delegated client-related tasks, the supervisor must ensure that the aide
    a. Is trained and able to demonstrate competency in carrying out the selected task and using equipment, if appropriate;
    b. Has been instructed on how to specifically carry out the delegated task with the specific client; and
    c. Knows the precautions, signs, and symptoms for the particular client that would indicate the need to seek assistance from the occupational therapist or occupational therapy assistant.
6. The supervision of the aide needs to be documented. Documentation includes information about frequency and methods of supervision used, the content of supervision, and the names and credentials of all persons participating in the supervisory process.

Summary

These guidelines about supervision, roles, and responsibilities are to assist in the appropriate utilization of occupational therapists, occupational therapy assistants, and occupational therapy aides and in the appropriate and effective provision of occupational therapy services. It is expected that occupational therapy services are delivered in accordance with applicable state and federal regulations, relevant workplace policies, the *Occupational Therapy Code of Ethics and Ethics Standards* (AOTA, 2010), and continuing competency and professional development guidelines. For information regarding the supervision of occupational therapy students, please refer to *Fieldwork Level II and Occupational Therapy Students: A Position Paper* (AOTA, 2012).

References

American Occupational Therapy Association. (2009). Guidelines for supervision, roles, and responsibilities during the delivery of occupational therapy services. *American Journal of Occupational Therapy, 63,* 797–803. http://dx.doi.org/10/5014/ajot.63.6.797

American Occupational Therapy Association. (2010). Occupational therapy code of ethics and ethics standards (2010). *American Journal of Occupational Therapy, 64*(6, Suppl.), S17–S26. http://dx.doi.org/10.5014/ajot.2010.64S17

American Occupational Therapy Association. (2012). Fieldwork level II and occupational therapy students: A position paper. *American Journal of Occupational Therapy, 66*(6, Suppl.), S75–S77. http://dx.doi.org/10.5014/ajot.2012.66S75

American Occupational Therapy Association. (2014). Occupational therapy practice framework: Domain and process (3rd ed.). *American Journal of Occupational Therapy, 68,* (Suppl. 1), S1–S48. http://dx.doi.org/10.5014/ajot.2014.682005

Additional Reading

American Occupational Therapy Association. (2010). Standards of practice for occupational therapy. *American Journal of Occupational Therapy, 64*(Suppl.), S106–S111. http://dx.doi.org/10.5014/ajot.2010.64S106

Authors

Sara Jane Brayman, PhD, OTR/L, FAOTA
Gloria Frolek Clark, MS, OTR/L, FAOTA
Janet V. DeLany, DEd, OTR/L
Eileen R. Garza, PhD, OTR, ATP
Mary V. Radomski, MA, OTR/L, FAOTA
Ruth Ramsey, MS, OTR/L
Carol Siebert, MS, OTR/L
Kristi Voelkerding, BS, COTA/L
Patricia D. LaVesser, PhD, OTR/L, *SIS Liaison*
Lenna Aird, *ASD Liaison*
Deborah Lieberman, MHSA, OTR/L, FAOTA, *AOTA Headquarters Liaison*

for

The Commission on Practice
Sara Jane Brayman, PhD, OTR/L, FAOTA, *Chairperson*

Adopted by the Representative Assembly 2004C24

Edited by the Commission on Practice 2014
Debbie Amini, EdD, OTR/L, CHT, FAOTA, *Chairperson*

Adopted by the Representative Assembly Coordinating Council (RACC) for the Representative Assembly, 2014.

Note. This document replaces the 2009 document *Guidelines for Supervision, Roles, and Responsibilities During the Delivery of Occupational Therapy Services,* previously published and copyrighted in 2009 by the American Occupational Therapy Association in the *American Journal of Occupational Therapy, 63,* 797–803. http://dx.doi.org/10.5014/ajot.63.6.797

Appendix G.

DECISION TABLE

Possible Action	Positive Outcomes	Negative Consequences
Take no action		

Appendix H.

Scope of Practice

Statement of Purpose

The purpose of this document is to

A. Define the scope of practice in occupational therapy by

1. Delineating the domain of occupational therapy practice and services provided by occupational therapists and occupational therapy assistants;

2. Delineating the dynamic process of occupational therapy evaluation and intervention services used to achieve outcomes that support the participation of clients in everyday life activities (occupations); and

3. Describing the education and certification requirements needed to practice as an occupational therapist and occupational therapy assistant;

B. Inform consumers, health care providers, educators, the community, funding agencies, payers, referral sources, and policymakers regarding the scope of occupational therapy.

Introduction

The occupational therapy scope of practice is based on the American Occupational Therapy Association (AOTA) documents *Occupational Therapy Practice Framework: Domain and Process* (AOTA, 2014b) and *Philosophical Base of Occupational Therapy* (AOTA, 2011b), which states that "the use of occupation to promote individual, community, and population health is the core of occupational therapy practice, education, research, and advocacy" (p. S65). Occupational therapy is a dynamic and evolving profession that is responsive to consumer and societal needs, to system changes, and to emerging knowledge and research.

This document is designed to support and be used in conjunction with the *Definition of Occupational Therapy Practice for the AOTA Model Practice Act* (AOTA, 2011a). Although this document may be a resource to augment state statutes and regulations that govern the practice of occupational therapy, it does not supersede existing laws and other regulatory requirements. Occupational therapists and occupational therapy assistants are required to abide by relevant statutes and regulations when providing occupational therapy services. State statutes and other regulatory requirements typically include statements about educational requirements to practice occupational therapy, procedures to practice occupational therapy legally within the defined area of jurisdiction, the definition and scope of occupational therapy practice, and supervision requirements for occupational therapy assistants.

It is the position of AOTA that a referral is not required for the provision of occupational therapy services, but referrals for such services are generally affected by laws and payment policy. AOTA's position is also that "an occupational therapist accepts and responds to referrals in compliance with state or federal laws, other regulatory and payer requirements, and AOTA documents" (AOTA 2010b, Standard II.2, p. S108). State laws and other regulatory requirements should be viewed as minimum criteria to practice occupational therapy. Ethical guidelines that ensure safe and effective delivery of occupational therapy services to clients always guide occupational therapy practice (AOTA, 2010a). Policies of payers such as insurance companies also must be followed.

Occupational therapy services may be provided by two levels of practitioners: (1) the occupational therapist and (2) the occupational therapy assistant, as well as by occupational therapy students under appropriate supervision (AOTA, 2012). Occupational therapists function as autonomous practitioners, are responsible for all aspects of occupational therapy service delivery, and are accountable for the safety and effectiveness of the occupational therapy service delivery process.

The occupational therapy assistant delivers occupational therapy services only under the supervision of and in partnership with the occupational therapist (AOTA, 2014a). When the term *occupational therapy practitioner* is used in this document, it refers to both occupational therapists and occupational therapy assistants (AOTA, 2011c).

Definition of Occupational Therapy

The *Occupational Therapy Practice Framework* (AOTA, 2014b) defines *occupational therapy* as

> the therapeutic use of everyday life activities (occupations) with individuals or groups for the purpose of enhancing or enabling participation in roles, habits, and routines in home, school, workplace, community, and other settings. Occupational therapy practitioners use their knowledge of the transactional relationship among the person, his or her engagement in valuable occupations, and the context to design occupation-based intervention plans that facilitate change or growth in client factors (body functions, body structures, values, beliefs, and spirituality) and skills (motor, process, and social interaction) needed for successful participation. Occupational therapy practitioners are concerned with the end result of participation and thus enable engagement through adaptations and modifications to the environment or objects within the environment when needed. Occupational therapy services are provided for habilitation, rehabilitation, and promotion of health and wellness for clients with disability- and non–disability-related needs. These services include acquisition and preservation of occupational identity for those who have or are at risk for developing an illness, injury, disease, disorder, condition, impairment, disability, activity limitation, or participation restriction. (p. S1)

Occupational Therapy Practice

Occupational therapists and occupational therapy assistants are experts at analyzing the client factors, performance skills, performance patterns, and contexts and environments necessary for people to engage in their everyday activities and occupations. The practice of occupational therapy includes

A. Evaluation of factors affecting activities of daily living (ADLs), instrumental activities of daily living (IADLs), rest and sleep, education, work, play, leisure, and social participation, including
   1. Client factors, including body functions (e.g., neuromuscular, sensory, visual, perceptual, cognitive) and body structures (e.g., cardiovascular, digestive, integumentary, genitourinary systems)
   2. Habits, routines, roles, and rituals
   3. Physical and social environments and cultural, personal, temporal, and virtual contexts and activity demands that affect performance
   4. Performance skills, including motor, process, and social interaction skills

B. Approaches to identify and select interventions, such as
   1. Establishment, remediation, or restoration of a skill or ability that has not yet developed or is impaired

2. Compensation, modification, or adaptation of activity or environment to enhance performance
3. Maintenance and enhancement of capabilities without which performance in everyday life activities would decline
4. Health promotion and wellness to enable or enhance performance in everyday life activities
5. Prevention of barriers to performance.

C. Interventions and procedures to promote or enhance safety and performance in ADLs, IADLs, rest and sleep, education, work, play, leisure, and social participation, for example,

1. Occupations and activities
    a. Completing morning dressing and hygiene routine using adaptive devices
    b. Playing on a playground with children and adults
    c. Engaging in driver rehabilitation and community mobility program
    d. Managing feeding, eating, and swallowing to enable eating and feeding performance.
2. Preparatory methods and tasks
    a. Exercises, including tasks and methods to increase motion, strength, and endurance for occupational participation
    b. Assessment, design, fabrication, application, fitting, and training in assistive technology and adaptive devices
    c. Design and fabrication of splints and orthotic devices and training in the use of prosthetic devices
    d. Modification of environments (e.g., home, work, school, community) and adaptation of processes, including the application of ergonomic principles
    e. Application of physical agent modalities and use of a range of specific therapeutic procedures (e.g., wound care management; techniques to enhance sensory, perceptual, and cognitive processing; manual therapy techniques) to enhance performance skills
    f. Assessment, recommendation, and training in techniques to enhance functional mobility, including wheelchair management
    g. Explore and identify effective tools for regulating nervous system arousal levels in order to participate in therapy and/or in valued daily activities.
3. Education and training
    a. Training in self-care, self-management, home management, and community or work reintegration
    b. Education and training of individuals, including family members, caregivers, and others.
4. Advocacy
    a. Efforts directed toward promoting occupational justice and empowering clients to seek and obtain resources to fully participate in their daily life occupations.
5. Group interventions
    a. Facilitate learning and skill acquisition through the dynamics of group or social interaction across the life span.

6. Care coordination, case management, and transition services
7. Consultative services to groups, programs, organizations, or communities.

Scope of Practice: Domain and Process

The scope of practice includes the domain and process of occupational therapy services. These two concepts are intertwined, with the *domain* defining the focus of occupational therapy, and the *process* defining the delivery of occupational therapy.

The *domain* of occupational therapy is the everyday life activities (occupations) that people find meaningful and purposeful. Within this domain, occupational therapy services enable clients to participate in their everyday life activities in their desired roles, contexts and environments, and life situations.

Clients may be individuals or persons, groups, or populations. The occupations in which clients engage occur throughout the life span and include

- ADLs (self-care activities);
- IADLs (activities to support daily life within the home and community that often require complex interactions, e.g., household management, financial management, child care);
- Rest and sleep (activities relating to obtaining rest and sleep, including identifying need for rest and sleep, preparing for sleep, and participating in rest and sleep);
- Education (activities to participate as a learner in a learning environment);
- Work (activities for engaging in remunerative employment or volunteer activities);
- Play (activities pursued for enjoyment and diversion);
- Leisure (nonobligatory, discretionary, and intrinsically rewarding activities); and
- Social participation (the ability to exhibit behaviors and characteristics expected during interaction with others within a social system).

Within their domain of practice, occupational therapists and occupational therapy assistants consider the repertoire of occupations in which the client engages, the performance skills and patterns the client uses, the contexts and environments influencing engagement, the features and demands of the activity, and the client's body functions and structures. Occupational therapists and occupational therapy assistants use their knowledge and skills to help clients conduct or resume daily life activities that support function and health throughout the life span. Participation in activities and occupations that are meaningful to the client involves emotional, psychosocial, cognitive, and physical aspects of performance. Participation in meaningful activities and occupations enhances health, well-being, and life satisfaction.

The domain of occupational therapy practice complements the World Health Organization's (WHO's) conceptualization of *participation and health* articulated in the *International Classification of Functioning, Disability and Health* (*ICF;* WHO, 2001). Occupational therapy incorporates the basic constructs of *ICF,* including environment, participation, activities, and body structures and functions, when providing interventions to enable full participation in occupations and maximize occupational engagement.

The *process* of occupational therapy refers to the delivery of services and includes evaluating, intervening, and targeting of outcomes. Occupation remains central to the occupational therapy process, which is client centered, involving collaboration with the client throughout each aspect of service delivery. During the evaluation, the therapist develops an occupational profile; analyzes the client's ability to carry out everyday life activities; and determines the client's occupational needs, strengths, barriers to participation, and priorities for intervention.

OCCUPATIONS	***CLIENT FACTORS***	***PERFORMANCE SKILLS***	***PERFORMANCE PATTERNS***	***CONTEXTS AND ENVIRONMENTS***
Activities of daily living (ADLs)* Instrumental activities of daily living (IADLs) Rest and sleep Education Work Play Leisure Social participation	Values, beliefs, and spirituality Body functions Body structures	Motor skills Process skills Social interaction skills	Habits Routines Rituals Roles	Cultural Personal Physical Social Temporal Virtual
*Also referred to as *basic activities of daily living (BADLs)* or *personal activities of daily living (PADLs)*.				

Exhibit 1. Aspects of the domain of occupational therapy.
All aspects of the domain transact to support engagement, participation, and health. This exhibit does not imply a hierarchy.

Source. From "Occupational Therapy Practice Framework: Domain and Process," by the American Occupational Therapy Association, 2014, *American Journal of Occupational Therapy, 68,* S4. Copyright © 2014 by the American Occupational Therapy Association. Used with permission.

Evaluation and intervention may address one or more aspects of the domain (Exhibit 1) that influence occupational performance. Intervention includes planning and implementing occupational therapy services and involves activities and occupations, preparatory methods and tasks, education and training, and advocacy. The occupational therapist and occupational therapy assistant in partnership with the occupational therapist utilize occupation-based theories, frames of reference, evidence, and clinical reasoning to guide the intervention (AOTA, 2014b).

The outcome of occupational therapy intervention is directed toward "achieving health, well-being, and participation in life through engagement in occupations" (AOTA, 2014b, p. S4). Outcomes of the intervention determine future actions with the client and include occupational performance, prevention (of risk factors, disease, and disability), health and wellness, quality of life, participation, role competence, well-being, and occupational justice (AOTA, 2014b).

Sites of Intervention and Areas of Focus

Occupational therapy services are provided to persons, groups, and populations. People served come from all age groups. Practitioners work with individuals one to one, in groups, or at the population level to address occupational needs and issues, for example, in mental health; work and industry; rehabilitation, disability, and participation; productive aging; and health and wellness.

Along the continuum of service, occupational therapy services may be provided to clients throughout the life span in a variety of settings. The settings may include, but are not limited to, the following:

- Institutional settings (inpatient; e.g., acute care, rehabilitation facilities, psychiatric hospitals, community and specialty-focused hospitals, nursing facilities, prisons),
- Outpatient settings (e.g., hospitals, clinics, medical and therapy offices),
- Home and community settings (e.g., residences, group homes, assisted living, schools, early intervention centers, day care centers, industry and business, hospice, sheltered workshops, transitional-living facilities, wellness and fitness centers, community mental health facilities), and
- Research facilities.

Education and Certification Requirements

To practice as an occupational therapist, the individual trained in the United States

- Has graduated from an occupational therapy program accredited by the Accreditation Council for Occupational Therapy Education (ACOTE®; 2012) or predecessor organizations;
- Has successfully completed a period of supervised fieldwork experience required by the recognized educational institution where the applicant met the academic requirements of an educational program for occupational therapists that is accredited by ACOTE or predecessor organizations;
- Has passed a nationally recognized entry-level examination for occupational therapists; and
- Fulfills state requirements for licensure, certification, or registration.

To practice as an occupational therapy assistant, the individual trained in the United States

- Has graduated from an occupational therapy assistant program accredited by ACOTE or predecessor organizations;
- Has successfully completed a period of supervised fieldwork experience required by the recognized educational institution where the applicant met the academic requirements of an educational program for occupational therapy assistants that is accredited by ACOTE or predecessor organizations;
- Has passed a nationally recognized entry-level examination for occupational therapy assistants; and
- Fulfills state requirements for licensure, certification, or registration.

AOTA supports licensure of qualified occupational therapists and occupational therapy assistants (AOTA, 2009). State and other legislative or regulatory agencies may impose additional requirements to practice as occupational therapists and occupational therapy assistants in their area of jurisdiction.

References

American Council for Occupational Therapy Education. (2012). 2011 Accreditation Council for Occupational Therapy Education (ACOTE®) standards. *American Journal of Occupational Therapy, 66*, S6–S74. http://dx.doi.org/10.5014/ajot.2012.66S6

American Occupational Therapy Association. (2009). Policy 5.3: Licensure. In *Policy manual* (2013 ed., pp. 60–61). Bethesda, MD: Author.

American Occupational Therapy Association. (2010a). Occupational therapy code of ethics and ethics standards (2010). *American Journal of Occupational Therapy, 64*(Suppl.), S17–S26. http://dx.doi.org/10.5014/ajot.2010.64S17

American Occupational Therapy Association. (2010b). Standards of practice for occupational therapy. *American Journal of Occupational Therapy, 64*(Suppl.), S106–S111. http://dx.doi.org/10.5014/ajot.2010.64S106

American Occupational Therapy Association. (2011a). *Definition of occupational therapy practice for the AOTA Model Practice Act.* Retrieved from http://www.aota.org/~/media/Corporate/Files/Advocacy/State/Resources/PracticeAct/Model%20Definition%20of%20OT%20Practice%20%20Adopted%2041411.ashx

American Occupational Therapy Association. (2011b). The philosophical base of occupational therapy. *American Journal of Occupational Therapy, 65*(Suppl.), S65. http://dx.doi.org/10.5014/ajot.2011.65S65

American Occupational Therapy Association. (2011c). Policy 1.44. Categories of occupational therapy personnel. In *Policy manual* (2013 ed., pp. 32–33). Bethesda, MD: Author.

American Occupational Therapy Association. (2012). Fieldwork level II and occupational therapy students: A position paper. *American Journal of Occupational Therapy*, 66(6, Suppl.), S75–S77. http://dx.doi.org/10.5014/ajot.2012.66S75

American Occupational Therapy Association. (2014a). Guidelines for supervision, roles, and responsibilities during the delivery of occupational therapy services. *American Journal of Occupational Therapy, 68*(Suppl. 3), S16–S22. http://dx.doi.org/10.5014/ajot.2014.686S03

American Occupational Therapy Association. (2014b). Occupational therapy practice framework: Domain and process (3rd ed.). *American Journal of Occupational Therapy, 68*(Suppl. 1), S1–S48. http://dx.doi.org/10.5014/ajot.2014.682006

World Health Organization. (2001). *International classification of functioning, disability and health.* Geneva: Author.

Authors

The Commission on Practice:
Sara Jane Brayman, PhD, OTR/L, FAOTA, *Chairperson*
Gloria Frolek Clark, MS, OTR/L, FAOTA
Janet V. DeLany, DEd, OTR/L
Eileen R. Garza, PhD, OTR, ATP
Mary V. Radomski, MA, OTR/L, FAOTA
Ruth Ramsey, MS, OTR/L
Carol Siebert, MS, OTR/L
Kristi Voelkerding, BS, COTA/L
Patricia D. LaVesser, PhD, OTR/L, *SIS Liaison*
Lenna Aird, *ASD Liaison*
Deborah Lieberman, MHSA, OTR/L, FAOTA, *AOTA Headquarters Liaison*

for

The Commission on Practice
Sara Jane Brayman, PhD, OTR/L, FAOTA, *Chairperson*, 2002–2005

Adopted by the Representative Assembly 2004C23

Edited by the Commission on Practice 2014
Debbie Amini, EdD, OTR/L, CHT, FAOTA, *Chairperson*

Adopted by the Representative Assembly Coordinating Council (RACC) for the Representative Assembly, 2014

Note. This document replaces the 2010 document *Scope of Practice,* previously published and copyrighted in 2010 by the American Occupational Therapy Association in the *American Journal of Occupational Therapy, 64*(6, Suppl.), S70–S77. http://dx.doi.org/10.5014/ajot.2010.64S70

CITATION INDEX

C

D

I

J

K

P

Q

R

S

T

U

V

W

Y

Z

SUBJECT INDEX

Note. Page numbers in *italic* indicate figures, tables, exhibits, vignettes, and case studies.

B

F

P

S

U

V

W

Y

Z